T0261658

Big Data Analysis and Artificial Intelligence for Medical Sciences

Big Data Analysis and Artificial Intelligence for Medical Sciences

Edited by

Bruno Carpentieri
Free University of Bozen-Bolzano
Bozen-Bolzano
Italy

Paola Lecca
Free University of Bozen-Bolzano
Bozen-Bolzano
Italy

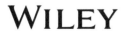

This edition first published 2024
© 2024 John Wiley & Sons Ltd.

All rights reserved. No part of this publication may be reproduced, stored in a retrieval system, or transmitted, in any form or by any means, electronic, mechanical, photocopying, recording or otherwise, except as permitted by law. Advice on how to obtain permission to reuse material from this title is available at http://www.wiley.com/go/permissions.

The right of Bruno Carpentieri and Paola Lecca to be identified as the author of the editorial material in this work has been asserted in accordance with law.

Registered Offices
John Wiley & Sons, Inc., 111 River Street, Hoboken, NJ 07030, USA
John Wiley & Sons Ltd, The Atrium, Southern Gate, Chichester, West Sussex, PO19 8SQ, UK

For details of our global editorial offices, customer services, and more information about Wiley products visit us at www.wiley.com.

Wiley also publishes its books in a variety of electronic formats and by print-on-demand. Some content that appears in standard print versions of this book may not be available in other formats.

Trademarks: Wiley and the Wiley logo are trademarks or registered trademarks of John Wiley & Sons, Inc. and/or its affiliates in the United States and other countries and may not be used without written permission. All other trademarks are the property of their respective owners. John Wiley & Sons, Inc. is not associated with any product or vendor mentioned in this book.

Limit of Liability/Disclaimer of Warranty
While the publisher and authors have used their best efforts in preparing this work, they make no representations or warranties with respect to the accuracy or completeness of the contents of this work and specifically disclaim all warranties, including without limitation any implied warranties of merchantability or fitness for a particular purpose. No warranty may be created or extended by sales representatives, written sales materials or promotional statements for this work. This work is sold with the understanding that the publisher is not engaged in rendering professional services. The advice and strategies contained herein may not be suitable for your situation. You should consult with a specialist where appropriate. The fact that an organization, website, or product is referred to in this work as a citation and/or potential source of further information does not mean that the publisher and authors endorse the information or services the organization, website, or product may provide or recommendations it may make. Further, readers should be aware that websites listed in this work may have changed or disappeared between when this work was written and when it is read. Neither the publisher nor authors shall be liable for any loss of profit or any other commercial damages, including but not limited to special, incidental, consequential, or other damages.

Library of Congress Cataloging-in-Publication Data applied for
Hardback ISBN 9781119846536

Cover Design: Wiley
Cover Image: © Yuichiro Chino/Getty Images

Set in 9.5/12.5pt STIXTwoText by Straive, Chennai, India
Printed and bound by CPI Group (UK) Ltd, Croydon, CR0 4YY

C9781119846536_020524

Contents

List of Contributors

Daniela Besozzi

Department of Informatics
Systems and Communication
University of Milano-Bicocca
Milano
Italy

and

Bicocca Bioinformatics Biostatistics and
Bioimaging Centre - B4
University of Milano-Bicocca
Vedano al Lambro
Italy

Federico Cabitza

Department of Computer Science
Systems and Communication
University of Milano-Bicocca
Milan
Italy

and

IRCCS Istituto Ortopedico Galeazzi
Milan
Italy

Barbara Di Camillo

Department of Information Engineering
University of Padova
Padua
Italy

and

Department of Comparative Biomedicine
and Food Science
University of Padova
Padua
Italy

Andrea Campagner

IRCCS Istituto Ortopedico Galeazzi
Milan
Italy

Angel Canal-Alonso

BISITE Research Group
University of Salamanca
Salamanca
Spain

and

Institute for Biomedical Research of
Salamanca
University of Salamanca
Salamanca
Spain

Bruno Carpentieri

Faculty of Engineering
Free University of Bozen-Bolzano
Bolzano
Italy

Paolo Cazzaniga

Department of Human and Social Sciences
University of Bergamo
Bergamo
Italy

and

Bicocca Bioinformatics Biostatistics and
Bioimaging Centre - B4
University of Milano-Bicocca
Vedano al Lambro
Italy

Yee W. Choon

Artificial Intelligence Lab
Institute for Artificial Intelligence and
Big Data
Universiti Malaysia Kelantan
Kota Bharu
Kelantan
Malaysia

and

Faculty of Data Science and Computing
Universiti Malaysia Kelantan
Kota Bharu
Kelantan
Malaysia

Juan M. Corchado

BISITE Research Group
University of Salamanca
Salamanca
Spain

and

Institute for Biomedical Research of
Salamanca
University of Salamanca
Salamanca
Spain

and

Air Institute
IoT Digital Innovation Hub
Salamanca
Spain

and

Department of Electronics
Information and Communication
Faculty of Engineering
Osaka Institute of Technology
Osaka
Japan

Mai Dabas

Department of Biomedical Engineering
Faculty of Engineering
Tel Aviv University
Tel Aviv
Israel

Luca Dedè

MOX - Dipartimento di Matematica
Politecnico di Milano
Milano
Italy

Víctor Duarte

BISITE Research Group
University of Salamanca
Salamanca
Spain

and

Air Institute
Salamanca
Spain

Stefania Fresca

MOX - Dipartimento di Matematica
Politecnico di Milano
Milano
Italy

Caro Fuchs

Department of Industrial Engineering and
Innovation Sciences
Eindhoven University of Technology
Eindhoven
The Netherlands

Chiara Gallese

Department of Electrical Engineering
Eindhoven University of Technology
Eindhoven
Netherlands

Amit Gefen

Department of Biomedical Engineering
Faculty of Engineering
Tel Aviv University
Tel Aviv
Israel

and

Skin Integrity Research Group (SKINT)
University Centre for Nursing and
Midwifery
Department of Public Health and Primary
Care
Ghent University
Ghent
Belgium

and

Department of Mathematics and Statistics
Faculty of Sciences, Hasselt University
Hasselt
Belgium

Thanh Trung Giang

Tay Bac University
VNU University of Engineering and
Technology
Hanoi
Vietnam

Alesandro Gómez

BISITE Research Group
University of Salamanca
Salamanca
Spain

and

Air Institute
IoT Digital Innovation Hub
Salamanca
Spain

Gerhard A. Holzapfel

Institute of Biomechanics
Graz University of Technology
Graz
Austria

and

Department of Structural Engineering
Norwegian University of Science and
Technology
Trondheim
Norway

Zhang N. Hor

Faculty of Computing
Universiti Teknologi Malaysia
Johor
Malaysia

Carlo Ierna

Radboud University Nijmegen
Faculty of Philosophy, Theology, and
Religious Studies
Center for the History of Philosophy and
Science
Nijmegen
The Netherlands

Paola Lecca

Faculty of Engineering
Free University of Bozen-Bolzano
Bolzano
Italy

Enrico Longato

Department of Information Engineering
University of Padova
Padua
Italy

Eleonora Lusito

San Raffaele Telethon Institute for Gene
Therapy (SR-Tiget)
IRCCS San Raffaele Scientific Institute
Milan
Italy

Hairudin A. Majid

Faculty of Computing
Universiti Teknologi Malaysia
Johor
Malaysia

Andrea Manzoni

MOX - Dipartimento di Matematica
Politecnico di Milano
Milano
Italy

Mohd S. Mohamad

Health Data Science Lab
Department of Genetics and Genomics
College of Medical and Health Sciences
United Arab Emirates University
Al Ain
Abu Dhabi
United Arab Emirates

and

Big Data Analytics Center
United Arab Emirates University
Al Ain
Abu Dhabi
United Arab Emirates

Thanh-Phuong Nguyen

Innovation Business Unit
Dennemeyer TechSys, Luxembourg
Luxembourg

Marco S. Nobile

Department of Environmental Sciences
Informatics and Statistics
Ca' Foscari University of Venice
Venice
Italy

and

Bicocca Bioinformatics Biostatistics and
Bioimaging Centre - B4
University of Milano-Bicocca
Vedano al Lambro
Italy

Gabriella Panuccio

Istituto Italiano di Tecnologia
Enhanced Regenerative Medicine
Genova
Italy

Quang Trung Pham

Tay Bac University
Sonla
Vietnam

Simone Rampelli

Unit of Microbiome Science and
Biotechnology
Department of Pharmacy and
Biotechnology
University of Bologna
Bologna
Italy

Muhammad A. Remli

Artificial Intelligence Lab
Institute for Artificial Intelligence and Big
Data
Universiti Malaysia Kelantan
Kota Bharu
Kelantan
Malaysia

and

Faculty of Data Science and Computing
Universiti Malaysia Kelantan
Kota Bharu
Kelantan
Malaysia

Seyed Shayan Sajjadinia

Faculty of Engineering
Free University of Bozen-Bolzano
Bozen-Bolzano
Italy

Simone Spolaor

Microsystems, Eindhoven University of
Technology
Eindhoven
The Netherlands

Narayan P. Subramaniyam

Faculty of Medicine and Health
Technology and BioMediTech Institute
Tampere University
Tampere
Finland

Erica Tavazzi

Department of Information Engineering
University of Padova
Padua
Italy

Dang Hung Tran

Hanoi National University of Education
Hanoi
Vietnam

Silvia Turroni

Unit of Microbiome Science and
Biotechnology
Department of Pharmacy and
Biotechnology
University of Bologna
Bologna
Italy

Martina Vettoretti

Department of Information Engineering
University of Padova
Padua
Italy

Preface

Our modern society is characterized by an unprecedented ability to generate vast amounts of data. The use of *big data* in science is driving the development of a new scientific paradigm. Smart search and learning computer algorithms are utilized to extract meaningful patterns from large datasets and generate new knowledge that can be applied to model the behavior of complex real-world systems much faster than by using traditional scientific laws and theories. The name of the new game is *machine learning, deep learning, and artificial intelligence*. These data-driven research methodologies are already paving the way for advanced discoveries in numerous scientific disciplines. In healthcare industry and research, the data-driven modeling approach is opening new frontiers, for example, enabling to produce more accurate diagnoses, to facilitate the design of drugs, to innovate treatment protocols and prevent diseases, to produce personalized treatments and reduce medical costs, thereby significantly advancing medical research.

Computational science, the scientific investigation and solution of complex problems in science and engineering through modeling and simulation on computers, may be considered the third pillar of science, complementing theory and experimenting. The conventional simulation approach refers to the theory-based approach in which a model is built using laws and predictive statements from physics, chemistry, biology, and other fields that describe the causal relationships between a set of controllable inputs and a set of target variables. The underlying physics is described by mathematical models such as systems of ordinary and/or partial differential equations. The model is then solved numerically unless a closed-form solution to the resulting set of equations is available, which is rarely the case in practice. Theory-based simulation models are generally very powerful in understanding the behavior of the system. However, they sometimes fail to accurately reveal the properties of a complex system due to lack of theory and simplified assumptions, large numbers of variables and parameters involved in the simulation and, sometimes, a lack of robust numerical solvers. In these circumstances, data-driven models can be used to identify correlations between two sets of controlled input and output variables without the need to explicitly describe their causal pips. Data-mining techniques, for instance, can be used to predict future data patterns by analyzing the properties of existing datasets. Genetic algorithms and artificial neural networks can map relationships between two datasets by reducing a cost or error function and then predicting the future behavior of the target system.

Several scientific disciplines, such as computer vision and image recognition, self-driving cars, natural language processing, website recommendations, solid-state materials science, finance, bioinformatics, and chemistry, to name a few, have adopted machine learning algorithms in the past decade or so. Thanks to their general applicability to different applications, data-driven models are computationally attractive for use in the medical sciences and the healthcare industry, where they are becoming increasingly popular. Examples of recent studies using data-driven neural network models include better image classification of coronary angiography X-rays, localization of brain tumors from MRI image slices, and strabismus recognition. Support vector machines have assisted in the detection of common pneumothorax by analyzing binary patterns in chest X-ray images, as well as in the prediction of fractures in hip bones and vertebrates using datasets acquired from random and cluster-based under-sampling methods. Blood pressure has been predicted using principal component analysis. The application of fuzzy logic and ontological reasoning allows for more precise, personalized recommendations of antidiabetic drugs for individual patients. Projects like IBM's Watson Oncology, Microsoft's Hanover, and Google's DeepMind are only a few examples of the many programs that companies are developing to leverage big data in the healthcare industry.

This book provides an overview of the current state of the art in the use of artificial intelligence in medicine and biology. It collects chapters written by international experts in the field of medical and biological research. Their studies are the result of years of interdisciplinary collaborations with clinicians as well as computer scientists, mathematicians, and engineers. The aim of the book is to demonstrate the efforts made in the fields of computational biology and medical sciences to design and implement robust, accurate, and efficient computer algorithms for modeling the behavior of complex biological systems much faster than using traditional modeling approaches solely based on theory. Through the authors' contributions in the various chapters, we aim to highlight the difference between traditional computational approaches to data processing (those of mathematical biology) and the new way knowledge is extracted from data, and the experiment-data-theory-model-validation cycle is being implemented. The style of the book is not that of a typical textbook. We believe that understanding these new trends, the difficulties that have arisen as a result of these changes, and the potential future directions these changes may take, directly through the authors' reports of scientific work expressed in simple but rigorous language, may add a remarkable breadth. It may be of great benefit not only to professional scholars but also to MSc or PhD program students who are the future and those who will take up the baton to continue the race in scientific and technological research.

Bolzano

8 July 2023

Bruno Carpentieri and *Paola Lecca*

The Editors

1

Introduction

Bruno Carpentieri and Paola Lecca

Faculty of Engineering, Computer Science and Artificial Intelligence Institute, Free University of Bozen-Bolzano, Bolzano, Italy

The concept of intelligent machines is frequently attributed to Alan Turing, who published a seminal paper titled "Computing Machinery and Intelligence" in 1950, in which he developed a simple test known as the "Turing test" to assess whether a machine can demonstrate human-like intelligence. Six years later, in 1956, during the Dartmouth Conference, an influential event in the history of AI, the term "artificial intelligence" (AI) was coined by emeritus Stanford Professor John McCarthy, known as the "Father of AI" to characterize "the science and engineering of creating intelligent machines." The Turing test has had a significant impact on the development of modern AI by establishing a standard for measuring progress in AI research. Nevertheless, AI encompasses a broader spectrum of methods, concepts, and technologies. Using techniques, such as machine learning (ML), natural language processing (NLP), computer vision, and others, entail the study and development of systems that can perform tasks that typically require human intelligence. Early basic AI systems relied on explicitly coded rules based on a simple set of "if, then" or symbolic reasoning approaches, in which particular conditions would trigger specific actions to make judgments and to perform tasks. These early models necessitated considerable manual rule programming, which was time-consuming and difficult to scale to complex problems. As a result of these limitations, widespread adoption of early AI models proved difficult, particularly in complicated domains such as medicine. Advances in AI research have led to the development of more sophisticated algorithms that function similarly to the human brain and have helped address some of these challenges and opened up new possibilities for AI applications. ML has evolved into a field known as deep learning (DL), which consists of techniques for creating and training artificial neural networks (ANNs) with multiple layers of interconnected nodes, also known as neurons, capable of learning and making decisions independently, similar to the human brain. These neural networks are inspired by the structure and operation of biological neural networks in the human brain, although they do not completely replicate the human brain's complexities and mechanisms. By iteratively adjusting the weights and biases of the interconnected neurons, DL algorithms are able to recognize complex patterns, extract meaningful representations from large amounts of raw data, and make decisions or predictions across multiple domains. This has produced

Big Data Analysis and Artificial Intelligence for Medical Sciences, First Edition.
Edited by Bruno Carpentieri and Paola Lecca.
© 2024 John Wiley & Sons Ltd. Published 2024 by John Wiley & Sons Ltd.

extraordinary progress in numerous fields, including computer vision, NLP, speech recognition, and medical sciences.

The significant breakthroughs of DL methods can be attributed to the early 2000s owing to the availability of large datasets, increased computational power, and advancements in parallel computing, in particular with the advent of graphics processing units (GPUs), which played a crucial role in training deep neural networks on a larger scale. DL is now a dominant approach at the forefront of AI research, with applications in a variety of disciplines. In the medical field, it has shown the potential to revolutionize healthcare and pave the way for personalized medicine (Gilvary et al. 2019). The use of predictive models, advanced data analytics, and DL algorithms can provide valuable insights for healthcare applications such as diagnosis, treatment selection, and therapy response prediction. The ability to analyze vast quantities of patient data, including medical records, genetic information, imaging data, and real-time sensor data, is one of the primary benefits of AI in medicine (Zeng et al. 2021; Liu et al. 2021b; Ahmad et al. 2021; Hamet and Tremblay 2017). This data can guide interventions and preventive measures to reduce risks and promote proactive healthcare, enhance clinical workflow, and procedure precision. On the basis of the analysis of multiple risk factors, it can be possible to assess an individual's likelihood of developing specific diseases. In the context of medicine and healthcare, however, data-driven models present significant computational challenges. When the model is too complex or the training dataset is too small relative to the model's capacity, it may begin to capture noise or oddities that are specific to the training data, and perform exceptionally well on the training data but poorly on new, unseen data. Such models are called "overfit." Noise and unpredictability are common features of complex healthcare datasets. A DL model that overfits to these details when applied to new patient data may produce erroneous or unreliable predictions. In healthcare, researchers are actively investigating methods to reduce overfitting and to ensure the robustness and dependability of DL models across diverse patient populations and situations. The availability of larger datasets, transfer learning techniques, and advances in model architecture and regularization methods are important factors to mitigate overfitting concerns and facilitate the adoption of DL in the medical field.

Convolutional neural networks (CNNs) were an additional significant advancement and a subclass of DL algorithms used in image processing that were designed specifically for analyzing visual data, such as images. Inspired by the structure and operation of the human visual cortex, they imitate the activity of networked neurons by employing layers of interconnected nodes, known as "convolutional layers," which learn spatial hierarchies of features from the input data. Convolutional layers apply filters or kernels to input images, extracting and preserving local features and spatial relationships. In subsequent layers, these extracted features are combined and further processed to capture increasingly complex patterns and structures. Typically, the final layers of a CNN are composed of fully connected layers and are responsible for making predictions based on the learned features. CNNs have revolutionized image processing and computer vision tasks, outperforming traditional machine learning approaches in image classification, object detection, segmentation, and other tasks. Their ability to automatically acquire features from raw image data has made them extremely valuable in numerous applications, including autonomous vehicles, surveillance and medical imaging, and others. One of the first successful CNN architectures was LeNet-5 (LeCun et al. 1998), introduced by Yann LeCun et al. in 1998, primarily designed for handwritten digit recognition. Other popular CNN models are AlexNet (Krizhevsky et al. 2017) (developed by Alex Krizhevsky et al.), that made a breakthrough in the field by significantly lowering error rates; VGGNet (Simonyan and Zisserman 2014) (developed at the University of Oxford by the Visual Geometry Group); GoogLeNet (Szegedy et al. 2015) (introduced by Christian Szegedy et al. from Google), that used parallel convolutional operations at different scales; ResNet (He et al. 2016) (proposed by Kaiming He et al.), that enabled the successful training of networks with hundreds or even thousands of layers; DenseNet (Huang et al. 2017) proposed by Gao Huang et al., and MobileNet (Howard et al. 2017) introduced by Andrew G. Howard et al. in 2017. These are only a few examples of popular CNN architectures. Numerous other CNN models have been developed over the years to address various applications, performance demands and computational constraints, and demonstrate great potential in the field of medicine. Their ability to analyze and interpret medical images, such as X-rays, computerized tomography (CT) scans, magnetic resonance imaging (MRI), and pathology slides, can assist in the diagnosis, planning of treatment, and monitoring of disease. In recent years, CNNs have been used for a variety of medical imaging applications, including image classification (classify medical images to identify different types of tumors, lesions, or diseases), segmentation (segment medical images to identify regions or specific structures of interest, such as organs, tumors, or blood vessels with the purpose of surgical planning, radiation therapy, disease progression study), object detection (for detecting abnormalities, nodules, or lesions within medical images), and disease prediction and prognosis (predict the likelihood of disease occurrence and its progression based on medical images and other clinical data), only to name a few.

As a result of these advancements, today, we are entering a new era in medicine in which risk assessment models can be implemented in clinical practice to improve diagnostic accuracy and operational efficiency. Kaul et al. coined the acronym "AIM" which stands for "Artificial Intelligence in Medicine" in a paper published in 2020 on gastrointestinal endoscopy, titled "History of artificial intelligence in medicine" (Kaul et al. 2020), an eloquent fact of the emergence of a new strand in computational science applied to the life sciences. According to Kaul and coauthors in that research, the critical advances came in the last two decades although AIM has undergone significant change during the last five decades. Watson, an open-domain question–answering system developed by IBM in 2007, competed against human contestants on the television game show Jeopardy! in 2011. Unlike conventional systems, which relied on either forward reasoning (following rules from data to conclusions), backward reasoning (following rules from conclusions to data), or manually created "if-then" rules, this technology, known as DeepQA (Ferrucci et al. 2010), used NLP and a variety of searches to analyze data over unstructured content and produce likely answers. This approach was less complicated and less expensive to use, and easier to maintain. Using IBM Watson, a novel RNA-binding protein that was changed in amyotrophic lateral sclerosis, was successfully discovered by Bakkar et al. in 2017. DeepQA technology could be applied to give evidence-based medicine solutions using data from a patient's electronic medical record and other electronic sources. This opened up new opportunities for evidence-based clinical decision-making. Digitalized medicine became more widely accessible thanks to advances in computer hardware and software, and AIM rapidly expanded as a result of this momentum. Chatbots were originally created for surface-level communication (Eliza), but NLP has transformed them into useful conversation-based interfaces. This technology was utilized to create Apple's Siri and Amazon's Alexa in 2011 and 2014, respectively. Mandy was launched in 2017 as an automated patient intake technology for a primary care practice, while Pharmabot was created in 2015 to assist with medication instruction for pediatric patients and their parents (Ni et al. 2017; Comendador et al. 2015).

The use of AI in the medical field is rapidly expanding. CardioAI (the first Arterys product (Arterys 2018)) analyses cardiac MRI and provides details like the cardiac ejection percent. The tool incorporates non-contrast CT pictures of the head, chest, and musculoskeletal systems, as well as liver and lung imaging. In 2017, the US Food and Drug Administration approved Arterys (currently acquired by Tempus Radiology) as the first clinical cloud-based DL application in healthcare. DL can help to locate lesions, make differential diagnoses, and generate automated medical reports. With fivefold cross-validation, Gargeya and Leng (2017) employed DL to screen for diabetic retinopathy in 2017, reaching a 94% sensitivity and 98% specificity (area under the curve). Esteva et al. similarly trained a CNN to differentiate between nonmelanoma and melanoma skin cancers, and the results indicate that the CNN's performance is comparable to that of specialists. Weng et al. (2017) demonstrated that a CNN can be utilized to predict cardiovascular risk in cohort populations. Astonishingly, AI has been found to improve the accuracy of cardiovascular risk prediction compared to the standard methodology specified by the American College of Cardiology. It was also used to consistently predict the progression of Alzheimer disease by analyzing amyloid imaging data and precisely predicting drug therapy response in this disease (Mathotaarachchi et al. 2017; Fleck et al. 2017).

The literature is so extensive, despite the recent emergence of AI in this field, that it is difficult to compile an exhaustive and summarizing compendium. There are numerous review and perspective articles, blog posts, and journal portfolios that discuss the medical applications of AI, see e.g. Liu et al. (2021b), Suh et al. (2022), Briganti and Le Moine (2020), and Malik et al. (2019). The majority of these meta-reviews identify four application areas: (i) disease diagnose; (ii) drug development; (iii) personalized therapies; and (iv) gene editing, as depicted in Figure 1.1 and suggested, for instance, by Markus Schmitt, head of data science at Data Revenue (https://datarevenue.com).

1.1 Disease Diagnoses

For accurate disease diagnosis, years of medical training are required. Even so, the process of diagnosis is frequently laborious and lengthy. In many fields, the demand for expertise greatly exceeds the available supply. Consequently, doctors are under pressure, and critical patient diagnoses are frequently delayed. Recent advances in machine learning, particularly in DL algorithms, have significantly enhanced the accuracy and accessibility of disease diagnosis. Using machine learning, algorithms can learn to recognize patterns in the same way that doctors do. An important distinction, however, is that learning algorithms require

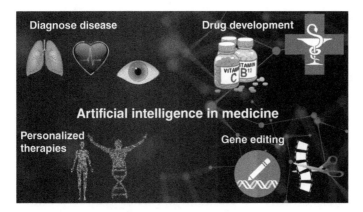

Figure 1.1 The four main applications of artificial intelligence in knowledge extraction and interpretation of biological and biochemical data for applications in the clinic and medicine. The rapid advancement of AI technologies will add further application domains in the near future, formalizing AI as an integral part of modern healthcare.

thousands of concrete examples. In addition, because robots cannot read between the lines in textbooks, these examples must be neatly digitalized. Consequently, machine learning (including DL) is particularly advantageous in fields where the diagnostic data a doctor considers has already been digitized, such as:

- utilizing CT images to diagnose strokes and lung cancer (Chiu et al. 2022; Aydín et al. 2021; Zhou and Xin 2022),
- evaluating the risk of sudden cardiac death or other heart disorders using cardiac MRI and electrocardiogram (ECG) data (Haq et al. 2020; Klein et al. 2022; Ledziński and Grześk 2023; Martínez-Sellés and Marina-Breysse 2023; Karatzia et al. 2022; Yasmin et al. 2021; Kabra et al. 2022; Madan et al. 2022; Argentiero et al. 2022; Jone et al. 2022),
- identifying skin disorders from photographic images (Goyal et al. 2020; Thieme et al. 2023; Son et al. 2021; Ahmad et al. 2023; Combalia et al. 2022; Liopyris et al. 2022; Nigar et al. 2022; Sreekala et al. 2022),
- and recognizing diabetic retinopathy in photographs of the eyes (Sheng et al. 2022; Huang et al. 2022; Padhy et al. 2019; Bader Alazzam et al. 2021; Lim et al. 2023; Mohan et al. 2022; Babenko et al. 2022; Muchuchuti and Viriri 2023; Sun et al. 2023).

Because there is a vast quantity of reliable data available in these medical areas, algorithms are enhancing their diagnostic capabilities to match those of specialists. The algorithm's ability to generate conclusions in a fraction of a second and its economic replicability on a global scale make up the difference. On this basis, it is anticipated that everyone, everywhere will soon have access to affordable radiological diagnostic services of the same high quality. More sophisticated AI diagnosis is being developed. Machine learning in diagnostics is still in its early stages; more ambitious systems will combine a number of data sources (such as CT, MRI, genomics, proteomics, patient data, and even handwritten documents) to evaluate an illness or its progression. It is important to recognize, however, that it is unlikely that AI will completely replace doctors. Instead,

AI tools will assist the doctors to focus on signal interpretation, e.g. to identify potentially malignant tumors and hazardous cardiac patterns.

1.2   Drug Development

Understanding a disease's fundamental causes (technically, "the pathways") and resistance mechanisms is the first step toward designing a treatment. This earliest stage of drug discovery is also known as "target identification." Methods for identifying targets, such as genes involved in disease pathophysiology, include genome-wide association studies (GWAS), risk gene identification, and data mining of published literature. The next phase is to identify effective disease targets (typically proteins). The amount of data available for identifying feasible target pathways has significantly expanded thanks to the widespread use of high-throughput methods like short hairpin RNA (shRNA) screening and deep sequencing. However, integrating a huge number and variety of data sources, and then identifying relevant patterns, remains difficult using traditional methods. All of the available data can be analyzed more easily by machine learning algorithms, which can even be trained to recognize good target proteins automatically (You et al. 2022; Zeng et al. 2020; Najm et al. 2021; Xu et al. 2021; Liu et al. 2021a; Dezsö and Ceccarelli 2020). After identifying a drug's target, the next stage is to find a substance that can interact with the target molecule in the appropriate manner. This entails screening a large number of candidate compounds for their affinity toward the target as well as their toxicity (unintended side effects). These substances may be synthetic, bioengineered, or natural.

It requires a significant amount of time to eliminate false positives and inaccuracies, which may result in a large number of undesired recommendations (false positives). Machine learning techniques can be beneficial in this scenario because they can be trained to predict the suitability of a molecule using structural fingerprints and molecular descriptors (Arnold 2023; Paul et al. 2021; Brown et al. 2020). Then, scientists rapidly sift through millions of potential molecules to identify the most promising candidates – those with the fewest adverse effects. Ultimately, this expedites the drug design process. Finally, it is important to note that machine learning may speed up clinical trials by autonomously selecting qualified applicants and ensuring the correct distribution among participant groups. Using algorithms, one can identify patterns that distinguish between excellent and bad candidates. In addition, they can serve as an early warning system for a clinical study that is not producing reliable results, allowing researchers to intervene sooner, and potentially save the development of the drug.

1.3   Personalized Medicine

Precision medicine is regarded as crucial for the treatment of complex diseases, including systemic autoimmune diseases such as rheumatoid arthritis (RA), systemic lupus erythematosus (SLE), and psoriatic arthritis (PsA). Despite the remarkable number of novel molecules being developed for the treatment of these diseases, the growing understanding of their pathogenesis, and the advances in early diagnosis, it is clear that the clinical and serological heterogeneity of these diseases, as well as the large number of comorbidities that can affect them, continue to limit the ability to tailor the treatment for these patients. There are often few therapy options available for these disorders, even when many organs are involved. Treat-to-target therapy is one of the available therapeutic modalities, and it remains the optimal approach for the majority of rheumatic disorders. However, patients have varying responses to medications and treatment plans. Therefore, there is an enormous potential for personalized care to lengthen patients' lives. One issue is that it is extremely difficult to determine which characteristics should influence therapy selection. ML can automate this tedious statistical work by cross-referencing similar patients and comparing their treatments and outcomes to determine a patient's likely response to a particular therapy (Peng et al. 2021; Fröhlich et al. 2018; Quazi 2022; Papadakis et al. 2019; Emmert-Streib and Dehmer 2019; Gaur et al. 2022; Sahu et al. 2022). The resultant outcome projections make it much simpler for clinicians to formulate the optimal treatment plan. In a recent perspective paper by Sebastiani et al. (2022), it is highlighted, for instance, that treatment and identification of immune-mediated disorders have undergone significant advancements over the past decade. For the treatment of these conditions, an increasing number of novel monoclonal antibodies and small compounds have been developed. Parallel to this, a large number of novel genetic or serological markers have been identified that enhance our ability to detect autoimmune diseases at an early stage. Due to advances in AI and ML, the treatment and follow-up of certain diseases, including cancer, have significantly improved over the past decade. However, the authors of Sebastiani et al. (2022) caution that our understanding of autoimmune systemic diseases is still quite limited. Despite the significant progress in our understanding, it is currently believed that we are still a long way from providing patients with true precision medicine.

1.4 Gene Editing

Clustered regularly interspaced short palindromic repeats (CRISPR), and more specifically the CRISPR-Cas9 system for gene editing, represents an important development in our ability to accurately and economically modify DNA, much like a surgeon. This technique uses short guide RNAs (sgRNA) to target and modify a specific region of DNA. However, the guide RNA can bind to multiple DNA sites, which may have undesired consequences (off-target effects). The careful selection of guide RNA with minimal negative side effects is one of the primary obstacles to the widespread use of the CRISPR system. ML techniques have been shown to make the best predictions for a specific sgRNA's level of guide-target interactions and off-target effects (Liu et al. 2020; Das et al. 2023; Vora et al. 2022; Fong and Wong 2023; Abadi et al. 2017; Aktas et al. 2019; Wang et al. 2020).

Aim of the book is to offer a portrait of the current state of the use of AI methodology in medicine and biology, of the new contributions in terms of techniques and algorithms, and of their integration with traditional disciplines and philosophies of thought typical of other fields such as mathematics and the more classical algorithmic approaches of computer science. Recently, AI techniques have now innervated these domains to the extent that they have become integral elements of them, described, narrated, and hence, conceptualized in terms of an AI-specific language and pattern of thought. The chapters dealing specifically with algorithmic techniques and methodological approaches address the following two consolidated topics.

1) **Data-driven and knowledge-driven modeling**: *Fuzzy Logic for Knowledge-Driven and Data-Driven Modeling in Biomedical Sciences* by Paolo Cazzaniga, Simone Spolaor, Caro Fuchs, Marco S. Nobile, and Daniela Besozzi; *Application of Machine Learning Algorithms to Diagnosis and Prognosis of Chronic Wounds* by Mai Dabas and Amit Gefen; *Deep Learning Techniques for Gene Identification in Cancer Prevention* by Eleonora Lusito; and *Deep Learning-Based Reduced Order Models for Cardiac Electrophysiology* by Stefania Fresca, Luca Dedè, and Andrea Manzoni.

2) **Data analytics: technologies and methods for data interpretation and new knowledge inference**: *Deep Learning for Network Biology* by Eleonora Lusito; *Analysis Pipelines and a Platform Solution for Next Generation Sequencing Data* by Víctor Duarte, Alesandro Gómez, and Juan Manuel Corchado; *The Potential of Microbiome Big Data in Precision Medicine: Predicting Outcomes Through Machine Learning* by Silvia Turroni and Simone Rampelli; *Hybrid Data-Driven and Numerical Modeling of Articular Cartilage* by Seyed Shayan Sajjadinia, Bruno Carpentieri, and Gerhard A. Holzapfel; *A Hybrid of Differential Evolution and Minimization of Metabolic Adjustment for Succinic and Ethanol Production* by Zhang Neng Hor, Mohd Saberi Mohamad, Yee Wen Choon, Muhammad Akmal Remli, and Hairudin Abdul Majid; *Predictive Patient Stratification Using Artificial Intelligence and Machine Learning* by Thanh-Phuong Nguyen, Thanh Trung Giang, Quang Trung Pham, and Dang Hung Tran.

There is no need to emphasize how the fields of data analytics and data modeling are intertwined and cooperate to accelerate industrial and decision-making processes in the fields of medicine, biology, pharmacology, and recently, medicinal chemistry (Struble et al. 2020; Bajorath 2021; Tyrchan et al. 2022). Alongside the relevant areas of data science in informatics and mathematics, the book contains an innovative counterpoint pertinent to the increasing support that AI techniques and methodologies are providing to the field of biomedical engineering, e.g. the chapter *Using AI to Steer Brain Regeneration: The Enhanced Regenerative Medicine Paradigm* by Gabriella Panuccio, Narayan Puthanmadam Subramaniyam, Angel Canal-Alonso, Juan Manuel Corchado, and Carlo Ierna. The book also offers new visions and perspectives on the current state of the art, performance, and industrial applications of AI techniques in the life sciences, e.g. in the chapters *Toward Better Ways to Assess Predictive Computing in Medicine: On Reliability, Robustness and Utility* by Federico Cabitza and Andrea Campagner; *Artificial Intelligence: From Drug Discovery to Clinical Pharmacology* by Paola Lecca.

Alongside the undisputed benefits that the use of AI is bringing to medicine and healthcare, there are also new problems. A recent review by Naik et al. (2022) outlines the most pressing ones stating that privacy and surveillance, interpretability of the results, bias or discrimination, and potentially the philosophical problem are among the legal and ethical issues that society faces as a result of AI (Ahmad et al. 2021; Gruson et al. 2019). As a result of their use, there are concerns that modern digital technologies will become a new source of inaccuracy and data breaches. The deployment of CNN architectures in medicine requires rigorous validation, regulatory compliance, and ethical considerations. Medical imaging datasets must be diverse, representative, and carefully curated to ensure the reliability and generalizability of AI models (Razmjooy and Rajinikanth 2022; Wang et al. 2021). Mistakes in process or protocol in the realm of healthcare can have disastrous effects for the patient who is the victim of the error. It is critical to remember this since patients come into contact with physicians at the most vulnerable times in their lives. Currently, there are no well-defined regulations in place to address the legal and ethical difficulties that may develop as a result of the usage of AI. There are now numerous papers addressing these ethical issues related to AI in various fields of application, to name but a few, we refer the reader to Bankins and Formosa (2023), and for the ethical and legal implication in medicine, we refer the reader also to Karimian et al. (2022), Farhud and Zokaei (2021), Gerke et al. (2020), and Rigby (2019). The chapter *Legal Aspects of AI in the Biomedical Field, The Role of Interpretable Models* by Chiara Gallese and the chapter *The Long Path to Usable AI* by Barbara Di Camillo, Enrico Longato, Erica Tavazzi, and Martina Vettoretti are specifically dedicated to these topics. However, context-specific legal and ethical issues are also mentioned in the chapters on technical advances and current uses of AI in medicine and biology, and proposal to face these challenges are discussed. Continued research and collaboration among specialists in medicine and DL, as well as ethical deployment of these models, can help to accelerate their acceptance and improve healthcare outcomes in the future.

Author Biographies

Bruno Carpentieri earned a Laurea Degree in Applied Mathematics from Bari University in 1997 and then pursued his PhD studies in Computer Science at Toulouse Institute of Technology, France. He has gained professional experience as a postdoctoral researcher at the University of Graz, as an Assistant Professor at the University of Groningen, and as a Reader at Nottingham Trent University. Since May 2017, he holds the position of Associate Professor in Applied Mathematics at the Faculty of Engineering, Free University of Bozen-Bolzano. His scientific interests include numerical linear algebra and high-performance computing, with applications in biomechanics, heart modelling, and cancer research.

Paola Lecca got a Master Degree in Theoretical Physics and a PhD in Computer Science and Telecommunication from University of Trento, Italy. She is Assistant Professor at the Faculty of Engineering of the Free University of Bozen-Bolzano (Italy). Her research lines include graph theory, dynamical networks modelling, and statistical inference. Paola Lecca has experience in applying these conceptual and algorithmic tools to bioinformatics and computational biology. Paola Lecca is Senior Professional Member of Association for Computing Machinery, New York USA, and member of the advisory board of the International Research Institute Foundation for Artificial Intelligence and Computer, Salamanca Spain.

References

Abadi, S., Yan, W.X., Amar, D., and Mayrose, I. (2017). A machine learning approach for predicting CRISPR-Cas9 cleavage efficiencies and patterns underlying its mechanism of action. *PLoS Computational Biology* 13 (10): e1005807.

Ahmad, Z., Rahim, S., Zubair, M., and Abdul-Ghafar, J. (2021). Artificial intelligence (AI) in medicine, current applications and future role with special emphasis on its potential and promise in pathology: present and future impact, obstacles including costs and acceptance among pathologists, practical and philosophical considerations. A comprehensive review. *Diagnostic Pathology* 16: 1–16.

Ahmad, N., Shah, J.H., Khan, M.A. et al. (2023). A novel framework of multiclass skin lesion recognition from dermoscopic images using deep learning and explainable AI. *Frontiers in Oncology* 13: 1151257.

Aktas, Ö., Dogan, E., and Ensari, T. (2019). CRISPR/CAS9 target prediction with deep learning. *2019 Scientific Meeting on Electrical-Electronics & Biomedical Engineering and Computer Science (EBBT)*, 1–5. IEEE.

Argentiero, A., Muscogiuri, G., Rabbat, M.G. et al. (2022). The applications of artificial intelligence in cardiovascular magnetic resonance - a comprehensive review. *Journal of Clinical Medicine* 11 (10): https://doi.org/10.3390/jcm11102866.

Arnold, C. (2023). Inside the nascent industry of AI-designed drugs. *Nature Medicine* 29: 1292–1295.

Arterys (2018). Cardio AI-AI Assisted Cardiac MRI Software Arterys — arterys.com. https://www.arterys.com/cardio-radiology-ai-platform (accessed 04 January 2024).

Aydín, N., Çelik, Ö., Aslan, A.F. et al. (2021). Detection of lung cancer on computed tomography using artificial intelligence applications developed by deep learning methods and the contribution of deep learning to the classification of lung carcinoma. *Current Medical Imaging* 17 (9): 1137–1141.

Babenko, B., Mitani, A., Traynis, I. et al. (2022). Detection of signs of disease in external photographs of the eyes via deep learning. *Nature Biomedical Engineering* 6: 1370–1383.

Bader Alazzam, M., Alassery, F., and Almulihi, A. (2021). Identification of diabetic retinopathy through machine learning. *Mobile Information Systems* 2021: 1–8.

Bajorath, J. (2021). State-of-the-art of artificial intelligence in medicinal chemistry. 7 (6): https://doi.org/10.2144/fsoa-2021-0030.

Bankins, S. and Formosa, P. (2023). The ethical implications of artificial intelligence (AI) for meaningful work. *Journal of Business Ethics* https://doi.org/10.1007/s10551-023-05339-7.

Briganti, G. and Le Moine, O. (2020). Artificial intelligence in medicine: today and tomorrow. *Frontiers in Medicine* 7: 27.

Brown, N., Ertl, P., Lewis, R. et al. (2020). Artificial intelligence in chemistry and drug design. *Journal of Computer-Aided Molecular Design* 34: 709–715.

Chiu, H.-Y., Chao, H.-S., and Chen, Y.-M. (2022). Application of artificial intelligence in lung cancer. *Cancers* 14 (6): https://doi.org/10.3390/cancers14061370.

Combalia, M., Codella, N., Rotemberg, V. et al. (2022). Validation of artificial intelligence prediction models for skin cancer diagnosis using dermoscopy images: the 2019 international skin imaging collaboration grand challenge. *The Lancet Digital Health* 4 (5): e330–e339.

Comendador, B.E.V., Francisco, B.M.B., Medenilla, J.S. et al. (2015). Pharmabot: a pediatric generic medicine consultant chatbot. *Journal of Automation and Control Engineering* 3 (2): 137–140. https://doi.org/10.12720/joace.3.2.137-140.

Das, J., Kumar, S., Mishra, D.C. et al. (2023). Machine learning in the estimation of CRISPR-Cas9 cleavage sites for plant system. *Frontiers in Genetics* 13: 1085332.

Dezsö, Z. and Ceccarelli, M. (2020). Machine learning prediction of oncology drug targets based on protein and network properties. *BMC Bioinformatics* 21: 1–12.

Emmert-Streib, F. and Dehmer, M. (2019). A machine learning perspective on personalized medicine: an automized, comprehensive knowledge base with ontology for pattern recognition. *Machine Learning and Knowledge Extraction* 1 (1): 149–156. https://doi.org/10.3390/make1010009.

Farhud, D.D. and Zokaei, S. (2021). Ethical issues of artificial intelligence in medicine and healthcare. *Iranian Journal of Public Health* https://doi.org/10.18502/ijph.v50i11.7600.

Ferrucci, D., Brown, E., Chu-Carroll, J. et al. (2010). Building Watson: an overview of the DeepQA project. *AI Magazine* 31 (3): 59–79.

Fleck, D.E., Ernest, N., Adler, C.M. et al. (2017). Prediction of lithium response in first-episode mania using the LITHium intelligent agent (LITHIA): pilot data and proof-of-concept. *Bipolar Disorders* 19 (4): 259–272. https://doi.org/10.1111/bdi.12507.

Fong, J.H.C. and Wong, A.S.L. (2023). Advancing CRISPR/Cas gene editing with machine learning. *Current Opinion in Biomedical Engineering* 100477. https://doi.org/10.1016/j.cobme.2023.100477.

Fröhlich, H., Balling, R., Beerenwinkel, N. et al. (2018). From hype to reality: data science enabling personalized medicine. *BMC Medicine* 16 (1): 1–15.

Gargeya, R. and Leng, T. (2017). Automated identification of diabetic retinopathy using deep learning. *Ophthalmology* 124 (7): 962–969. https://doi.org/10.1016/j.ophtha.2017.02.008.

Gaur, N., Dharwadkar, R., and Thomas, J. (2022). Personalized therapy using deep learning advances. In: *Deep Learning for Targeted Treatments: Transformation in Healthcare* (ed. R. Malviya, G. Ghinea, R.K. Dhanaraj, et al.), 171–197. https://doi.org/10.1002/9781119857983.ch6.

Gerke, S., Minssen, T., and Cohen, G. (2020). Ethical and legal challenges of artificial intelligence-driven healthcare. In: *Artificial Intelligence in Healthcare*, 295–336. Elsevier. https://doi.org/10.1016/b978-0-12-818438-7.00012-5.

Gilvary, C., Madhukar, N., Elkhader, J., and Elemento, O. (2019). The missing pieces of artificial intelligence in medicine. *Trends in Pharmacological Sciences* 40 (8): 555–564. https://doi.org/10.1016/j.tips.2019.06.001. https://www.sciencedirect.com/science/article/pii/S0165614719301312. Special Issue: Rise of Machines in Medicine.

Goyal, M., Knackstedt, T., Yan, S., and Hassanpour, S. (2020). Artificial intelligence-based image classification methods for diagnosis of skin cancer: challenges and opportunities. *Computers in Biology and Medicine* 127: 104065. https://doi.org/10.1016/j.compbiomed.2020.104065.

Gruson, D., Helleputte, T., Rousseau, P., and Gruson, D. (2019). Data science, artificial intelligence, and machine learning: opportunities for laboratory medicine and the value of positive regulation. *Clinical Biochemistry* 69: 1–7. https://doi.org/10.1016/j.clinbiochem.2019.04.013.

Hamet, P. and Tremblay, J. (2017). Artificial intelligence in medicine. *Metabolism* 69: S36–S40. https://doi.org/10.1016/j.metabol.2017.01.011. https://www.sciencedirect.com/science/article/pii/S002604951730015X. Insights Into the Future of Medicine: Technologies, Concepts, and Integration.

Haq, I.-U., Haq, I., and Xu, B. (2020). Artificial intelligence in personalized cardiovascular medicine and cardiovascular imaging. *Cardiovascular Diagnosis and Therapy* 11 (3). https://cdt.amegroups.com/article/view/41252.

He, K., Zhang, X., Ren, S., and Sun, J. (2016). Deep residual learning for image recognition. *Proceedings of the IEEE Conference on Computer Vision and Pattern Recognition*, 770–778.

Howard, A.G., Zhu, M., Chen, B. et al. (2017). MobileNets: efficient convolutional neural networks for mobile vision applications. *arXiv preprint arXiv:1704.04861*.

Huang, G., Liu, Z., Van Der Maaten, L., and Weinberger, K.Q. (2017). Densely connected convolutional networks. *Proceedings of the IEEE Conference on Computer Vision and Pattern Recognition*, 4700–4708.

Huang, X., Wang, H., She, C. et al. (2022). Artificial intelligence promotes the diagnosis and screening of diabetic retinopathy. *Frontiers in Endocrinology* 13: 946915.

Jone, P.-N., Gearhart, A., Lei, H. et al. (2022). Artificial intelligence in congenital heart disease: current state and prospects. *JACC: Advances* 1 (5): 100153. https://doi.org/10.1016/j.jacadv.2022.100153.

Kabra, R., Israni, S., Vijay, B. et al. (2022). Emerging role of artificial intelligence in cardiac electrophysiology. *Cardiovascular Digital Health Journal* 3 (6): 263–275. https://doi.org/10.1016/j.cvdhj.2022.09.001.

Karatzia, L., Aung, N., and Aksentijevic, D. (2022). Artificial intelligence in cardiology: hope for the future and power for the present. *Frontiers in Cardiovascular Medicine* 9: 945726.

Karimian, G., Petelos, E., and Evers, S.M.A.A. (2022). The ethical issues of the application of artificial intelligence in healthcare: a systematic scoping review. *AI and Ethics* 2 (4): 539–551. https://doi.org/10.1007/s43681-021-00131-7.

Kaul, V., Enslin, S., and Gross, S.A. (2020). History of artificial intelligence in medicine. *Gastrointestinal Endoscopy* 92 (4): 807–812. https://doi.org/10.1016/j.gie.2020.06.040.

Klein, C.J., Ozcan, I., Attia, Z.I. et al. (2022). Electrocardiogram-artificial intelligence and immune-mediated necrotizing myopathy: predicting left ventricular dysfunction and clinical outcomes. *Mayo Clinic Proceedings: Innovations, Quality & Outcomes* 6 (5): 450–457. https://doi.org/10.1016/j.mayocpiqo.2022.08.003.

Krizhevsky, A., Sutskever, I., and Hinton, G.E. (2017). ImageNet classification with deep convolutional neural networks. *Communications of the ACM* 60 (6): 84–90.

LeCun, Y., Bottou, L., Bengio, Y., and Haffner, P. (1998). Gradient-based learning applied to document recognition. *Proceedings of the IEEE* 86 (11): 2278–2324.

Ledziński, Ł. and Grześk, G. (2023). Artificial intelligence technologies in cardiology. *Journal of Cardiovascular Development and Disease* 10 (5): https://doi.org/10.3390/jcdd10050202.

Lim, J.I., Regillo, C.D., Sadda, S.V.R. et al. (2023). Artificial intelligence detection of diabetic retinopathy: subgroup comparison of the eyeart system with ophthalmologists' dilated examinations. *Ophthalmology Science* 3 (1): 100228. https://doi.org/10.1016/j.xops.2022.100228.

Liopyris, K., Gregoriou, S., Dias, J., and Stratigos, A.J. (2022). Artificial intelligence in dermatology: challenges and perspectives. *Dermatology and Therapy* 12: 2637–2651.

Liu, Q., Cheng, X., Liu, G. et al. (2020). Deep learning improves the ability of sgRNA off-target propensity prediction. *BMC Bioinformatics* 21 (1): 1–15.

Liu, G., Singha, M., Pu, L. et al. (2021a). GraphDTI: a robust deep learning predictor of drug-target interactions from multiple heterogeneous data. *Journal of Cheminformatics* 13: 1–17.

Liu, P.-r., Lu, L., Zhang, J.-y. et al. (2021b). Application of artificial intelligence in medicine: an overview. *Current Medical Science* 41 (6): 1105–1115.

Madan, N., Lucas, J., Akhter, N. et al. (2022). Artificial intelligence and imaging: opportunities in cardio-oncology. *American Heart Journal Plus: Cardiology Research and Practice* 15: 100126. https://doi.org/10.1016/j.ahjo.2022.100126.

Malik, P., Pathania, M., Rathaur, V.K. et al. (2019). Overview of artificial intelligence in medicine. *Journal of Family Medicine and Primary Care* 8 (7): 2328.

Martínez-Sellés, M. and Marina-Breysse, M. (2023). Current and future use of artificial intelligence in electrocardiography. *Journal of Cardiovascular Development and Disease* 10 (4): https://doi.org/10.3390/jcdd10040175.

Mathotaarachchi, S., Pascoal, T.A., Shin, M. et al. (2017). Identifying incipient dementia individuals using machine learning and amyloid imaging. *Neurobiology of Aging* 59: 80–90. https://doi.org/10.1016/j.neurobiolaging.2017.06.027.

Mohan, S., Gaur, R., and Raman, R. (2022). Using artificial intelligence in diabetic retinopathy. *IHOPE Journal of Ophthalmology* 1 (3): 71–78.

Muchuchuti, S. and Viriri, S. (2023). Retinal disease detection using deep learning techniques: a comprehensive review. *Journal of Imaging* 9 (4): https://doi.org/10.3390/jimaging9040084.

Naik, N., Hameed, B.M.Z., Shetty, D.K. et al. (2022). Legal and ethical consideration in artificial intelligence in healthcare: who takes responsibility? *Frontiers in Surgery* 9: https://doi.org/10.3389/fsurg.2022.862322.

Najm, M., Azencott, C.-A., Playe, B., and Stoven, V. (2021). Drug target identification with machine learning: how to choose negative examples. *International Journal of Molecular Sciences* 22 (10): https://doi.org/10.3390/ijms22105118.

Ni, L., Lu, C., Liu, N., and Liu, J. (2017). MANDY: towards a smart primary care chatbot application. In: *Knowledge and Systems Sciences. KSS 2017*, Communications in Computer and Information Science, vol. 780 (ed. J. Chen, T. Theeramunkong, T. Supnithi, and X. Tang). Singapore: Springer.

Nigar, N., Umar, M., Shahzad, M.K. et al. (2022). A deep learning approach based on explainable artificial intelligence for skin lesion classification. *IEEE Access* 10: 113715–113725. https://doi.org/10.1109/ACCESS.2022.3217217.

Padhy, S.K., Takkar, B., Chawla, R., and Kumar, A. (2019). Artificial intelligence in diabetic retinopathy: a natural step to the future. *Indian Journal of Ophthalmology* 67 (7): 1004.

Papadakis, G.Z., Karantanas, A.H., Tsiknakis, M. et al. (2019). Deep learning opens new horizons in personalized medicine. *Biomedical Reports* 10 (4): 215–217.

Paul, D., Sanap, G., Shenoy, S. et al. (2021). Artificial intelligence in drug discovery and development. *Drug Discovery Today* 26 (1): 80.

Peng, J., Jury, E.C., Dönnes, P., and Ciurtin, C. (2021). Machine learning techniques for personalised medicine approaches in immune-mediated chronic inflammatory diseases: applications and challenges. *Frontiers in Pharmacology* 12: 720694.

Quazi, S. (2022). Artificial intelligence and machine learning in precision and genomic medicine. *Medical Oncology* 39 (8): 120.

Razmjooy, N. and Rajinikanth, V. (ed.) (2022). *Frontiers of Artificial Intelligence in Medical Imaging. 2053–2563.* IOP Publishing. ISBN: 978-0-7503-4012-0 https://doi.org/10.1088/978-0-7503-4012-0.

Rigby, M.J. (2019). Ethical dimensions of using artificial intelligence in health care. *AMA Journal of Ethics* 21 (2): E121–E124. https://doi.org/10.1001/amajethics.2019.121.

Sahu, M., Gupta, R., Ambasta, R.K., and Kumar, P. (2022). Artificial intelligence and machine learning in precision medicine: a paradigm shift in big data analysis. In: *Precision Medicine, Progress in Molecular Biology and Translational Science*, Chapter 3, vol. 190 (ed. D.B. Teplow), 57–100. Academic Press https://doi.org/10.1016/bs.pmbts.2022.03.002.

Sebastiani, M., Vacchi, C., Manfredi, A., and Cassone, G. (2022). Personalized medicine and machine learning: a roadmap for the future. *Journal of Clinical Medicine* 11 (14): https://doi .org/10.3390/jcm11144110.

Sheng, B., Chen, X., Li, T. et al. (2022). An overview of artificial intelligence in diabetic retinopathy and other ocular diseases. *Frontiers in Public Health* 10: 971943.

Simonyan, K. and Zisserman, A. (2014). Very deep convolutional networks for large-scale image recognition. *arXiv preprint arXiv:1409.1556.*

Son, H.M., Jeon, W., Kim, J. et al. (2021). AI-based localization and classification of skin disease with erythema. *Scientific Reports* 11 (1): 5350.

Sreekala, K., Rajkumar, N., Sugumar, R. et al. (2022). Skin diseases classification using hybrid AI based localization approach. *Computational Intelligence and Neuroscience* 2022: 6138490.

Struble, T.J., Alvarez, J.C., Brown, S.P. et al. (2020). Current and future roles of artificial intelligence in medicinal chemistry synthesis. *Journal of Medicinal Chemistry* 63 (16): 8667–8682.

Suh, H.-J., Son, J., and Kang, K. (2022). Application of artificial intelligence in the practice of medicine. *Applied Sciences* 12 (9): https://doi.org/10.3390/app12094649.

Sun, G., Wang, X., Xu, L. et al. (2023). Deep learning for the detection of multiple fundus diseases using ultra-widefield images. *Ophthalmology and Therapy* 12 (2): 895–907.

Szegedy, C., Liu, W., Jia, Y. et al. (2015). Going deeper with convolutions. *Proceedings of the IEEE Conference on Computer Vision and Pattern Recognition*, 1–9.

Thieme, A.H., Zheng, Y., Machiraju, G. et al. (2023). A deep-learning algorithm to classify skin lesions from mpox virus infection. *Nature Medicine* 29 (3): 738–747.

Tyrchan, C., Nittinger, E., Gogishvili, D. et al. (2022). Approaches using AI in medicinal chemistry. In: *Computational and Data-Driven Chemistry Using Artificial Intelligence*, Chapter 4 (ed. T. Akitsu), 111–159. Elsevier. ISBN: 978-0-12-822249-2 https://doi.org/10 .1016/B978-0-12-822249-2.00002-5.

Vora, D.S., Verma, Y., and Sundar, D. (2022). A machine learning approach to identify the importance of novel features for CRISPR/Cas9 activity prediction. *Biomolecules* 12 (8): https://doi.org/10.3390/biom12081123.

Wang, J., Zhang, X., Cheng, L., and Luo, Y. (2020). An overview and metanalysis of machine and deep learning-based CRISPR gRNA design tools. *RNA Biology* 17 (1): 13–22. https://doi .org/10.1080/15476286.2019.1669406. PMID: 31533522.

Wang, S., Cao, G., Wang, Y. et al. (2021). Review and prospect: artificial intelligence in advanced medical imaging. *Frontiers in Radiology* 1: https://doi.org/10.3389/fradi.2021.781868.

Weng, S.F., Reps, J., Kai, J. et al. (2017). Can machine-learning improve cardiovascular risk prediction using routine clinical data? *PLoS ONE* 12 (4): e0174944. https://doi.org/10.1371/journal.pone.0174944.

Xu, L., Ru, X., and Song, R. (2021). Application of machine learning for drug–target interaction prediction. *Frontiers in Genetics* 12: 680117.

Yasmin, F., Shah, S.M., Naeem, A. et al. (2021). Artificial intelligence in the diagnosis and detection of heart failure: the past, present, and future. *RCM* 22 (4): 1095–1113. https://doi.org/10.31083/j.rcm2204121.

You, Y., Lai, X., Pan, Y. et al. (2022). Artificial intelligence in cancer target identification and drug discovery. *Signal Transduction and Targeted Therapy* 7 (1): 156.

Zeng, X., Zhu, S., Lu, W. et al. (2020). Target identification among known drugs by deep learning from heterogeneous networks. *Chemical Science* 11: 1775–1797. https://doi.org/10.1039/C9SC04336E.

Zeng, D., Cao, Z., and Neill, D.B. (2021). Artificial intelligence–enabled public health surveillance— from local detection to global epidemic monitoring and control. In: *Artificial Intelligence in Medicine*, 437–453. Elsevier.

Zhou, J. and Xin, H. (2022). Emerging artificial intelligence methods for fighting lung cancer: a survey. *Clinical eHealth* 5: 19–34. https://doi.org/10.1016/j.ceh.2022.04.001.

2

Fuzzy Logic for Knowledge-Driven and Data-Driven Modeling in Biomedical Sciences

Paolo Cazzaniga[1,5], Simone Spolaor[2], Caro Fuchs[3], Marco S. Nobile[4,5] and Daniela Besozzi[6,5]

[1] *Department of Human and Social Sciences, University of Bergamo, Bergamo, Italy*
[2] *Microsystems, Eindhoven University of Technology, Eindhoven, The Netherlands*
[3] *Department of Industrial Engineering and Innovation Sciences, Eindhoven University of Technology, Eindhoven, The Netherlands*
[4] *Department of Environmental Sciences, Informatics and Statistics, Ca' Foscari University of Venice, Venice, Italy*
[5] *Bicocca Bioinformatics Biostatistics and Bioimaging Centre - B4, University of Milano-Bicocca, Vedano al Lambro, Italy*
[6] *Department of Informatics, Systems and Communication, University of Milano-Bicocca, Milano, Italy*

2.1 Introduction

In the field of biomedical sciences, mathematical models facilitate the analysis, comprehension, and control of the mechanisms that govern the functioning of cells and organisms (Brady and Enderling 2019; Anderson and Rejniak 2007; Edelstein-Keshet 2005; Bar-Yam 1997). As such, modeling outcomes can support laboratory experiments to clarify and understand the emergent behaviors of cellular processes under both physiological and perturbed conditions, possibly leading to the identification of novel treatments or laying the foundation for precision medicine interventions.

The definition of a correct and accurate model, which gives a precise and appropriate description of the biological reality, represents a challenging task that relies on observations of the system, as well as on quantitative and qualitative measurements performed under various conditions, along with the process of selecting the fundamental variables that must be included in the model itself. There exist two different strategies for the formalization of mathematical models, based either on domain knowledge or on data, which most of the times are only partially available to work on the scientific question of interest. Following a knowledge-driven modeling approach, the experts first identify the processes that govern the behavior of the observed system; then, using domain-specific knowledge about these processes, the structure of the model can be defined by using a mathematical formalism of choice (e.g. ordinary differential equations (ODEs)). By contrast, the data-driven modeling approach exploits computational tools to automatically derive the structure of a model from data; in this case, models are constructed by relying only on the analysis of the available data, without making any assumptions about the underlying mechanisms.

When modeling real-world systems, there are two main difficulties that must be addressed. First, classic mechanistic modeling approaches require both the identification

Big Data Analysis and Artificial Intelligence for Medical Sciences, First Edition.
Edited by Bruno Carpentieri and Paola Lecca.
© 2024 John Wiley & Sons Ltd. Published 2024 by John Wiley & Sons Ltd.

of the model's equations, and acceptably accurate values for their parameters. Second, models automatically derived by means of machine learning (ML) approaches, such as artificial neural networks (Graupe 2013), provide black box solutions whose functioning can hardly be interpreted by domain experts. These limitations are often encountered in biomedical research, where cellular and physiological data are generally scarce, qualitative in nature, and the interpretability of the model's prediction is essential to take informed decisions (e.g. on the therapy that a patient has to undertake).

To overcome such limitations, we describe in this chapter alternative modeling strategies based on fuzzy logic, and we show how these can be applied to the biomedical domain. Fuzzy logic allows for obtaining models with a high degree of interpretability, thanks to the use of linguistic terms and to the flexibility of fuzzy sets in handling heterogeneous types of data. Moreover, fuzzy logic allows for exploiting both quantitative and qualitative data, providing a description of the system in a precise yet approximate way with respect to the physical reality, as it can deal with uncertain or imprecise information (Zadeh 1973). Lastly, the obtained model can be easily interpreted by domain experts, and no precise, numerical parameterization is required to describe the dynamics of the system under investigation.

In this chapter, we describe some general-purpose computational methods, based on fuzzy logic, that we designed to facilitate the modeling and analysis of heterogeneous complex systems in biomedical research. In particular, in the context of the knowledge-driven strategy, we describe dynamic fuzzy models (Nobile et al. 2020) – which allow for predicting the emergent behaviors of highly heterogeneous systems in unperturbed and perturbed conditions – and FuzzX (Spolaor et al. 2019) – a framework suitable for the analysis of hybrid mechanistic/fuzzy logic models. In the context of the data-driven strategy, we describe pyFUME (Fuchs et al. 2020b), a computational tool for automatically estimating fuzzy inference systems from data. To showcase the benefit of these modeling and computational methods, we show three applications related to (i) the identification of minimal drug combinations capable of maximizing apoptotic death in cancer cells, (ii) the analysis of oscillatory regimes in a hybrid model of signal transduction pathway in yeast, and (iii) the assessment of tremor severity in a neurological disorder. Thanks to the use of the main concepts of fuzzy logic (linguistic terms, fuzzy sets and fuzzy rules written in human-comprehensible language), these models are characterized by a high level of interpretability, which makes their application suitable in biomedical sciences.

2.2   Fuzzy Logic

Fuzzy logic is an extension of multivalued logic, specifically designed to deal with approximate reasoning (Zadeh 1965, 1988), and regarded as the first attempt to formalize in a mathematical framework the way humans "compute" with words (Zadeh 1999). In the last decades, it has been applied in various research fields, including process control and modeling of complex systems, information retrieval, pattern recognition, classification and regression tasks, and decision-making (Zadeh 1973; Yen and Langari 1999; Klir and Yuan 1995).

What distinguishes fuzzy logic from classic logic is that fuzzy logic statements (or fuzzy rules) can assume "to a certain degree" either the value true or false. This characteristic derives from the introduction of fuzzy sets (Zadeh 1965), which represent an extension of classic sets aimed at providing a means to represent vague, non-crisp concepts, and to describe sets having not well defined boundaries.

The numerous advantages of fuzzy logic stem from the fact that this mathematical framework connects the qualitative world of words to the quantitative world of measures. In fact, fuzzy logic can be exploited to: (i) increase the interpretability of computational models; (ii) provide cost-effective approximations of complex system behaviors, even in the absence of precise quantitative information; and (iii) model a wide variety of phenomena and concepts that are not amenable of precise measurements. Non-crisp concepts and uncertainty in measurements are especially common in medical studies and in cellular biology, where researchers deal with extremely complex systems, like cells or whole organisms, and data is often available only in a qualitative form and for limited parts of the system (e.g. MRI images, gene expression, and physiological data of patients).

In this section, we describe the essential concepts related to fuzzy logic that are necessary to understand the methods and applications presented in this chapter.

2.2.1 Fuzzy Sets

Differently from classic set theory, where an object can either belong or not to a given set – intuitively, these sets are characterized by crisp borders – in fuzzy sets the definition of ordinary set is extended such that its boundaries are not sharp. So doing, an element can belong to a fuzzy set to "a certain degree" (Zadeh 1965). This concept can be formalized as follows: given a universe of discourse $\mathcal{U}$, together with any generic element $u \in \mathcal{U}$, a fuzzy set A is characterized by a so-called membership function $\mu_A : \mathcal{U} \rightarrow [0, 1]$, which maps u to its degree of membership. Stated otherwise, $\mu_A(u)$ is the degree of membership of the element u to the fuzzy set A. If A is an ordinary set, then its membership function $\mu_A(u)$ will assume only the values 1 or 0.

Fuzzy sets are useful to represent concepts of human reasoning that cannot be represented by crisp sets. Figure 2.1 provides an example of this scenario, by presenting a partition of the concept of "water temperature" using crisp and fuzzy sets. In Figure 2.1a, two crisp sets are used to partition the temperature of water into the sets "cold" and "hot," with a clear threshold between them set at 30 °C. In Figure 2.1b, two fuzzy sets are employed to partition the same range of temperatures. The fuzzy partition has a smooth and continuous transition from "cold" to "hot," not requiring any crisp threshold and thus providing a representation of water temperature that is closer to human perception.

Although several interpretations of fuzzy sets exist, in this chapter, fuzzy sets represent the degree of similarity to a prototype object or condition (Dubois and Prade 1997); no higher-order fuzzy sets (e.g. type-2 fuzzy sets) will be considered (Mendel and John 2002).

2.2.2 Linguistic Variables

Another fundamental concept in fuzzy logic, strictly related to fuzzy sets, is known as linguistic variable. Linguistic variables connect the quantitative world of measures to the qualitative world of human reasoning, since, differently from common numerical variables, they can assume as values words or sentences in some natural or artificial language

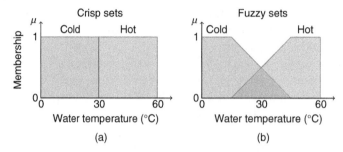

Figure 2.1 Comparison between crisp sets (a) and fuzzy sets (b) to represent the concept of water temperature.

(Zadeh 1975). For example, in Figure 2.1 the concept of "water temperature" is represented with a linguistic variable that partitions the universe of discourse into two fuzzy sets, "cold" and "hot," connecting quantitative values of temperature to how humans perceive and describe them.

A linguistic variable l can be defined as a quadruple $l = \{X, \mathcal{U}, \Lambda, M\}$, where:

- X is the name of the linguistic variable;
- $\mathcal{U}$ is the universe of discourse in which X has meaning;
- $\Lambda = \{\lambda_1, \ldots, \lambda_k\}$ is the term set of X, which includes the k linguistic values that l can assume;
- $M = \{\mu_{\lambda_1}, \ldots, \mu_{\lambda_k}\}$ is the set of fuzzy sets in which $\mathcal{U}$ is partitioned; each term $\lambda \in \Lambda$ is associated with a single fuzzy set $\mu \in M$.

For the sake of clarity, and to avoid an excess of notation, we point out that: (i) μ can be used to denote both the fuzzy set and its membership function, since a fuzzy set is defined by its membership function; (ii) we can refer to a linguistic variable l by using its name X.

We highlight that, despite the original definition of linguistic variables takes into account linguistic hedges (e.g. "very," "less") (Zadeh 1975), the works presented in this chapter do not deal with such objects.

2.2.3 Fuzzy Rules

In classic logic, IF-THEN rules are used to express implications and represent some form of knowledge about the represented object. These rules can be extended into fuzzy IF-THEN rules for the purpose of fuzzy set-based approximate reasoning (Dubois and Prade 1996). Fuzzy IF-THEN rules are logic statements in which the antecedent, or both the antecedent and the consequent, contain fuzzy sets rather than crisp sets. Different definitions of fuzzy implication can be found in the literature (Dubois and Prade 1996), but generally, fuzzy rules are defined by an expression in the form:

IF X IS λ THEN Y IS z,

where X and Y are the names of linguistic variables, λ is a term of X, and z is either a term of Y, a crisp value, or a function of the variables appearing in the antecedent. In general, the antecedent of a fuzzy rule can be any well-formed logic expression (for example, formed by means of the logic operators AND, OR, NOT). A set of fuzzy rules is known as a "fuzzy rule base."

It is worth noting that fuzzy rules give a rough description of the relationship between the variables appearing in the antecedent and in the consequent of the rules. In fact, fuzzy antecedents in fuzzy rules provide the basis for an interpolation mechanism, as explained in Section 2.2.4.

2.2.4 Fuzzy Inference Systems

Taken together, linguistic variables and a fuzzy rule base are the foundations of a Fuzzy Inference System (FIS) (Cherkassky 1998). A FIS maps a given input to an output by means of fuzzy logic. A common architecture of a FIS is shown in Figure 2.2, and it can be described as follows:

1) fuzzification of crisp values and evaluation of their membership degree;
2) inference of rule conclusions (i.e. rule evaluations) and their aggregation into a single output;
3) defuzzification (if required) of the fuzzy rules' output into a single crisp value.

The term fuzzification refers to the process to determine the degree to which an input data belongs to a fuzzy set, by exploiting the membership functions, while defuzzification refers the process to determine a crisp value from the output of the aggregated fuzzy sets.

The knowledge base, which is the ensemble of linguistic variables and the rule base, is exploited in each passage of the inference process. When knowledge-driven approaches are employed, the knowledge base is generally built by domain experts of the system that is under investigation. However, during the last decades several methods were developed to automatically build the knowledge base starting from a given dataset (Wang and Mendel 1992).

Several types of FIS exist in the literature, and the choice of one over the others ultimately affects the conclusions that can be drawn during fuzzy inference. All works presented in this chapter employs one of the most common and successful interpretation of

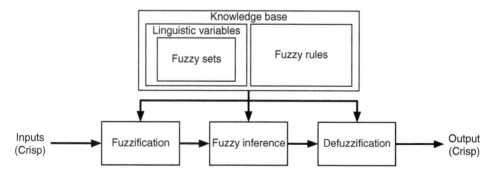

Figure 2.2 General architecture of a fuzzy inference system. The knowledge base comprising linguistic variables and fuzzy rules is exploited in each phase of the inference process, which includes fuzzification, fuzzy inference, and defuzzification.

fuzzy inference: the Takagi Sugeno Kang (also known as TSK or Sugeno) method (Takagi and Sugeno 1985). The Sugeno inference method is characterized by the fact that the consequent appearing in the fuzzy rules is a function of the variables appearing in the antecedent. Sugeno FIS are classified according to the order of such functions: e.g. a zero-order Sugeno FIS employs constant functions (i.e. a crisp value) in the consequents of its fuzzy rules, while a first-order Sugeno FIS employs linear functions. Contrary to other methods, there is no need for defuzzification since the evaluation of the rules returns only crisp values. Moreover, Sugeno FIS were proven to be universal approximators (Wang 1992; Castro and Delgado 1996), their output surface was proven to be continuous Takács (2004), and they are computationally less demanding compared to other types of FIS.

Although used in several practical applications, sometimes the definition of a multiple-input/single-output FIS might not be sufficient, especially if the variables to be modeled are strongly interdependent. To overcome this limitation, the output of a FIS can be fed as input to a downstream one, in order to "connect" more than one FIS, and create a fuzzy inference network (FN). Some examples of FNs are showcased in Section 2.3.

2.2.5 Simpful

Despite the success of fuzzy logic in many research fields, general-purpose software that implement fuzzy sets and fuzzy logic based methods are still limited in number and scope, outdated or not open-source. To overcome these limitations we developed Simpful (Spolaor et al. 2020), a user-friendly, open-source and general-purpose Python library for fuzzy logic. All the models and methods presented in what follows were implemented using Simpful.

Simpful was specifically designed to simplify the definition, analysis, and interpretation of fuzzy models. To achieve this, Simpful provides a lightweight application programming interface (API) that allows the users to intuitively define all the components necessary to implement a FIS (e.g. fuzzy sets, linguistic variables). One of its most distinctive features is that fuzzy rules are specified by means of strings of text, simplifying both the definition and the interpretation of the model. Simpful indeed facilitates the comprehensibility of the model by avoiding any complex syntax, and by encoding the rule base as logic statements written in natural language.

Currently, Simpful supports the definition of arbitrarily shaped membership functions and complex fuzzy rules consisting of several clauses, fuzzy inference based on either Sugeno (of any order) (Sugeno 1985) or Mamdani (Mamdani and Assilian 1975) methods, the definition of FN, methods for fuzzy aggregation, and plotting facilities. The library is freely available, under GPL license, on GitHub: https://github.com/aresio/simpful. Simpful can also be installed by using the PyPI facility via: `pip install simpful`.

2.3 Knowledge-Driven Modeling

In the definition of a model following a knowledge-driven approach, the domain experts generally identify both the components and the processes that are involved in the system of interest and govern its behavior. This domain-specific knowledge is then used to specify all functional, mechanistic or logic connections necessary to build the model structure.

According to this approach, a system can be mathematically formalized by means of mechanism-based (Wilkinson 2009) or logic-based (Le Novère 2015) modeling strategies. The former strategy requires the accurate setting of all quantitative parameters (e.g. kinetic rates and molecular amounts, in the case of biological models) related to the interactions between the system components. Such values are generally not available in the literature, or are difficult to measure by means of *ad hoc* experiments, thus hampering the applicability of simulation and analysis tools. In addition, in many life sciences applications, the components and processes of a biological system are often measured and described in a qualitative manner.

To overcome these limitations, the logic-based modeling strategy represents an effective alternative, as it allows for describing and studying biomedical systems even if only qualitative data are available (Wynn et al. 2012; Zañudo and Albert 2015). In particular, the modeling approaches exploiting fuzzy logic, capable of dealing with any uncertainty ascribable to the system (Yen and Langari 1999; Nobile et al. 2020), can be used to define mathematical models formalized as fuzzy inference networks, as described in Section 2.2.

Fuzzy logic has been exploited in a variety of applications concerning the biomedical sciences, including the modeling and simulation of signaling pathways (Aldridge et al. 2009), gene regulatory networks (Küffner et al. 2010), and the automatic inference of network models (Morris et al. 2016; Keller et al. 2016). The definition of a novel dynamic fuzzy modeling approach, and its application for the investigation of programmed cell death processes in cancer cells, are described in Sections 2.3.1 and 2.3.2, respectively.

Mechanism-based and logic-based modeling approaches can be combined to capture different features of complex systems, lead to a better investigation of dynamic behaviors, and leverage any available quantitative or qualitative data. So doing, hybrid models consisting in a quantitative (or mechanistic) module and a qualitative (or logic) module, which can reciprocally control each other's dynamics, can thus be defined (Spolaor et al. 2019). A novel hybrid framework that exploits fuzzy logic, and its application for the analysis of a signal transduction pathway, are presented in Sections 2.3.3 and 2.3.4, respectively.

2.3.1 Dynamic Fuzzy Modeling

In this section, we present a modeling and simulation method that we conceived to analyze heterogeneous biomedical systems—whose components can range from single molecules to cellular processes and phenotypes—and that relies on a knowledge-driven approach based on fuzzy logic (Nobile et al. 2020).

This method, known as *dynamic fuzzy models* (DFMs), allows for carrying out dynamical simulations of the temporal evolution of the system, without requiring any precise quantitative parameterization concerning the state or the abundance of the components. In a DFM, linguistic variables and linguistic terms (e.g. low, medium, and high) are associated with each component of the system to provide a qualitative description of all the possible states that the components can reach over time (Aldridge et al. 2009), and to handle the uncertainty of the state of the variables by means of the membership functions associated with

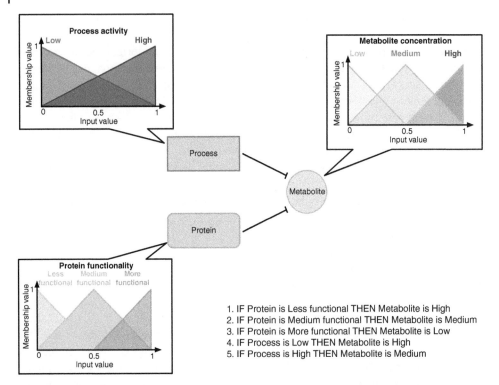

1. IF Protein is Less functional THEN Metabolite is High
2. IF Protein is Medium functional THEN Metabolite is Medium
3. IF Protein is More functional THEN Metabolite is Low
4. IF Process is Low THEN Metabolite is High
5. IF Process is High THEN Metabolite is Medium

Figure 2.3 The linguistic variables, together with their associated term sets and membership functions, as specified for three different kinds of components of a generic biological system: cellular process activity, protein functionality, and metabolite concentration. The component Metabolite is under negative regulation by both components process and protein, as represented by the blunt-ended arrow. The five fuzzy rules describe the regulation of the Metabolite according to the linguistic terms of the regulating components.

each linguistic term. Fuzzy rules describing the behavior of DFMs can be defined starting from linguistic variables and terms, as schematized in Figure 2.3.

DFMs include *inner* and *outer* variables: the former can either appear as antecedent or as consequent in fuzzy rules, while the latter represent *input* and *output* variables. In particular, input variables can only appear as antecedents in fuzzy rules, and refer to the components of the system that govern the dynamics evolution by means of user-defined functions or perturbations; output variables can only appear as consequents in fuzzy rules, and refer to the observable components of the system. The state of all variables (excluding the input variables) change according to the synchronous application of the fuzzy rules defined in the DFM, evaluated exploiting the zero-order Sugeno method (Sugeno 1985). The Sugeno inference is iteratively applied to obtain the temporal dynamics of the system, until the simulation reaches the maximum number of steps set by the user.

The simulation and analysis of DFMs can be realized by using FUMOSO (FUzzy MOdels SimulatOr) (Nobile et al. 2020), an open-source and cross-platform software that, thanks to a Graphical user interface, allows the user to specify several settings, such as the simulation time, the state of all variables, and the functions driving the state change of input variables. The user can also define and apply perturbations to any chosen variable during the simulations, in order to mimic a desired behavior of the system or to explore the emergent behavior under different scenarios; in this case, during the perturbation interval, the Sugeno inference is disabled for the variables included in the perturbation and their state is updated by using a time-dependent arbitrary function.

The analysis of the dynamics of DFMs by means of FUMOSO can be aided by the application of global optimization algorithms to automatically identify an optimal perturbation, which can be intuitively defined as the set of variables perturbations that leads to a desired behavior of the DFM (i.e. the objective of the analysis). Global optimization algorithms indeed allow for realizing an effective and efficient exploration of the huge search space of possible perturbations, whose dimension grows exponentially with the number of perturbed variables.

2.3.2 Application 1: Maximizing Cancer Cells Death with Minimal Drug Combinations

As an example of DFM and of the application of FUMOSO, we describe here a model developed to investigate death and survival processes of K-ras induced cancer cells displaying the typical Warburg effect (Nobile et al. 2020; Spolaor et al. 2021). The Warburg effect, or aerobic glycolysis, is a metabolic hallmark of malignancy. It has been observed that cancer cells might acquire the ability to survive in environmental conditions characterized by glucose starvation thanks to the activation of compensatory signaling pathways (Palorini et al. 2016; Huang et al. 2019) and alternative metabolic routes (Zaugg et al. 2011; Ye et al. 2015).

The DFM, depicted in Figure 2.4, describes cancer cell death processes occurring upon glucose starvation, along with a pathway centered on mitochondria—involving reactive oxygen species (ROS), adenosine triphosphate (ATP) depletion, and calcium (Ca^{2+}) overloading (Taylor et al. 2008)—and with the pathway related to the endoplasmic reticulum (ER)-stress, which is associated with the reduction of *N*-glycosylation and cell attachment, leading to the activation of the unfolded protein response (UPR) and to cell death (Hetz and Papa 2018). The DFM also includes two major survival mechanisms, namely, mitochondrial activity rewiring and autophagy. The complete list of fuzzy rules and all the information of this DFM can be found in Nobile et al. (2020).

FUMOSO was exploited to simulate the dynamics of the DFM, to the aim of experimentally validating the model against data obtained from cell cultures grown in different glucose availability, and under the inactivation or hyperactivation of protein kinase A (PKA) (Nobile et al. 2020). Figure 2.5 shows an example of simulated dynamics of the main observable output variables in unperturbed conditions, which were shown to be in agreement with the experimental data. The dynamics were generated by reporting, for each time step, the values of the variables corresponding to the system phenotypes, as obtained from the simulation of the DFM.

The optimization analysis performed with FUMOSO allowed for identifying the minimal set of simultaneous perturbations that need to be carried out to maximize proapoptotic processes, suggesting novel therapeutic treatments (Nobile et al. 2020; Spolaor et al. 2021). For instance, Figure 2.6 shows the effects of a double perturbation consisting in UPR activation

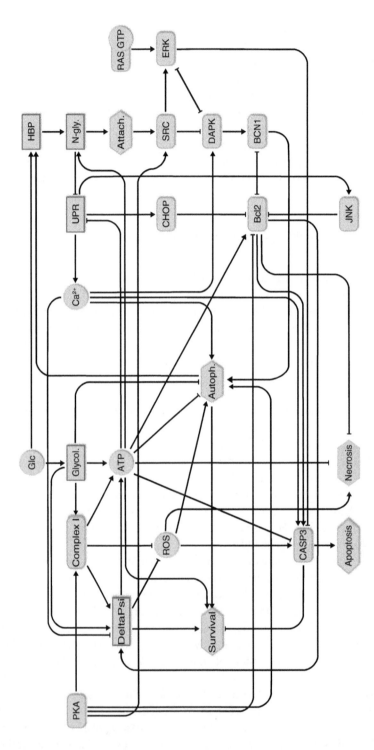

Figure 2.4 DFM describing cell death and survival of cancer cells upon glucose starvation. Circles represent metabolites and ions, rounded rectangles represent proteins, squared rectangles represent pathways or cellular processes, hexagons represent the system phenotypes related to cell death. Positive and negative regulations are pictured as arrows and blunt-ended arrows, respectively. Glucose, Ras-GTP and PKA are input variables; survival, autophagy, apoptosis and necrosis are output variables, while the remaining are inner variables.

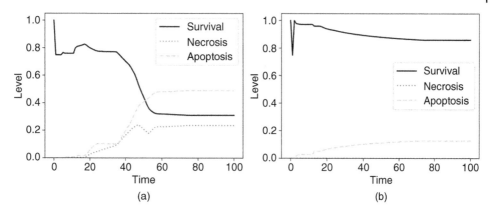

Figure 2.5 Dynamics of the three main model output (Apoptosis, Necrosis, and Survival) under unperturbed conditions, in the case of low (a) and high (b) PKA expression.

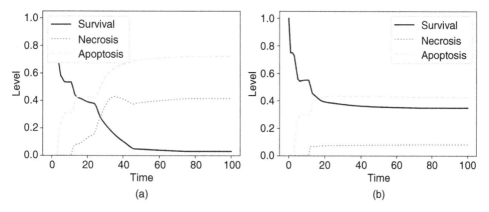

Figure 2.6 Dynamics of the three main model output (Apoptosis, Necrosis, and Survival) upon UPR activation and autophagy inhibition, in the case of low (a) and high (b) PKA expression.

coupled with autophagy inhibition, which eventually increase the value of Apopstosis while reducing Survival.

2.3.3 FuzzX: A Hybrid Mechanistic-Fuzzy Modeling and Simulation Engine

FuzzX (Fuzzy-mechanistic modeling of compleX systems) is a general-purpose methodology for hybrid modeling that couples the quantitative description and analysis of well-known and detailed processes, along with other phenomena whose functioning is not well characterized and can only be described by means of linguistic concepts (Spolaor et al. 2019). The modeling of complex systems that simultaneously exploits qualitative and quantitative approaches could be beneficial in a vast range of applications, since precise and quantitative data is not always readily available for all system components and interactions that must be included in the model. As a matter of fact, the integration of uncertain and qualitative information with precise and quantitative data allows for defining comprehensive mathematical models involving all processes occurring in the system, and for better describing its emergent behaviors.

In FuzzX, the mechanistic (quantitative) module of a hybrid model can be formalized with any fully parameterized modeling formalism, such as ODEs, Markov jump processes or algebraic equations. The variables included in this module can be used as input for those present in the qualitative module, whose description is given as a fuzzy inference network (Chang and Lee 1999; Yaakob et al. 2017). Fuzzy rules can control either variables or parameters of the mechanistic module. In particular, FuzzX is capable to overcome different limitations of other hybrid modeling approaches, as it allows for dynamically integrating a detailed quantitative model with a qualitative fuzzy rule base system, accurately describing emergent phenomena thanks to the possibility of including regulatory feedbacks and stochastic processes, and to the correct synchronization of the qualitative and quantitative modules during the simulation.

In FuzzX, a hybrid model Ω is formalized by specifying a mechanistic module $\mathcal{M}$ and a fuzzy module $\mathcal{F}$, where $\mathcal{M} = \langle \mathcal{V}^{\mathrm{M}}, \theta^{\mathrm{M}}, \mathcal{P} \rangle$ consists in three disjoint sets corresponding to variables, parameters and mechanistic processes governing the functioning of Ω, respectively, and $\mathcal{F} = \langle \mathcal{V}^{\mathrm{F}}, \mathcal{R} \rangle$ consists in two disjoint sets corresponding to linguistic variables and fuzzy rules, respectively. An interface between $\mathcal{M}$ and $\mathcal{F}$ is also defined, to allow the *communication* between the two modules; the interface is formally defined as the set $\mathcal{I} = (\mathcal{V}^{\mathrm{M}} \cap \mathcal{V}^{\mathrm{F}}) \cup (\theta^{\mathrm{M}} \cap \mathcal{V}^{\mathrm{F}})$. Figure 2.7 provides a graphical representation of the two modules and the interface of a hybrid model Ω, as defined in FuzzX.

The sets of mechanistic and fuzzy variables are denoted in Ω as $\mathcal{V}^{\mathrm{M}} = \{x_1^{\mathrm{M}}, \ldots, x_m^{\mathrm{M}}\}$ and $\mathcal{V}^{\mathrm{F}} = \{x_1^{\mathrm{F}}, \ldots, x_j^{\mathrm{F}}\}$, respectively. The states of the mechanistic and fuzzy modules at time t (and, overall, the state of the system Ω) are denoted by $\mathbf{X}^{\mathrm{M}}(t) = (x_1^{\mathrm{M}}(t), \ldots, x_m^{\mathrm{M}}(t))$ and $\mathbf{X}^{\mathrm{F}}(t) = (x_1^{\mathrm{F}}(t), \ldots, x_j^{\mathrm{F}}(t))$, respectively. Considering that the variables in $\mathcal{V}^{\mathrm{M}}$ assume values in the set

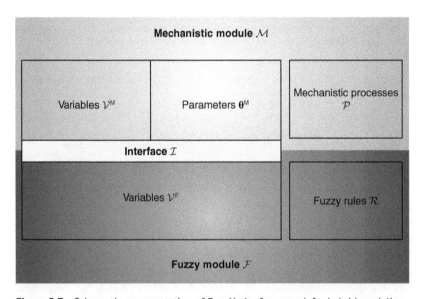

Figure 2.7 Schematic representation of FuzzX, the framework for hybrid modeling.

$\mathcal{X}_M$, defined according to the mathematical formalism used to describe $\mathcal{M}$, and the variables in $\mathcal{V}^F$ assume values in $\mathbb{R}$, it is possible to define the functions used to update the state of the two modules. The first function, $U^M : \mathcal{X}_M^m \rightarrow \mathcal{X}_M^m$, maps the state $\mathbf{X}^M(t)$ of $\mathcal{M}$ into the next state $\mathbf{X}^M(t+1)$, according to the parameterization in θ^M and the mechanistic processes in $\mathcal{P}$, that is, it describes the temporal evolution of the processes of Ω that are described in mechanistic detail. The second function, $U^F : \mathbb{R}^f \rightarrow \mathbb{R}^f$, maps the state $\mathbf{X}^F(t)$ of $\mathcal{F}$ into the next state $\mathbf{X}^F(t+1)$, by considering the fuzzy rules in $\mathcal{R}$, that is, represents the evolution of processes that are known at a higher level of abstraction.

A simulation step of Ω is realized by first applying U^M for a user-defined time interval of length $\Delta \in \mathbb{R}^+$ to calculate the dynamics of the mechanistic module, and then using U^F to perform a fuzzy inference. The application of U^M and U^F on the elements of $\mathcal{I}$ allows the two modules to interact; the value of Δ indicates how often the two modules will interact with each other. The simulation terminates as soon as a user-defined time limit $t_{max} \in \mathbb{R}^+$ is reached, which corresponds to the execution of $k = \lceil \frac{t_{max}}{\Delta} \rceil$ simulation steps.

2.3.4 Application 2: Analyzing Oscillatory Regimes in Signal Transduction Pathways

As an example of the application of FuzzX, we present the hybrid model of the Ras/cAMP/PKA signal transduction pathway in the yeast *Saccharomyces cerevisiae*, which is a network of finely regulated biochemical reactions that control metabolism and cell cycle in response to extracellular nutrients and stress conditions (Thevelein 1994; Thevelein and de Winde 1999). Such regulations are carried out through the activation of the PKA protein that, in turn, regulates a plethora of downstream target proteins.

In the hybrid model (schematized in Figure 2.8), we denote with C the active form of PKA, whose activation is mediated by the chemical bond with the "second messenger" molecule cAMP—acting as a glucose-signal transducer—which is synthesized by protein Cyr1 and degraded by protein Pde1. Cyr1 activity is controlled by protein Ras2 that can either be inactive (when it is bound to molecule GDP, i.e. Ras2-GDP), or active (when it is bound to molecule GTP, i.e. Ras2-GTP). The transition between the inactive and active states of Ras2 is regulated by Cdc25 and Ira2 proteins. PKA regulates proteins Cdc25, Ira2 and Pde1 through positive and negative feedback mechanisms that ensure, under certain conditions, the establishment of stable oscillatory regimes in the dynamics of Ras2-GTP, cAMP, and C (Garmendia-Torres et al. 2007; Pescini et al. 2012; Besozzi et al. 2012).

The hybrid model of this pathway was built by formalizing the mechanistic module as a reaction-based model (Besozzi 2016) comprising 10 reactions. The components belonging to the fuzzy module consist in 8 linguistic variables and 16 fuzzy rules, while the interface between the two modules consists in the species Ras2-GTP.

Figure 2.9 shows the dynamics of the interface species Ras2-GTP and of the linguistic variables Cyr1, cAMP, C, and Pde1 belonging to the fuzzy module, simulated with $\Delta = 10$. The hybrid model is capable of correctly reproducing the stable oscillations that characterize the behavior of the biochemical pathway, as already shown in Pescini et al. (2012), with a computational effort considerably smaller than that required by the simulations with a classic stochastic simulation algorithm (Spolaor et al. 2019).

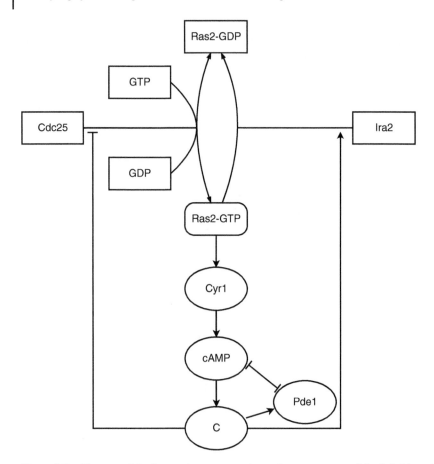

Figure 2.8 Diagram of the interactions among the main components of the hybrid model of the Ras/cAMP/PKA pathway. Variables belonging to the mechanistic module are represented by rectangles, variables belonging to the fuzzy module are represented by ellipses, while the interface species (Ras2-GTP) is represented as rounded rectangle. Positive and negative regulations are pictured as arrows and blunt-ended arrows, respectively.

2.4 Data-Driven Modeling

Data play a major role in all applications related to biomedical sciences, including healthcare. As a way of example, new knowledge is acquired through clinical trials in which statistical analysis of collected data provides insights in the efficiency of new treatment methods, and epidemiological studies can affect healthcare policy making. Also, in the treatment of individual patients data play a relevant role; for instance, clinicians collect data using the hypothetico-deductive approach (Shortliffe et al. 2014) to support or falsify the hypothesised diagnosis, to track the health status of patients, and determine treatment efficiency over prolonged periods of time.

With the introduction of electronic health records, these data are now more easily stored, accessed, and shared between health care providers, which now have access to vast amounts of diverse data to base their judgements on patients under treatments. While these immense

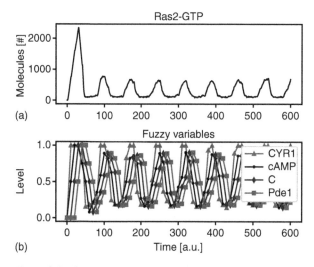

Figure 2.9 Dynamics of five key components in the Ras/cAMP/PKA pathway: the Ras2-GTP species belonging to the interface between the two modules of the hybrid model (a), and the 4 fuzzy variables (b).

amounts of data might overwhelm healthcare providers, it does enable the use of large-scale data analytics. The data deluge has caused an increase in the development and application of ML methods. Among these methods, in the last decades FISs carved out their own niche as (light) grey box models, which are considered more interpretable and transparent than other commonly employed methods, such as artificial neural networks.

To facilitate the development of FISs based on data, we recently introduced the Python package pyFUME (Fuchs et al. 2020b). In this section, we first describe pyFUME along with its main functionalities; afterwards, we demonstrate its usefulness by presenting a real-world application aimed at assessing tremor severity in essential tremor (ET) patients, based on data gathered using smartphone sensors.

2.4.1 pyFUME: Automatic Generation of Fuzzy Inference Systems

Although commercially distributed alternatives are available, software able to assist practitioners and researchers in each step of the estimation of a FIS from data are still limited in scope and applicability. This is especially true when looking at software developed in Python, a programming language that quickly gained popularity among data scientists and it is often considered their language of choice. To fill this gap, pyFUME (Fuchs et al. 2020b), a Python library for automatically estimating FISs from data was recently presented.

pyFUME contains a set of classes and methods to estimate the antecedent sets and the consequent parameters of a Sugeno FIS from data, and then create an executable FIS exploiting the Simpful library (Spolaor et al. 2020). pyFUME helps practitioners to effortlessly create FISs out of data thanks to its easy-to-use interface. At the same time, it gives researchers who want to fine-tune each step of the estimation process the flexibility to fully customize the internal pipeline and/or create personalized processing modules. The pyFUME package gives as an output—besides the executable model object—a file containing the Simpful code, which has the advantage that the generated FIS is presented in an easy to read syntax. The generated model can be visually analyzed using Simpful's plot facilities.

pyFUME can assist the user in all the steps of the creation of a FIS. It can load the data from a .*csv*-file, split the data in training and testing datasets (supporting both the hold-out and the k-fold cross validation method), and it can impute missing values with the mean of the K-nearest-neighbor data points. After this, feature selection can be performed using several approaches, such as sequential forward selection or a more advanced approach based a Fuzzy Self-Tuning PSO (FST-PSO) (Nobile et al. 2018). The latter approach has the added advantage to also optimize the number of rules of the FIS, if requested by the user. Once, the data have been prepared and relevant features have been selected, the model building can begin. The user can choose to cluster the data in the input–output space by means of Fuzzy C-Means (FCM) clustering (Bezdek 1981), Gustafson–Kessel clustering (Gustafson and Kessel 1979), or an approach based on FST-PSO (Nobile et al. 2018; Fuchs et al. 2019). Afterward, the antecedent sets (using the method described in Fuchs et al. (2018)) and the consequent parameters (as described in Babuška (2000)) of a zero- or first-order Sugeno FIS, can be estimated. Currently, pyFUME supports Gaussian, double Gaussian, and sigmoidal membership functions (Klir and Yuan 1995). The developed model can then be simplified using the graph-based simplification approach presented in Fuchs et al. (2020a), which detects and automatically drops highly overlapping antecedent sets from the rule base. Finally, the model can be evaluated in terms of performance by calculating the root mean squared error (RMSE), mean squared error (MSE), mean absolute error (MAE), or the mean absolute percentage error (MAPE), either on the internally separated test dataset or on an externally provided dataset.

An example of one of the predefined pipeline is schematized in Figure 2.10, showing how pyFUME's classes are linked to train a model using the hold-out method. In this example, no data imputation or model simplification is performed. The exact methods (e.g. the exact

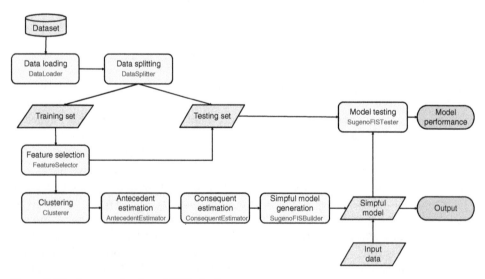

Figure 2.10 An example of a pyFUME pipeline.

feature selection or clustering method) that are used in each pyFUME block can be specified by the user, otherwise default options are employed.

pyFUME is implemented in the Python 3 language. It depends on NumPy (Oliphant 2007), Scipy (Jones et al. 2001) and Simpful (Spolaor et al. 2020), and can be downloaded from GitHub at: https://github.com/CaroFuchs/pyFUME. pyFUME can also be installed by using the PyPI facility: `pip install pyFUME`.

2.4.2 Application 3: Assessing Tremor Severity in Neurological Disorders

To show the effectiveness of pyFUME, we present an application where it was used to investigate tremor severity in ET patients. The data-driven model is aimed at helping clinicians to more objectively assess the severity of the patient's tremor, as well as increasing the inter-rater reliability among clinicians. More details and background on this study can be found in Zamora et al. (2019) and Fuchs et al. (2021).

ET is a neurological disorder that causes involuntary trembling, especially in the patient's hands; despite being a non-dangerous condition, it can worsen over time and become severe in some individuals. Tremor severity assessment is an important step for the diagnosis and treatment decision-making of this disease. Traditionally, tremor severity is measured with qualitative rating scales, such as the Quality of life in Essential Tremor (QUEST) score, or the Essential Tremor Rating Scale (ETRS) score. Since, these scales are subjective in nature, attention has shifted to computerized tremor analysis.

Here, we present the FIS developed to map the relationship between sensor measurements and QUEST/ETRS scores. To avoid the use of expensive and dedicated hardware to measure tremors, we exploited TREMOR12 (Kubben et al. 2016), a smartphone application developed by clinicians from the Maastricht University Medical Center. Twenty participants (11 men, 9 women), who were all diagnosed with ET, took part in the experiment. The tremor data were collected by strapping smartphones to the wrists of ET patients. The participants were asked to perform five different tests; specifically, the tremor was recorded: (i) during rest while the arm was resting on the table, (ii) while both arms were stretched forward with the hand palms facing down, (iii) while both hands were held in front of the chest with the hand palm down and elbows sideways, (iv) while the participant picked up a glass of water from the table, brought the glass toward the mouth, and put it back on the table, and (v) while the participant moved their index finger to their own nose and subsequently to the index finger of the researcher. The resulting raw sensor data was preprocessed to remove any artifact due to patient's intentional movement, and features (i.e. scalar real values that can be used in the modeling phase) were extracted from the sensor data.

Finally, the data were exploited to automatically build a transparent, interpretable, and succinct FIS for the severity assessment of ET, by means of pyFUME coupled with FST-PSO to identify optimal cluster structure in data, reducing the possibility of a premature convergence to sub-optimal models (Nobile et al. 2018; Fuchs et al. 2019). All other settings for pyFUME were kept on default (for more information, see Fuchs et al. (2021)).

Two FISs were trained: one to map the sensor data to the ETRS score, and one to the QUEST score. Since, both models are similar in nature, here we focus only on the ETRS model. Information on the QUEST model can be found in Fuchs et al. (2021). The model to determine the patient's ETRS score consists of the two following rules:

- RULE1: IF (dominantFrequency IS high) AND (dominantMagnitude IS
  any value) AND (signalPeriod IS any value) AND (powerGrowth IS
  any value) THEN (ETRS score = 27.8 * dominantFrequency -42.4 *
  dominantMagnitude +22.4 * signalPeriod + 23.3 * powerGrowth
  + 8.7)
- RULE 2: IF (dominantFrequency IS low) AND (dominantMagnitude IS
  low) AND (signalPeriod IS medium) AND (powerGrowth IS medium)
  THEN (ETRS Score = -10.8 * dominantFrequency + 53.5 *
  dominantMagnitude - 18.2 * signalPeriod + 14.0 * powerGrowth
  + 58.5)

The linguistic terms as used in the rules are defined by their membership functions, shown in Figure 2.11.

With an MAE of 1.85, the developed model outperforms a multiple regression line (R^2 = 0.58, MAE = 8.44). Our FIS also performs better than the decision tree presented in Zamora et al. (2019), which was trained on the same dataset and has an MAE of 6.41.

It is worth mentioning that the developed model could help clinicians monitor their ET patients. For instance, the model could be used to measure the effect of deep brain simulation (DBS) on the patient's tremors. DBS requires the surgical placement of a neurostimulator that sends electrical impulses trough electrodes to specific brain nuclei, in order to suppress the patient's tremor. After the placement of the neurostimulator, the optimal patient-specific settings for stimulation should be determined, which is "an ad hoc empirical process, with associated difficulties of time, expense, and patient discomfort" (Kuncel and Grill 2004). The immediate feedback of sensor data and ML could ease this process.

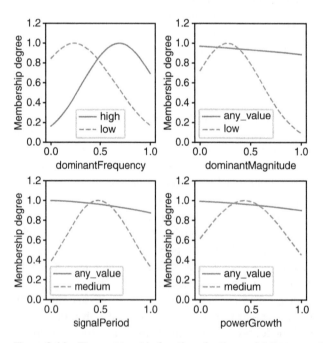

Figure 2.11 The membership functions for the model that maps the sensor data to the ETRS score.

Ultimately, this could lead to self-learning neurostimulators, in which the settings of the stimulation are adjusted automatically based on real-time feedback.

The use of sensor data from wearables, combined with models produced by ML algorithms, can also be useful for patients treated in different ways. For example, they can be used to find the correct dosage for ET patients treated with medication, or measure the effectiveness of magnetic resonance guided focused ultrasound.

2.5 Discussion

In this chapter, we discussed two alternative strategies for the definition of mathematical models, either based on domain knowledge or on available data, to tackle research problem pertaining the biomedical sciences. In the knowledge-driven approach, the model is defined relying on specific information about the components—and their mutual regulation—involved in the system under investigation; in the data-driven approach, on the contrary, computational strategies as ML are employed to automatically construct the model from the available data, without any *a priori* information to drive the modeling process. In both cases, fuzzy logic can be profitably exploited, since its application is independent from the modeling approach employed; moreover, fuzzy logic can be coupled with computational intelligence methods, to obtain mathematical models characterized by a high level of interpretability, thus making its application suitable in difficult real-world scenarios such as medicine (Barro and Marin 2001).

To corroborate our standpoint, we described two knowledge-driven computational methods capable of addressing critical issues that often arise in the modeling of complex systems. Specifically, knowledge-driven modeling based on fuzzy logic can deal with the multilevel nature that is typical of biomedical systems—e.g. molecules, cells, tissues, organs, and organisms—as well as with the lack of quantitative data, which limits the precise (numerical) parameterization of the model. These approaches are particularly suitable for the modeling and simulation of heterogeneous systems, and for the integration of multiple data types generated from different measurement platforms (e.g. imaging techniques and transcriptional data) using knowledge-based rules. In this context, we showed that the analysis of dynamic fuzzy logic models can be coupled with optimization algorithms (e.g. simulated annealing), for instance to uncover new potential therapeutic targets when applied to investigate complex biomedical systems, thus reducing the costs and facilitating the design of *ad hoc* laboratory experiments. Moreover, we showed that hybrid models, albeit requiring less precise information with respect to a fully mechanistic model, allow for the description of complex behaviors even when detailed mechanistic information is not available.

For what concerns the data-driven modeling approaches, we described a strategy based on pyFUME, a Python package specifically developed for the automatic creation of interpretable FIS from data. These models consist of fuzzy rules, which make the FIS transparent and open to interpretation. The interpretability property can be leveraged to validate the developed models with the help of domain experts, and to direct the attention of researchers to previously unknown relationships in the data. Interpretability and explainability are indispensable features in biomedical sciences and healthcare—for instance, for the development of reliable clinical decision support systems—and can help to make ML models compliant with (privacy) legislation (Sutton et al. 2020; Amann et al. 2022).

We envision that fuzzy models can provide human-comprehensible explanations to complex behaviors and patterns arising in several systems that are subject of study in the biomedical field. In the future, we plan to develop new methods to bridge the gap between knowledge-driven and data-driven approaches, in order to exploit, at the same time, the available data and the knowledge of domain experts.

Author Biographies

Paolo Cazzaniga received the MSc and PhD in Computer Science from the University of Milano-Bicocca, Italy, in 2005 and 2010, respectively. From February 2011 to May 2021, he was Assistant Professor at the University of Bergamo, Italy; since June 2021, he is Associate Professor at the University of Bergamo, Italy. He is a member of SYSBIO.IT Centre of Systems Biology, Italy, and of the Bicocca Bioinformatics, Biostatistics and Bioimaging (B4) research center, Milan, Italy. His research interests range from the interdisciplinary field of Systems Biology to simulation algorithms, evolutionary computation, swarm intelligence, natural computing, and GPU computing.

Simone Spolaor obtained his Master Degree in Molecular Biotechnology and Bioinformatics from the University of Milan, Italy, in 2016, and his PhD in Computer Science at the University of Milano-Bicocca, Italy, in 2020. During his PhD, he developed computational techniques to simulate and analyze complex biochemical systems, with a focus on methods based on fuzzy logic. Currently, he is a Post doc in the Neuromorphic Engineering Group at the Eindhoven University of Technology. His scientific interests include Systems and Synthetic Biology, complex systems simulation, bio-inspired algorithms, and intelligent matter.

Caro Fuchs pursues her PhD degree at the Department of Industrial Engineering and Innovation Sciences of the Eindhoven University of Technology (TU/e) and at the Jheronimus Academy of Data Science (JADS). Her research interests include interpretable decision support systems, data analysis, ML, and computational modeling methods, with a special focus on fuzzy inference systems. She mainly applies her research in the healthcare domain.

Marco S. Nobile received his PhD in Computer Science from the University of Milano-Bicocca, Italy. He is currently Associate Professor with the Department of Environmental Sciences, Informatics and Statistics of the Ca' Foscari University of Venice. Prof. Nobile is Senior Member of IEEE and belongs to the Bioinformatics and Bioengineering Technical Committee, where he leads the Task Force on advanced representation in biological and medical search and optimization. He is also Associate Editor of IEEE Transactions on Artificial Intelligence. Prof. Nobile's main research interests are Computational Intelligence and Interpretable AI, applied to biomedical problems.

Daniela Besozzi received the MS in Mathematics from the University of Insubria, Italy, in 2000 and the PhD in Computer Science from the University of Milano, Italy, in 2004.

From December 2002 to September 2015, she was Assistant Professor at the Department of Computer Science, University of Milano, Italy. Since October 2015, she is Associate Professor at the Department of Informatics, Systems and Communication, University of Milano-Bicocca, Italy. She is member of Bicocca Bioinformatics, Biostatistics and Bioimaging (B4) research center, and of SYSBIO/ISBE.IT Centre of Systems Biology. Her research interests include mathematical modeling, systems biology, bioinformatics, computational intelligence, and evolutionary computation.

References

Aldridge, B.B., Saez-Rodriguez, J., Muhlich, J.L. et al. (2009). Fuzzy logic analysis of kinase pathway crosstalk in TNF/EGF/insulin-induced signaling. *PLoS Computational Biology* 5 (4): e1000340. https://doi.org/10.1371/journal.pcbi.1000340.

Amann, J., Vetter, D., Blomberg, S.N. et al. and on behalf of the Z-Inspection initiative(2022, 2022). To explain or not to explain? Artificial intelligence explainability in clinical decision support systems. *PLOS Digital Health* 1 (2): 1–18. https://doi.org/10.1371/journal.pdig .0000016.

Anderson, A. and Rejniak, K. (2007). *Single-Cell-Based Models in Biology and Medicine.* Springer Science & Business Media. https://doi.org/10.1007/978-3-7643-8123-3.

Babuška, R. (2000). *Fuzzy Modelling and Identification Toolbox*, Version 3. Delft, The Netherlands: Control Engineering Laboratory, Faculty of Information Technology and Systems, Delft University of Technology.

Barro, S. and Marin, R. (2001). *Fuzzy Logic in Medicine*, Studies in Fuzziness and Soft Computing. Physica-Verlag HD. ISBN: 9783790814293. https://doi.org/10.1007/978-3-7908-1804-8.

Bar-Yam, Y. (1997). *Dynamics of Complex Systems*, vol. 213. Reading, MA: Addison-Wesley https://doi.org/10.1201/9780429034961.

Besozzi, D. (2016). Reaction-based models of biochemical networks. In: *Pursuit of the Universal. 12th Conference on Computability in Europe, CiE 2016, Proceedings*, volume 9709 of LNCS, Switzerland (ed. A. Beckmann, L. Bienvenu, and N. Jonoska), 24–34. Springer International Publishing. https://doi.org/10.1007/978-3-319-40189-8_3.

Besozzi, D., Cazzaniga, P., Pescini, D. et al. (2012). The role of feedback control mechanisms on the establishment of oscillatory regimes in the Ras/cAMP/PKA pathway in *S. cerevisiae.* *EURASIP Journal on Bioinformatics and Systems Biology* 2012 (1): 10. https://doi.org/10 .1186/1687-4153-2012-10.

Bezdek, J.C. (1981). Models for pattern recognition. In: *Pattern Recognition with Fuzzy Objective Function Algorithms*, 1–13. Springer. https://doi.org/10.1007/978-1-4757-0450-11.

Brady, R. and Enderling, H. (2019). Mathematical models of cancer: when to predict novel therapies, and when not to. *Bulletin of Mathematical Biology* 81 (10): 3722–3731. https://doi .org/10.1007/s11538-019-00640-x.

Castro, J.L. and Delgado, M. (1996). Fuzzy systems with defuzzification are universal approximators. *IEEE Transactions on Systems, Man, and Cybernetics, Part B (Cybernetics)* 26 (1): 149–152. https://doi.org/10.1109/3477.484447.

Chang, P. and Lee, S.E. (1999). Fuzzy decision networks and deconvolution. *Computers & Mathematics with Applications* 37 (11-12): 53–63. https://doi.org/10.1016/S0898-1221(99)00143-1.

Cherkassky, V. (1998). Fuzzy inference systems: a critical review. In: *Computational Intelligence: Soft Computing and Fuzzy-Neuro Integration with Applications*, 177–197. Springer. https://doi.org/10.1007/978-3-642-58930-0_10.

Dubois, D. and Prade, H. (1996). What are fuzzy rules and how to use them. *Fuzzy Sets and Systems* 84 (2): 169–185. https://doi.org/10.1016/0165-0114(96)00066-8.

Dubois, D. and Prade, H. (1997). The three semantics of fuzzy sets. *Fuzzy Sets and Systems* 90 (2): 141–150. https://doi.org/10.1016/S0165-0114(97)00080-8.

Edelstein-Keshet, L. (2005). *Mathematical Models in Biology*. SIAM. https://doi.org/10.1137/1.9780898719147.

Fuchs, C., Wilbik, A., and Kaymak, U. (2018). Towards more specific estimation of membership functions for data-driven fuzzy inference systems. *2018 IEEE International Conference on Fuzzy Systems (FUZZ-IEEE)*, 1–8. IEEE. https://doi.org/10.1109/FUZZ-IEEE.2018.8491524.

Fuchs, C., Spolaor, S., Nobile, M.S., and Kaymak, U. (2019). A swarm intelligence approach to avoid local optima in fuzzy c-means clustering. *2019 IEEE International Conference on Fuzzy Systems (FUZZ-IEEE)*, 1–6. IEEE. https://doi.org/10.1109/FUZZ-IEEE.2019.8858940.

Fuchs, C., Spolaor, S., Nobile, M.S., and Kaymak, U. (2020a). A graph theory approach to fuzzy rule base simplification. *International Conference on Information Processing and Management of Uncertainty in Knowledge-Based Systems*, 387–401. Springer. https://doi.org/10.1007/978-3-030-50146-4_29.

Fuchs, C., Spolaor, S., Nobile, M.S., and Kaymak, U. (2020b). pyFUME: a Python package for fuzzy model estimation. *2020 IEEE International Conference on Fuzzy Systems (FUZZ-IEEE)*, 1–8. IEEE. https://doi.org/10.1109/FUZZ48607.2020.9177565.

Fuchs, C., Nobile, M.S., Zamora, G. et al. (2021). Tremor assessment using smartphone sensor data and fuzzy reasoning. *BMC Bioinformatics* 22 (2): 1–17. https://doi.org/10.1186/s12859-021-03961-8.

Garmendia-Torres, C., Goldbeter, A., and Jacquet, M. (2007). Nucleocytoplasmic oscillations of the yeast transcription factor Msn2: evidence for periodic PKA activation. *Current Biology* 17 (12): 1044–1049. https://doi.org/10.1016/j.cub.2007.05.032.

Graupe, D. (2013). *Principles of Artificial Neural Networks*, vol. 7. World Scientific https://doi.org/10.1142/8868.

Gustafson, D.E. and Kessel, W.C. (1979). Fuzzy clustering with a fuzzy covariance matrix. *1978 IEEE Conference on Decision and Control*, 761–766. IEEE. https://doi.org/10.1109/CDC.1978.268028.

Hetz, C. and Papa, F.R. (2018). The unfolded protein response and cell fate control. *Molecular Cell* 69: 169–181. https://doi.org/10.1016/j.molcel.2017.06.017.

Huang, C., Li, Y., Li, Z. et al. (2019). LIMS1 promotes pancreatic cancer cell survival under oxygen-glucose deprivation conditions by enhancing HIF1A protein translation. *Clinical Cancer Research*. https://doi.org/10.1158/1078-0432.CCR-18-3533. Published OnlineFirst.

Jones, E., Oliphant, T.E., Peterson, P. et al. (2001). SciPY: open source scientific tools for python. https://www.scipy.org.

Keller, R., Klein, M., Thomas, M. et al. (2016). Coordinating role of RXRα in downregulating hepatic detoxification during inflammation revealed by fuzzy-logic modeling. *PLoS Computational Biology* 12 (1): e1004431. https://doi.org/10.1371/journal.pcbi.1004431.

Klir, G.J. and Yuan, B. (1995). *Fuzzy Sets and Fuzzy Logic: Theory and Applications*. Upper Saddle River, NJ: https://doi.org/10.1021/ci950144a.

Kubben, P.L., Kuijf, M.L., Ackermans, L.P.C.M. et al. (2016). TREMOR12: an open-source mobile app for tremor quantification. *Stereotactic and Functional Neurosurgery* 94 (3): 182–186. https://doi.org/10.1159/000446610.

Küffner, R., Petri, T., Windhager, L., and Zimmer, R. (2010). Petri nets with fuzzy logic (PNFL): reverse engineering and parametrization. *PLoS ONE* 5 (9): e12807. https://doi.org/10.1371/journal.pone.0012807.

Kuncel, A.M. and Grill, W.M. (2004). Selection of stimulus parameters for deep brain stimulation. *Clinical Neurophysiology* 115 (11): 2431–2441. https://doi.org/10.1016/j.clinph.2004.05.031.

Le Novère, N. (2015). Quantitative and logic modelling of molecular and gene networks. *Nature Reviews Genetics* 16 (3): 146–158. https://doi.org/10.1038/nrg3885.

Mamdani, E.H. and Assilian, S. (1975). An experiment in linguistic synthesis with a fuzzy logic controller. *International Journal of Man-Machine Studies* 7 (1): 1–13. https://doi.org/10.1016/S0020-7373(75)80002-2.

Mendel, J.M. and John, R.I. (2002). Type-2 fuzzy sets made simple. *IEEE Transactions on Fuzzy Systems* 10 (2): 117–127. https://doi.org/10.1109/91.995115.

Morris, M.K., Clarke, D.C., Osimiri, L.C., and Lauffenburger, D.A. (2016). Systematic analysis of quantitative logic model ensembles predicts drug combination effects on cell signaling networks. *CPT: Pharmacometrics & Systems Pharmacology* 5 (10): 544–553. https://doi.org/10.1002/psp4.12104.

Nobile, M.S., Cazzaniga, P., Besozzi, D. et al. (2018). Fuzzy self-tuning PSO: a settings-free algorithm for global optimization. *Swarm and Evolutionary Computation* 39: 70–85. https://doi.org/10.1016/j.swevo.2017.09.001.

Nobile, M.S., Votta, G., Palorini, R. et al. (2020). Fuzzy modeling and global optimization to predict novel therapeutic targets in cancer cells. *Bioinformatics* 36 (7): 2181–2188. https://doi.org/10.1093/bioinformatics/btz868.

Oliphant, T.E. (2007). Python for scientific computing. *Computing in Science & Engineering* 9 (3): 10–20. https://doi.org/10.1109/MCSE.2007.58.

Palorini, R., Votta, G., Pirola, Y. et al. (2016). Protein Kinase A activation promotes cancer cell resistance to glucose starvation and *anoikis*. *PLoS Genetics* 12 (3): e1005931. https://doi.org/10.1371/journal.pgen.1005931.

Pescini, D., Cazzaniga, P., Besozzi, D. et al. (2012). Simulation of the Ras/cAMP/PKA pathway in budding yeast highlights the establishment of stable oscillatory states. *Biotechnology Advances* 30 (1): 99–107. https://doi.org/10.1016/j.biotechadv.2011.06.014.

Shortliffe, E.H., Shortliffe, E.H., Cimino, J.J., and Cimino, J.J. (2014). *Biomedical Informatics: Computer Applications in Health Care and Biomedicine*. Springer. https://doi.org/10.1007/978-1-4471-4474-8.

Spolaor, S., Nobile, M.S., Mauri, G. et al. (2019). Coupling mechanistic approaches and fuzzy logic to model and simulate complex systems. *IEEE Transactions on Fuzzy Systems*. https://doi.org/10.1109/TFUZZ.2019.2921517.

Spolaor, S., Fuchs, C., Cazzaniga, P. et al. (2020). Simpful: a user-friendly Python library for fuzzy logic. *International Journal of Computational Intelligence Systems* 13 (1): 1687–1698. https://doi.org/10.2991/ijcis.d.201012.002.

Spolaor, S., Scheve, M., Firat, M. et al. (2021). Screening for combination cancer therapies with dynamic fuzzy modeling and multi-objective optimization. *Frontiers in Genetics* 12: https://doi.org/10.3389/fgene.2021.617935.

Sugeno, M. (1985). *Industrial Applications of Fuzzy Control*. New York: Elsevier Science Inc. ISBN: 0444878297.

Sutton, R.T., Pincock, D., Baumgart, D.C. et al. (2020). An overview of clinical decision support systems: benefits, risks, and strategies for success. *npj Digital Medicine* 3 (1): 1–10. https://doi.org/10.1038/s41746-020-0221-y.

Takács, M. (2004). Critical analysis of various known methods for approximate reasoning in fuzzy logic control. *5th International Symposium of Hungarian Researchers on Computational Intelligence*. Hungary Budapest.

Takagi, T. and Sugeno, M. (1985). Fuzzy identification of systems and its applications to modeling and control. *IEEE Transactions on Systems, Man, and Cybernetics* 1: 116–132. https://doi.org/10.1109/TSMC.1985.6313399.

Taylor, R.C., Cullen, S.P., and Martin, S.J. (2008). Apoptosis: controlled demolition at the cellular level. *Nature Reviews Molecular Cell Biology* 9 (3): 231. https://doi.org/10.1038/nrm2312.

Thevelein, J.M. (1994). Signal transduction in yeast. *Yeast* 10: 1753–1790. https://doi.org/10.1002/yea.320101308.

Thevelein, J.M. and de Winde, J.H. (1999). Novel sensing mechanisms and targets for the cAMP-protein kinase A pathway in the yeast *Saccharomyces cerevisiae*. *Molecular Microbiology* 33: 904–918. https://doi.org/10.1046/j.1365-2958.1999.01538.x.

Wang, L.-X. (1992). Fuzzy systems are universal approximators. *[1992 Proceedings] IEEE International Conference on Fuzzy Systems*, 1163–1170. IEEE, 1992. https://doi.org/10.1109/FUZZY.1992.258721.

Wang, L.-X. and Mendel, J.M. (1992). Generating fuzzy rules by learning from examples. *IEEE Transactions on Systems, Man, and Cybernetics* 22 (6): 1414–1427. https://doi.org/10.1109/21.199466.

Wilkinson, D.J. (2009). Stochastic modelling for quantitative description of heterogeneous biological systems. *Nature Reviews Genetics* 10 (2): 122–133. https://doi.org/10.1038/nrg2509.

Wynn, M.L., Consul, N., Merajver, S.D., and Schnell, S. (2012). Logic-based models in systems biology: a predictive and parameter-free network analysis method. *Integrative Biology* 4 (11): 1323–1337. https://doi.org/10.1039/c2ib20193c.

Yaakob, A.M., Serguieva, A., and Gegov, A. (2017). FN-TOPSIS: fuzzy networks for ranking traded equities. *IEEE Transactions on Fuzzy Systems* 25 (2): 315–332. https://doi.org/10.1109/TFUZZ.2016.2555999.

Ye, P., Liu, Y., Chen, C. et al. (2015). An mTORC1-Mdm2-Drosha axis for miRNA biogenesis in response to glucose- and amino acid-deprivation. *Molecular Cell* 57 (4): 708–720. https://doi.org/10.1016/j.molcel.2014.12.034.

Yen, J. and Langari, R. (1999). *Fuzzy Logic: Intelligence, Control, and Information*, vol. 1. Upper Saddle River, NJ: Prentice Hall.

Zadeh, L.A. (1965). Fuzzy sets. *Information and Control* 8 (3): 338–353. https://doi.org/10.1016/S0019-9958(65)90241-X.

Zadeh, L.A. (1973). Outline of a new approach to the analysis of complex systems and decision processes. *IEEE Transactions on Systems, Man, and Cybernetics* SMC-3 (1): 28–44. https://doi.org/10.1109/TSMC.1973.5408575.

Zadeh, L.A. (1975). The concept of a linguistic variable and its application to approximate reasoning— I. *Information Sciences* 8 (3): 199–249. https://doi.org/10.1016/0020-0255(75)90036-5.

Zadeh, L.A. (1988). Fuzzy logic. *Computer* 21 (4): 83–93. https://doi.org/10.1109/2.53.

Zadeh, L.A. (1999). Fuzzy logic = computing with words. In: *Computing with Words in Information/Intelligent Systems 1*, 3–23. Springer https://doi.org/10.1109/91.493904.

Zamora, G., Fuchs, C., Degeneffe, A. et al. (2019). A smartphone-based clinical decision support system for tremor assessment. *International Meeting on Computational Intelligence Methods for Bioinformatics and Biostatistics*, 3–12. Springer, 2019. https://doi.org/10.1007/978-3-030-63061-4_1.

Zañudo, J.G.T. and Albert, R. (2015). Cell fate reprogramming by control of intracellular network dynamics. *PLoS Computational Biology* 11 (4): e1004193. https://doi.org/10.1371/journal.pcbi.1004193.

Zaugg, K., Yao, Y., Reilly, P.T. et al. (2011). Carnitine palmitoyltransferase 1C promotes cell survival and tumor growth under conditions of metabolic stress. *Genes & Development* 25 (10): 1041–1051. https://doi.org/10.1101/gad.1987211.

3

Application of Machine Learning Algorithms to Diagnosis and Prognosis of Chronic Wounds

Mai Dabas[1] and Amit Gefen[1,2,3]

[1]*Department of Biomedical Engineering, Faculty of Engineering, Tel Aviv University, Tel Aviv, Israel*
[2]*Skin Integrity Research Group (SKINT), University Centre for Nursing and Midwifery, Department of Public Health and Primary Care, Ghent University, Ghent, Belgium*
[3]*Department of Mathematics and Statistics, Faculty of Sciences, Hasselt University, Hasselt, Belgium*

3.1 Background

3.1.1 Chronic Wounds

Chronic wounds (CWs), such as pressure ulcers/injuries, venous leg ulcers, and diabetic foot ulcers (DFU), are defined as wounds that fail to progress through an orderly and timely reparation often due to a stall in the inflammatory phase of healing (Izadi and Ganchi 2005). Other wounds, which are traumatic in origin, such as burns and surgical wounds, may become infected and shift to chronicity. As all wound types have the potential to become hard to heal, and there is no clear consensus concerning the time duration of a wound that defines chronicity, CW are typically classified by combining their etiological cause, clinical diagnosis, and treatment protocol (Leaper and Durani 2008; Werdin et al. 2008; Martin and Nunan 2015). As the number of patients with CW consistently increases with the global aging of populations and the spread of chronic diseases, such as diabetes and obesity [and under the influence of the coronavirus 2019 disease (COVID-19)], healthcare professionals face the growing challenge of providing safe and effective care to all their patients simultaneously (Whitney et al. 2006).

3.1.2 Implementation of AI Methodologies in Wound Care and Management

An uprising and highly promising scientific approach for improving wound care and management for patients with CW is the development and clinical implementation of artificial intelligence (AI) technologies (Anisuzzaman et al. 2021). The use of AI in healthcare involves machine learning (ML) algorithms and software that mimic human cognition and action in the analysis, presentation, comprehension, and interpretation of complex medical and healthcare data.

Pressure ulcers/injuries, for example, appear to be very good candidates for effective application of AI-powered wound care, both in risk assessment and in early diagnosis aspects. With regards to risk assessment, Xu et al. (2022) published a retrospective cohort

Big Data Analysis and Artificial Intelligence for Medical Sciences, First Edition.
Edited by Bruno Carpentieri and Paola Lecca.
© 2024 John Wiley & Sons Ltd. Published 2024 by John Wiley & Sons Ltd.

study where they had developed a risk assessment tool that analyzed the electronic health records (EHRs) of 618 patients in an intensive care unit (ICU), through an ML algorithm comprising logistic regression and a random forest classifier with a cross-validation technique (Xu et al. 2022). They concluded that their ML algorithm can successfully substitute the traditional Braden risk assessment (Braden and Bergstrom 1988) process in the ICU setting, by automatically monitoring and processing the EHRs. In the context of early detection, Lustig et al. (2022) reported an ML algorithm that was trained using a database comprising six consecutive daily subepidermal moisture (SEM) measurements recorded from 173 patients in acute and post-acute care settings, which demonstrated strong predictive power in forecasting heel deep tissue injury (DTI) events the next day, based on the weighted trend of the acquired day-to-day SEM data (Lustig et al. 2022). Indeed, Raju et al. (2015) suggested earlier that prediction of pressure ulcers can be performed more effectively by utilizing data science, and more specifically, data mining modeling, to support and augment the Braden risk assessments conducted by nurses, and it appears that this approach is successfully maturing now, as demonstrated in the aforementioned articles (Raju et al. 2015).

Accordingly, AI-powered wound care is potentially able to reduce the workload on specialists, increase the accessibility to specific relevant medical expertise, and expand the potential of remote (tele-) wound treatment or management. Specifically, using a variety of textual and image data, collected from either new or already-available medical records and imaging modalities (as relevant to the affected body area), AI-based methodologies and algorithms may be able to provide clinical decision-support in wound diagnosis, prognosis, and management, and even contribute to the prevention of CW.

3.2 Clinical Visual Assessment of Wounds Supported by Artificial Intelligence

In order to examine a CW, the development of infection in an acute wound, or the progress or healing process of wounds in general, physicians and nurses perform frequent clinical visual assessments (VAs). Two main tasks that ML algorithms tend to perform efficiently in this aspect are classification and segmentation. In classification tasks, the AI algorithms acquire a wound image as an input and distinguish between predefined sets of classes, e.g. class I and class II. In segmentation tasks, AI algorithms also obtain an image as an input but classify each pixel therein to labels such as granulation versus necrotic tissues. It then becomes possible to present regions of the classified tissues per their specific labels or superimpose those with a picture of the entire wound. These types of models can assist in recognition of wound tissues and distinguish those from healthy skin by means of binary classifications, which determine whether an image (analyzed in a classification task) or a pixel of an image (in a segmentation task) represents healthy skin or wound tissues. Such classification and segmentation tasks require image datasets which can be acquired using multiple imaging methods, e.g. digital cameras, smartphones in healthcare facilities, through infrared, Raman spectroscopy (RS), and optical coherence tomography (OCT) techniques, hyperspectral and multispectral imaging or extracted from available online databases. The images are first labeled by expert physicians, manually or using software to establish a ground truth, and then preprocessed and fed into the developed algorithms for training and evaluation of the algorithm performances.

There are many types of ML classifiers available for these tasks such as support vector machine (SVM), logistic regression (LR), multilayer perceptron (MLP), radial basis function (RBF) kernel, random forest (RF), and k-nearest neighbors (KNN) (Mitchell 1997). The following models are defined as classic classifiers which can be employed to perform the classification of healthy versus wound tissues. An example for MLP and RBF classifiers implementation in CW was presented by Song and Sacan (2012), who used 92 DFU digital color images, labeled by experts to identify the wound region; these images were then split into a training set of 78 images and a test set of 14 images (Song and Sacan 2012). Song and colleagues compared the performances of the MLP method and RBF method in the task of wound area segmentation and found that the RBF was more accurate for this task (85.7% accuracy by RBF versus 71.4% by MLP) and required a shorter training period (1.7 seconds by RBF versus 12.6 seconds by MLP). Chen et al. (2018) studied a dataset of 131 surgical wound images acquired using different smartphones/tablets and labeled by clinical experts (Chen et al. 2018). They developed an algorithm for wound detection and assessment based on classic ML techniques and found that the combined KNN and RF classifiers achieved the highest accuracy (90%). Those examples demonstrate that the mentioned algorithms can be implemented separately or can be combined into an integrated model mostly providing better accuracy.

Other than using basic ML methods mentioned above, another promising approach is developing algorithms based on deep neural networks (DNNs) (Schulz and Behnke 2012). DNNs are neural networks with multiple hidden layers which allow learning from raw data without the necessity of hand-crafted features. They also provide better accuracy for more complex problems and, therefore, address a broad spectrum of problems (Santosh et al. 2022). After comparing the algorithm performances with the basic ML methods, it was shown that DNNs generally achieve better results than the basic ML methods (Kamath et al. 2018). For example, Sevik et al. (2019) developed an algorithm for distinguishing between skin and burn areas on burn wound images taken by technicians in emergency services (Şevik et al. 2019). They used 105 images acquired in hospital conditions and compared the segmentation and classification tasks performed using traditional computer vision and ML techniques, with those of a more advanced deep learning (DL) technique having a multi-class pixelwise segmentation architecture (commonly known as the "Seg-Net'") (Badrinarayanan et al. 2015). Sevik and colleagues found that the fully automated DL system had a greater F-score relative to the classic techniques and was, therefore, superior to most of the existing methods in the area of tissue health (i.e. healthy skin versus burn) classification. Specifically, the F-score of the DL architecture was 0.85, whereas the F-score of the best classic architecture was 0.74.

Other algorithms can be developed to distinguish between the different types of tissues within a CW and to correctly classify them. These algorithms may enable to automatically identify necrotic tissues, granulation tissue, and slough and healing tissues. An example of such implementation was demonstrated by Garcia-Zapirain et al. (2018), who used a database of 193 images to develop a system for automatic segmentation and detection of tissues inside a pressure ulcer/injury (Garcia-Zapirain et al. 2018). Their algorithm consisted of two main steps using a 3-dimensional (3D) convolutional neural network (CNN) model (a CNN model applied on a 3D dataset, such as a series of 2D images taken through time or space (Yang et al. 2018)). In the first step, the 3D CNN model was used to distinguish the external pressure ulcer/injury boundaries using the preprocessed images as an input. In the second step, a deeper 3D CNN model was designed to segment the internal boundaries of the necrotic, granulation, and slough tissues from the background. They compared the performances of their algorithm to two traditional computer vision segmentation techniques, the fuzzy c-means (FCM) (Bezdek 1984) and the linear combination of discrete Gaussians (LCDG) (Elnakib et al. 2016), and found that their approach has reached the highest AUC for classification of all the three aforementioned tissue types. Specifically, the average AUC of their algorithm was 95%, while the other two tested computer vision techniques reached substantially lower AUC values of 69% and 77%. Accordingly, their layered CNN approach contributed another tier to the role of AI in VAs.

Another potential capability that AI methodologies may provide for supporting a VA process is in identifying the type of the wound that is under assessment, objectively and automatically. Kavitha et al. (2017) proposed a method to perform an automatic, binary classification between pressure ulcers/injuries and leg ulcers (Kavitha et al. 2017). They suggested a pipeline process for the wound image analysis that included preprocessing of the digital wound images (e.g. color correction, noise removal, and color homogenization), segmentation, feature extraction, and, finally, classification of the CW type. Using 59 wound images, they trained and evaluated their algorithm. They found that the accuracy of their classification process was 83.1% using the MLP classifier, which is relatively high.

Another example for classification task was detailed in Lustig et al. (2022) study, which aimed to develop an AI-powered classification algorithm to diagnose and predict the formation of heel DTIs based on a daily-collected database of SEM measurements (Lustig et al. 2022). SEM data, which are established biophysical marker of pressure ulcer formation, were collected using a commercial SEM scanner (Bruin Biometrics LLC, Los Angeles, CA, United States). Classification algorithm was developed to identify patients who eventually developed heel DTI among patients who did not, using SEM measurements (Figure 3.1). Furthermore, a prediction algorithm was designed to predict whether a heel DTI will occur. The classification algorithm gained 79% accuracy and 90% sensitivity, whereas the prediction algorithm gained an average accuracy of 77% and average sensitivity of 80%. These results point out the potential clinical utility of SEM measurements, integrated with AI classification methodologies, to early detect DTIs and pressure ulcers/injuries.

Assessment of the wound severity and depth and identifying the presence of infection and ischemia are also possible using AI methodologies, by training these algorithms to obtain quantitative information and measurements concerning the wound size or to detect and assess wound infection and/or ischemia.

3.2.1 Predicting the Formation and Progress of Wounds Based on Electronic Health Records

The practice of acquiring and regularly updating EHRs, clinical background notes, records of examination results, physician assessments, medical procedures, and clinical notes, in general, generates large (textual and numerical) databases of patient and population conditions. Traditionally, physicians and nurses have used manual scoring tools to identify patients at risk of developing wounds. The currently available AI methods can support this process and provide considerably more rapid and objective risk assessments, by

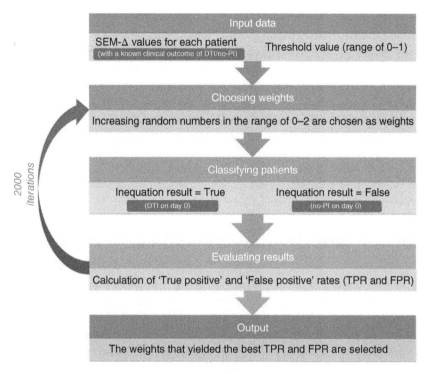

Figure 3.1 Flow chart of the ML algorithm training for heel DTI classification. Source: Reproduced from Lustig et al. 2022.

computationally analyzing the large amounts of accumulated data in EHRs. Predictive models which are based on generalizable features (such as data from EHRs) can provide more in-depth information about the risk of patients to develop a new wound and/or the likelihood of an existing wound to deteriorate, which in turn, facilitates informed clinical decision-making concerning preventative or treatment interventions (Jung et al. 2016).

Many research studies published over time aimed to develop predictive models for wound formation and evolution based on categorical and quantitative information that has been collected from clinical notes and EHRs. Goodwin and Demner-Fushman (2020) aimed to develop a generalizable model capable of leveraging clinical notes to predict healthcare-associated diseases 24–96 hours in advance and specifically the onset of hospital-acquired pressure ulcers/injuries (Goodwin and Demner-Fushman 2020). They developed a recurrent additive network for temporal risk prediction (CANTRIP), based on natural language processing (NLP) methodologies, using 35,218 clinical reports of patient cases. This CANTRIP algorithm, operating on text alone, obtained AUC of 74–87% and specificity of 77–85% which is promising. Of note is that shallow models (where there are less layers in the neural network structure) typically exhibit poorer performances with respect to all the relevant metrics that are commonly used for assessment of the algorithm performances (sensitivity and specificity, AUC, etc.).

Chun et al. (2021) aimed to establish a model that predicts seven-day clinical outcomes in children with a pressure ulcer/injury (Chun et al. 2021). They included 152 patients with a category-I pressure ulcer/injury or a suspected DTI and divided this cohort into two groups, namely, those who demonstrated healing versus children who presented delayed healing. The patients were followed for seven days, and their pressure ulcers/injuries were analyzed by their characteristics, demographics, treatment, clinical situation, vital signs, and blood test results. Using the collected data, a prediction model was constructed by RF (including a so-called "eXtreme Gradient Boosting" ML approach (Chen and Guestrin 2016)). The best prediction model, trained and tested using RF with 10 variables, achieved an accuracy, sensitivity, specificity, and AUC of 0.82, 0.80, 0.84, and 0.89, respectively. The most influential variables, in order of importance, were the serum creatinine level, the red blood cell count, and the hematocrit reading. This model, which is unique in being specific to the pediatric population, may allow to improve the quality of care and clinical outcomes in children with pressure ulcers/injuries.

3.2.2 Predicting the Formation and Evolution of Wounds Based on a Dynamic Evaluation of Wound Characteristics and Relevant Physiological Measures

Chronic and acute wounds both change over time. Changes in peri-wound skin and the appearance of the wound bed, together with physiological measures such as the skin and wound tissue temperatures, the exudate production, its contents, and biophysical and biochemical properties may indicate healthy healing or, alert that the wound is shifting into infection, chronicity or both. By using AI methodologies, it may be possible to predict the potential path of progression of a wound (toward either healthy healing or chronicity) in advance, using data of temporal and dynamic measures, and to clinically intervene accordingly. Martinez-Jiménez et al. (2018), for example, aimed to determine if temperature differences between a burn region and the healthy skin of a patient, assessed by infrared thermography, could be used to predict the treatment modality of spontaneous healing by re-epithelization, skin grafting, or amputations (Martínez-Jiménez et al. 2018). In the algorithm development step, they recorded the temperature differences between the burns and healthy skin tissues of patients during the first three days after injury and then categorized the patients according to one of the three aforementioned treatment modalities. A prediction model, based on the above burn-skin temperature differences, was developed using a recursive partitioning RF ML algorithm. They found that their algorithm correctly predicted into which treatment category a certain patient would eventually fall, with 85.4% accuracy.

The use of AI algorithms such as the above may contribute to predicting the severity of the injury and the clinical outcome and will, therefore, guide clinical decision-making, and optimize institutional healthcare resources. In particular, the use of adequate AI algorithms as adjunct to clinical judgment has the potential to prevent or at least mitigate potentially devastating consequences of inadequate treatment procedures.

An example for the development of AI algorithm based on an integrated database is presented by Kim et al. (2020), who built an ML model to predict the healing of DFU, using both EHRs and an image database (Kim et al. 2020). In their research, both hand-crafted color texture features and DL-based features were extracted from the wound images. For prediction, SVM and RF models were trained, and the results showed that models built from hand-crafted imaging features alone outperformed models built with clinical or DL features alone. These results suggested that the use of only hand-crafted image features and raw clinical attributes, which provide more intuitive insights to both clinicians and patients, can yield adequate wound healing predictions.

Another approach for preventing the formation and progression of pressure ulcers/injuries associated with prolonged bed stays is to detect the body position and evaluate whether a monitored patient has remained in a certain posture for a long period of time. Prolonged bed rests without repositioning may lead to pressure ulcers/injuries (Alinia et al. 2020; Matar et al. 2020; Wong et al. 2020); accordingly, developing a model that automatically detects movement in bed can be used for scheduling postural changes for patients, which contributes to effectively using nursing labor and time.

For example, Matar et al. (2020) suggested an autonomous method for classifying four in-bed lying postures using data from textile-made pressure sensors embedded under the bedsheet (Matar et al. 2020). Data collected from twelve adult subjects were implemented in a supervised artificial neural network model for the in-bed posture classification. The classification model reached high prediction scores, with accuracy of 97% and a Cohen's Kappa coefficient (a measure of inter-rater reliability) of 0.972. Apart from preventing pressure ulcers/injuries associated with prolonged stays in bed, an autonomous method of in-bed posture monitoring such as the above can also be used in several other medical fields where in-bed posture identification is much needed, such as in sleep studies and postsurgical (recovery from anesthesia) procedures.

3.2.3 Feasible Implementation of AI Solutions For Wound Care Delivery and Management

Many published studies show promising results regarding wound care and management and have the potential to improve wound care delivered to patients who suffer from CW by using AI methodologies. However, it appears that many of those studies mainly presented ML models which are still far from being available for implementation in real life due to various reasons, such as ML models that did not consider the backend processes required for implementation, or in the absence of sufficient details concerning the software and/or hardware for the implementation (e.g. where it was unclear if a mobile phone or a tablet can run the algorithm and provide the desired outputs). On the contrary, other studies describe end-to-end automatic systems in which data acquisition, data processing, and final results can all be obtained and can be integrated by software updates to existing electronics in the hardware systems or devices that are already in use by healthcare professionals during their daily routine of clinical practice. Hence, those suggested models can potentially be practiced by healthcare providers and clinicians in healthcare facilities "as is."

For example, Lustig et al. (2022) demonstrated in their study (which was also described in short in the Background Section above) the feasibility of such potential integration by developing an ML algorithm for early detection of heel DTI, based on data collected by the commercial SEM scanner (Bruin Biometrics LLC, Los Angeles, CA, United States); the SEM scanner is a medical device which is currently being used clinically, on a daily basis, by care providers in many healthcare facilities worldwide (Lustig et al. 2022).

Zahia et al. (2020) described an end-to-end nonintrusive system which automatically retrieves quantitative information of a pressure injury, such as the depth, area, volume, and major and minor axes of the wound under observation, using a 2D image and a 3D mesh of the wound (Zahia et al. 2020). The 2D wound image was obtained by means of a tablet camera, and the 3D wound mesh was acquired through an easy-to-use structure sensor mounted on the tablet. CNN algorithms were then used to automatically detect and segment the wound area from the 2D image, then the segmentation results were combined with the 3D wound mesh, and the quantitative information associated with the wound was automatically computed. During their research, Zahia et al. showed that caregivers could capture the 2D images and the 3D meshes efficiently, and the acquisition time ranged from one to two minutes in total, which is clinically feasible. This system appears to be approachable and easy to use by healthcare providers using a simple tablet and a mounted sensor, in addition to the short time it takes to collect the relevant data which enables the clinicians to manage their time with their patients more effectively.

Nonetheless, real-life implementation of AI technologies in healthcare is subjected to many obstacles. One of the main barriers is the absence of regulations concerning the safety and efficacy of AI systems in the medical field. Related to that are growing concerns regarding data privacy and cybersecurity. Furthermore, the medical environment is currently not compatible to automated data exchange and for continuous supply and update of the data for further development and improvement of AI systems (F et al. 2017). However, we believe that following the substantial growth in medical research regarding integration of AI methodologies in wound care and management, feasible implementation of AI technologies in the wound care field would eventually become available.

3.2.4 Types of Data Modalities for Diagnosis, Detection, and Prediction of Chronic Wounds

Many data types, i.e. clinical notes, image datasets, EHRs, and experimental measurements, are used for model construction for the purpose of different tasks, such as wound/tissue type classification, prediction, and diagnosis.

One of the main utilities of ML algorithms in wound care is to build a predictive model to provide wound prognosis or an automated advice concerning the required treatment or to calculate the likelihood of the wound to heal. A variety of data types and modalities can be used for this purpose, including EHRs, image datasets, spatial/temporal dynamic data, or a combination of several modalities, to build more reliable databases for model construction, training, and evaluation.

Wound assessment and diagnosis can be obtained by different data modalities, such as image datasets, EHRs, and experimental results when image datasets are the most frequently used modality in this case. As an example, WoundSeg is a DNN developed and presented by Liu et al. (2018), and its main goal is to locate and segment CW automatically in images (Xiaohui et al. 2017). The WoundSeg algorithm, developed based on a dataset of wound images, includes a computationally efficient wound segmentation based on a MobileNets model (a CNN containing depth-wise separable convolutions, to build a light-weight DNN (Howard et al. 2017)), as well as data augmentation and post-processing. The WoundSeg model presented by Xiaohui and colleagues showed promising results (98% accuracy and 93% precision) which are considered to position this model as an alternative approach for replacing the traditional empirical and manual wound area measurements.

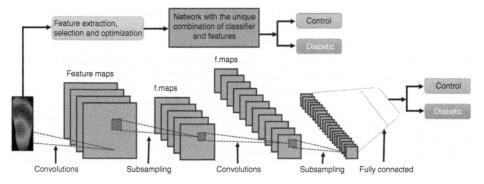

Figure 3.2 Example for deep leaning-based image classification pipeline. The pipeline consists of feature extraction, selection and optimization, and then classification between the control and diabetic patients. Source: Reproduced from Khandakar et al. 2021/Elsevier/CC BY 4.0.

Classification task (see example in Figure 3.2), which allows to classify wound etiologies, wound tissue types, healthy and infected skin, and wound severity stages, is mostly based on image datasets collected by digital cameras, and less frequently on experimental results or EHRs.

Alzubaidi et al. (2019) presented such classifier named DFU_QUTNet, a deep CNN which proposes automatic classification of healthy skin and DFU from color images (Alzubaidi et al. 2019).

The structure of this network allows to extract a variety of features from different layers of the network and to combine and feed them inside a classifier to get a final classification prediction. The suggested DFU_QUTNet model achieved F-score of 94.5% and outperformed other state-of-the-art CNN networks which are commonly used for such classification tasks (such as GoogleNet (Szegedy et al. 2014), VGG-16 (Simonyan and Zisserman 2014), and AlexNet (Krizhevsky et al. 2012)).

3.3 Smartphone and Tablet Use in Wound Diagnosis and Management

The outbreak of the COVID-19 has brought the topic of telemedicine into a sharp focus. In the context of pressure ulcers/injuries, the need for tele-healthcare is often associated with limited access to elderly care facilities, in view of the risk of COVID-19 infection to the facilities, and the increased susceptibility of elderly residents in long-term care settings to both pressure ulcers/injuries and COVID-19. Bioengineering contributions in this regard may focus on ML algorithms that provide AI consultation systems to expert healthcare professionals, through smartphone/tablet application software. This can lead to development of big databases of nursing home resident data that will reveal the extrinsic and intrinsic factors affecting the risk of pressure ulcers/injuries or the likelihood of their healing in these individuals for particular settings or institutes (including under the effects of COVID-19). The availability of such AI-based consultation tools may also have an overall positive effect on the standard of care that aged-care residents are receiving as a collective, as well as individually (e.g. if specific measures are taken to mitigate the injury risk).

The data collected by AI systems through smartphones/tablets may include EHRs, Vas, additional physiological measures that indicate susceptibility or early signs of a forming pressure ulcer/injury such as changes in SEM, infrared thermography or ultrasound measurements, and any relevant risk factors, including ones that can be mitigated by adequate interventions. Based on data mining and ML algorithms employing the collected big data, AI systems can then offer clinicians the specific measures that have been proven to be successful in other similar cases. Such AI systems may further incorporate all the published recommendations in the 2019 International Guideline for Pressure Ulcer/Injury Prevention and Treatment (Padula et al. 2019). Hence, effectively, AI systems will facilitate machine-based, real-time consultation, as adjunct to the expert clinical judgment and experience, which will be the most advanced and up-to-date comprehensive synthesis of all the available and contemporary medical knowledge regarding pressure ulcer/injury prevention and treatment, including in individuals affected by COVID-19. All of that will be available at the click of a button and will be delivered instantaneously to the cellular devices that healthcare professionals typically use in their daily work already.

In fact, from a hardware and software technology perspective, smartphones and tablets are already mature for implementation of AI systems. Their design features include powerful processors, multiple high-resolution cameras, and communication capabilities, particularly including wireless connection to cloud computing. Therefore, smartphones and tablets are very likely to play a major role in the growing impact of AI in wound diagnosis and management, as they facilitate image and textual data collection, potential integration of physiological sensors, fast data analysis supported by cloud computing, and friendly user interfaces. In particular, acquiring image data using smartphone cameras does not require special proficiencies and, therefore, can be done by healthcare professionals during their routine care of patients (many clinicians regularly document the wound healing of their patients using smartphones already). Acquiring such visual data in real-life scenarios, under hospital conditions, and by unprofessional photographers also provides realistic settings and data for the AI algorithms to cope with, which is a challenge.

Shenoy et al. (2019) have implemented their wound image classification network called "Deepwound" on a mobile application that can assist physicians and patients in postoperative wound surveillance (Shenoy et al. 2019). They collected 1335 diverse smartphone wound images containing nine different wound types and conditions, ranged from open wounds with infections to closed wounds with sutures. They then generated a model called "Deepwound," a combination of three separate models that are based on the VGG-16 CNN architecture after modifications. The mobile application presented in their article, called "Theia," is a suggested way to deliver the "Deepwound" model to patients and care providers, by classifying every image that a user acquires into one of nine possible categories (wound and tissue types), such as granulation tissue, open wound, and sutures. The "Deepwound" model performances were evaluated through parameters of accuracy, sensitivity, specificity, and F-score. Classification of wounds closed by tape strips obtained the best-combined accuracy, sensitivity, AUC, and F-score of 0.97, 0.82, 0.95, and 0.85, respectively, whereas the drainage classification achieved the best sensitivity score of 0.98. The Shenoy et al. (2019) approach further facilitates remote monitoring of patients, ease of communication with the medical team, and early identification of wound infections. Their mobile application can also generate comprehensive medical reports that can be used for the purpose of billing insurers, thus saving the cost of a clinician time.

Another interesting approach is described in Chen et al. (2018) study, which proposed a surgical wound assessment system for self-care, based on an image database acquired by smartphone cameras (Chen et al. 2018). This system enabled patients to capture their surgical wounds by using mobile devices and upload these images for further analysis of wound segmentation, skin and wound area detection, and wound assessment (state and symptoms).

The Chen and colleagues approach achieved an accuracy rate of 90% for wound state assessment and 91% for symptom assessment, using a KNN classifier. The case studies examined in this paper showed that the suggested system could detect and assess multiple symptoms of surgical wounds, and the results further demonstrated that this system may support healthcare professionals in obtaining robust surgical wound assessments, which in turn improves cost-effective usage of medical resources.

3.4   Conclusions

The implementation and application of AI methodologies in wound care and management was examined and discussed in this chapter. A strong positive impact and prospect of novel AI methodologies in the wound care arena was revealed, specifically showing that the implementation of computerized ML algorithms in the diagnosis of acute and CW has the potential to improve the wound care delivered to hospitalized patients and aged-care residents, particularly by enabling clinicians, healthcare professionals, and nurses to allocate their time more efficiently.

ML models based on imaging data, which are widely used in the wound care field, are considered to be relatively narrow in terms of the task type the ML algorithm is trained to perform. That said, focusing on implementation of ML in CW care and management, the tasks are relatively coherent and invariable, and can be categorized as classification or prediction tasks. Classification of CW by means of ML typically requires an imaging model for detection of the wound and its etiology and/or segmentation of the wound and the tissues within. As for prediction tasks, ML models can be taught to predict the potential path of progression of a wound (i.e. toward healing, or stagnation and chronicity). Given the successful performance of ML in these aspects as presented above, we expect that these tasks can be supported by ML, first perhaps as adjunct to clinical judgment and then as a robo-advisor where wound care specialty is not immediately available or accessible.

Many AI algorithms are developed and evaluated for classification and segmentation of the wound area based on datasets of wound images. SVM, LR, and RF are the most commonly classification models used for such purposes. In order to evaluate those models, statistical measures, such as sensitivity, specificity, accuracy, and F-score, are calculated based on the models' results and the ground truth provided by healthcare specialists or caregivers. Other AI methodologies can be implemented to support visual skin or wound assessments, for discrimination between different wound types such as pressure ulcers/injuries versus leg ulcers or burns, or for determination of the wound severity, depth, and the presence and stage of infection. Another approach is to apply these AI methodologies for risk assessments, i.e. to predict the probability of a certain patient to develop a CW based on their clinical records or images acquired at different time points, or to identify the wound based on textural EHRs and NLP methodologies, a promising approach for prevention and early detection of wounds.

An innovative approach for AI-powered wound care is through telemedicine and tele-healthcare, using smartphones/tablets for collecting skin or wound images and possibly other (patho-)physiological measures, which become the inputs for the AI-based system. This appears to be a promising approach for AI-based remote consultation. In such remote consultation, the AI algorithm provides immediate automated advice to the local healthcare professional (as a "robo-advisor"), but the medical information can also be transferred via cloud computing to a remote human expert who can further guide the local clinician (with the AI system serving as an adjunct to the clinical judgments of both). The prospect of such AI systems relies on the fact that caregivers and healthcare professionals are already experienced in using mobile apps and in acquiring image data by means of their personal smartphones; hence, no specific expertise or training is needed (in fact, numerous wound care clinicians use their cell phone cameras for documenting the healing of the wounds that they treat, as part of their daily routine). Integration of AI-powered wound care algorithms with cloud computing using smartphones as a platform hardware is,therefore, a practical and promising way forward. While many wound care clinicians already use their smartphones/tablets for wound documentation on a daily basis, the use of smartphones/tablets for other purposes, such as remote consultation and image collection, would be naturally and easily implemented by practicing clinicians.

As for other novel approaches described above, such as predicting the formation and progress of wounds or supporting the clinical VA of wounds using AI technology – along with the progression of AI methodologies and their applications in the wound care arena, their accessibility among clinicians and health professionals is soon to come and will be done by implementation of computerized algorithms in handheld diagnostic devices or bedside terminals in healthcare facilities or even during home hospitalization.

Even though the topic of implementation of AI in clinical practice is in its early days, we believe that the methodologic issues highlighted above (such as utilization of smartphones/tablets for remote consultation, and NLP methodologies for wound identification based on EHRs) can potentially improve wound care delivery, and might optimize clinicians and healthcare professionals working time.

Acronyms

AUC	area under the curve
AI	artificial intelligence
BW	burn wound
CW	chronic wounds
CNN	convolutional neural network
DL	deep learning
DNN	deep neural network

DFU	diabetic foot ulcer
EHR	electronic health record
KNN	k-nearest neighbors
ML	machine learning
MLP	multi-layer perceptron
NLP	natural language processing
NN	neural network
OCT	optical coherence tomography
PU	pressure ulcer
RS	Raman spectroscopy
RF	random forest
ROC	receiver operating curve
RGB	red-green-blue
ROI	region of interest
SEM	subepidermal Moisture
SVM	support vector machine
SSI	surgical site infection

Author Biographies

Mai Dabas received a BSc in Biomedical Engineering from Tel Aviv University in Tel Aviv, Israel, in 2021. Since 2021, she has been a master's student at the Department of Biomedical Engineering of the Faculty of Engineering at the Tel Aviv University. Her master's work focuses on the contribution of image processing and ML tools to wounds treatment and prevention.

Amit Gefen, PhD, is currently a full and the Berman chair professor, with the Department of Biomedical Engineering at the Faculty of Engineering of Tel Aviv University. His research interests are in studying normal and pathological effects of biomechanical factors on the structure and function of cells, tissues, and organs, with emphasis on applications in wound research. Dr. Gefen has published more than 300 articles in peer-reviewed international journals, many of which are on CW and their prevention, and he has edited several relevant books. Dr. Gefen is a previous president of the European Pressure Ulcer Advisory Panel (EPUAP, www.epuap.org), a member of the World Council of Biomechanics, a fellow of the International Academy of Medical and Biological Engineering and the European Alliance for Medical and Biological Engineering and Science and was recently named among the top-ranked 100 scientists in biomedical engineering worldwide according to the Elsevier and Stanford global ranking.

References

Alinia, P., Samadani, A., Milosevic, M. et al. (2020). Pervasive lying posture tracking. *Sensors* 20 (20): 5953. https://doi.org/10.3390/S20205953.

Alzubaidi, L., Fadhel, M.A., Oleiwi, S.R. et al. (2019). DFU_QUTNet: diabetic foot ulcer classification using novel deep convolutional neural network. *Multimedia Tools and Applications* 79 (21): 15655–15677. https://doi.org/10.1007/s11042-019-07820-w.

Anisuzzaman, D. M., C Wang, B Rostami et al. (2021) 'Image-based artificial intelligence in wound assessment: a systematic review', *Advances in Wound Care* 11, 12 687-709 https://home.liebertpub.com/wound. https://doi.org/10.1089/WOUND.2021.0091.

Badrinarayanan, V., Handa, A. and Cipolla, R. (2015). SegNet: A Deep Convolutional Encoder-Decoder Architecture for Robust Semantic Pixel-Wise Labelling. https://arxiv.org/abs/1505.07293v1 (accessed 20 July 2021).

Bezdek, J.C. (1984). FCM: the fuzzy c-means clustering algorithm. *Computers & Geosciences* 10 (3): 191–203.

Braden & Bergstrom (1988). *Braden Risk Assessment Tool.* https://www.sahealth.sa.gov.au/wps/wcm/connect/b24a8480438d09be9e63dfbc736a4e18/2010maybradenrisktool.pdf?MOD=AJPERES&CACHEID=ROOTWORKSPACE-b24a8480438d09be9e63dfbc736a4e18-nwLnylK (accessed 2 October 2022).

Chen, T. and Guestrin, C. (2016). XGBoost: a scalable tree boosting system'. In: *Proceedings of the ACM SIGKDD International Conference on Knowledge Discovery and Data Mining*, 13–17 August 2016, 785–794. https://doi.org/10.1145/2939672.2939785.

Chen, Y.-W.W., Hsu, J.T., Hung, C.C. et al. (2018). Surgical wounds assessment system for self-care. *IEEE Transactions on Systems, Man, and Cybernetics: Systems* 50 (12): 5076–5091. https://doi.org/10.1109/TSMC.2018.2856405.

Chun, X., Pan, L., Lin, Y. et al. (2021). A model for predicting 7-day pressure injury outcomes in paediatric patients: a machine learning approach. *Journal of Advanced Nursing* 77 (3): 1304–1314. https://doi.org/10.1111/JAN.14680.

Elnakib, A., Casanova, M.F., Soliman, A. et al. (2016). Analysis of 3D corpus callosum images in the brains of autistic individuals. *IGI Global* 159–184. https://doi.org/10.4018/978-1-4666-8828-5.ch008.

Garcia-Zapirain, B., Elmogy, M., El-Baz, A. et al. (2018). Classification of pressure ulcer tissues with 3D convolutional neural network. *Medical & biological engineering & computing* 56 (12): 2245–2258. https://doi.org/10.1007/s11517-018-1835-y.

Goodwin, T.R. and Demner-Fushman, D. (2020). A customizable deep learning model for nosocomial risk prediction from critical care notes with indirect supervision. *Journal of the American Medical Informatics Association : JAMIA* ocaa004. https://doi.org/10.1093/jamia/ocaa004.

Howard, A.G., Zhu, M., Chen, B. et al. (2017). Efficient convolutional neural networks for mobile vision applications. *Computer Vision and Pattern Recognition* arXiv:1704.04861. https://arxiv.org/abs/1704.04861.

Izadi, K. and Ganchi, P. (2005). Chronic wounds. *Clinics in Plastic Surgery* 32 (2): 209–222. https://doi.org/10.1016/j.cps.2004.11.011.

Jung, K., Covington, S., Sen, C.K. et al. (2016). Rapid identification of slow healing wounds. *Wound Repair and Regeneration* 24 (1): 181–188. https://doi.org/10.1111/wrr.12384.

Kamath, S., Sirazitdinova, E., and Deserno, T.M. (2018). Machine learning for mobile wound assessment. In: *Medical Imaging 2018: Imaging Informatics for Healthcare, Research, and Applications* (ed. S. Kamath, E. Sirazitdinova, and T.M. Deserno), 1057917. Surathkal, India: National Institute of Technology Karnataka, SPIE https://doi.org/10.1117/12.2293704.

Kavitha, I., Suganthi, S.S., and Ramakrishnan, S. (2017). Analysis of chronic wound images using factorization based segmentation and machine learning methods. In: *2017 International Conference on Computational Biology and Bioinformatics, ICCBB 2017*, 74–78. Association for Computing Machinery (ACM International Conference Proceeding Series) https://doi.org/10.1145/3155077.3155092.

Khandakar, A., Chowdhury, M.E., Reaz, M.B. et al. (2021). A machine learning model for early detection of diabetic foot using thermogram images. *Computers in Biology and Medicine* 137: 104838. https://doi.org/10.1016/J.COMPBIOMED.2021.104838.

Kim, R.B., Gryak, J., Mishra, A. et al. (2020). Utilization of smartphone and tablet camera photographs to predict healing of diabetes-related foot ulcers. *Computers in Biology and Medicine* 126: 104042. https://doi.org/10.1016/J.COMPBIOMED.2020.104042.

Krizhevsky, A., Sutskever, I., and Hinton, G.E. (2012). ImageNet classification with deep convolutional neural networks. In: *Advances in Neural Information Processing Systems* (ed. F. Pereira et al.). Curran Associates Inc. https://proceedings.neurips.cc/paper/2012/file/c399862d3b9d6b76c8436e924a68c45b-Paper.pdf.

Leaper, D.J. and Durani, P. (2008). Topical antimicrobial therapy of chronic wounds healing by secondary intention using iodine products. *International Wound Journal* 5 (2): 361–368. https://doi.org/10.1111/J.1742-481X.2007.00406.X.

Lustig, M., Schwartz, D., Bryant, R. et al. (2022). A machine learning algorithm for early detection of heel deep tissue injuries based on a daily history of subepidermal moisture measurements. *International Wound Journal* 19 (6): 1339–1348. https://doi.org/10.1111/iwj.13728.

Martin, P. and Nunan, R. (2015). Cellular and molecular mechanisms of repair in acute and chronic wound healing. *British Journal of Dermatology* 173 (2): 370–378. https://doi.org/10.1111/BJD.13954.

Martínez-Jiménez, M.A., Ramirez-GarciaLuna, J.L., Kolosovas-Machuca, E.S. et al. (2018). Development and validation of an algorithm to predict the treatment modality of burn wounds using thermographic scans: prospective cohort study. *PloS one* 13 (11): e0206477–e0206477. https://doi.org/10.1371/journal.pone.0206477.

Matar, G., Lina, J.M.J.-M., and Kaddoum, G. (2020). Artificial neural network for in-bed posture classification using bed-sheet pressure sensors. *IEEE Journal of Biomedical and Health Informatics* 24 (1): 101–110. https://doi.org/10.1109/JBHI.2019.2899070.

Mitchell, T.M. (1997). *Machine Learning*. McGraw-Hill Science/Engineering/Math http://www.cs.cmu.edu/~tom/files/MachineLearningTomMitchell.pdf.

Padula, W.V., Pronovost, P.J., Makic, M.B.F. et al. (2019). Value of hospital resources for effective pressure injury prevention: a cost-effectiveness analysis. *BMJ quality & safety* 28 (2): 132–141. https://doi.org/10.1136/bmjqs-2017-007505.

Raju, D., Su, X., Patrician, P.A. et al. (2015). Exploring factors associated with pressure ulcers: a data mining approach. *International Journal of Nursing Studies* 52 (1): 102–111. https://doi.org/10.1016/J.IJNURSTU.2014.08.002.

Santosh, K., Das, N., and Ghosh, S. (2022). *Deep Learning Models for Medical Imaging, Deep Learning Models for Medical Imaging*. Academic Press https://doi.org/10.1016/B978-0-12-823504-1.00011-8.

Schulz, H. and Behnke, S. (2012). Deep learning: layer-wise learning of feature hierarchies. *KI-Künstliche Intelligenz* 26: 357–363. https://doi.org/10.1007/s13218-012-0198-z.

Şevik, U., Karakullukçu, E., Berber, T. et al. (2019). Automatic classification of skin burn colour images using texture-based feature extraction. *IET Image Processing* 13 (11): 2018–2028. https://doi.org/10.1049/iet-ipr.2018.5899.

Shenoy, V.N., Foster, E., Aalami, L. et al. (2019, 2018). Deepwound: automated postoperative wound assessment and surgical site surveillance through convolutional neural networks. In: *IEEE International Conference on Bioinformatics and Biomedicine, BIBM 2018*. Cupertino High School, Cupertino, CA, United States (ed. S. H. et al.), 1017–1021. Institute of Electrical and Electronics Engineers Inc. https://doi.org/10.1109/BIBM.2018.8621130.

Simonyan, K. and Zisserman, A. (2014). Very deep convolutional networks for large-scale image recognition. *Computer and Information Sciences* https://doi.org/10.48550/ARXIV .1409.1556.

Song, B. and Sacan, A. (2012). Automated wound identification system based on image segmentation and Artificial Neural Networks. In: *2012 IEEE International Conference on Bioinformatics and Biomedicine (BIBM)*, 4–7 October 2012, School of Biomedical Engineering, Drexel University, Philadelphia, PA, United States BT. IEEE, 4 pp. https://doi .org/10.1109/BIBM.2012.6392633.

Szegedy, C., Liu, W., Jia, Y. et al. (2014). Going deeper with convolutions, *CoRR*, abs/1409.4. http://arxiv.org/abs/1409.4842.

Werdin, F., Tenenhaus, M., and Rennekampff, H.-O. (2008). Chronic wound care. *The Lancet* 372 (9653): 1860–1862. https://doi.org/10.1016/S0140-6736(08)61793-6.

Whitney, J., Phillips, L., Aslam, R. et al. (2006). Guidelines for the treatment of pressure ulcers. *Wound Repair and Regeneration* 14 (6): 663–679. https://doi.org/10.1111/J.1524-475X.2006 .00175.X.

Wong, G., Gabison, S., Dolatabadi, E. et al. (2020). Toward mitigating pressure injuries: detecting patient orientation from vertical bed reaction forces. *Journal of Rehabilitation and Assistive Technologies Engineering* https://doi.org/10.1177/2055668320912168 7: 205566832091216.

Xiaohui, L., Wang, C., Li, F. et al. (2017). A framework of wound segmentation based on deep convolutional networks'. In: *10th International Congress on Image and Signal Processing, BioMedical Engineering and Informatics, CISP-BMEI 2017* (ed. Q. S. et al.), 1–7. National Laboratory for Parallel and Distributed Processing, National University of Defense Technology, Changsha, China: Institute of Electrical and Electronics Engineers Inc. (Proceedings - 2017 10th International Congress on Image and Signal Processing, BioMedical Engineering and Informatics, CISP-BMEI 2017) https://doi.org/10.1109/CISP-BMEI.2017.8302184.

Xu, J., Chen, D., Deng, X. et al. (2022). Development and validation of a machine learning algorithm–based risk prediction model of pressure injury in the intensive care unit. *International Wound Journal* 19: 1637–1649. https://doi.org/10.1111/IWJ.13764.

Yang, Z., Yabansu, Y.C., Al-Bahrani, R. et al. (2018). Deep learning approaches for mining structure-property linkages in high contrast composites from simulation datasets. *Computational Materials Science* 151: 278–287. https://doi.org/10.1016/J.COMMATSCI.2018 .05.014.

Zahia, S., Garcia-Zapirain, B., and Elmaghraby, A. (2020). Integrating 3D model representation for an accurate non-invasive assessment of pressure injuries with deep learning. *Sensors* 20 (10): 2933. https://doi.org/10.3390/S20102933.

4

Deep Learning Techniques for Gene Identification in Cancer Prevention

Eleonora Lusito

San Raffaele Telethon Institute for Gene Therapy (SR-Tiget), IRCCS San Raffaele Scientific Institute, Milan, Italy

4.1 The Next-Generation Era of Cancer Investigation

4.1.1 Cancer at Its First Definitions

Since its first definition, cancer has been described as an abnormal cell proliferation. The terms carcinos and carcinoma were introduced for the first time by the Greek physician Hippocrates (460–370 BC) to refer to the proliferating mass of a crab, likely because the finger-like spreading projections resemble the shape of a crab. The Greek term was subsequently translated into the Latin word cancer by the Roman physician Celsus (28–50 BC) and the Greek physician Galen (130–200 AD) used for the first time the word oncos (Di Lonardo et al. 2015). Beyond the initial coarse description, as physicians developed a greater understanding of the human body, they gained more insights into the structural and physical features of cancer with therapeutic implications. The Scottish John Hunter (1728–1793), the father of the surgery, was the first to introduce the surgical resection as the major therapeutic option based on the physical properties like the density and the mobility of the tumor mass (Androutsos et al. 2007). The subsequent use of the modern microscope in medicine in the 19th century with direct observation of the cellular features, allowed a more detailed description of the neoplasm and opened to new therapeutic perspectives. In 1863, Rudolph Virchow identified white blood cells (leukocytes) in cancerous tissue, making the first connection between inflammation and cancer, while in 1902, Theodor Boveri proposed that malignant tumors arise from single cells that have chromosome damage and suggested that chromosome alterations cause the cells to divide uncontrollably. In 1909, Paul Ehrlich for the first time introduced the hypothesis that the immune system plays a major role in surveillance against tumors, a concept that is at the basis of anticancer immunotherapy (Faguet 2015). In 1903, five years later from the discovery of radium and polonium by Marie and Pierre Curie, S.W. Goldberg, and Efim London for the first time used the radium to eradicate basal cell carcinoma of the skin from two patients (Mould 2007), and in 1932, the more conservative and less disfiguring radical mastectomy

Big Data Analysis and Artificial Intelligence for Medical Sciences, First Edition.
Edited by Bruno Carpentieri and Paola Lecca.
© 2024 John Wiley & Sons Ltd. Published 2024 by John Wiley & Sons Ltd.

for breast cancer was introduced (Loukas et al. 2011). In 1941, Charles Huggins introduced the hormonal treatment of breast and prostate cancer after demonstrating that cancer cells require chemical signals to grow and survive (Huggins and Hodges 2002; Huggins and Dao 1953). Although many key landmark discoveries have been done during the past 250 years in cancer research and care of which only a few have been listed here, the greatest advances in the comprehension of the molecular basis of the disease, its progression, and treatment as well as early detection, arise from the last five decades of an unprecedented technological development.

4.1.2 Attempts to Sequence Nucleic Acids Over the Years

The milestone discovery of the double-helix structure of the DNA by James Watson and Francis Crick in 1953 from X-ray crystallographic data produced by Rosalind Franklin and Maurice Wilkins, represents the founding of modern biology. Since that moment, many scientific efforts have been done to gain even more insights into the molecular basis of living matter. One of the first was the identification of the sequence, i.e. the order, of the nucleotides in the DNA and RNA, the two nucleic acids in which the information about proteins and other molecules required for a vital cell is encoded. Due to the difficulties to obtain the sequence of the long DNA molecule, initial attempts were done on the most readily available populations of pure RNA species like microbial ribosomal or transfer RNA (rRNA and tRNA, respectively). The genomes of single-stranded RNA bacteriophages (ssRNA phage) have also simplified the efforts to determine the first genomic sequences with respect to the eukaryotic double-stranded DNA (Heather and Chain 2016). In 1965, Frederick Sanger and colleagues developed a technique based on the detection of ^{32}P-radiolabeled partial-digestion fragments after two-dimensional fractionation that allowed to measure the nucleotide composition and position of rRNA from Escherichia coli (Sanger et al. 1965). From this pioneering technique, many attempts have been done to improve the sequencing. Ray Wu and Dale Kaiser, for example, used the DNA polymerase and radioactive nucleotides to fill the 5′ overhanging "cohesive" ends of the Enterobacteria phage λ (Wu and Kaiser 1968; Wu 1970). With this approach, while measuring the incorporation of the nucleotides, they were able to predict the sequence. On the same path, in 1977, Frederick Sanger developed the "chain-termination" or dideoxy technique that marked the way nucleic acids are sequenced today (Sanger et al. 1977). This procedure makes use of the standard deoxynucleoside triphosphates dATP, dCTP, dGTP, and dTTP (dNTPs) that are the normal substrates for DNA polymerizing enzymes (i.e. the nucleotides), a single-stranded DNA template, a DNA polymerase that synthetizes the DNA during the polymerase chain reaction (PCR), and modified nucleotides, the dideoxynucleotides ddNTPs, that are chemical analogs of dNTPs. Unlike dNTPs, ddNTPs lack the 3′ hydroxyl group (3′-OH) that is required for the extension of DNA chains, and therefore cannot form the phosphodiester bond with the 5′ phosphate of the adjacent nucleotide as shown in Figure 4.1.

Mixing radiolabeled ddNTPs into a DNA extension reaction at a fraction of the concentration of standard dNTPs results in DNA strands of each possible length being produced. With four parallel reactions each with a different ddNTP base on four lanes of a polyacrylamide gel followed by autoradiography, it is possible to obtain the nucleotide

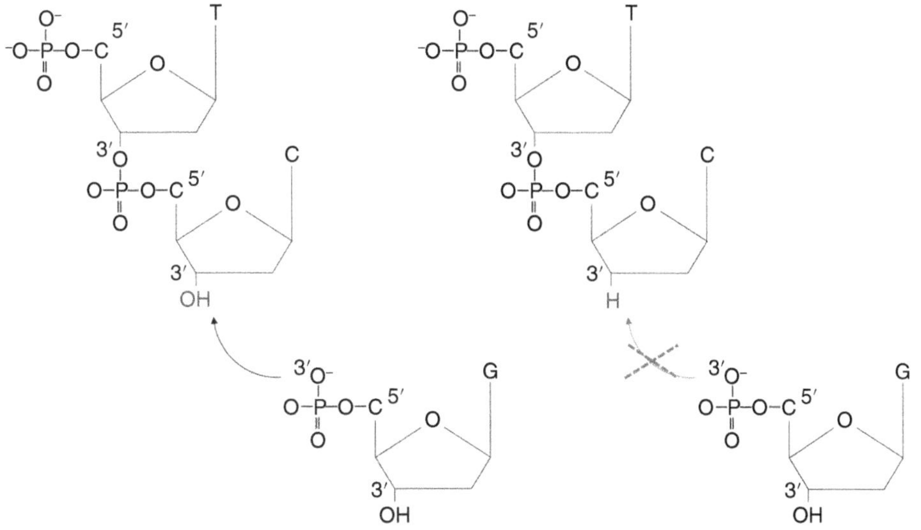

Figure 4.1   The chemical basis of chain termination sequencing. Three types of nucleotides are shown: a Thymine (T) a Cytosine (C), and a Guanine (G). Nucleotides are composed of a pentose carbon sugar, a nitrogenous base (here, a T or a C or a G), and a phosphate. In a normal nucleotide or dNTP (on the left), the 3rd carbon of the sugar has an –OH group that allows the binding to the next nucleotide during the template synthesis. In the presence of ddNTPs (on the right) the lack of oxygen prevents the next nucleotide from binding, and the chain termination occurs. During the elongation of the molecule, when a ddNTP is added instead of a dNTP, the entire process is stopped.

sequence (Figure 4.2). A radioactive band is in fact, expected to appear at the corresponding lane of the gel. The combination of the radioactive bands allows to predict the order of the nucleotides from anywhere in the sequence overcoming the limitation of sequencing only the end terminus of small genomes. This revolutionary technique for DNA sequencing called "first generation sequencing" that allowed the completion of the human genome in 2001 (Venter et al. 2001), has been extensively used over the years for its accuracy, robustness, and ease of use and is currently adopted in clinical practice for targeted sequencing of clinically relevant germline mutations. Many improvements have been made to it, mainly focused on the attempt to automate the entire process although its application is limited by the inherent low-throughput and high costs.

4.1.3   From the First to the Third-Generation Sequencing

From the first generation, sequencing technology has made considerable progress up to now. The massively parallel sequencing widely used today, i.e. the NGS introduced in the late 20th and early 21st has replaced the Sanger sequencing (Sanger et al. 1977) for its features of ultra-high throughput, scalability, and speed although the general biochemical principle remains the same. The basic NGS process involves the fragmentation of DNA/RNA into multiple pieces of genomic material that is firstly massively amplified by the PCR to increase the sensitivity of the sequencing process and then sequenced in parallel. Millions to billions of DNA reads are generated by the sequencer with lengths between 25 and 400 base pairs (bps). These reads are shorter than those generated by the

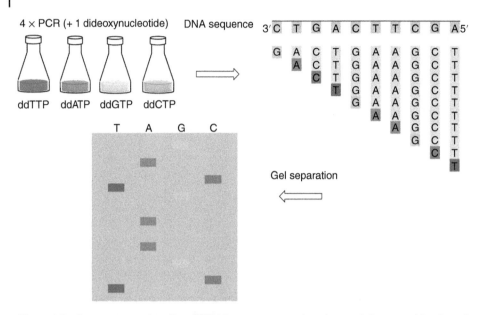

Figure 4.2 Sanger sequencing. Four PCR mixes are prepared, each containing a combination of normal nucleotides and one dideoxynucleotide (ddA, ddT, ddC, or ddG). Each PCR generates terminating fragments for the specific ddNTP in the mix that are subsequently separated with the gel electrophoresis. The base sequence is determined after ordering the fragments according to their length.

traditional Sanger sequencing (from 300 to 750 bp), a feature that makes the reconstruction of the entire sequence challenging (Rizzo and Buck 2012). Recently developed NGS technologies like PacBio and Nanopore (Kingan et al. 2019; Jain et al. 2015) address this issue by producing and massively sequencing reads longer than 750 bp (Athanasopoulou et al. 2021). This is the "third generation sequencing" in contrast with the "second generation sequencing" made by short reads. The increased length of the sequenced reads is not the only feature that makes the third generation sequencing particularly promising. The direct sequencing of the single molecules without the DNA amplification makes this technology more accurate and powerful. One of the major issues, in fact, of the PCR enrichment phase, is the introduction of errors with respect to the original sequence due to the polymerase activity, a confounding factor particularly relevant when looking for the presence of biologically meaningful genomic variations.

4.1.4 Applications of NGS in Clinical Oncology

Deep sequencing of the genome of any organism represents an unprecedented opportunity to elucidate the genetic basis of the phenotypes of living cells and to understand how specific diseases, such as cancer, form. In humans, over the years, it allowed to isolate key genes that maintain the functional equilibrium and that when altered, cause abnormal and tumor-promoting cellular behaviors like uncontrolled cell proliferation, the ability to invade adjacent tissues, escape immune control, and revert the differentiation status (Nones and Patch 2020; Amaddeo et al. 2012). More than just increasing the basic knowledge of cancer, the most natural consequence of a deep understanding of the disease, is the identification of more effective therapies tailored to the genomic profile of individuals (Fusco et al. 2022). The information on the genomic features of a cancer patient can, in fact, support the medical decisions at the primary line of intervention but also the identification of additional strategies in the presence of relapse and resistance to the standard treatments (Qin 2019; Lips et al. 2015; Li et al. 2020). Despite the great potential and general interest for the public health worldwide in this direction, the direct application of NGS to guide cancer therapy in medical practice is hindered by the clinical interpretation of the generated data, for example, the functional role of a mutation or a list of mutations and its interference with the therapy, a hurdle that still needs to be overcome. Conversely, the use of NGS in cancer diagnosis and prognosis is now widely accepted with different applications ranging from the definition of gene expression panels to targeted sequencing, to whole exome and whole genome sequencing (WES and WGS, respectively) (Park et al. 2014; Lowes et al. 2016; Rusch et al. 2018). Tumor subtypes with different clinical outcomes that in the past were identified based predominantly on morphological features, now are jointly confirmed by the NGS-measured expression of a panel of molecular biomarkers. The best known and Food and Drug Administration (FDA) approved kits that make use of targeted RNA-NGS technology are the MammaPrint® (MP) and the BluePrint® (BP), two molecular tests that classify breast cancer patients into low and high risk according to the expression of 70 prognostic genes (the MP kit) and into luminal-, HER2-, and basal-type based on the expression of 80-gene signature for subtyping (the BP kit) (van de Vijver et al. 2002; Glas et al. 2006; van't Veer et al. 2002; Cardoso et al. 2016; Piccart et al. 2021; Krijgsman et al. 2012; Whitworth et al. 2014; Whitworth et al. 2017; Mittempergher et al. 2020). Another important application of NGS in clinical oncology is for early detection and prevention. In liquid biopsy, NGS is applied to sequence circulating tumor DNA (ctDNA) molecules that are DNA fragments released by tumor cells. It is a noninvasive way to monitor the appearance of a tumor and represents a valuable tool to predict the risk of recurrence and to allow its early detection. Targeted NGS-based tests are also widely used for hereditary cancer risk assessment. Based on the presence of germline cancer-causing mutations on a list of marker genes identified through population-based sequencing profiling, they classify individuals according to their susceptibility to cancer thus promoting prevention interventions.

4.2 Deep Learning Approaches for Genomic Variants Identification in Cancer

4.2.1 Cancer Causing Factors

The neoplastic transformation from a normal cell requires the co-occurrence of a series of genetic and epigenetic alterations in key cellular metabolic and regulatory processes (Hanahan and Weinberg 2011; Hanahan 2022; Baylin and Jones 2016; Orsolic et al. 2022). Although the tissue of origin of the tumor and the microenvironment impact on the development and progression of the disease in a context-dependent manner, all cancer cells exhibit common traits, the so-called cancer hallmarks, that are: selective growth and proliferative advantage, altered stress response that promote overall survival, vascularization, invasion and metastasis, metabolic rewiring, and immune modulation (Hanahan 2022). The accumulation of random but functional somatic mutations in the DNA during cell replication is the most direct determinant of cancer. Additional risk factors can contribute to cancer susceptibility, like the exposure to environmental factors, i.e. carcinogens that damage the DNA, some types of viral infections such as human papillomavirus (HPV), the inheritance of cancer-causing genetic changes present in the germ cells, and the increasing age of individuals (Takeshima and Ushijima 2019). It has been recently shown that while the higher incidence of cancer in older individuals is due to the accumulation of somatic mutations and epigenetic changes during their lifetime, patients who develop cancer at a younger age carry higher content of germline variants that when occur in a protein-coding region, can impact on protein function (Qing et al. 2020; Murff et al. 2004).

4.2.2   The Contribution of Germline Alterations to Cancer

Large-scale cancer genome sequencing projects have confirmed that most cancers harbor few highly recurrent somatic mutations along with many less frequent ones (Raphael et al. 2014; Kumar et al. 2020; Brown et al. 2019; Hess et al. 2019). All individuals also carry hundreds of common and rare high-functional impact germline variants that contribute to disease susceptibility. Although poorly investigated for many years where researchers focused more on somatic mutations, several studies have recently associated mutations in high-penetrance genes like BRCA1, BRCA2, PTEN, TP53, KRAS, ATM, and APC to cancer, thus highlighting that germline mutations also impact on tumor evolution (O'Shaughnessy et al. 2020; Copson et al. 2018; Kleihues et al. 1997; Nichols et al. 2001). Genome-Wide Association Studies (GWAS) have also identified many low-penetrance germline variants (~1300 cancer risk single nucleotide polymorphisms, SNPs) associated with slightly increased risk of cancer development (Carter et al. 2017) acting by rising the overall mutation rate (Jendrzejewski et al. 2019; Li et al. 2018). Although germline variations play an important role in cancer risk and susceptibility, they can explain a small minority of cancers if compared with somatic mutations.

4.2.3   Somatic Mutations and Cancer

Somatic mutations are changes that occur in the genomes (i.e. at DNA level) of all dividing cells, normal and neoplastic. When fixed over several DNA replications in a subset of genes called "cancer genes" at checkpoints of regulatory and signaling pathways, causes cancer by conferring an evolutionary advantage. Cancer somatic mutations are classified as "Drivers" and "Passengers." The first confers growth and survival advantage and are indeed positively selected during the clonal expansion from the progenitor cell where they arise. They usually occur in genes called oncogenes and tumor suppressor genes. Passenger mutations are not evolutionary selected, and their presence alone is not sufficient to confer any selective growth advantage compared to drivers (Bozic et al. 2010). Although they are not considered crucial for cancer progression, it is thought that their co-occurrence could elicit an effect comparable to that of the drivers and that they can cooperate with the latter to promote tumorigenicity (Kumar et al. 2020). Mutations occur in all cancers, but mutational signatures differ between cancer types and patients according to the genetic diversity of individuals.

4.2.4 Calling Variants from Sequence Data

Mutated genomic regions (germline or somatic) and genes are identified through targeted panel, whole exome, or whole genome DNA sequencing. In a typical NGS experiment, millions of sequences are generated by the sequencer from the targeted/disease samples and from the normal samples or from the parents for germline alterations identification, with which they are compared. Sequence data processing is performed with sophisticated bioinformatics tools that first align the sequenced reads to the reference genome to find their genomic location and then identify sequence variations that comprise SNPs, small/large insertions and/or deletions (INDELs), and structural variants. This last phase is called "variant calling." The computational identification of biologically relevant variants is not an easy task and is affected by several confounders like the properties of the sequencing instrument, the presence of errors introduced with sample handling, library preparation and PCR enrichment, and the accuracy of the sequence aligners (Ma et al. 2019). Many available methods successfully distinguish between true mutations and experimental errors although their application is limited to the widely used short reads sequencing technology (Bentley et al. 2008; Bentley 2006; Goodwin et al. 2016) for which they are designed. They cannot be directly applied to the analysis of data generated by the emerging long-reads technology (Pollard et al. 2018) for which they need to be adapted. High sensitivity and accuracy of variant calling are not exclusively achievable by sophisticated analytical tools able to deal with different sources of variations. The most straightforward approach is to increase the sequencing read depth (Ajay et al. 2011; Meynert et al.; 2013) that, according to the Lander/Waterman equation (Lander and Waterman 1988), is given by LN/G, where L is the read length, N is the number of reads and G is the haploid genome length. The higher the number of aligned reads, the higher the confidence of the base call. Increasing the coverage allows to reduce the number of missed true variants (false negatives) and to reduce the number of the ones erroneously classified as such (false positives). Although it comes intuitively that increasing the coverage would result in an increased confidence in variant detection, different reasons prevent to perform high coverage sequencing. Among the others, the most common is the high cost of sequencing. Independently form the abovementioned issues, a good variant caller must, ultimately, be able to distinguish uninformative sources of variation from DNA alterations with putative biological impact.

4.2.5 Computational Approaches for Variant Discovery

Traditional tools for variant calling are genome analysis toolkit (GATK) HaplotypeCaller and Platypus (McKenna et al. 2010; Rimmer et al. 2014). They are based on local de novo assembly in an active region, i.e. in a region where multiple reads of a target genome disagree with the reference. The basic principle is a dynamic reassembly of the reads in a region whenever signs of variation of the target with respect to the reference are found. This procedure improves the accuracy of the variant caller, especially in the presence of regions with different types of variants close to each other. Although they reach high sensitivity for detecting single nucleotide variants (SNVs)/indels they are more prone to errors in low coverage regions. The recently developed deep learning-based variant callers overcome this limitation by turning the variant calling into an image classification task able to identify mutations regardless of the proximity of them and of the sequencing coverage of a particular region (Khazeeva et al. 2022; Poplin et al. 2018; Cai et al. 2019). From the reads aligned to the reference genome, they first produce pileup image tensors and then classify each of them for the presence of candidate variants, using CNNs (O'Shea and Nash 2015).

4.2.6 Convolutional Neural Networks (CNNs): Basic Principles

CNNs are a class of deep learning methods. They are more often used for classification and become dominant in various computer vision (CV) tasks. Compared with traditional CV, they replace the manual extraction of the relevant features from input images that will be used for the training, with an end-to-end learning. A deep learning model is "trained" on the given images annotated only for the classes of objects and extracts the most descriptive and relevant features while discovering underlying patterns in the data. Compared with the manual annotation, CNNs allow to deal with classification tasks with increasing number of classes to classify. Three major building blocks form CNNs (Figure 4.3) and are at the basis of their superior performance compared with traditional neural networks: the convolution layer(s), the pooling layer(s), and fully connected (FC) layer(s). The convolutional layer is the core of a CNN and takes most of the computational resources. It requires input data, a feature detector (known also as a filter or a kernel), and a feature map. The feature detector is a two-dimensional (2D) array of weights, which scans a part of the input image. It moves across the receptive fields of the image and checks if the feature is present. The pooling layer performs the down sampling. It reduces the number of parameters in the input. As for the convolutional layer, it sweeps a filter across the entire input, but without any weight. Finally, the FC layer performs the task of classification based on the features extracted through the previous layers and their different filters. To classify inputs, it usually uses a softmax activation function (Goodfellow et al. 2016) that produces a probability from *0* to *1* while

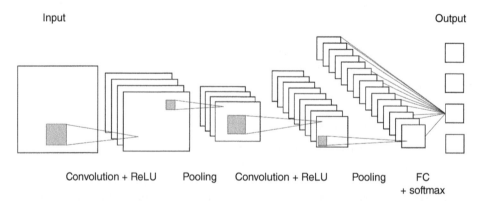

Input   Output

Convolution + ReLU   Pooling   Convolution + ReLU   Pooling   FC
+ softmax

Figure 4.3   The major components of a convolutional neural network (CNN). The schematic representation of a CNN with two hidden layers each consisting into a convolution and pooling. Additional layers are the input, the output, and the fully connected layer (FC). ReLU is the activation function. It sets all negative values to *0* while maintaining the remaining constant, thus allowing it to deal with nonlinear relationships. Softmax is an activation layer used for classification and is applied to the last layer of the network. It converts the output of the FC layer into probabilities. Red squares represent filters used to create the feature maps.

convolutional pooling layers use the rectified linear unit (ReLU) function to account for nonlinearity. The use of multiple building blocks allows the CNN to learn spatial hierarchies of features automatically and adaptively through backpropagation.

4.2.7 Application of CNNs to Variant Calling

To identify variants among 6 billion letters of "A," "C," "G," and "T" that represent the four types of bases found in a DNA molecule: adenine (A), cytosine (C), guanine (G), and thymine (T), three requirements are essentials: (i) the correct location of a read in the genome, (ii) the correct alignments between the mapped reads to the reference genome, and (iii) the correct statistics used to identify the variants from the alignments. While for steps (i) and (ii) a good aligner is sufficient, for step (iii) different algorithms are available. Here, recently proposed methods based on deep neural networks (DNNs) will be discussed. Compared with traditional methods based on probabilistic models of sequencing errors to determine the likelihood of a variation (Luo et al. 2017; Hoffmann et al. 2014; Lähnemann et al. 2021), deep learning-based approaches showed an increased sensitivity and accuracy although the cost of a high number of parameters to be estimated. Among deep learning tools, CNNs reached a great attention. They treat the genetic variants identification task as an image classification problem and for this, they represent an innovative approach. In a simple CNN model applied to genomic data for variant calling, sequence alignments are firstly converted into "pile-up" images. The different colors and alpha channels are used to encode the read sequences, the per base quality, and the genomic strand of a read. The red blue green (RGB) pixel-encoded image, is the input of the CNN. For the regression and classification tasks, each variant is modeled with some categorical variables that capture the features of each candidate. Usually, they are:

- the alternate base at a SNP (A, C, T, or G), or the reference base otherwise
- the zygosity of the variant (i.e. homozygote or heterozygote)
- the variant type (i.e. SNP, INDEL)
- the length of an INDEL

The number of variables may vary depending on the prior information available, but the four reported above represent the minimum set of information required to infer the presence of a genomic variation and to classify it. The variable that identifies the "alternate base," assumes four different values depending on the base found at each position of the target genome, i.e. the genome to be investigated, with respect to the reference. The variable "zygosity" represents the zygosity of the variation. Each variant, in fact, can be heterozygous with respect to the reference allele or homozygous for the alternate allele. In the first case, only one of the two alleles differs from the reference while in the second, both alleles differ. The homozygosity with the reference means that there is not variation in that portion of the genome. The variable "variant type" represents the type of the variant. A SNP is a variation of a single base in a certain stretch of DNA. These variations occur normally throughout a person's DNA. They occur almost once in every 1,000 nucleotides on average, which means there are roughly 4 to 5 million SNPs in a person's genome. Most SNPs have no effects on health or development. They can be used as biological markers to locate genes that are associated with a certain disease and may help to predict an individual's response to drugs, susceptibility to environmental factors such as toxins, and risk of developing diseases. They are also used to track the inheritance of disease genes within families. INDELs are variations in which the DNA sequence is changed by adding one or more nucleotides. If they occur at a genetic locus, the final gene product, i.e. the protein, may not function properly. The length of the INDEL ranges from *0* to *n* or greater, where *n* is usually established to be 3 or 4 based on experimental evidence. A length equal to *0* means the absence of the INDEL and hence a perfect match with the reference. For a CNN-based identification of variants, each categorical variable is mapped into a binary vector usually using one-hot encoding (OHE) also called "dummy encoding." This allows the input to be numeric.

4.2.8 A Typical CNN Architecture for Variant Calling

A typical CNN architecture (Figure 4.4) for variant calling is the following and contains:

(1) a multidimensional tensor, i.e. the "pile-up" image. It is built after the alignment from the following inputs: a binary alignment and map (BAM) file that contains aligned sequences of the sample genome, the reference genome, and a browser extensible data (BED) text file that contains information on the genomic regions as coordinates and associated annotations. The shape of the tensor is normally *33 × 4 × 4* (height by width by arrays). The first dimension, "*33*," is given by the candidate variation, plus (usually)

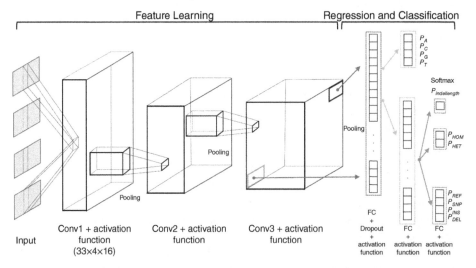

Figure 4.4 A typical CNN architecture for variant calling. A typical CNN architecture for variant calling is reported. Source: Adapted from Luo et al. (2019). From the left to the right: a multidimensional tensor of sequencing read alignments as input, three convolution hidden layers (Conv1, Conv2 and Conv3) for feature learning with activation function and pooling, and three FC layers highlighted with red, yellow, and blue boxes for regression and classification: the first for the alternative allele predictions and the second and third for the zygosity, variant type and indel length predictions. Dropout refers only to the first FC layer. For the first convolution layer the dimension (height × width × filters) is reported in parenthesis. Cuboid boxes represent CNN filters and the arrows the flow of the prediction/learning process across subsequent layers.

16bps that flank it on both sides of the sequence, i.e. to the left and to the right. The length of the flanking region is arbitrary. Its function is to include a sufficiently large portion of the genome to capture the background noise. It is optimized to reach high prediction accuracy while ensuring high computational efficiency. The second dimension, "*4*," corresponds to the count of "A," "C," "G," and "T" and their frequencies on the reads. Finally, the third dimension corresponds to four different ways of counting so that *4* arrays of shape *33 × 4* are created in which the first tensor encodes the reference sequence (i.e. the nonvariant), the second the inserted sequence(s), the third the deleted BP(s), and the fourth, the alternative allele(s). The tensors from the second to the fourth, use the relative count against the first, i.e. the reference. In a simpler model, substitutions and insertions can be seen in the same array although it becomes an issue to recapitulate the allele of the inserted sequence;

(2) Convolution and pooling layers in a variable number depending on how deep the network is. They are used for dimensionality reduction and feature learning. In a simple architecture with three convolutional and pooling layers, each pooling layer summarizes the features generated by the convolutional layer immediately before;

(3) Two or more FC layers to perform the regression and the classification. Usually, the first computes the alternative allele predictions while the second computes the zygosity, the variant type, and the INDEL length. *N* different outputs are generated for the INDEL length: an INDEL with a length between *0* and *nbps* or more or equal to *n*.

The frequently used CNN architecture in variant calling is Inception-v3 (Szegedy et al. 2015) that is a model based on a sparsely connected architecture in the convolutional layers instead of a fully connected architecture, particularly useful when dealing with a high number of parameters.

4.2.9 The Activation Function

The most important element in a neural network (NN) is the activation function. Based on its values, a neuron will be activated or not and transferred to the next layer. Also known as transfer function (TF), it is a node at the end or between NNs. It was introduced to overcome the inability of a classifier, whose essence is a linear equation, to deal with the classification problem of non-linear systems. Common activation functions also used for variant calling-CNNs, include sigmoid, tanh, ReLU, and softplus (Nwankpa et al. 2018) and are shown in Figure 4.5. The curve of the sigmoid function whose formula is: $f(x) = 1/1+e^{-x}$ is a common nonlinear activation function.

Although this function was extensively used at the early age of deep learning, today, it is not, because of its soft saturability: as from Figure 4.5, the slope of the graph tends to be zero when the input is very large or very small. Consequently, the derivative values in these regions are very small and converge to *0*, an effect known as "the vanishing gradient." When they are small there is minimal learning while when they are *0* there is no learning. In a slow learning condition, the optimization algorithm whose role is to minimize the error, can stall in local minimum values and reach maximum performance. The updated version of the sigmoid function is the tanh function whose formula is as follows:

$$f(x) = 1 - e^{-2x}/1 + e^{-2x}.$$

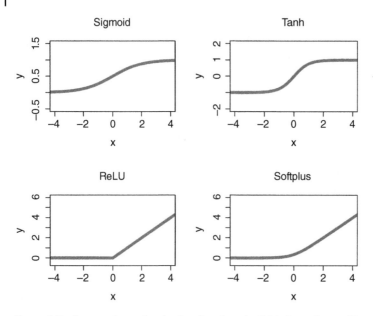

Figure 4.5 Commonly used activation functions in CNNs for variant calling. Representative plots of the behavior of sigmoid, tanh, ReLU, and softplus functions based on the features of input data.

It is a symmetric function centered on 0. The convergence rate of this function is higher compared to the sigmoid, but the problem of gradient diffusion remains unsolved. A widely diffused function is ReLU (Agarap 2018) defined as:

$$f(x) = \max (0, x).$$

It is a piecewise linear function that outputs the input directly if it is positive, otherwise, it will output 0. This function provides a solution to the gradient diffusion problem although forcing some data to be 0 can introduce sparsity. Moreover, since the derivative is always 0 when the input value is negative, neurons are always in the off-state as 0 gradients flow through them. Consequently, dead neurons are generated. This issue is usually solved by enforcing a small gradient flow through the network with a variation of the ReLU called the Leaky ReLU (LReLU) (Maas et al. 2013; Xu et al. 2015). Another widely used function is the softplus. It has small reservations about values less than 0, which will decrease the possibility of neuronal death although it requires more computation than ReLU. Its formula is as follows:

$$f(x) = \ln(1 + e^x).$$

Recently, the scaled exponential linear unit (SELU) (Klambauer et al. 2017) function has been introduced. It is a variant of the ReLU. Its equation is as follows:

$$SELU(x) = \lambda \begin{cases} x, & \text{if } x > 0, \\ \alpha e^x - \alpha, & \text{if } x \le 0. \end{cases}$$

As from the formula, if the input value is greater than 0 the output value is x multiplied by lambda (λ and α are two constants of value 10,505 and 16,732, respectively), while if it is less than or equal to 0, the function goes up to 0. The SELU is self-normalizing the

NN and its application allows to perform batch normalization (BN) of hidden layers while reducing computational costs. It, in fact, uses the Banach fixed-point theorem to internally ensure convergence to zero mean, and unit variance in each hidden layer thus replacing the standard BN, that requires to include an additional external implicit layer at the cost of an increased computational complexity. Due to its characteristics and particularly for self-normalization, the SELU function is widely used in CNNs for variant calling. Despite the high number of features to be learned, its application allows the model to converge fast and efficiently.

4.2.10 Dropout and L1–L2 Regularization

Another key component of a CNN particularly relevant for an efficient deep learning-based variant caller is the dropout layer. It is a mask that nullifies the contribution of some neurons towards the next layer (Figure 4.6) while leaving unmodified the others. The use of the dropout layers is a strategy that together with the normalization, prevents the overfitting of training data and is useful with features that are not independent (Srivastava et al. 2014). It, in fact, improves the generalization performance of the model by making the learning features not heavily correlated.

If not used, the first batch of training samples greatly influences the learning, and the features that appear only in later samples or batches, cannot be learned. In variant calling, the use of the dropout is crucial because although more than 3 million labeled truth-curated variants are available for training, the scarcity of some labels, particularly referred to variants with long indel length, leads to overfitting of the model favoring abundantly labeled data. The dropout, instead, mitigates the class imbalance. The way a dropout ignores some nodes during the training is probabilistic. Each node is randomly ignored with a probability of p. The activations of the remaining nodes are then summarized, and the sum is magnified by $1/p$. In this way, during the training up to $1 \div (1-p)^n$ subnetworks are created. The dropout can be ideally applied to any hidden layer of the training. Usually, it is applied to the FC (dense) layers but it can also be applied to the convolutional layers after the activation function of each of them. Although this last application can be adopted, it is important to notice that the use of the dropout after the convolutional layer, slides the filter over the width and height of the input image thus generating a 2D activation map that can lose some important features. Apart from the dropout, the regularization is achieved

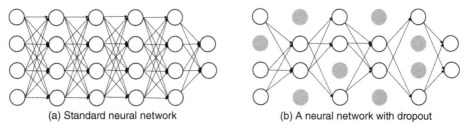

(a) Standard neural network   (b) A neural network with dropout

Figure 4.6 Neural network dropout. A schematic representation of a neural network with dropout (b) compared with a standard neural network (a). Circles represent nodes and arrows the connections from the output of one artificial neuron to the input of the subsequent one. Grey circles represent inactivated nodes during the dropout process.

also with the application of L1 and L2 techniques (Ng 2004). Both consist of adding a regularization term to the cost function to reduce the overfitting of models characterized by high variance. The L1 is also called Lasso regularization and is as follows:

$$\text{Cost function} = \text{Loss} + \lambda/2m^* \, \Sigma \|w\|,$$

while the L2 is the Ridge regularization and is as follows:

$$\text{Cost function} = \text{Loss} + \lambda/2m^* \, \Sigma \|w\|^2,$$

where λ is the regularization parameter and is the hyperparameter whose value in a CNN is optimized to get better results, m is the number of parameters and w is the weights. In L1, the absolute value of the weights is penalized, and they may be reduced to 0. This regularization is frequently used to compress the model, especially in the presence of many features. In L2, the penalty is equal to the square of the absolute magnitude of the weights. Features with 0 coefficients are hence avoided and all of them are used. This type of regularization can deal with multicollinearity problems by penalizing insignificant weights. Given the nature of the data, for a variant caller, the L2 is usually the best choice particularly because of the high collinearity of the features that must be learned.

4.2.11 Advantages of Deep Learning Over the Existing Techniques

Variant calling is the first step before relating the genotypes to a phenotype for the presence of a genomic alteration. As previously stated, because sequencing techniques have intrinsic errors, the challenge for a variant caller is to accurately predict the variant from the short reads that align to the locus while distinguishing it from a sequencing error. The advantage of using a CNN-deep learning approach to infer variations in the genome, is the possibility to use an image as input, that captures more information as a whole, than sequenced features analyzed individually. Its better performance with respect to algorithms based on probabilistic models was widely demonstrated in benchmark studies and relies on its ability to identify variations in difficult-to-call regions of DNA that are characterized by the presence of repetitive or tandem-duplicated sequences and with low-coverage sequencing data (Barbitoff et al. 2022). One of the classical approaches, the widely used GATK proposed in 2010 (Van der Auwera et al. 2013; De Pristo et al. 2011; McKenna et al. 2010), is based on a statistical framework that combines logistic regression, hidden Markov models, and Gaussian mixture models. It outputs sequencing statistics based on counting reads with alternative sequences in a genomic position and has been shown to generate less accurate results with respect to deep learning-based methods. GATK accuracy, in fact, depends on the coverage of the sequencing while methods based on deep learning show high precision and better accuracy in SNPs and localized indels calling irrespectively of sequence coverage. This represents an advantage when and where it is not possible to reach high sequencing coverage for technical or economic reasons. It has also been shown that at low coverage GATK calls more $A > T$, $C > A$, $G > T$, and $T > A$ substitutions than expected from the distribution of variants in the human genome while the false positives (i.e. the erroneously called variations) and false negatives (i.e. the erroneously called non-variations) from deep learning tools seem to be independent from the base change. Given these global considerations, the identification of relevant mutations particularly in cancer, can benefit from deep learning-based methods especially for the presence of low-frequency and often not harmful variations that serve as confounders.

4.2.12 Residual Neural Networks (ResNet)-Inspired CNN in Genomic Variants Detection

A modified implementation of CNN for variant calling is the ResNet inspired CNN (Szegedy et al. 2015). The major advantage of using a ResNet architecture is that it overcomes the "vanishing gradient problem" of deep networks thus allowing to build CNNs with up to thousands of convolutional layers for more accurate predictions. During the training, as the gradient is backpropagated to earlier layers, repeated multiplication may make the gradient infinitely small. Therefore, as the network goes deeper its performance gets rapidly saturated and the accuracy of the predictions decreases after reaching a maximum. ResNet deals with this effect by introducing the so-called "identity shortcut connections." Based on the identity mapping, they allow to skip some layers of the network in the forward step of an input. Two distant layers can then be linked without involving the set of layers between them as shown in Figure 4.7.

Mathematically, it consists of approximating a residual function $F(x): = H(x) - x$ instead of $H(x)$ where $H(x)$ is the underlying mapping to be fit by the stacked layers, and x denotes the input to the first of these layers. The theoretical justification comes from the universal approximation theorem (Hornik et al. 1989): if multiple nonlinear layers can asymptotically approximate complicated functions, they can asymptotically approximate also the residual functions given that the input and the output are of the same dimensions. The original function thus becomes:

$$F(x) + x.$$

Figure 4.7 Identity shortcut connection of a ResNet. A schematic representation of the identity shortcut connection. An identity mapping is performed and subsequently added to the convolutional layers' stack outputs. In this way, a link between two distant layers is established without involving the layers between them. $F(x)$ is the output of the previous block while x is the output of the current block. $F(x) + x$ is the residual mapping with $F(x) = H(x) - x$.

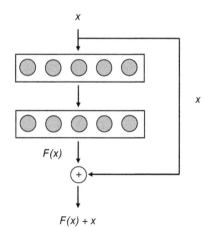

During the training, if the residual network learns the identity mapping with optimal weights, all the solvers can push the weights of the multiple nonlinear layers to 0. In this way corrections are not required, (x) is set to 0 and the network can use the shortcut path to perform the identity mapping. In real cases, it is unlikely that identity mappings are optimal, but the skip-connections at least facilitate the solver to find a more suitable weight with reference to an identity mapping than to learn a completely new one. The advantage of using a ResNet-inspired CNN architecture in variant calling is that it allows to increase in the network depth (Liu et al. 2019). This is particularly relevant to achieve high accuracy predictions, especially in the case of poorly detectable mutations present in poorly sequenced regions (i.e. difficult-to-sequence regions with high GC-content [between 70% and 80%], various repeats, with hairpin structures), with low-quality sequencing data and in the presence of contaminants that affect the sample purity. A typical ResNet-CNN architecture for variant calling is shown in Figure 4.8 and is composed of a user-defined number of convolutional layers and an equal number of shortcut identity connections (Sahraeian et al. 2019). Inputs are received by the first convolutional layer and can be aligned reads transformed into pileup image tensors or a matrix consisting of a reference channel, tumor, and normal frequency channels, coverage and position channels, and additional channels summarizing the alignment features. The output of the first layer is given to n subsequent blocks that contain other convolutional layers and shortcut identity connections. Each block also includes BN and pooling layers. A FC layer then receives the output of the last block. The resulting feature vector is then fed to two softmax classifiers and a regressor. The first classifier predicts and outputs probabilities of the mutation type from the four classes of nonsomatic, single nucleotide variation, INDEL while the second predicts the length of the mutation. The regressor also predicts the position (i.e. the locus in the genome) of the mutations in the matrix to ensure the right call for them.

4.3 Deep Learning in Cancer Transcriptomics

4.3.1 Gene Expression and Cancer

The most common effect of changes in DNA sequence is the direct or indirect gene expression alteration that reflects into gain or loss of protein activities and ultimately into aberrant signaling pathways (Gerstung et al. 2015). The ways a mutation occurring in a protein-coding region can impact gene expression are different. Some mutations introduce premature stop codon that causes the reduced dosage of mRNA transcript while others affect protein activities by changing the amino acid sequences (Reva et al. 2011). Genetic changes are not the exclusive events that modulate gene expression. Epigenetic processes, including DNA methylation, histone modification, and various RNA-mediated processes, also impact on it by turning genes "on" and "off." Given the synergistic effects they could have on gene expression, the integration of mutational profiles with epigenetic and transcriptomic characterizations can undoubtedly offer a better understanding of the mechanisms at the basis of cancer.

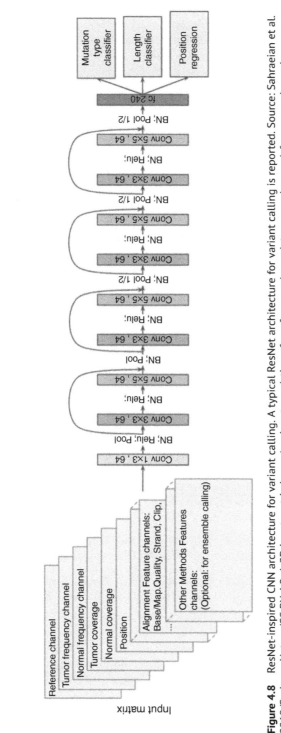

Figure 4.8 ResNet-inspired CNN architecture for variant calling. A typical ResNet architecture for variant calling is reported. Source: Sahraeian et al. 2019/Springer Nature/CC BY 4.0. A 3D input matrix is used as input consisting of a reference channel, tumor and normal-frequency channels, coverage and position channels, and additional channels that summarize the features of the alignment. Different convolutional layers with shortcut identity connections, pooling (Pool), and BN are used for the learning phase while softmax classifiers and a regressor are used on the FC layer to predict the mutation type, size, and position.

4.3.2 Analytical Approaches to Deal with Gene Expression Data

From the analytical perspective, dealing with gene expression is significantly challenging because of the high dimensionality and complexity of data to be analyzed. The traditional approach based on differential gene expression analysis between conditions like tumors versus normals, early stage versus advanced tumors, pharmacologically treated versus untreated tumors, and many others, led to the identification of relevant cancer driver genes whose transcriptional changes are still used in clinical practice to profile individuals for the presence of the disease and to define the prognosis (Cronin et al. 2007; Buyse et al. 2006; Lu et al. 2010). Although this analytical strategy allowed to reach relevant findings in the field, it suffers from a major limitation. Only genes whose expression changes linearly across conditions can be easily detected with respect to nonlinear ones resulting to be not statistically significant although functionally associated with the condition. Moreover, traditional statistical learning techniques, suffer from the curse of dimensionality, a phenomenon related to the characteristic of high-dimensional data like the transcriptomic ones, in which messenger RNA (mRNA) levels of thousands of genes are measured over a limited number of samples (Duda et al. 2001; Ransohoff et al. 2005). The large number of variables with unknown but complex correlation structures engenders issues like singularity and overfitting that affect the accuracy and generalization of the predictions made by standard statistical methods. Dimensionality reduction techniques, a set of methods that allow to extract the meaningful part of high-dimensional and noisy expression data while removing multicollinearity, are efficiently used to stem this effect. Common strategies include the supervised selection of genes that best predict a desired outcome based on univariate measurements such as t-test and rank test, a weighted combination of genes that represent the total variation of the data, the Principal Component Analysis (PCA), the partial least squares (PLS), machine learning-based algorithms like LASSO and random forest (RF) and many others (Wang and van der Laan 2011; Ghosh 2002; Nguyen and Rocke 2002; Huang and Pan 2003; Efron et al. 2004; Hedenfalk et al. 2001; Dettling and Bühlmann 2003). Among deep neural networks, stacked denoising autoencoders (SDAEs) (Vincent et al. 2010) and variational autoencoders (VAEs) (Kingma and Welling 2022; Kingma and Welling 2019) are widely used tools for representation learning from gene expression data due to their ability to perform dimensionality reduction while learning linear but also nonlinear relationships.

4.3.3 Stacked Denoising Autoencoders (SDAEs) for Dimensionality Reduction

An autoencoder (AE) is a type of unsupervised feedforward NN whose goal is to reduce data dimensions while learning how to ignore the noise (Baldi 2012). From the encoded lower dimensional representation, it then learns how to reconstruct data to a representation that is as close to the original input as possible. Unlike traditional CNNs, which model data by minimizing inaccurate class predictions, AEs model them including learning through data reconstruction. The architecture of a typical AE contains three major components: an encoder a code and a decoder as shown in Figure 4.9. The encoder compresses the input and produces the code that is the lower-dimensional representation of the input, and the decoder reconstructs the output from the low-dimensional representation. The code is also called "the latent-space representation" and is a compact summary of the input.

Input   Reconstructed data

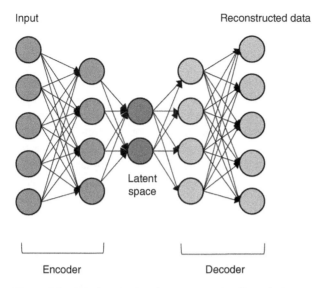

Encoder   Decoder

Figure 4.9 Building blocks of an autoencoder. The principal components of an autoencoder are reported. Gray circles represent the input and the encoder that is a fully connected ANN whose function is to compress input data to produce the code, represented with dark gray circles and called "latent space." From the code, the decoder (light gray circles) which has a similar ANN structure to the encoder, reconstructs the input.

A stacked denoising AE is a collection of AEs in each layer of a multi-layer NN, in which some noise is added, or some input values are stochastically masked (Figure 4.10) to prevent the network from learning the identity function, an event that happens when there are more hidden nodes than in the input.

The encoder of an AE is a non-linear function of the form:

$$f_\theta(x) = \sigma(Wx + b),$$

with parameters $\theta = \{W,b\}$ (i.e. the weight and bias respectively) and σ that is the activation function. The matrix W has dimensions: $d' \times d$ where d refers to the initial

Figure 4.10 The denoising autoencoder. The input x is stochastically corrupted through q_D. The encoder maps the corrupted input to y through f_θ and the decoder reconstructs x through $g_{\theta'}$ to give z. The reconstruction error is measured by the loss $L_H(x, z)$.

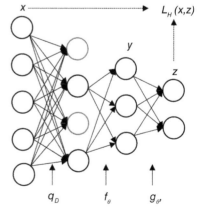

high-dimensional matrix and d' to the lower-dimensional encoding. The bias vector b is of dimension d'. The decoder can be expressed as:

$$z = g_{\theta'}(y) = \sigma(W'y + b').$$

Z is not an exact reconstruction of the input but is rather a set of parameters of a distribution $p(X|Z = z)$ that, with high probability may regenerate x. The encoder of a SDAE decreases the dimensionality of input data stack-by-stack by smoothing the loss of information. Depending on the architecture and deepness of a SDAE, the computational complexity may become high. A pretraining phase of the parameters represents a valuable strategy to reduce it and to ensure a better generalization on a specific task of interest. Moreover, it allows to deal with the vanishing gradient issue of very DNNs consisting of a loss of error information while propagating back to the earlier layers with a minimal update of the weights. The greedy layer-wise pretraining, an unsupervised algorithm proposed by Hinton et al. (2006) for deep belief networks (DBNs), proved to be powerful for these purposes. It trains each layer in a sequential way while feeding lower layers' results to the upper layers (Figure 4.11). In this way, each layer is optimized at a time greedily and learns a higher-level representation of the layer below (where the weights are fixed), in an unsupervised way since the training criterion does not depend on the labels. After the pre-training, the trained model can be fine-tuned with a supervised method.

By aggregating locally optimal solutions, the problem of training a deep network is solved and an overall good enough global solution is reached. The parameters that are calculated in the pretraining are used for the supervised fine-tuning of the entire training set where they are updated. As for CNNs for variant calling, in the case of SDAEs applied to gene expression data analysis, a dropout regularization can also be included during the training. By randomly removing fractions of hidden units the model is simplified and the overfitting is prevented. Corrupted input values can also be used together with the unmodified ones to test the robustness of the model and its ability to recover clean inputs despite the confounders.

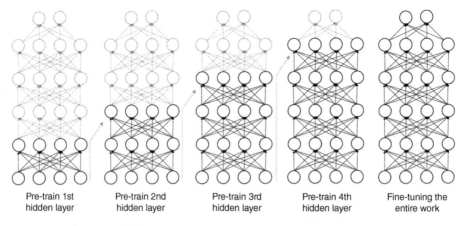

| Pre-train 1st hidden layer | Pre-train 2nd hidden layer | Pre-train 3rd hidden layer | Pre-train 4th hidden layer | Fine-tuning the entire work |

Figure 4.11 The greedy layer-wise pretraining. A representation of the greedy layer-wise pretraining strategy of a deep autoencoder. Gray nodes indicate layers not enrolled during the fine-tuning. Gray arrows indicate the flow of the output of single-layer pretraining from the previous layer to the upper layers to produce a new representation of data.

4.3.4 The Variational Autoencoder (VAE)

Additional widely used artificial neural network techniques to learn meaningful latent space from transcriptomic data are VAEs (Figure 4.12). They are data-driven unsupervised deep generative models (DGMs) introduced by Kingma and Welling in 2013 and used in many contexts (Kingma and Welling 2022). They belong to the family of probabilistic graphical models and variational Bayesian methods. The core of a VAE is the autoencoding framework which, similarly to SDAEs, learns latent representations through data compression and nonlinear activation functions. The major difference with respect to the traditional AEs is that VAEs are stochastic and learn the distribution of explanatory features over samples while traditional AEs are deterministic and are trained by minimizing the reconstruction error. They hence probabilistically describe an observation in the latent space and output a probability distribution for each latent attribute instead of generating a single value. VAEs have proven to be particularly efficient in dealing with continuous latent variables or parameters having an intractable posterior distribution. Supposing a dataset $X = \{x^{(i)}\}^N_{i=1}$ consisting of N independent identically distributed (i.i.d.) samples of some continuous or discrete variable x and assuming that data are generated by some random process involving an unobserved continuous random variable z, intractability happens in the following cases: when the marginal likelihood cannot be differentiated because its integral $p(x) = \int p(z)p(x|z)dz$ is intractable and when, the true posterior density $p(z|x) = p(x|z)p(z)/p(x)$ is intractable due to high latent dimensionality. In this case, the EM algorithm to find local maximum likelihood parameters cannot be applied. In this context, a VAE transforms an inference problem into an optimization one by approximating $p(z|x)$ by another tractable distribution $q(z|x)$, a variational distribution, whose parameters let it

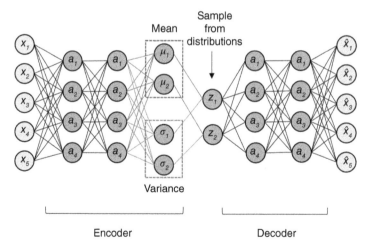

Figure 4.12 The basic architecture of a variational autoencoder. The building blocks of a typical VAE are shown. From the left to the right, light gray circles represent input data, dark gray circles the nodes of the encoder layers, and light gray and dark gray boxes enclose the nodes in the bottleneck layer that represent the parameters (mean and variance) of the probability distribution of the latent space (the output of the encoder) from which, by sampling, the input (light gray circles) is reconstructed by the decoder (dark gray circles).

to be very similar to $p(z|x)$. To ensure that $q(z|x)$ is similar to $p(z|x)$ the Kullback–Leibler (KL) divergence between the two distributions is minimized by maximizing the following:

$$E_{q(z|x)} \log p(x \mid z) - KL(q(z \mid x) \| p(z)),$$

where the first term represents the reconstruction likelihood while the second ensures that the learned distribution q is similar to the true prior distribution p that is assumed to follow a unit Gaussian distribution. The q distribution is used to infer the putative hidden variables, i.e. the latent state that generates the observations. In a VAE architecture, the encoder learns a mapping from x to z while the decoder learns a mapping from z back to x. As previously stated, a VAE does not directly outputs values for the latent state but instead, it outputs parameters describing a distribution for each dimension in the latent space. It, hence, learns two distinct latent representations: a mean and a standard deviation vector encoding. Considering the simple case in which it is assumed that the covariance matrix has only nonzero values on the diagonal, the decoder will then generate a latent vector by sampling from these Gaussian distributions to reconstruct the original output as shown in Figure 4.12.

While doing this, a reparameterization trick is required and used to perform backpropagation otherwise not feasible, in the presence of a random sampling process. It consists of random sampling a parameter ε from a unit Gaussian (Figure 4.13) and then shifting and scaling it by the latent distribution's mean μ and variance σ, respectively.

By doing this, the parameters can be optimized despite the random sampling. VAEs showed their great advantage over classical AEs with large datasets where the batch optimization is too costly and sampling-based solutions like Monte Carlo EM are too slow due to the sampling loop per datapoint they require. They have been typically applied

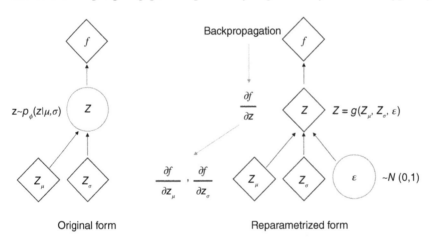

Original form   Reparametrized form

Figure 4.13 The reparameterization trick. The reparameterization trick for a VAE is shown on the right and the original form on the left. Light gray circles are stochastic nodes whereas black diamonds are deterministic nodes (i.e. input and weights). Z_μ and Z_σ are the parameters that the network tries to learn. During the training, the input is mapped to two latent variables Z_μ and Z_σ from which the decoder reconstructs the original input. The issue of impossible backpropagation in the presence of stochasticity (original form) is solved by turning the random node into a deterministic one through ε (reparametrized form). The new sampling operation becomes $z = g(z_\mu, z_\sigma, \varepsilon)$.

to image data with remarkable generative capacity and modeling flexibility (Chen et al. 2018; Asaoka et al. 2020; Elbattah et al. 2021; Ternes et al. 2022). VAEs applied to modeling gene expression data, allow to automatically engineer of nonlinear relationships between mRNA measurements, in a low dimensional space thus ignoring uninformative sources of variations while preserving the biologically meaningful ones (Way and Greene 2018; Simidjievski et al. 2019; Grønbech et al. 2020). Due to their ability to approximate irregular latent spaces with stochastic inference, VAEs have been proved to be powerful tools also for the unsupervised integration of heterogeneous data sources (Hira et al. 2021; Ma and Zhang 2019).

4.3.5 VAEs to Integrate Gene Expression and Methylation Data

4.3.5.1 DNA Methylation: the Epigenetic Regulation of Gene Expression

DNA methylation is a biological process of eukaryotic cells by which methyl (CH_3) groups are added to the DNA molecule, often to the fifth carbon atom of a cytosine ring. These modified cytosine residues usually lie next to a guanine base (CpG methylation) and the result is two methylated cytosines positioned diagonally to each other on opposite strands of DNA (Figure 4.14).

DNA methylation is one of the heritable epigenetic marks, i.e. not encoded in the DNA sequence. It is a stable repressive mark catalyzed by DNA methyltransferases (DNMTs) and is the key player in epigenetic silencing of transcription (Jin et al. 2011). DNA methylation regulates the chromatin status via the interaction of DNMTs with other modifications and with the components of the machinery that mediate those marks. Epigenetic modifications like DNA methylation, are fundamental for mammalian development and cell proliferation. They can be altered in mature mammals due to the occurrence of random or environmental factors (Lam et al. 2012; Nilsson et al. 2015; Milagro et al. 2012; Casillas et al. 2003). The disruption of epigenetic processes results in altered transcriptional states that ultimately can cause malignant cellular transformation. Compared to normal cells, the genomes of cancer cells are hypomethylated (Gama-Sosa et al. 1983; Feinberg and Vogelstein 1983; De Capoa et al. 2003; Seifert et al. 2007; Cadieux et al. 2006; Sharma et al. 2010). Hypermethylation occurs by silencing the genes, often tumor-suppressors, involved in tumor cell invasion, cell cycle control, DNA repair, and other tumorigenic mechanisms thus favoring the growth and spread of cancer (Akiyama et al. 2003; Ballestar et al. 2003; Brueckner et al. 2005; Esteller et al. 1999). It can be detected early in the course of the disease and can serve as a biomarker for cancer prevention and early diagnosis. Methylated DNA impacts gene expression in two

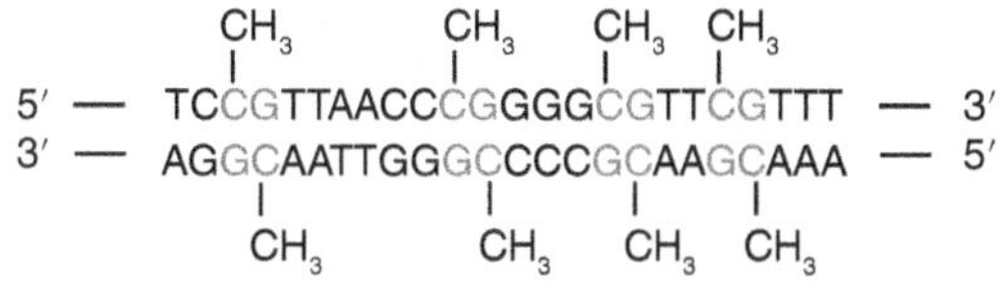

Figure 4.14 DNA methylation. The two strands of a DNA molecule with methylated cytosines (CH_3 -C) are shown in light gray together with an adjacent guanine base (G) are shown. The other bases of the DNA molecule not involved in DNA methylation are shown in black. 3′ and 5′ represent the ends of the DNA and refer to the number of carbon atoms in a deoxyribose sugar molecule to which a phosphate group bonds.

different ways: it physically impedes the binding of transcriptional proteins to the genes avoiding the synthesis of mRNA and through the binding of methyl-CpG-binding domain (MBD) proteins, histone deacetylases and other chromatin remodeling proteins that are recruited to modify histones thereby forming compact and not accessible chromatin (i.e. the heterochromatin) that prevents the transcription (Moore et al. 2013). When gene expression data are generated, the molecular events responsible for the modulation of mRNA levels cannot be directly inferred. Transcriptomic changes can, in fact, result from abnormal methylation of DNA or from mutations, two molecular events that give rise to a final common phenotype. It then becomes intuitive that the integration of high-throughput data that measure these two events can support and favor, at least to some extent, the elucidation of the determinants of complex and multifaced diseases like cancer and allow patients' classification based on distinctive molecular traits that serve as proxies of clinical outcome. In the following paragraph the application of VAEs to integrate and relate gene expression with methylation data will be discussed, leaving out the mutational data for simplicity. At least in principle, any type of data can be integrated using VAEs although at the cost of computational complexity and interpretability of the results.

4.3.5.2 Preprocessing Input Data of Different Sources

In a deep learning framework that uses VAEs to integrate gene expression and methylation sequencing data from cancer samples, these two types of inputs are given to the encoder, and latent features are learned (Hira et al. 2021; Seal et al. 2020). In this type of analysis, normal samples can be used together with tumor samples in matched conditions to infer distinctive disease features, or conversely, only cancer samples can be used when normal samples are not available, are of bad quality, or of a small sample size. In this second case, de novo subtypes can be identified from samples of the same tumor type or by comparing different tumor types. While transcriptomic data refer to the count of mRNA molecules of expressed exons, i.e. the genes, methylation data are reported for each chromosome of the individual. Before running the VAE, a preprocessing of data is performed to improve the accuracy of the predictions and the overall performance of the NN. It includes the filtering of genes expressed in less than a certain percentage (usually 10%) of the entire set of data, a procedure that allows to remove unwanted sources of variation and to reduce the sparsity of data, features of gene expression data, that impact on the efficiency of the encoding without a gain of biological knowledge. Data are further harmonized so that missing values are replaced with the mean of corresponding molecular features. Gene expression data are first expressed as $\log_2$ Fragments Per Kilobase of transcript per Million (FPKM) and then normalized to the range of *0* and *1* to be consistent with methylation data that are expressed in percentage.

4.3.5.3 A VAE Architecture for Multimodal Data

The first layer of the encoder of a VAE used to integrate transcriptional and methylation datasets is usually composed by one FC block for gene expression data and different FC blocks for methylation features according to their targeting chromosome. The strategy to split the methylation data allows to reduce the number of parameters to be estimated in the FC layers and hence the computer memory required for the training. It prevents also from overfitting the methylation data and reduces the imbalance between the dimensionality

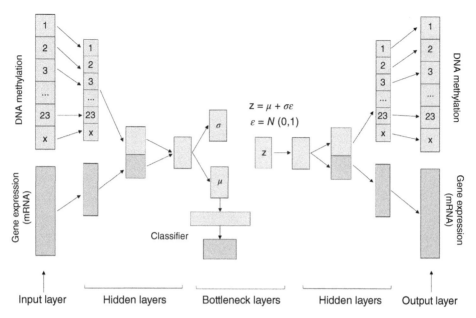

Figure 4.15 A VAE architecture for DNA methylation and gene expression data integration. Source: Adapted from Hira et al. (2021). A schematic representation of a VAE architecture used to integrate different sources of data from (Hira et al. 2021). It consists of an encoder and a decoder composed of two hidden layers. The bottleneck layer is composed of two layers that encode the parameters (μ and σ of the Gaussian distribution) of the probability distribution of the latent space and a 2-layered ANN-based classifier for supervised latent features learning. Different FC blocks (in light gray) are used for methylation data (one for each chromosome from 1 to 23 + x) and one for gene expression (in gray). The latent feature vector z is reported together with the distribution of ε.

of the two data types. Based on this structure, the first hidden layer serves to capture the intra-chromosome relationships whereas inter-chromosome relationships are captured through a second hidden layer as shown in Figure 4.15. The two equally sized vectors, one for gene expression and one for methylation are concatenated in the second hidden layer and encoded to a multi-omics vector. A final hidden layer of the encoder fully connects the two output layers and represents the mean μ and the standard deviation σ of the variational distribution $q(z|x)$ of the latent variable z given the input sample x.

As explained before, the reparameterization trick is required to make the sampling phase differentiable and to allow backpropagation. It is given by $z = \mu + \sigma\varepsilon$ where ε is a random variable sampled from the unit normal distribution $\mathcal{N}(0, I)$. The bottleneck layer, i.e. the layer in which z, μ, and σ are estimated is normally set to 128 hidden nodes. Its output can be used not only for dimensionality reduction purposes but also for classification. The structure of the decoder is similar to the encoder. It takes the latent variable z as input and outputs a reconstructed vector x' which consists of both, DNA methylation and the gene expression profile. To perform the classification of input samples from the output of the encoder, i.e. the vector μ, a classification network is usually included in the entire architecture. The dimension of the output of the classifier is n for the tumor type classification with n, the number of different tumors included in the analysis, and $n+1$ when normal samples are also included. A regularization of the classifier is usually added to encourage the network to identify latent features that can be additionally used for classification. This is required because the latent features extracted by the bottleneck layer of the encoder represent intrinsic characteristics of data not necessarily related to the samples' classification. The major goal of the encoder, is, in fact, the accurate reconstruction of the input, a task that can be easily disjoint for classification purposes. To this aim, a combination of VAE and classification loss can be written as follows:

$$\mathcal{L}_{\text{vae}} = \frac{1}{M} \sum_{j=1}^{M} CE(x_{mj} x'_{mj}) + CE(x_e x'_e) + \mathcal{L}_{\text{KL}},$$

while the classification loss becomes:

$$\mathcal{L}_{\text{class}} = CE(y, y'),$$

where

- x_e is the gene expression profile of the input sample x and x'_e is the reconstructed gene expression vector
- x_{mj} are the 23 input vectors that contain the molecular features of DNA methylation according to the chromosome they refer to, with j that represents the index of the corresponding chromosome
- M is the number of chromosomes
- CE is the binary cross-entropy between the input vectors and the reconstructed vectors
- $\mathcal{L}_{\text{KL}}$ is the KL divergence between the learned distribution and a unit Gaussian distribution given by: $\mathcal{L}_{\text{KL}} = D_{KL} (\mathcal{N}(\mu, \sigma) || \mathcal{N}(0, I))$
- Y is the ground truth label of a given sample x while the label predicted by the classifier is y'.

The total loss can be defined as the sum of the loss of VAE and the loss of the classifier and is:

$$\mathcal{L}_{\text{total}} = \alpha \mathcal{L}_{\text{vae}} + \beta \alpha \mathcal{L}_{\text{class}},$$

where α and β are two parameters that weight the two loss functions during the training.

Additional components of a VAE for integration tasks, in common with other NNs, are BN and activation functions that are included in each FC block. ReLU is usually used for most hidden layers whereas the sigmoid is applied to the output layer of the decoder. Finally, the softmax regularization is used in the classification network to the lower dimensional latent representation to generate the probabilities over the predicted output categories. The application of VAEs to integrate gene expression and methylation data for dimensionality reduction and classification is only one of all possible applications. Additional high-throughput datasets, can, in fact, be used to infer biological knowledge. A relevant aspect when performing integration analyses is that as the input increases in sample size and data type, the preprocessing and normalization steps, before running a VAE, become essential to limit the impact of the data sources-related intrinsic heterogeneity and noise.

4.4 Conclusions

The growing application of deep learning methods in oncology proves their ability to successfully deal with the complexity of cancer data to address challenging tasks like patient diagnosis and classification, prognosis, and treatment decisions. Although they are increasing the deepness of our knowledge of cancer, the biological and medical interpretation of the results they generate from the "-omics," represents a limiting step for a more real application of them into the clinic, an aspect not strictly related to deep learning techniques but also to the intrinsic complexity of the disease. There is no doubt, however, that accurate predictions can support and complement the existing and well-established knowledge to improve the clinical management of patients and to assist cancer researchers. To this aim, some improvements are needed to make DL techniques more robust with respect to the data on which predictions are made. Input data are often multimodal. They come from transcriptomic, epigenomic, proteomic and many other "-omics". Together with the intrinsic diversity of high-throughput platforms, they carry a variability related to the genetic heterogeneity of individuals and to the customized experimental procedures of different laboratories (e.g. the protocols used to generate a sequence library for transcriptomic studies). A good DL model must efficiently deal with systemic sources of variation, but also with random measurement errors not always efficiently moldable. Another relevant issue which slows down the successful application of these methods in oncology is the lack of a representative number of annotated reference datasets for model training to achieve a significant generalization performance. In cancer research, this is often related to good quality sample availability (i.e. with enough not-degraded molecules to be measured), eligible for high-throughput molecular profiling. Transfer learning methods have been recently proposed as powerful tools to make accurate predictions in the absence of large datasets, although with some limitations. Finally, DL tools should be able to estimate the uncertainty in their predictions and demand to the experts the final decision when it becomes critical. Despite the mentioned critical aspects that need to be considered for further developments, DL methods still retain the potential to positively impact cancer care. As new throughput data and more powerful and general DL tools will be generated, the supportive role of DL to allow precision oncology will become increasingly substantial.

Acronyms

AE	autoencoder
ANN	artificial neural network
ASGD	asynchronous stochastic gradient algorithm
BAM	binary alignment and map
BED	browser extensible data
BN	batch normalization
BP	BluePrint
bps	base pairs
CE	cross entropy
CNNs	convolutional neural networks
ctDNA	circulating tumor DNA
CV	computer vision
dATP	deoxy denosine triphosphate
DBNs	deep belief networks
dCTP	deoxycytidine triphosphate

DDAs	Drug-Disease Associations
DDIs	drug–drug interactions
ddNTP	dideoxynucleotides triphosphates
DGMs	deep generative models
dGTP	deoxyguanosine triphosphate
DL	deep learning
DNA	deoxyribonucleic acid
DNMT	DNA methyltransferases
dNTP	deoxynucleoside triphosphate
DTIs	drug–target interactions
dTTP	deoxythymidine triphosphate
EM	expectation maximization
FC	fully connected
FDA	Food and Drug Administration
FPKM	fragments per kilobase million
GATK	genome analysis toolkit
GCNs	graph convolutional networks
GNNs	graph neural networks
GRIs	gene regulatory interactions
GWAS	Genome-Wide Association Studies
HPV	human papillomavirus
INDELs	insertions and/or deletions
KL	Kullback–Leibler
LReLU	leaky ReLU
LSTM	long short-term memory
MBD	methyl binding domain
MP	MammaPrint
MRI	magnetic resonance imaging
mRNA	messenger RNA
NGS	next generation sequencing
OHE	one-hot encoding
PCA	principal component analysis
PCR	polymerase chain reaction
PLS	partial least squares
PPIs	protein–protein interactions
PPINs	protein–protein interaction networks
ReLU	rectified linear unit
ResNet	residual neural network
RF	random forest
RGB	red green blue
RN	relational network
RNA	ribonucleic acid
rRNA	ribosomal RNA
SDAEs	stacked denoising autoencoders
SELU	scaled exponential linear unit

SNPs	single-nucleotide polymorphisms
SNVs	single nucleotide variants
ssRNA	single-stranded RNA
SVM	support vector machine
TFs	transcription factors
TF	transfer function
tRNA	transfer RNA
VAEs	variational autoencoders
WES	whole exome sequencing
WGS	whole genome sequencing

Author Biographies

Eleonora Lusito is a postdoctoral fellow in computational biology at San Raffaele Telethon Institute for Gene Therapy in Milano (Italy). She has a background in molecular biology, bioinformatics, and biostatistics. After dedicating her PhD to the inference of clinically relevant gene regulatory networks in breast cancer, she moved to the deconvolution of the transcriptional plasticity of myeloid cells in pathologic conditions with diagnostic and therapeutic implications. She is an experienced researcher in the application of deep learning methods to "-omics" data at single cell level. She is first author and co-author of publications in high-impact journals.

References

Agarap, A.F. (2018). Deep Learning using Rectified Linear Units (ReLU). ArXiv: 1803.08375v2, [cs.NE]. https://arxiv.org/abs/1803.08375.

Ajay, S.S., Parker, S.C.J., Abaan, H.O. et al. (2011). Accurate and comprehensive sequencing of personal genomes. *Genome Research* 21 (9): 1498–1505. https://doi.org/10.1101/gr.123638 .111.

Akiyama, Y., Watkins, N., Suzuki, H. et al. (2003). GATA-4 and GATA-5 transcription factor genes and potential downstream antitumor target genes are epigenetically silenced in colorectal and gastric cancer. *Molecular and Cellular Biology* 23 (23): 8429–8439. https://doi .org/10.1128/MCB.23.23.8429-8439.2003.

Amaddeo, G., Guichard, C., Imbeaud, S., and Zucman-Rossi, J. (2012). Next-generation sequencing identified new oncogenes and tumor suppressor genes in human hepatic tumors. *Oncoimmunology* 1 (9): 1612–1613. https://doi.org/10.4161/onci.21480.

Androutsos, G., Vladimiros, L., and Diamantis, A. (2007). John Hunter (1728- 1793): founder of scientific surgery and precursor of oncology. *Journal of BUON* 12 (3): 421–427.

Asaoka, R., Murata, H., Matsuura, M. et al. (2020). Improving the structure-function relationship in glaucomatous visual fields by using a deep learning-based noise reduction approach. *Ophthalmology Glaucoma* 3 (3): 210–217. https://doi.org/10.1016/j.ogla.2020.01 .001.

Athanasopoulou, K., Boti, M.A., Adamopoulos, P.G. et al. (2021). Third-generation sequencing: the spearhead towards the radical transformation of modern genomics. *Life (Basel)* 12 (1): 30. https://doi.org/10.3390/life12010030.

Baldi, P. (2012). Autoencoders, unsupervised learning, and deep architectures. In: *Proceedings of ICML Workshop on Unsupervised and Transfer Learning, PMLR*, vol. 27, 37–49.

Ballestar, E., Paz, M.F., Valle, L. et al. (2003). Methyl-CpG binding proteins identify novel sites of epigenetic inactivation in human cancer. *The EMBO Journal* 22 (23): 6335–6345. https://doi.org/10.1093/emboj/cdg604.

Barbitoff, Y.A., Abasov, R., Tvorogova, V.E. et al. (2022). Systematic benchmark of state-of-the-art variant calling pipelines identifies major factors affecting accuracy of coding sequence variant discovery. *BMC Genomics* 23 (1): 155. https://doi.org/10.1186/s12864-022-08365-3.

Baylin, S.B. and Jones, P.A. (2016). Epigenetic determinants of cancer. *Cold Spring Harbor Perspectives in Biology* 8 (9): a019505.

Bentley, D.R. (2006). Whole-genome re-sequencing. *Current Opinion in Genetics & Development* 16 (6): 545–552. https://doi.org/10.1016/j.gde.2006.10.009.

Bentley, D.R., Balasubramanian, S., Swerdlow, H.P. et al. (2008). Accurate whole human genome sequencing using reversible terminator chemistry. *Nature* 456 (7218): 53–59. https://doi.org/10.1038/nature07517.

Bozic, I., Antal, T., Ohtsuki, H. et al. (2010). Accumulation of driver and passenger mutations during tumor progression. *Proceedings of the National Academy of Sciences of the United States of America* 107 (43): 18545–18550. https://doi.org/10.1073/pnas.1010978107.

Brown, A.L., Li, M., Goncearenco, A., and Panchenko, A.R. (2019). Finding driver mutations in cancer: Elucidating the role of background mutational processes. *PLoS Computational Biology* 15 (4): e1006981. https://doi.org/10.1371/journal.pcbi.1006981.

Brueckner, B., Boy, R.G., Siedlecki, P. et al. (2005). Epigenetic reactivation of tumor suppressor genes by a novel small-molecule inhibitor of human DNA methyltransferases. *Cancer Research* 65 (14): 6305–6311. https://doi.org/10.1158/0008-5472.CAN-04-2957.

Buyse, M., Loi, S., van't Veer, L. et al. (2006). Validation and clinical utility of a 70-gene prognostic signature for women with node-negative breast cancer. *Journal of the National Cancer Institute* 98 (17): 1183–1192. https://doi.org/10.1093/jnci/djj329.

Cadieux, B., Ching, T.-T., VandenBerg, S.R., and Costello, J.F. (2006). Genome-wide hypomethylation in human glioblastomas associated with specific copy number alteration, methylenetetrahydrofolate reductase allele status, and increased proliferation. *Cancer Research* 66 (17): 8469–8476. https://doi.org/10.1158/0008-5472.CAN-06-1547.

Cai, L., Wu, Y., and Gao, J. (2019). DeepSV: accurate calling of genomic deletions from high-throughput sequencing data using deep convolutional neural network. *BMC Bioinformatics* 20 (1): 665. https://doi.org/10.1186/s12859-019-3299-y.

de Capoa, A., Musolino, A., Della Rosa, S. et al. (2003). DNA demethylation is directly related to tumour progression: evidence in normal, pre-malignant and malignant cells from uterine cervix samples. *Oncology Reports* 10 (3): 545–549.

Cardoso, F., van't Veer, L.J., Bogaerts, J. et al. (2016). 70-Gene signature as an aid to treatment decisions in early-stage breast cancer. *The New England Journal of Medicine* 375 (8): 717–729. https://doi.org/10.1056/NEJMoa1602253.

Carter, H., Marty, R., Hofree, M. et al. (2017). Interaction landscape of inherited polymorphisms with somatic events in cancer. *Cancer Discovery* 7 (4): 410–423. https://doi.org/10.1158/2159-8290.CD-16-1045.

Casillas, M.A. Jr., Lopatina, N., Andrews, L.G., and Tollefsbol, T.O. (2003). Transcriptional control of the DNA methyltransferases is altered in aging and neoplastically-transformed human fibroblasts. *Molecular and Cellular Biochemistry* 252 (1-2): 33–43. https://doi.org/10.1023/a:1025548623524.

Chen, S., Meng, Z., and Zhao, Q. (2018). Electrocardiogram recognization based on variational autoencoder. In: *Machine Learning and Biometrics*, vol. 7634. IntechOpen.

Copson, E.R., Maishman, T.C., Tapper, W.J. et al. (2018). Germline BRCA mutation and outcome in young-onset breast cancer (POSH): a prospective cohort study. *The Lancet Oncology* 19 (2): 169–180. https://doi.org/10.1016/S1470-2045(17)30891-4.

Cronin, M., Sangli, C., Liu, M.L. et al. (2007). Analytical validation of the oncotype DX genomic diagnostic test for recurrence prognosis and therapeutic response prediction in node-negative, estrogen receptor-positive breast cancer. *Clinical Chemistry* 53 (6): 1084–1091. https://doi.org/10.1373/clinchem.2006.076497.

De Pristo, M.A., Banks, E., Poplin, R. et al. (2011). A framework for variation discovery and genotyping using next-generation DNA sequencing data. *Nature Genetics* 43 (5): 491–498. https://doi.org/10.1038/ng.806.

Dettling, M. and Bühlmann, P. (2003). Boosting for tumor classification with gene expression data. *Bioinformatics* 19 (9): 1061–1069. https://doi.org/10.1093/bioinformatics/btf867.

Di Lonardo, A., Nasi, S., and Pulciani, S. (2015). We should not forget the past. *Journal of Cancer* 6 (1): 29–39. https://doi.org/10.7150/jca.10336.

Duda, R.O., Hart, P.E., and Stork, D.G. (2001). *Pattern Classification*, 2e. New York: Wiley.

Efron, B., Hastie, T., Johnstone, I., and Tibshirani, R. (2004). Least Angle Regression. ArXiv: 0406456v2, [math.ST]. https://arxiv.org/abs/math/0406456.

Elbattah, M., Loughnane, C., Guérin, J.-L. et al. (2021). Variational autoencoder for image-based augmentation of eye-tracking data. *Journal of Imaging* 7 (5): 83. https://doi.org/10.3390/jimaging7050083.

Esteller, M., Hamilton, S.R., Burger, P.C. et al. (1999). Inactivation of the DNA repair gene O6-methylguanine-DNA methyltransferase by promoter hypermethylation is a common event in primary human neoplasia. *Cancer Research* 59 (4): 793–797.

Faguet, G.B. (2015). A brief history of cancer: Age-old milestones underlying our current knowledge database. *International Journal of Cancer* 136 (9): 2022–2036. https://doi.org/10.1002/ijc.29134.

Feinberg, A.P. and Vogelstein, B. (1983). Hypomethylation distinguishes genes of some human cancers from their normal counterparts. *Nature* 301 (5895): 89–92. https://doi.org/10.1038/301089a0.

Fusco, M.J., Knepper, T.C., Balliu, J. et al. (2022). Evaluation of targeted next-generation sequencing for the management of patients diagnosed with a cancer of unknown primary. *The Oncologist* 27 (1): e9–e17. https://doi.org/10.1093/oncolo/oyab014.

Gama-Sosa, M.A., Slagel, V.A., Trewyn, R.W. et al. (1983). The 5-methylcytosine content of DNA from human tumors. *Nucleic Acids Research* 11 (19): 6883–6894. https://doi.org/10.1093/nar/11.19.6883.

Gerstung, M., Pellagatti, A., Malcovati, L. et al. (2015). Combining gene mutation with gene expression data improves outcome prediction in myelodysplastic syndromes. *Nature Communications* 6: 5901. https://doi.org/10.1038/ncomms6901.

Ghosh, D. (2002). Singular value decomposition regression models for classification of tumors from microarray experiments. *Pacific Symposium on Biocomputing* 18–29.

Glas, A.M., Floore, A., Delahaye, L.J.M.J. et al. (2006). Converting a breast cancer microarray signature into a high-throughput diagnostic test. *BMC Genomics* 7: 278. https://doi.org/10 .1186/1471-2164-7-278.

Goodfellow, I., Bengio, Y., and Courville, A. (2016). *Deep learning*. MIT Press http://www .deeplearningbook.org.

Goodwin, S., McPherson, J.D., and McCombie, W.R. (2016). Coming of age: ten years of next-generation sequencing technologies. *Nature Reviews. Genetics* 17 (6): 333–351. https:// doi.org/10.1038/nrg.2016.49.

Grønbech, C.H., Vording, M.F., Timshel, P.N. et al. (2020). scVAE: variational auto-encoders for single-cell gene expression data. *Bioinformatics* 36 (16): 4415–4422. https://doi.org/10.1093/ bioinformatics/btaa293.

Hanahan, D. (2022). Hallmarks of cancer: new dimensions. *Cancer Discovery* 12 (1): 31–46. https://doi.org/10.1158/2159-8290.CD-21-1059.

Hanahan, D. and Weinberg, R.A. (2011). Hallmarks of cancer: the next generation. *Cell* 144 (5): 646–674. https://doi.org/10.1016/j.cell.2011.02.013.

Heather, J.M. and Chain, B. (2016). The sequence of sequencers: the history of sequencing DNA. *Genomics* 107 (1): 1–8. https://doi.org/10.1016/j.ygeno.2015.11.003.

Hedenfalk, I., Duggan, D., Chen, Y. et al. (2001). Gene-expression profiles in hereditary breast cancer. *The New England Journal of Medicine* 344 (8): 539–548. https://doi.org/10.1056/ NEJM200102223440801.

Hess, J.M., Bernards, A., Kim, J. et al. (2019). Passenger hotspot mutations in cancer. *Cancer Cell* 36 (3): 288–301.e14. https://doi.org/10.1016/j.ccell.2019.08.002.

Hinton, G.E., Osindero, S., and Teh, Y.-W. (2006). A fast learning algorithm for deep belief nets. *Neural Computation* 18 (7): 1527–1554. https://doi.org/10.1162/neco.2006.18.7.1527.

Hira, M.T., Razzaque, M.A., Angione, C. et al. (2021). Integrated multi-omics analysis of ovarian cancer using variational autoencoders. *Scientific Reports* 11 (1): 6265. https://doi.org/ 10.1038/s41598-021-85285-4.

Hoffmann, S., Stadler, P.F., and Strimmer, K. (2014). A Simple Data-Adaptive Probabilistic Variant Calling Model. ArXiv: 1405.5251, [q-bio.GN]. https://arxiv.org/abs/1405.5251.

Hornik, K., Stinchcombe, M., and White, H. (1989). Multilayer feedforward networks are universal approximators. *Neural Networks* 2 (5): 359–366. https://doi.org/10.1016/0893-6080(89)90020-8.

Huang, X. and Pan, W. (2003). Linear regression and two-class classification with gene expression data. *Bioinformatics* 19 (16): 2072–2078. https://doi.org/10.1093/bioinformatics/ btg283.

Huggins, C. and Dao, T.L.Y. (1953). Adrenalectomy and oophorectomy in treatment of advanced carcinoma of the breast. *Journal of the American Medical Association* 151 (16): 1388–1394.

Huggins, C. and Hodges, C.V. (2002). Studies on prostatic cancer: I. The effect of castration, of estrogen and of androgen injection on serum phosphatases in metastatic carcinoma of the prostate. *The Journal of Urology* 168 (1): 9–12. https://doi.org/10.1016/s0022-5347(05)64820-3.

Jain, M., Fiddes, I.T., Miga, K.H. et al. (2015). Improved data analysis for the MinION nanopore sequencer. *Nature Methods* 12 (4): 351–356. https://doi.org/10.1038/nmeth.3290.

Jendrzejewski, J.P., Sworczak, K., Comiskey, D.F., and de la Chapelle, A. (2019). Clinical implications of GWAS variants associated with differentiated thyroid cancer. *Endokrynologia Polska* 70 (5): 423–429. https://doi.org/10.5603/EP.a2019.0027.

Jin, B., Li, Y., and Robertson, K.D. (2011). DNA methylation: superior or subordinate in the epigenetic hierarchy? *Genes & Cancer* 2 (6): 607–617. https://doi.org/10.1177/1947601910393957.

Khazeeva, G., Sablauskas, K., van der Sanden, B. et al. (2022). DeNovoCNN: a deep learning approach to de novo variant calling in next generation sequencing data. *Nucleic Acids Research* 50 (17): e97. https://doi.org/10.1093/nar/gkac511.

Kingan, S.B., Urban, J., Lambert, C.C. et al. (2019). A high-quality genome assembly from a single, field-collected spotted lanternfly (*Lycorma delicatula*) using the PacBio Sequel II system. *Gigascience* 8 (10): giz122. https://doi.org/10.1093/gigascience/giz122.

Kingma, D.P. and Welling, M. (2019). An Introduction to Variational Autoencoders. ArXiv: 1906.02691v3, [cs.LG]. https://arxiv.org/abs/1906.02691.

Kingma, D.P. and Welling, M. (2022). Auto-Encoding Variational Bayes. ArXiv: 1312.6114v11, [stat.ML]. https://arxiv.org/abs/1312.6114.

Klambauer, G., Unterthiner, T., Mayr, A., and Hochreiter, S. (2017). Self-Normalizing Neural Networks. ArXiv: 1706.02515v5, [cs.LG]. https://arxiv.org/abs/1706.02515.

Kleihues, P., Schäuble, B., zur Hausen, A. et al. (1997). Tumors associated with p53 germline mutations: a synopsis of 91 families. *The American Journal of Pathology* 150 (1): 1–13.

Krijgsman, O., Roepman, P., Zwart, W. et al. (2012). A diagnostic gene profile for molecular subtyping of breast cancer associated with treatment response. *Breast Cancer Research and Treatment* 133 (1): 37–47. https://doi.org/10.1007/s10549-011-1683-z.

Kumar, S., Warrell, J., Li, S. et al. (2020). Passenger mutations in more than 2,500 cancer genomes: overall molecular functional impact and consequences. *Cell* 180 (5): 915–927.e16. https://doi.org/10.1016/j.cell.2020.01.032.

Lähnemann, D., Köster, J., Fischer, U. et al. (2021). Accurate and scalable variant calling from single cell DNA sequencing data with ProSolo. *Nature Communications* 12 (1): 6744. https://doi.org/10.1038/s41467-021-26938-w.

Lam, L.L., Emberly, E., Fraser, H.B. et al. (2012). Factors underlying variable DNA methylation in a human community cohort. *Proceedings of the National Academy of Sciences of the United States of America* 109 (Suppl 2): 17253–17260. https://doi.org/10.1073/pnas.1121249109.

Lander, E.S. and Waterman, M.S. (1988). Genomic mapping by fingerprinting random clones: a mathematical analysis. *Genomics* 2 (3): 231–239. https://doi.org/10.1016/0888-7543(88)90007-9.

Li, N., Rowley, S.M., Thompson, E.R. et al. (2018). Evaluating the breast cancer predisposition role of rare variants in genes associated with low-penetrance breast cancer risk SNPs. *Breast Cancer Research* 20 (1): 3. https://doi.org/10.1186/s13058-017-0929-z.

Li, B., Brady, S.W., Ma, X. et al. (2020). Therapy-induced mutations drive the genomic landscape of relapsed acute lymphoblastic leukemia. *Blood* 135 (1): 41–55. https://doi.org/10.1182/blood.2019002220.

Lips, E.H., Michaut, M., Hoogstraat, M. et al. (2015). Next generation sequencing of triple negative breast cancer to find predictors for chemotherapy response. *Breast Cancer Research* 17 (1): 134. https://doi.org/10.1186/s13058-015-0642-8.

Liu, Z., Yao, Y., Wei, Q. et al. (2019). Res2s2aM: deep residual network-based model for identifying functional noncoding SNPs in trait-associated regions. *Pacific Symposium on Biocomputing* 24: 76–87.

Loukas, M., Tubbs, R.S., Mirzayan, N. et al. (2011). The history of mastectomy. *The American Surgeon* 77 (5): 566–571.

Lowes, L.E., Bratman, S.V., Dittamore, R. et al. (2016). Circulating tumor cells (CTC) and cell-free DNA (cfDNA) workshop 2016: scientific opportunities and logistics for cancer clinical trial incorporation. *International Journal of Molecular Sciences* 17 (9): 1505. https://doi.org/10.3390/ijms17091505.

Lu, T.-P., Tsai, M.-H., Lee, J.-M. et al. (2010). Identification of a novel biomarker, SEMA5A, for non-small cell lung carcinoma in nonsmoking women. *Cancer Epidemiology, Biomarkers & Prevention* 19 (10): 2590–2597. https://doi.org/10.1158/1055-9965.EPI-10-0332.

Luo, R., Schatz, M.C., and Salzberg, S.L. (2017). 16GT: a fast and sensitive variant caller using a 16-genotype probabilistic model. *Gigascience* 6 (7): 1–4. https://doi.org/10.1093/gigascience/gix045.

Luo, R., Sedlazeck, F.J., Lam, T.W., and Schatz, M.C. (2019). A multi-task convolutional deep neural network for variant calling in single molecule sequencing. *Nature Communications* 10 (1): 998. https://doi.org/10.1038/s41467-019-09025-z.

Ma, T. and Zhang, A. (2019). Integrate multi-omics data with biological interaction networks using Multi-view Factorization AutoEncoder (MAE). *BMC Genomics* 20 (Suppl 11): 944. https://doi.org/10.1186/s12864-019-6285-x.

Ma, X., Shao, Y., Tian, L. et al. (2019). Analysis of error profiles in deep next-generation sequencing data. *Genome Biology* 20 (1): 50. https://doi.org/10.1186/s13059-019-1659-6.

Maas, A.L., Hannun, A.Y., and Ng, A.Y. (2013). Rectifier nonlinearities improve neural network acoustic models. In: *Proceedings of the 30th International Conference on Machine Learning*, vol. 30, 3.

McKenna, A., Hanna, M., Banks, E. et al. (2010). The genome analysis toolkit: a mapreduce framework for analyzing next-generation DNA sequencing data. *Genome Research* 20 (9): 1297–1303. https://doi.org/10.1101/gr.107524.110.

Meynert, A.M., Bicknell, L.S., Hurles, M.E. et al. (2013). Quantifying single nucleotide variant detection sensitivity in exome sequencing. *BMC Bioinformatics* 14: 195. https://doi.org/10.1186/1471-2105-14-195.

Milagro, F.I., Gómez-Abellán, P., Campión, J. et al. (2012). CLOCK, PER2 and BMAL1 DNA methylation: association with obesity and metabolic syndrome characteristics and monounsaturated fat intake. *Chronobiology International* 9: 1180–1194. https://doi.org/10.3109/07420528.2012.719967.

Mittempergher, L., Delahaye, L.J., Witteveen, A.T. et al. (2020). Performance characteristics of the BluePrint® breast cancer diagnostic test. *Translational Oncology* 13 (4): 100756. https://doi.org/10.1016/j.tranon.2020.100756.

Moore, L.D., Le, T., and Fan, G. (2013). DNA methylation and its basic function. *Neuropsychopharmacology* 38 (1): 23–38. https://doi.org/10.1038/npp.2012.112.

Mould, R.F. (2007). Priority for radium therapy of benign conditions and cancer. *Current Oncology* 14 (3): 118–122. https://doi.org/10.3747/co.2007.120.

Murff, H.J., Spigel, D.R., and Syngal, S. (2004). Does this patient have a family history of cancer? An evidence-based analysis of the accuracy of family cancer history. *JAMA* 292 (12): 1480–1489. https://doi.org/10.1001/jama.292.12.1480.

Ng, A.Y. (2004). Feature selection, L 1 vs. L 2 regularization, and rotational invariance. In: *ICML '04: Proceedings of the twenty-first international conference on Machine learning.* https://doi.org/10.1145/1015330.1015435.

Nguyen, D.V. and Rocke, D.M. (2002). Tumor classification by partial least squares using microarray gene expression data. *Bioinformatics* 18 (1): 39–50. https://doi.org/10.1093/bioinformatics/18.1.39.

Nichols, K.E., Malkin, D., Garber, J.E. et al. (2001). Germ-line p53 mutations predispose to a wide spectrum of early-onset cancers. *Cancer Epidemiology, Biomarkers & Prevention* 10 (2): 83–87.

Nilsson, E., Matte, A., Perfilyev, A. et al. (2015). Epigenetic alterations in human liver from subjects with type 2 diabetes in parallel with reduced folate levels. *The Journal of Clinical Endocrinology and Metabolism* 100 (11): E1491–E1501. https://doi.org/10.1210/jc.2015-3204.

Nones, K. and Patch, A.M. (2020). The impact of next generation sequencing in cancer research. *Cancers (Basel)* 12 (10): 2928. https://doi.org/10.3390/cancers12102928.

Nwankpa, C., Ijomah, W., Gachagan, A., and Marshall, S. (2018). Activation Functions: Comparison of trends in Practice and Research for Deep Learning. ArXiv: 1811.03378, [cs.LG]. https://arxiv.org/abs/1811.03378.

Orsolic, I., Carrier, A., and Esteller, M. (2022). Genetic and epigenetic defects of the RNA modification machinery in cancer. *Trends in Genetics* 39 (1): 74–88. https://doi.org/10.1016/j.tig.2022.10.004.

O'Shaughnessy, J., Brezden-Masley, C., Cazzaniga, M. et al. (2020). Prevalence of germline BRCA mutations in HER2-negative metastatic breast cancer: global results from the real-world, observational BREAKOUT study. *Breast Cancer Research* 22 (1): 114. https://doi.org/10.1186/s13058-020-01349-9.

O'Shea, K. and Nash, R. (2015). An Introduction to Convolutional Neural Networks. ArXiv:1511.08458, [cs.NE]. https://arxiv.org/abs/1511.08458.

Park, J.Y., Kricka, L.J., Clark, P. et al. (2014). Clinical genomics: when whole genome sequencing is like a whole-body CT scan. *Clinical Chemistry* 60 (11): 1390–1392. https://doi.org/10.1373/clinchem.2014.230276.

Piccart, M., van't Veer, L.J., Poncet, C. et al. (2021). 70-Gene signature as an aid for treatment decisions in early breast cancer: updated results of the phase 3 randomised MINDACT trial with an exploratory analysis by age. *The Lancet Oncology* 22 (4): 476–488. https://doi.org/10.1016/S1470-2045(21)00007-3.

Pollard, M.O., Gurdasani, D., Mentzer, A.J. et al. (2018). Long reads: their purpose and place. *Human Molecular Genetics* 27 (R2): R234–R241. https://doi.org/10.1093/hmg/ddy177.

Poplin, R., Chang, P.-C., Alexander, D. et al. (2018). A universal SNP and small-indel variant caller using deep neural networks. *Nature Biotechnology* 36 (10): 983–987. https://doi.org/10.1038/nbt.4235.

Qin, D. (2019). Next-generation sequencing and its clinical application. *Cancer Biology & Medicine* 16 (1): 4–10. https://doi.org/10.20892/j.issn.2095-3941.2018.0055.

Qing, T., Mohsen, H., Marczyk, M. et al. (2020). Germline variant burden in cancer genes correlates with age at diagnosis and somatic mutation burden. *Nature Communications* 11 (1): 2438. https://doi.org/10.1038/s41467-020-16293-7.

Ransohoff, D.F. (2005). Bias as a threat to the validity of cancer molecular-marker research. *Nature Reviews. Cancer* 5 (2): 142–149. https://doi.org/10.1038/nrc1550.

Raphael, B.J., Dobson, J.R., Oesper, L., and Vandin, F. (2014). Identifying driver mutations in sequenced cancer genomes: computational approaches to enable precision medicine. *Genome Medicine* 6 (1): 5. https://doi.org/10.1186/gm524.

Reva, B., Antipin, Y., and Sander, C. (2011). Predicting the functional impact of protein mutations: application to cancer genomics. *Nucleic Acids Research* 39 (17): e118. https://doi.org/10.1093/nar/gkr407.

Rimmer, A., Phan, H., Mathieson, I. et al. (2014). Integrating mapping-, assembly- and haplotype-based approaches for calling variants in clinical sequencing applications. *Nature Genetics* 46 (8): 912–918. https://doi.org/10.1038/ng.3036.

Rizzo, J.M. and Buck, M.J. (2012). Key principles and clinical applications of "next-generation" DNA sequencing. *Cancer Prevention Research (Philadelphia, Pa.)* 5 (7): 887–900. https://doi.org/10.1158/1940-6207.CAPR-11-0432.

Rusch, M., Nakitandwe, J., Shurtleff, S. et al. (2018). Clinical cancer genomic profiling by three-platform sequencing of whole genome, whole exome and transcriptome. *Nature Communications* 9 (1): 3962. https://doi.org/10.1038/s41467-018-06485-7.

Sahraeian, S.M.E., Liu, R., Lau, B. et al. (2019). Deep convolutional neural networks for accurate somatic mutation detection. *Nature Communications* 10 (1): 1041. https://doi.org/10.1038/s41467-019-09027-x.

Sanger, F., Brownlee, G.G., and Barrell, B.G. (1965). A two-dimensional fractionation procedure for radioactive nucleotides. *Journal of Molecular Biology* 13 (2): 373–398. https://doi.org/10.1016/s0022-2836(65)80104-8.

Sanger, F., Nicklen, S., and Coulson, A.R. (1977). DNA sequencing with chain-terminating inhibitors. *Proceedings of the National Academy of Sciences of the United States of America* 74 (12): 5463–5467. https://doi.org/10.1073/pnas.74.12.5463.

Seal, D.B., Das, V., Goswami, S., and De, R.K. (2020). Estimating gene expression from DNA methylation and copy number variation: A deep learning regression model for multi-omics integration. *Genomics* 112 (4): 2833–2841. https://doi.org/10.1016/j.ygeno.2020.03.021.

Seifert, H.-H., Schmiemann, V., Mueller, M. et al. (2007). In situ detection of global DNA hypomethylation in exfoliative urine cytology of patients with suspected bladder cancer. *Experimental and Molecular Pathology* 82 (3): 292–297. https://doi.org/10.1016/j.yexmp.2006.08.002.

Sharma, G., Mirza, S., Parshad, R. et al. (2010). CpG hypomethylation of MDR1 gene in tumor and serum of invasive ductal breast carcinoma patients. *Clinical Biochemistry* 43 (4–5): 373–379. https://doi.org/10.1016/j.clinbiochem.2009.10.009.

Simidjievski, N., Bodnar, C., Tariq, I. et al. (2019). Variational autoencoders for cancer data integration: design principles and computational practice. *Frontiers in Genetics* 10: 1205. https://doi.org/10.3389/fgene.2019.01205.

Srivastava, N., Hinton, G., Krizhevsky, A. et al. (2014). Dropout: a simple way to prevent neural networks from overfitting. *Journal of Machine Learning Research* 15 (56): 1929–1958.

Szegedy, C., Vanhoucke, V., Ioffe, S., et al. (2015). Rethinking the Inception Architecture for Computer Vision. ArXiv: 1512.00567v3, [cs.CV]. https://arxiv.org/abs/1512.00567.

van't Veer, L.J., Dai, H., van de Vijver, M.J. et al. (2002). Gene expression profiling predicts clinical outcome of breast cancer. *Nature* 415 (6871): 530–536. https://doi.org/10.1038/415530a.

Takeshima, H. and Ushijima, T. (2019). Accumulation of genetic and epigenetic alterations in normal cells and cancer risk. *NPJ Precision Oncology* 3: 7. https://doi.org/10.1038/s41698-019-0079-0.

Ternes, L., Dane, M., Gross, S. et al. (2022). A multi-encoder variational autoencoder controls multiple transformational features in single-cell image analysis. *Communications Biology* 5 (1): 255. https://doi.org/10.1038/s42003-022-03218-x.

Van der Auwera, G.A., Carneiro, M.O., Hartl, C. et al. (2013). From FastQ data to high confidence variant calls: the genome analysis toolkit best practices pipeline. *Current Protocols in Bioinformatics* 43 (1110): 11.10.1–11.10.33. https://doi.org/10.1002/0471250953.bi1110s43.

Venter, J.C., Adams, M.D., Myers, E.W. et al. (2001). The sequence of the human genome. *Science* 291 (5507): 1304–1351. https://doi.org/10.1126/science.1058040.

van de Vijver, M.J., He, Y.D., van't Veer, L.J. et al. (2002). A gene-expression signature as a predictor of survival in breast cancer. *The New England Journal of Medicine* 347 (25): 1999–2009. https://doi.org/10.1056/NEJMoa021967.

Vincent, P., Larochelle, H., Lajoie, I. et al. (2010). Stacked denoising autoencoders: learning useful representations in a deep network with a local denoising criterion. *Journal of Machine Learning Research* 11: 3371–3408. https://doi.org/10.5555/1756006.1953039.

Wang, H. and van der Laan, M.J. (2011). Dimension reduction with gene expression data using targeted variable importance measurement. *BMC Bioinformatics* 12: 312. https://doi.org/10.1186/1471-2105-12-312.

Way, G.P. and Greene, C.S. (2018). Extracting a biologically relevant latent space from cancer transcriptomes with variational autoencoders. *Pacific Symposium on Biocomputing* 23: 80–91.

Whitworth, P., Stork-Sloots, L., de Snoo, F.A. et al. (2014). Chemosensitivity predicted by BluePrint 80-gene functional subtype and MammaPrint in the Prospective Neoadjuvant Breast Registry Symphony Trial (NBRST). *Annals of Surgical Oncology* 21 (10): 3261–3267. https://doi.org/10.1245/s10434-014-3908-y.

Whitworth, P., Beitsch, P., Mislowsky, A. et al. (2017). Chemosensitivity and endocrine sensitivity in clinical luminal breast cancer patients in the prospective neoadjuvant breast registry symphony trial (NBRST) predicted by molecular subtyping. *Annals of Surgical Oncology* 24 (3): 669–675. https://doi.org/10.1245/s10434-016-5600-x.

Wu, R. (1970). Nucleotide sequence analysis of DNA. I. Partial sequence of the cohesive ends of bacteriophage lambda and 186 DNA. *Journal of Molecular Biology* 51 (3): 501–521. https://doi.org/10.1016/0022-2836(70)90004-5.

Wu, R. and Kaiser, A.D. (1968). Structure and base sequence in the cohesive ends of bacteriophage lambda DNA. *Journal of Molecular Biology* 35 (3): 523–537. https://doi.org/10.1016/s0022-2836(68)80012-9.

Xu, B., Wang, N., Chen, T., and Li, M. (2015). Empirical Evaluation of Rectified Activations in Convolutional Network. ArXiv: 1505.00853, [cs.LG]. https://arxiv.org/abs/1505.00853.

5

Deep Learning for Network Biology

Eleonora Lusito

San Raffaele Telethon Institute for Gene Therapy (SR-Tiget), IRCCS San Raffaele Scientific Institute, Milano, Italy

5.1 Types of Interactions Between Genes and Their Products

The genes and their products can interact in different ways and according to different contexts, directly or indirectly through the activity of biological or chemical intermediates like drugs. The major types of interactions will be described and are shown in Figure 5.1:

- Protein–protein interactions (PPIs) refer to physical interactions between proteins. They are essential for most of the processes of a cell (Dai et al. 2018; Sukenik et al. 2017; Schweppe et al. 2017). PPIs are often graphically and mathematically represented with diagrams (i.e. protein–protein interaction networks, PPINs), where the nodes represent the proteins that interact and the edges, the interactions, and the type. The thickness of the edges encodes the strength of the interaction, and hence, how much it is required for a particular biological function.
- Gene regulatory interactions (GRIs) refer to the mechanisms by which genes interact with each other through their products, to control a specific cell function often in response to extracellular signals. Regulatory interactions occur at the level of the DNA with epigenetic modifications, at the level of the transcription through the activity of transcription factors (TFs) and cofactors, and with posttranscriptional/translational modifications (Srikanth et al. 2020; Zeller et al. 2006; Sullivan et al. 2018; Artyomov et al. 2010). Graphically, as for PPINs, the nodes represent the genes while the connections are the regulatory relationships.
- Metabolic networks refer to metabolic and chemical reactions (Waller et al. 2020; Spirin et al. 2006). The nodes in a network diagram are the metabolites that can be the intermediates or the final products of a metabolic reaction. In a network diagram, the edges represent the flow of metabolites from the source to the target. Metabolic networks are usually represented by a small metabolic reaction, a simpler representation, given the complexity of them.
- Drug–drug interactions (DDIs) refer to the interactions among different drugs. They are widely adopted by clinicians to establish the most effective combination of

Big Data Analysis and Artificial Intelligence for Medical Sciences, First Edition.
Edited by Bruno Carpentieri and Paola Lecca.
© 2024 John Wiley & Sons Ltd. Published 2024 by John Wiley & Sons Ltd.

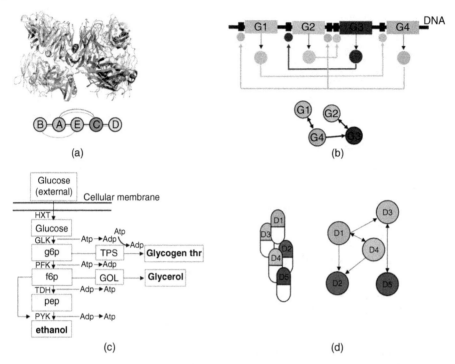

Figure 5.1 Types of biological and pharmacological interactions. The schematic representation of three types of biological interactions and one pharmacological interaction: (a) a multimeric heteroprotein complex from Peterson et al. (2018) as representative of PPIs. Interactions between different subunits are summarized in the diagram where nodes are colored according to the subunit and lines according to the type of interaction, i.e. in the naïve structure (black lines) or referred to the complex model (gray lines); (b) a toy representation of a GRI network where genes are indicated as rectangles (G1–G4) on a DNA strand and their products as dots (i.e. proteins) that interact with gene regulatory regions on DNA (black rectangles). The diagram is a schematic representation of the interactions; (c) the metabolic network of *S. cerevisiae* for ethanol production (modified from Wu et al. 2011). Intermediates and final products are reported, with the latter in bold. Enzymes and energy-molecules required and produced are outside the boxes; and (d) an example of a DDI network, where the interaction between drugs is shown with different gray shades is represented in the diagram with bidirectional arrows for reciprocal interactions and unidirectional arrows for exclusive interactions.

pharmacological treatments (Udrescu et al. 2016; Feng et al. 2020; Takeda et al. 2017). Clinically, significant DDIs occur when a drug impacts the efficacy or safety of another, taken concomitantly. Mechanisms of DDI include competitive protein-binding but can also occur when two drugs have opposing mechanism of action, overlapping side effects profiles, and similar therapeutic effects. In a graph representation, nodes are the drug compounds while the edges represent the relationships between them and their strength.

Although the metabolic reprogramming is essential to cancer cells to support the increased energy request for the continuous growth and proliferation, metabolic networks will not be discussed in the following paragraphs for simplicity. GRIs instead, will be discussed in the context of multimodal interactions with PPINs.

5.2   Deep Learning Methods with Graph-input Data

Deep learning methods designed to perform inference on graph inputs are called: GNNs. They adapt standard neural network methods to the graph domain. Classical deep learning methods operate on vector data and graphs cannot be directly converted into them. GNNs, instead, allow to deal with non-Euclidean data. Among different GNNs, graph-embedding techniques (Xu 2020) and graph convolutional networks (GCNs) (Kipf and Welling 2017) are widely used to model biological and PPIs.

5.2.1   Graph Embedding

The basic principle of network embedding that learns low-dimensional latent (i.e. hidden) feature representations of nodes or links in a network, is that the similarity in the embedding space should reflect the similarity in the network (Nelson et al. 2019; Gao et al. 2020; Liu et al. 2018). Let us consider $G = (V, E)$, as the set of vertices V, with $|V| = n$, and the set of edges E, where $e_{ij} \in E$ indicates an edge between v_i and v_j (Figure 5.2). Each graph G can be represented by its adjacency matrix $A \in \mathbb{R}^{n \times n}$. If the graph is unweighted and undirected, any edge e_{ij} is denoted by "1" at A_{ij} and A_{ji}. Graphs with node attributes, store these values in an additional matrix $X \in \mathbb{R}_{n \times d}$, where d is the dimension of them. If G is a weighted graph,

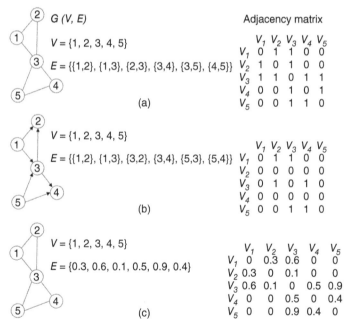

Figure 5.2   Types of graphs for interaction representation and their corresponding adjacency matrix. From the top to the bottom: (a) an unweighted and undirected graph with vertices (*V*) connected by edges (*E*) represented with a line; (b) an unweighted and directed graph with vertices connected by edges represented with an arrow; and (c) a weighted and undirected graph with vertices connected by edges represented with lines. The values of the adjacency matrix of this graph type are the weights.

the entry for edge e_{ij} in A will be the edge weight w_{ij}, and if G is a directed graph, an edge e_{ij} does not imply an edge e_{ji}, meaning that A is not necessarily symmetric.

5.2.1.1 Random Walk-Based Graph Embedding

In a hidden layer of a graph-deep neural network, a stochastic "random walk" Markov process performed on each node of the interactions graph, can learn the latent embedding, i.e. the similarity of the vertices, and allows to vectorize this information into a low dimension (Figure 5.3). (Huang et al. 2021; Perozzi et al. 2014; Grover and Leskovec 2016). Short-random walks allow to learn local structures of a graph, better capture community information, and parallelize simultaneous exploration of different regions of the entire graph thus reducing the computational complexity. Computations can be further reduced by establishing, for each node, a fixed number of random walks with a predefined length. The embedding that is learned, is used for node or graph classification and link prediction tasks (Figure 5.3). After the generation of multiple random walks from each node, in skip-gram-based embedding models (Mikolov et al. 2013), a skip-gram objective function is optimized. It maximizes the probability of predicting the nodes that surround a node in the random walk. Formally, it minimizes the following problem:

$$ -\log P(\{v_{i-w}, \ldots, v_{i-1}, v_{i+1}, \ldots, v_{i+w}\} | \Phi_i), $$

where $\Phi : V \mapsto \mathbb{R}^{|V| \times d}$ maps each vertex v into a d-dimensional space, resulting in a matrix of size $|V| \times d$, and w is the size of the context window surrounding a node v_i.

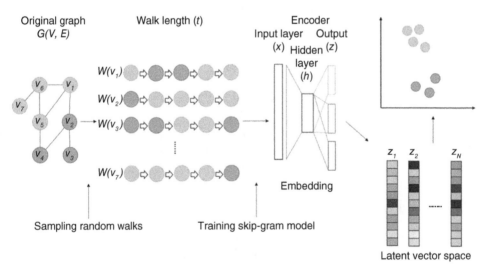

Figure 5.3 Random walk-based graph embedding. A schematic representation of random walk-based graph embedding. From the left to the right: the original graph, G (V, E), with two classes of nodes (light and dark gray circles). A random walk process is applied to first generate node contexts for each node on which an embedding model is applied to encode a low-dimensional, continuous representation (i.e. a vector) in the latent space. The learned node embedding features can be used for downstream tasks, such as node classification.

Figure 5.4 Random walk with search bias. A random walk from node t to node v with search bias α is represented. Source: Adapted from Paudel et al. 2019. p and q represent the return hyperparameter and the inout hyperparameter, respectively.

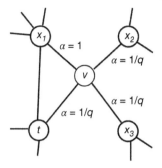

An extension of the basic idea of random walk introduces parameters to weight and control the bias of a depth-first search or a breadth-first search. Low-dimensional representations for nodes in a graph are hence learned by optimizing a neighborhood-preserving objective. Given a simple network as in Figure 5.4.

After transitioning to node v from t, the return hyperparameter, p, and the inout hyperparameter, q, control the probability of a walk staying inward revisiting nodes (t), staying close to the preceding nodes (x_1), or moving outward farther away (x_2, x_3).

5.2.1.2 Proximity-Based Graph Embedding

Another approach particularly useful for directed/undirected, weighted, and huge networks with millions of nodes and billions of edges is based on the optimization of an objective function that preserves global and local network structures (i.e. first-order and second-order proximities). Local structures are represented by the observed links which capture the first-order proximity between the vertices. Since the first-order proximity in real-world data is not sufficient to preserve the global network structure as a complement, the second-order proximity between the vertices, which is determined by the shared neighborhood structures, is considered. The idea behind is that nodes with shared neighbors are likely to be similar. To optimize the objective in this embedding learning, negative sampling is used (Yang et al. 2021). The objective optimization is a computationally expensive task especially for large-scale networks because it requires the summation over all the vertices when calculating the conditional probability: $p(\cdot|v_i)$. The negative sampling alleviates this problem by predicting the probability of the nodes to be neighbors instead of the probability of two nodes to be nearby. Computationally, it performs a sampling of multiple negative edges according to some noisy distribution for each edge (i,j). The following objective function is then specified for each edge:

$$\log \sigma \left(\overrightarrow{u_j'^T} \cdot \overrightarrow{u_j} \right) + \sum_{i=1}^{K} E_{vn \sim Pn(v)} \left[\log \sigma \left(-\overrightarrow{u_n'^T} \cdot i \right) \right],$$

where $\sigma(x) = 1/(1 + \exp(-x))$ is the sigmoid function and $\overrightarrow{u_j'^T}$ and $\overrightarrow{u_j}$ are two vectors, the first represents v_i treated as a context and the second as a vertex. The first term models the observed edges, the second term, the negative edges drawn from the noise distribution, and K is the number of negative edges. The equation above is then optimized with the asynchronous stochastic gradient algorithm (ASGD) (Zheng et al. 2020) that in each step samples a mini-batch of edges and then updates the model parameters. Because the gradient is multiplied by the weight of the edge, this becomes an issue in the presence of weights of edges with high variance. In this case, the scales of the gradients diverge, and to find a good learning rate becomes a complex task. With a large learning rate based on edges with small weights, it results into the explosion of the gradients on edges with large weights. The gradients are instead, too small in the presence of a learning rate based on edges with large weights. Conversely, the problem is not posed if the weights of all edges are equal. In this case, the learning rate is established with the edge-sampling algorithm (Ahmed et al. 2011) that unfolds a weighted edge into multiple binary edges. In this way, an edge with weight w is unfolded into w binary edges. The related memory issues that arise when the weights of the edges are very large are solved by sampling from the original edges so that the sampled edges are treated as binary with the sampling probabilities proportional to the original edge weights. This edge-sampling treatment allows the overall objective function to remain the same. The problem remains in the case of sampling the edges according to their variable weights. In this case, it is possible to calculate the sum of the weights over the set of edges between the vertices E:

$$w_{sum} = \sum_{i=1}^{|E|} w_i ,$$

as first step and then to sample a random value in the range of $[o, w_{sum}]$ to evaluate in which interval into the range of: $(\sum_{j=0}^{i-1} w_j, \sum_{j=0}^{i} w_j)$ the random value falls into. The "alias table" method by Li et al. (2014) is then used to draw a sample and is based on the weights of the edges. It takes a constant $O(1)$ time during drawing samples from the same discrete distribution. Beyond the specific approach that can be adapted to perform graph embedding, once the latent network structure is learned it can be used for graph classification and link prediction tasks like drug–disease associations (DDAs) (Zhao et al. 2021), DDI (Karim et al. 2019, Yu et al. 2021) and PPI predictions (Xiao and Deng 2020; Nasiri et al. 2021).

5.2.2 Graph Convolutional Networks (GCNs)

GCNs are CNNs applied to work with graph-structured data. While standard CNNs, to learn relevant features, leverage the spatial information through a set of images defined on the same regular grid, they cannot be directly used on graph inputs because the ordering of a graph's adjacency matrix is arbitrary. One of the strategies to address this issue is to use a spectral convolution over the graph (Chung 1997; Defferrard et al. 2016; Ma et al. 2019). Spectral methods build a convolution by creating a spectral filter defined in the Fourier domain using the graph Laplacian. Since the eigen decomposition of the graph Laplacian to find the orthogonal components that make the graph is computationally complex, spatial methods have been subsequently developed. The basic idea behind them is to learn an embedding for each node by aggregating its neighborhood in each successive layer, as shown in Figure 5.5.

For the aggregation phase, a permutation-invariant function, like the sum of the mean, is usually used. In this way, the issue of the arbitrary ordering of the adjacency matrix is addressed and a standard CNN can then be used. The kth layer in the network corresponds to incorporating the k-hop neighborhood of a given node. The seminal example of GCNs is the spatial-based method proposed by Kipf and Welling in 2017. Originally, this

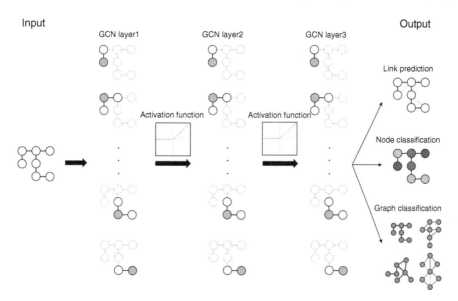

Figure 5.5 The architecture of a spatial-based GCN. The major components of a spatial-based GCN are shown. Three hidden layers for the convolution of the graph input are shown. Spatial features are used to learn from the graph for link prediction, node, and graph classification purposes.

approach was used to perform node classification via semi-supervised learning, but it can be generalized to classify high-order structures in the graph and to the graph itself. In their approach, a propagation layer for the network is defined where each layer incorporates information for that node's k-hop neighborhood and node features. The forward propagation of a two-layer network then takes the form:

$$Z = f(X, A) = \text{softmax}(A\hat{\sigma}\,(A\hat{X}\,W^{(0)})W^{(1)}),$$

where $\hat{A} \in \Re^{n \times n}$ is the normalized adjacency matrix (Kipf and Welling 2017) with added self-loops and results from the sum of the original adjacency matrix A and the identity matrix I_N. $AX \in \Re^{n \times d}$ is the feature matrix containing node attributes of all n nodes, $W^{(i)}$ are the weights from the ith layer and σ is the activation function like ReLU $= \max(.,$ $0)$. The softmax activation function is defined as $1/z\,[\exp(x_i)]$ with $Z = \sum_i \exp(x_i)$. The output of the model, i.e. Z, represents the class probabilities for each node so that $Z \in \Re^{n \times c}$ with $c =$ number of classes. If h is the number of hidden units, then $W^{(0)} \in \Re^{n \times h}$ and $W^{(1)} \in \Re^{n \times c}$. A more generalizable and computationally efficient alternative is the one proposed by Hamilton et al. (2018). Node classification and link prediction are achieved by sampling from the set of a node's neighbors instead of taking the entire neighborhood. Then, an aggregation function is learned, based on the mean, max, or long short-term memory (LSTM) (Hochreiter and Schmidhuber 1997). The node correspondence problem can also be addressed by imposing an ordering upon the graph. This is the easiest way to use a more traditional CNN structure (Niepert et al. 2016). A common fixed-size representation for all the graphs is used rather than the full graph. The entries in the grid are filled by the j most important nodes in a graph according to some predefined importance measure, as well as the k closest neighbors of each of the j nodes. In this way, graphs of different sizes are standardized to the same size grid. Then, a standard CNN filter can be applied. Independently from the method used, the training of the network is done by iteratively calculating a task-specific loss function over all relevant samples (i.e. the nodes with labels or the graphs). The gradient of the weights (W) is calculated and adjusted according to a predefined update equation. As for graph embedding, GCNs can be used to produce various outputs: for predicting new edges in the input network (Bonner et al. 2019; Huang et al. 2020), classifying individual nodes in the input graph, or classifying the entire input graph (Hu et al. 2019; Jin et al. 2020; Hou et al. 2022). For the graph classification task, the sum over all nodes is an additional and required step to map the output from $\mathbb{R}^{n \times c}$ to $\mathbb{R}^c$ where c indicates the class.

5.3 Applications of GNNs to Infer Biological and Pharmacological Interactions

5.3.1 Proteomics

GNNs are applied in proteomic, to predict if two proteins will interact (Jha et al. 2022; Zhou et al. 2022; Koca et al. 2022), the function of a given protein (Gligorijević et al. 2021; Zhao et al. 2022; Baldassarre et al. 2021) and its 3D structure (Jing et al. 2021; Xia et al. 2022). The first application is a link prediction task while the second is a classification. In the first case, in a protein graph where edges between nodes represent known protein interactions, the goal is to predict if other pairs of proteins will interact each other. Compared with machine learning (ML)-based existing methods, that use the primary structure of amino acid sequences to vectorize a protein and perform classification (Yang et al. 2010; Guo et al. 2008; Zhou et al. 2011), deep learning tools like GCNs, allow to directly incorporate the network information thus resulting in better predictions (Baranwal et al. 2020; Li et al. 2021). For classification purposes instead, the input is a PPI network where only the function of some nodes is known, and the goal is to classify the unknown nodes' function. To this aim, different strategies have been proposed. One of them uses multiple representations of the same PPIN where each network contains different information but the same set of nodes (Choi et al. 2021; Liu et al. 2020; Lei et al. 2019; Gligorijevic et al. 2018; Cao et al. 2016). With methods like the random walk (Xia et al. 2020), a vector representation of each node is then created and a positive point-wise mutual information matrix for each of the adjacency matrices is used as the input of a multimodal deep autoencoder. With this approach, many PPIs are given as input and all the available information can be easily integrated giving a low-dimensional vector. The protein function classification is finally performed using a support vector machine (SVM). Overall, the application of deep learning techniques in proteomics has reached a lot of attention in the last years, particularly in oncology, for the identification of critical nodes, i.e. relevant proteins that can be molecularly targeted. Moreover, the deconvolution of the functional as well as structural relationships between proteins is fundamental to predict the spread of the activating or inhibiting effects of one or more chemical compounds over the entire network for drug response predictions.

5.3.2 Drug Development and Repurposing

GNNs for drug discovery and repurposing are used to develop novel drug candidates and to identify new therapeutic uses of available compounds (Lim et al. 2019; Peng et al. 2020; Ding et al. 2021; Zhou et al. 2019; Popova et al. 2018; Maragakis et al. 2020). They are also used to investigate the properties of the potential drug candidates, i.e. the toxicity like the carcinogenicity, the distribution, and the metabolism (Yang et al. 2019; Liu et al. 2019; Aliper et al. 2016). In a GNN framework, the computational prediction of drug–target interactions (DTIs) is a link prediction task. Depending on data availability, a heterogeneous network composed of drugs, proteins (i.e. the targets), genomic information, and diseases is used as input to reach accurate predictions (Shao et al. 2022; Li et al. 2022). In a network diagram, all of them are represented as nodes of different types. Edges between nodes exist if they are connected by a relationship. The edge label is determined based on the type of the interaction that can be DDI, protein–protein similarities, drug–protein and PPIs, drug–disease, and drug–protein side effects interactions. A GCN is used to learn the embedding of the heterogeneous network. Representations are then taken as input by the decoder to capture the interactions. The output of this procedure is the estimated likelihood of the presence of an edge between pairs of nodes. When GCNs are used to predict the interactions between drug–targets like a ligand and a receptor, the nodes correspond to the residues. Each node is connected to the k closest other nodes determined by the mean distance between their atoms (Jha et al. 2022). Rather than simply predict whether a pair of proteins interact, this analysis predicts where, specifically, on the protein, the interaction will occur. In addition to the graph molecular structure also the non-covalent interactions among different molecules can be considered as input to infer pharmacologically relevant connections. Apart from the link prediction purposes, GNN are also applied in drug discovery, to investigate the properties of candidate new compounds (Cai et al. 2022; Jiang et al. 2021). This is the case of graph classification or regression in which whether a drug has certain properties is assessed. The properties of a compound usually refer to the absorption, distribution, metabolism, solubility, and toxicity. All of them are represented as graphs and the prediction of the pharmacological activity is based on the properties of other known drugs. By combining a GCN and an attention mechanism it is also possible to predict the stability of chemical compounds from their graph representation (Li et al. 2019). The molecular structure is captured at a local level while an attention mechanism learns the global graph information. The features that cause the instability of the molecule are hence captured and can be used to drive an efficient improvement of the compound.

5.3.3 Drug–Drug Interaction Prediction

A recent application of GCNs is to polypharmacy defined as the combination of different drugs to increase the benefits of the pharmacological treatment, particularly in the presence of complex diseases. Although promising in its final aim, the use of multiple medications can lead to interactions among coadministrated drugs resulting in toxicity and undesired effects (Maggiore et al. 2014; Woopen et al. 2016; Justice et al. 2021). From a deep learning perspective, the prediction of the side effects due to the combination of different drugs, is a link prediction task in which uni/multimodal graphs built combining PPIs, DDIs, and drug–protein interaction networks are used as input (Chen et al. 2020; He et al. 2022; Deng et al. 2020). As for drug discovery and repurposing, the node embedding is performed by the encoder, and the decoder outputs the final polypharmacy side effects model. The presence of interactions among the drugs is identified as well as the type of the interaction. The addition of PPI networks improves the accuracy of the predictions because most of the drug combinations have no common targets. Graph-based deep learning approaches for DDIs are also used to predict synergistic effects of drug combinations especially in cancer (Jiang et al. 2020; Wang et al. 2022; Jin et al. 2021). The problem is formulated as previously, as a link prediction task. A GCN encoder followed by a matrix decoder is used to predict the synergistic score among pairs of drugs starting from a multifeatured network. The integration, in the input network, of patients-related clinical information allows, at least in principle, a personalized treatment based on recorded favorable or adverse effects and DDI predictions.

5.3.4 Disease Classification and Outcome Prediction

The application of graph-based deep learning techniques to perform cancer subtype classification, diagnosis, and disease progression/outcome prediction, is still in early phase. However, some attempts have been made and will be listed and briefly explained:

- a combination of spectral clustering and CNNs has been used to predict different cancer types from PPI networks integrated with gene expression data (Matsubara et al. 2019; Chuang et al. 2021). In this approach, a Laplacian transformation (Qin and Gao 2010) is used to map PPI networks into 2D space. Convolutional and pooling layers are then added to the spectral 2D space after mapping gene expression data on it and generate a feature vector that serves as input for n hidden neural networks that output the prediction scores. The mapping of the PPI network to a spectral 2D space while preserving the topology, allows to generate an input that is compatible with the image-based inputs of standard CNNs. This integrated approach allowed to reach high accuracy while predicting tumor types and features with prognostic implications.
- A combination of GCN and a relational network (RN) on PPI networks and gene expression data has been used for breast cancer subtype classification (Rhee et al. 2018). In this approach, gene expression profiles are first mapped on the graph structure of the PPI networks for each sample. Graph convolution is then applied to capture localized patterns and a relation network is used to rationalize the associations between the graph nodes. The outputs of the graph convolution layer and the RN are merged to produce the final classification of breast cancer samples based on the known subtypes: Luminal A/B, Her2, and Basal (Dai et al. 2015). This hybrid approach has been demonstrated to capture the relevant features of breast cancer and can successfully classify the patients based on the combination of two different data sources that unveil embedded patterns in data and neural network techniques.
- A framework that combines GCN and matrix factorization has been used to discover disease–gene associations from different data sources (Choi and Lee 2021; Han et al. 2019; Zhang et al. 2019). In this approach, first, latent features are extracted from diseases and genes by running PCA on each of the following inputs/relations stored in repositories: disease features and gene features data that include gene expression and Connectivity Maps (www.broadinstitute.org/cmap), functional gene association data (i.e. functional gene networks) and gene orthology data of disease–gene associations from different nonhuman species. The extracted features of the two classes in their similarity graphs, represent the input of GCNs for embedding learning. An inner product (i.e. the matrix factorization) is subsequently used to combine the embeddings obtained for diseases and genes separately and to finally get a preference score matrix. Model optimization consists in

to minimizing the difference between the predicted scores and the disease–gene associations already known. The strategy of coupling GCNs with matrix factorization allows to learn nonlinear relationships from data while combining two different types of information, one on genes and one on diseases.

Apart from the examples discussed above, at present, the major application of GNNs for patient classification and disease outcome prediction for medical interventions, refers to biomedical images. A graph representation of multimodal neuroimages for GCNs is, for example, used to classify patients with Parkinson disease (Safai et al. 2022), or equivalently, a graph mapping on magnetic resonance imaging (MRI) is used to predict the presence of multiple sclerosis and to classify patients (Marzullo et al. 2019). A lot of work still needs to be done to bind the deepness of high-throughput molecular profiling with the analytical power of sophisticated tools like GNNs. The inherent complex and heterogeneous nature of multimodal "-omics" data, often sparse and noisy with strong class imbalance affects and slows the progress and the success of network-based deep learning applications with diagnostic and therapeutic readouts.

Author Biography

Eleonora Lusito is a postdoctoral fellow in computational biology at San Raffaele Telethon Institute for Gene Therapy in Milano (Italy). She has a background in molecular biology, bioinformatics, and biostatistics. After dedicating her Ph.D. to the inference of clinically relevant gene regulatory networks in breast cancer, she moved to the deconvolution of the transcriptional plasticity of myeloid cells in pathologic conditions with diagnostic and therapeutic implications. She is an experienced researcher in the application of deep learning methods to "-omics" data at single-cell level. She is the first author and coauthor of publications on high-impact journals.

References

Ahmed, N., Neville, J., and Kompella, R.R. (2011). *Network Sampling via Edge-based Node Selection with Graph Induction*. Purdue e-pubs. Department of Computer Science Technical Reports.

Aliper, A., Plis, S., Artemov, A. et al. (2016). Deep learning applications for predicting pharmacological properties of drugs and drug repurposing using transcriptomic data. *Molecular Pharmaceutics* 13 (7): 2524–2530. https://doi.org/10.1021/acs.molpharmaceut.6b00248.

Artyomov, M.N., Meissner, A., and Chakraborty, A.K. (2010). A model for genetic and epigenetic regulatory networks identifies rare pathways for transcription factor induced pluripotency. *PLoS Computational Biology* (5): e1000785. https://doi.org/10.1371/journal.pcbi.1000785.

Baldassarre, F., Hurtado, D.M., Elofsson, A., and Azizpour, H. (2021). GraphQA: protein model quality assessment using graph convolutional networks. *Bioinformatics* 37 (3): 360–366. https://doi.org/10.1093/bioinformatics/btaa714.

Baranwal, M., Magner, A., Elvati, P. et al. (2020). A deep learning architecture for metabolic pathway prediction. *Bioinformatics* 36: 8, 2547–2553. https://doi.org/10.1093/bioinformatics/btz954.

Bonner, S., Atapour-Abarghouei, A., Jackson, P.T.G. et al. (2019). Temporal neighbourhood aggregation: predicting future links in temporal graphs via recurrent variational graph convolutions. In: *IEEE International Conference on Big Data (Big Data)*, 5336–5345. https://doi.org/10.1109/BigData47090.2019.9005545.

Cai, H., Zhang, H., Zhao, D. et al. (2022). FP-GNN: a versatile deep learning architecture for enhanced molecular property prediction. *Briefings in Bioinformatics* 23 (6): bbac408. https://doi.org/10.1093/bib/bbac408.

Cao, S., Lu, W., and Xu, Q. (2016). Deep neural networks for learning graph representations. In: *Proceedings of the Thirtieth AAAI Conference on Artificial Intelligence*, Palo Alto, California, 1145–1152. The AAAI Press.

Chen, X., Liu, X., and Wu, J. (2020). GCN-BMP: investigating graph representation learning for (DDI) prediction task. *Methods* 179: 47–54. https://doi.org/10.1016/j.ymeth.2020.05.014.

Choi, W. and Lee, H. (2021). Identifying disease-gene associations using a convolutional neural network-based model by embedding a biological knowledge graph with entity descriptions. *PLoS One* 16 (10): e0258626. https://doi.org/10.1371/journal.pone.0258626.

Choi, K., Lee, Y., Kim, C., et al. (2021). An Effective GCN-based Hierarchical Multi-label classification for Protein Function Prediction. ArXiv: 2112.02810, [cs.AI]. https://arxiv.org/abs/2112.02810).

Chuang, Y.-H., Huang, S.-H., Hung, T.-M. et al. (2021). Convolutional neural network for human cancer types prediction by integrating protein interaction networks and omics data. *Scientific Reports* 11 (1): 20691. https://doi.org/10.1038/s41598-021-98814-y.

Chung, F.R. (1997). *Spectral Graph Theory*, vol. 92. American Mathematical Soc.

Dai, X., Li, T., Bai, Z. et al. (2015). Breast cancer intrinsic subtype classification, clinical use and future trends. *American Journal of Cancer Research* 5 (10): 2929–2943.

Dai, L., Zhao, T., Bisteau, X. et al. (2018). Modulation of protein-interaction states through the cell cycle. *Cell* 173 (6): 1481–1494.e13. https://doi.org/10.1016/j.cell.2018.03.065.

Defferrard, M., Bresson, X., and Vandergheynst, P. (2016). Convolutional Neural Networks on Graphs with Fast Localized Spectral Filtering. ArXiv: 1606.09375v3, [cs.LG]. https://arxiv.org/abs/1606.09375.

Deng, Y., Xu, X., Qiu, Y. et al. (2020). A multimodal deep learning framework for predicting drug-drug interaction events. *Bioinformatics* 36 (15): 4316–4322. https://doi.org/10.1093/bioinformatics/btaa501.

Ding, Y., Tang, J., and Guo, F. (2021). Identification of drug-target interactions via multi-view graph regularized link propagation model. *Neurocomputing* 461: 618–631. https://doi.org/10.1016/j.neucom.2021.05.100.

Feng, Y.-H., Zhang, S.-W., and Shi, J.-Y. (2020). DPDDI: a deep predictor for drug-drug interactions. *BMC Bioinformatics* (1): 419. https://doi.org/10.1186/s12859-020-03724-x.

Gao, X., Chen, J., Zhan, Z., and Yang, S. (2020). Learning heterogeneous information network embeddings via relational triplet network. *Neurocomputing* 412: 31–41. https://doi.org/10.1016/j.neucom.2020.06.043.

Gligorijevic, V., Barot, M., and Bonneau, R. (2018). deepNF: deep network fusion for protein function prediction. *Bioinformatics* 34: 22, 3873–3881. https://doi.org/10.1093/bioinformatics/bty440.

Gligorijević, V., Renfrew, P.D., Kosciolek, T. et al. (2021). Structure-based protein function prediction using graph convolutional networks. *Nature Communications* 12 (1): 3168. https://doi.org/10.1038/s41467-021-23303-9.

Grover, A. and Leskovec, J. (2016). node2vec: Scalable Feature Learning for Networks. ArXiv: 1607.00653, [cs.SI]. https://arxiv.org/abs/1607.00653.

Guo, Y., Yu, L., Wen, Z., and Li, M. (2008). Using support vector machine combined with auto covariance to predict protein-protein interactions from protein sequences. *Nucleic Acids Research* 36 (9): 3025–3030. https://doi.org/10.1093/nar/gkn159.

Hamilton, W.L., Ying, R., and Leskovec, J. (2018). Inductive Representation Learning on Large Graphs. ArXiv: 1706.02216v4, [cs.SI]. https://arxiv.org/abs/1706.02216.

P. Han, P. Yang, P. Zhao, S. Shang, Y. Liu, J. Zhou, and P. Kalnis. GCN-MF: disease-gene association identification by graph convolutional networks and matrix factorization. *KDD '19: Proceedings of the 25th ACM SIGKDD International Conference on Knowledge Discovery & Data Mining.* 705-713, 2019. https://doi.org/10.1145/3292500.3330912.

He, C., Liu, Y., Li, H. et al. (2022). Multi-type feature fusion based on graph neural network for drug-drug interaction prediction. *BMC Bioinformatics* 23 (1): 224. https://doi.org/10.1186/s12859-022-04763-2.

Hochreiter, S. and Schmidhuber, J. (1997). Long short-term memory. *Neural Computation* 9 (8): 1735–1780. https://doi.org/10.1162/neco.1997.9.8.1735.

Hou, Y., Jia, S., Lun, X., et al. (2022). GCNs-Net: A Graph Convolutional Neural Network Approach for Decoding Time-resolved EEG Motor Imagery Signals. ArXiv: 2006.08924v4, [eess.SP]. https://arxiv.org/abs/2006.08924.

Hu, F., Zhu, Y., Wu, S., et al. (2019). Hierarchical Graph Convolutional Networks for Semi-supervised Node Classification. ArXiv: 1902.06667v4, [cs.SI]. https://arxiv.org/abs/1902.06667.

Huang, K., Xiao, C., Glass, L.M. et al. (2020). SkipGNN: predicting molecular interactions with skip-graph networks. *Scientific Reports* 10 (1): 21092. https://doi.org/10.1038/s41598-020-77766-9.

Huang, Z., Silva, A., Singh, A. et al. (2021). A Broader Picture of Random-walk Based Graph Embedding. ArXiv: 2110.12344, [cs.LG]. https://arxiv.org/abs/2110.12344.

Jha, K., Saha, S., and Singh, H. (2022). Prediction of protein-protein interaction using graph neural networks. *Scientific Reports* 12 (1): 8360. https://doi.org/10.1038/s41598-022-12201-9.

Jiang, P., Huang, S., Fu, Z. et al. (2020). Deep graph embedding for prioritizing synergistic anticancer drug combinations. *Computational and Structural Biotechnology Journal* 18: 427–438. https://doi.org/10.1016/j.csbj.2020.02.006.

Jiang, D., Wu, Z., Hsieh, C.-Y. et al. (2021). Could graph neural networks learn better molecular representation for drug discovery? A comparison study of descriptor-based and graph-based models. *Journal of Cheminformatics* 13 (1): 12. https://doi.org/10.1186/s13321-020-00479-8.

Jin, H., Shi, Z., Peruri, A., and Zhang, X. (2020). Certified robustness of graph convolution networks for graph classification under topological attacks. In: *NIPS'20: Proceedings of the 34th International Conference on Neural Information Processing Systems*, vol. 709, 8463–8474.

Jin, W., Stokes, J.M., Eastman, R.T. et al. (2021). Deep learning identifies synergistic drug combinations for treating COVID-19. *Proceedings of the National Academy of Sciences of the United States of America* 118 (39): e2105070118. https://doi.org/10.1073/pnas.2105070118.

Jing, B., Eismann, S., Soni, P.N., and Dror, R.O. (2021). Equivariant Graph Neural Networks for 3D Macromolecular Structure. ArXiv: 2106.03843v2, [cs.LG]. https://arxiv.org/abs/2106.03843.

Justice, A.C., Gordon, K.S., Romero, J. et al. (2021). Polypharmacy-associated risk of hospitalisation among people ageing with and without HIV: an observational study. *Lancet Healthy Longevity* 2 (10): e639–e650. https://doi.org/10.1016/S2666-7568(21)00206-3.

Karim, M.R., Cochez, M., Jares, J.B. et al. (2019). Drug-Drug Interaction Prediction Based on Knowledge Graph Embeddings and Convolutional-LSTM Network. ArXiv: 1908.01288, [cs.LG]. https://arxiv.org/abs/1908.01288.

Kipf, T.N. and Welling, M. (2017). Semi-Supervised Classification with Graph Convolutional Networks. ArXiv: 1609.02907v4, [cs.LG]. https://arxiv.org/abs/1609.02907.

Koca, M.B., Nourani, E., Abbasoğlu, F. et al. (2022). Graph convolutional network based virus-human protein-protein interaction prediction for novel viruses. *Computational Biology and Chemistry* 101: 107755. https://doi.org/10.1016/j.compbiolchem.2022.107755.

Lei, H., Wen, Y., You, Z. et al. (2019). Protein-protein interactions prediction via multimodal deep polynomial network and regularized extreme learning machine. *IEEE Journal of Biomedical and Health Informatics* 23 (3): 1290–1303. https://doi.org/10.1109/JBHI.2018.2845866.

Li, A.Q., Ahmed, A., Ravi, S., and Smola, A.J. (2014). Reducing the sampling complexity of topic models. In: *KDD '14: Proceedings of the 20th ACM SIGKDD International Conference on Knowledge Discovery And Data Mining*, 891–900. https://doi.org/10.1145/2623330.2623756.

Li, X., Yan, X., Gu, Q. et al. (2019). Chemical stability prediction with an attention-based graph convolution network. *Journal of Chemical Information and Modeling* 59 (3): 1044–1049. https://doi.org/10.1021/acs.jcim.8b00672.

Li, G., Müller, M., Qian, G., et al. (2021). DeepGCNs: Making GCNs Go as Deep as CNNs. ArXiv: 1910.06849v3, [cs.CV] (). https://arxiv.org/abs/1910.06849.

Li, M., Cai, X., Li, L. et al. (2022). Heterogeneous graph attention network for drug-target interaction prediction. In: *CIKM '22: Proceedings of the 31st ACM International Conference on Information & Knowledge Management*, 1166–1176. https://doi.org/10.1145/3511808.3557346.

Lim, J., Hwang, S.-Y., Moon, S. et al. (2019). Scaffold-based molecular design with a graph generative model. *Chemical Science* 11 (4): 1153–1164. https://doi.org/10.1039/c9sc04503a.

Liu, N., Huang, X., Li, J., and Hu, X. (2018). On interpretation of network embedding via taxonomy induction. In: *KDD '18: Proceedings of the 24th ACM SIGKDD International Conference on Knowledge Discovery & Data Mining*, 1812–1820. https://doi.org/10.1145/3219819.3220001.

Liu, K., Sun, X., Jia, L. et al. (2019). Chemi-Net: a molecular graph convolutional network for accurate drug property prediction. *International Journal of Molecular Sciences* 20 (14): 3389. https://doi.org/10.3390/ijms20143389.

Liu, L., Zhu, X., Ma, Y. et al. (2020). Combining sequence and network information to enhance protein-protein interaction prediction. *BMC Bioinformatics* 21 (Suppl 16): 537. https://doi.org/10.1186/s12859-020-03896-6.

Ma, Y., Hao, J., Yang, Y., et al. (2019). Spectral-based Graph Convolutional Network for Directed Graphs. ArXiv: 1907.08990, [cs.LG]. https://arxiv.org/abs/1907.08990.

Maggiore, R.J., Dale, W., Gross, C.P. et al. (2014). Polypharmacy and potentially inappropriate medication use in older adults with cancer undergoing chemotherapy: effect on chemotherapy-related toxicity and hospitalization during treatment. *Journal of the American Geriatrics Society* 62 (8): 1505–1512. https://doi.org/10.1111/jgs.12942.

Maragakis, P., Nisonoff, H., Cole, B., and Shaw, D.E. (2020). A deep-learning view of chemical space designed to facilitate drug discovery. *Journal of Chemical Information and Modeling* 60 (10): 4487–4496. https://doi.org/10.1021/acs.jcim.0c00321.

Marzullo, A., Kocevar, G., Stamile, C. et al. (2019). Classification of multiple sclerosis clinical profiles via graph convolutional neural networks. *Frontiers in Neuroscience* 13: 594. https://doi.org/10.3389/fnins.2019.00594.

Matsubara, T., Ochiai, T., Hayashida, M. et al. (2019). Convolutional neural network approach to lung cancer classification integrating protein interaction network and gene expression profiles. *Journal of Bioinformatics and Computational Biology* 17 (3): 1940007. https://doi.org/10.1142/S0219720019400079.

Mikolov, T., Chen, K., Corrado, G., and Dean, J. (2013). Efficient Estimation of Word Representations in Vector Space. ArXiv: 1301.3781, [cs.CL]. https://arxiv.org/abs/1301.3781.

Nasiri, E., Berahmand, K., Rostami, M., and Dabiri, M. (2021). A novel link prediction algorithm for protein-protein interaction networks by attributed graph embedding. *Computers in Biology and Medicine* 137: 104772. https://doi.org/10.1016/j.compbiomed.2021.104772.

Nelson, W., Zitnik, M., Wang, B. et al. (2019). To embed or not: network embedding as a paradigm in computational biology. *Frontiers in Genetics* 10: 381. https://doi.org/10.3389/fgene.2019.00381.

Niepert, M., Ahmed, M., and Kutzkov, K. (2016). Learning Convolutional Neural Networks for Graphs. ArXiv: 1605.05273v4, [cs.LG]. https://arxiv.org/abs/1605.05273.

Paudel, R., Muncy, T., and Eberle, W. (2019). Detecting DoS attack in smart home IoT devices using a graph-based approach. In: *IEEE International Conference on Big Data (Big Data)*, 5249–5258. Los Angeles, CA, USA: https://doi.org/10.1109/BigData47090.2019.9006156.

Peng, J., Li, J., and Shang, X. (2020). A learning-based method for drug-target interaction prediction based on feature representation learning and deep neural network. *BMC Bioinformatics* 21 (Suppl 13): 394. https://doi.org/10.1186/s12859-020-03677-1.

Perozzi, B., Al-Rfou, R., and Skiena, S. (2014). DeepWalk: Online Learning of Social Representations. ArXiv: 1403.6652, [cs.SI]. https://arxiv.org/abs/1403.6652.

Peterson, L.X., Togawa, Y., Esquivel-Rodriguez, J. et al. (2018). Modeling the assembly order of multimeric heteroprotein complexes. *PLoS Computational Biology* 14 (1): e1005937. https://doi.org/10.1371/journal.pcbi.1005937.

Popova, M., Isayev, O., and Tropsha, A. (2018). Deep reinforcement learning for de novo drug design. *Science Advances* 4 (7): eaap7885. https://doi.org/10.1126/sciadv.aap7885.

Qin, G. and Gao, L. (2010). Spectral clustering for detecting protein complexes in protein–protein interaction (PPI) networks. *Mathematical and Computer Modelling* 52 (11–12). https://doi.org/10.1016/j.mcm.2010.06.015.

Rhee, S., Seo, S., and Kim, S. (2018). Hybrid Approach of Relation Network and Localized Graph Convolutional Filtering for Breast Cancer Subtype Classification. ArXiv: 1711.05859v3, [cs.CV]. https://arxiv.org/abs/1711.05859.

Safai, A., Vakharia, N., Prasad, S. et al. (2022). Multimodal brain connectomics-based prediction of Parkinson's disease using graph attention networks. *Frontiers in Neuroscience* 15: 741489. https://doi.org/10.3389/fnins.2021.741489.

Schweppe, D.K., Chavez, J.D., Lee, C.F. et al. (2017). Mitochondrial protein interactome elucidated by chemical cross-linking mass spectrometry. *Proceedings of the National Academy of Sciences of the United States of America* 114 (7): 1732–1737. https://doi.org/10.1073/pnas.1617220114.

Shao, K., Zhang, Y., Wen, Y. et al. (2022). DTI-HETA: prediction of drug-target interactions based on GCN and GAT on heterogeneous graph. *Briefings in Bioinformatics* 23 (3): bbac109. https://doi.org/10.1093/bib/bbac109.

Spirin, V., Gelfand, M.S., Mironov, A.A., and Mirny, L.A. (2006). A metabolic network in the evolutionary context: multiscale structure and modularity. *Proceedings of the National Academy of Sciences of the United States of America* 103 (23): 8774–8779. https://doi.org/10.1073/pnas.0510258103.

Srikanth, S., Ramachandran, S., and Mohan, S. (2020). Construction of the gene regulatory network identifies MYC as a transcriptional regulator of SWI/SNF complex. *Scientific Reports* 10 (1): 158. https://doi.org/10.1038/s41598-019-56844-7.

Sukenik, S., Ren, P., and Gruebele, M. (2017). Weak protein-protein interactions in live cells are quantified by cell-volume modulation. *Proceedings of the National Academy of Sciences of the United States of America* 26: 6776–6781. https://doi.org/10.1073/pnas.1700818114.

Sullivan, K.D., Galbraith, M.D., Andrysik, Z., and Espinosa, J.M. (2018). Mechanisms of transcriptional regulation by p53. *Cell Death and Differentiation* 1: 133–143. https://doi.org/10.1038/cdd.2017.174.

Takeda, T., Hao, M., Cheng, T. et al. (2017). Predicting drug-drug interactions through drug structural similarities and interaction networks incorporating pharmacokinetics and pharmacodynamics knowledge. *Journal of Cheminformatics* 9: 16. https://doi.org/10.1186/s13321-017-0200-8.

Udrescu, L., Sbârcea, L., Topîrceanu, A. et al. (2016). Clustering drug-drug interaction networks with energy model layouts: community analysis and drug repurposing. *Scientific Reports* 6: 32745. https://doi.org/10.1038/srep32745.

Waller, T.C., Berg, J.A., Lex, A. et al. (2020). Compartment and hub definitions tune metabolic networks for metabolomic interpretations. *Gigascience* 9 (1): giz137. https://doi.org/10.1093/gigascience/giz137.

Wang, X., Zhu, H., Jiang, Y. et al. (2022). PRODeepSyn: predicting anticancer synergistic drug combinations by embedding cell lines with protein-protein interaction network. *Briefings in Bioinformatics* 23 (2): bbab587. https://doi.org/10.1093/bib/bbab587.

Woopen, H., Richter, R., Ismaeel, F. et al. (2016). The influence of polypharmacy on grade III/IV toxicity, prior discontinuation of chemotherapy and overall survival in ovarian cancer. *Gynecologic Oncology* 140 (3): 554–558. https://doi.org/10.1016/j.ygyno.2016.01.012.

Wu, W.-H., Wang, F.-S., and Chang, M.-S. (2011). Multi-objective optimization of enzyme manipulations in metabolic networks considering resilience effects. *BMC Systems Biology* 5: 145. https://doi.org/10.1186/1752-0509-5-145.

Xia, F., Liu, J., Nie, H., et al. (2020). Random Walks: A Review of Algorithms and Applications. ArXiv: 2008.03639, [cs.SI]. https://arxiv.org/abs/2008.03639.

Xia, C., Feng, S.-H., Xia, Y. et al. (2022). Fast protein structure comparison through effective representation learning with contrastive graph neural networks. *PLoS Computational Biology* 18 (3): e1009986. https://doi.org/10.1371/journal.pcbi.1009986.

Xiao, Z. and Deng, Y. (2020). Graph embedding-based novel protein interaction prediction via higher-order graph convolutional network. *PLoS One* 15 (9): e0238915. https://doi.org/10.1371/journal.pone.0238915.

Xu, M. (2020). Understanding graph embedding methods and their applications. ArXiv: 2012.08019, [cs.LG]. https://arxiv.org/abs/2012.08019.

Yang, L., Xia, J.-F., and Gui, J. (2010). Prediction of protein-protein interactions from protein sequence using local descriptors. *Protein and Peptide Letters* 17 (9): 1085–1090. https://doi.org/10.2174/092986610791760306.

Yang, K., Swanson, K., Jin, W. et al. (2019). Analyzing learned molecular representations for property prediction. *Journal of Chemical Information and Modeling* 59 (8): 3370–3388. https://doi.org/10.1021/acs.jcim.9b00237.

Yang, Z., Zhou, C., Yang, H., et al. (2021). Understanding Negative Sampling in Graph Representation Learning. ArXiv: 2005.09863, [cs.LG]. https://arxiv.org/abs/2005.09863.

Yu, Y., Huang, K., Zhang, C. et al. (2021). SumGNN: multi-typed drug interaction prediction via efficient knowledge graph summarization. *Bioinformatics* 207: https://doi.org/10.1093/bioinformatics/btab207.

Zeller, K.I., Zhao, X.D., Lee, C.W.H. et al. (2006). Global mapping of c-Myc binding sites and target gene networks in human B cells. *Proceedings of the National Academy of Sciences of the United States of America* 103 (47): 17834–17839. https://doi.org/10.1073/pnas.0604129103.

Zhang, J., Hu, X., Jiang, Z. et al. (2019). Predicting disease-related RNA associations based on graph convolutional attention network. In: *Proceedings of the 2019 IEEE International Conference on Bioinformatics and Biomedicine (BIBM)*, 177–182. Red Hook, NY: Curran Associates.

Zhao, B.-W., You, Z.-H., Wong, L. et al. (2021). MGRL: predicting drug-disease associations based on multi-graph representation learning. *Frontiers in Genetics* 12: 657182. https://doi.org/10.3389/fgene.2021.657182.

Zhao, C., Liu, T., and Wang, Z. (2022). PANDA2: protein function prediction using graph neural networks. *NAR Genomics and Bioinformatics* 4 (1): lqac004. https://doi.org/10.1093/nargab/lqac004.

Zheng, S., Meng, Q., Wang, T., et al. (2020). Asynchronous Stochastic Gradient Descent with Delay Compensation. ArXiv: 1609.08326v6. https://arxiv.org/abs/1609.08326.

Zhou, Y.Z., Gao, Y., and Zheng, Y.Y. (2011). Prediction of protein-protein interactions using local description of amino acid sequence. *Communications in Computer and Information Science* 202: 254–262. https://doi.org/10.1007/978-3-642-22456-0_37.

Zhou, Z., Kearnes, S., Li, L. et al. (2019). Optimization of molecules via deep reinforcement learning. *Scientific Reports* 9 (1): 10752. https://doi.org/10.1038/s41598-019-47148-x.

Zhou, H., Wang, W., Jin, J. et al. (2022). Graph neural network for protein-protein interaction prediction: a comparative study. *Molecules* 27 (18): 6135. https://doi.org/10.3390/molecules27186135.

6

Deep Learning-Based Reduced Order Models for Cardiac Electrophysiology

Stefania Fresca, Luca Dedè and Andrea Manzoni

MOX - Dipartimento di Matematica, Politecnico di Milano, Piazza Leonardo da Vinci 32, I-20133 Milano, Italy

6.1 Overview of Cardiac Physiology

The heart is a double pump comprises four chambers: two atria, the left atrium (LA) and the right atrium (RA), and two ventricles, the left ventricle (LV) and the right ventricle (RV), see Figure 6.1. The atrioventricular septum separates the atria from the ventricles; blood flows from the former to the latter through the tricuspid valve in the right part and through the mitral valve in the left part of the heart (Jarvik 2004). Non-oxygenated blood enters the RA through the superior and inferior venae cavae and gets pumped first into the RV, then through the pulmonary valve into the pulmonary circulation, where it is oxygenated by the lungs. Through the pulmonary veins the oxygenated blood coming from the lungs enter the left part of the heart, from which the blood is pumped again into the aorta and to the systemic circulation of the body (Altman and Dittmer 1971; Opie 2004).

Muscle contraction and relaxation represent the pump function of the heart. In particular, tissue contraction is triggered by electrical signals self-generated in the heart and propagated through the myocardium thanks to the excitability of the cardiac cells, the cardiomyocites, see, e.g. Colli Franzone et al. (2014) and Klabunde (2011). When suitably stimulated, cardiomyocytes produce a variation of the potential across the cellular membrane, called *transmembrane potential*. Its time evolution is usually referred to as *action potential* (AP), involving a depolarization and a polarization in the early stage of every heartbeat. The AP is generated by several ion channels (e.g. calcium, sodium, and potassium) that open and close, and by the resulting ionic currents crossing the membrane. Five phases of the AP are identified (see Figure 6.2) (Colli Franzone et al. 2014). During phase 0 (depolarization), the Na^+ ionic channels of the sarcolemma, the lipid membrane that encloses cardiomyocytes, open, allowing a free flow of positive ions into the cell. Consequently, the transmembrane potential passes from a negative resting value of -84 mV to positive values. We denote with phase 1 the rapid decrease of potential due to an outward flow of K^+ and Cl^- ions, occurring after the inactivation of the Na^+ channels. Phase 2 is characterized by the balance of an inward current – caused by the transit of Ca^{2+} – and an outward current – caused by the transit of K^+, that maintains the potential almost constant ("plateau" phase). The repolarization of the cell – phase 3 – is a consequence of the closing of the Ca^{2+} channels. At this

Big Data Analysis and Artificial Intelligence for Medical Sciences, First Edition.
Edited by Bruno Carpentieri and Paola Lecca.
© 2024 John Wiley & Sons Ltd. Published 2024 by John Wiley & Sons Ltd.

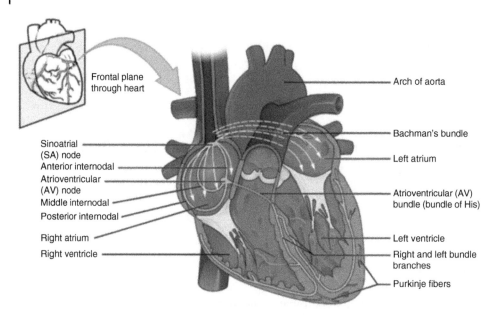

Frontal plane
through heart

Arch of aorta

Bachman's bundle

Sinoatrial
(SA) node

Left atrium

Anterior internodal

Atrioventricular
(AV) node

Atrioventricular (AV)
bundle (bundle of His)

Middle internodal

Posterior internodal

Right atrium

Left ventricle

Right ventricle

Right and left bundle
branches

Purkinje fibers

Figure 6.1 Anatomy of the anterior view of a frontal section of the heart. Source: Davis et al. 2019/with permission of Elsevier.

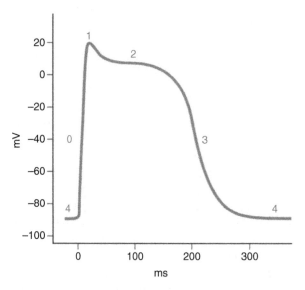

Figure 6.2 Evolution of the transmembrane potential versus time during the AP. The following phases are highlighted: (0) the depolarization phase, when the cascade effect of electrochemical reactions drives the opening of the ionic channels on the membrane, ultimately causing a spike in the potential which switches sign; (1) the short repolarization phase, when the potential shortly decreases immediately after the spike; (2) the plateau phase, when the net flux of electric charge due to the ions flowing inward/outward with respect to the cell membrane is zero; (3) the repolarization phase, when the channels, the ionic concentrations and the potential slowly return to the rest configuration; and (4) the resting phase, when the potential remains at its rest value of approximately $v = -90$ mV until the cell is stimulated.

stage, the outward current is still due to the flow of K^+ that causes the potential to return to negative values of $-80/-85$ mV. During phase 4 the potential remains constant value of -84 mV. Some of the K^+ ionic channels remain open, in order to guarantee the correct concentrations of ions outside and inside the cell. The cardiomyocyte stays in the resting phase until the next electric stimulation.

The electrical signal propagates from one cardiomyocite to those nearby because of the gap junctions located at the binding sites of adjacent cells. The electric excitation of the heart starts in the RA at the sinoatrial node (Brooks and Lu 1972), the natural pacemaker of the heart because of the ability of its cells to autonomously excite themselves, and travels across the atrial cardiac tissue. The signal travels from the RA to the LA through four muscular bundles (Sakamoto et al. 2005): the Bachmann's bundle, the anterior septum, the posterior septum and the coronary sinus musculature. When the excitation front reaches the atrioventricular node, located at the basis of the RA, the signal is transmitted from the atria to the ventricles after a delay of about 100 ms, due to the slow conduction characterizing the cells in this area, as it travels along the bundle of His and Purkinje fibers (Dzialowski and Crossley 2015). Such delay is important to establish the synchronized contraction of atria and ventricles and to determine the right cardiac rhythm.

6.1.1 Atrial Tachycardia and Atrial Fibrillation

Heart rhythm alterations (arrhythmias) affect millions of individuals in the world (Alonso and Bengtson 2014), and consist in conditions in which the heartbeat is irregular. There are two major types of arrhythmias involving the upper chambers (atria) of the heart: atrial tachycardia (AT) and fibrillation. AT occurs when the atrial pacing is too fast but usually regular, at rate higher than 100 beats per minute. ATs may be classified into two broad categories: focal and macro-re-entrant ATs (García-Cosío et al. 2012). Focal ATs are defined as arrhythmias that arise from a circumscribed site of early activation and propagate to the atria in a centrifugal pattern. In macro-re-entrant ATs, atrial activation occurs in a continuous, uninterrupted manner because of a wavefront rotating around an obstacle consisting in anatomical structures (venous or valvular orifices), scars, or areas of functional block. Atrial fibrillation (AF) is the most common type of cardiac arrhythmia, affecting the 2% of world population (Morillo et al. 2017), and verifies when the heart electrical signal propagates in a rapid and irregular way throughout the atria (Nishida and Nattel 2014). During AF, atrial cells fire at rates up to 200–600 times per minute with respect to 60–80 beats per minute in healthy conditions at rest.

The mechanisms sustaining AT and AF have not been clearly identified yet, however, macro-reentry and reentry breakup can be seen as cellular mechanisms associated to these dysfunctions (Nattel 2002). Reentry is a cellular mechanism where the electric signal does not complete the normal circuit, but rather follows an alternative path looping back upon itself and developing a self-perpetuating rapid and abnormal activation. Re-entries can be divided into two major types: anatomical and functional reentries (Colli Franzone et al. 2014). In the first case, re-entries develop around an anatomical obstacle, such as fibrosis, scar or slow conduction regions (Boyle et al. 2018; Saha et al. 2018). AT may be maintained by stable macro reentry whereas, during an AF episode, multiple coexisting unstable re-entries can be observed, that is a single spiral wave is fragmented into a spatiotemporally chaotic pattern comprising many wavelets of various sizes, the so-called reentry breakup. The major determinant of reentry behavior, breakup or not, is the action potential duration (APD) restitution (Clayton and Taggart 2005).

Several treatment options of AT and AF are available, including drug therapy, but the available drugs are not specific for atrial electrical activity and can have profound effects on ventricular electrophysiology (EP), cardioversion, and catheter ablation (Narayan et al. 2012a). The latter is a procedure used to destroy the arrhythmia driving tissue (Narayan et al. 2012b). A series of catheters are put into a blood vessel in the arm, groin, or neck. The wires are guided into the heart and a special system sends radiofrequency energy which destroys small areas of heart tissue. Catheter ablation normally consists in isolating the pulmonary veins (PVs) by burning tissue and destroying rotors cores, but it is still to be proved that ablating the tips is useful (Allessie and de Groot 2014; Narayan and Jalife 2014). Identifying the optimal target of ablation is far from being trivial, and the issue remains open and stands as the focus of several efforts by the scientific community.

Numerical simulations can play a great role in the cardiac EP context in order to improve the current available knowledge of heart electrical function/dysfunction, provide quantitative clinical responses in a noninvasive way and contribute substantially to the development of personalized approaches in medicine thus supporting clinicians' decisions in the prevention, diagnosis, and treatment of arrhythmias.

6.1.2 Mathematical Models for Cardiac Electrophysiology

The electrical activation of the heart, which drives its contraction, is the result of two processes (Quarteroni et al. 2017, 2019; Colli Franzone et al. 2014): the generation of ionic currents through the cellular membrane producing a local AP, at the microscopic scale; and the propagation of the AP from cell to cell in the form of a transmembrane potential, at the macroscopic scale. This latter process can be described by means of partial differential equations (PDEs), suitably coupled with systems of ordinary differential equations (ODEs) modeling the ionic currents in the cells.

In order to model the propagation of the electric signal in the heart, a spatio-temporal phenomenon, we may consider the so-called Bidomain equations (Colli Franzone et al. 2014; Geselowitz and Miller III 1983) in a domain $\Omega \subset \mathbb{R}^d$, with $d = 2, 3$, representing a portion of the myocardium, considered as a continuum composed by two interpenetrating domains, the intra- and the extracellular spaces. Each point $\mathbf{x} \in \Omega$ is associated with the intracellular potential u_i, the extracellular potential u_e, and the transmembrane potential $u = u_i - u_e$.

Coupling the nonlinear diffusion-reaction equation of the Bidomain model for the transmembrane potential $u = u(\mathbf{x}, t)$ and the diffusion equation for the extracellular potential $u_e = u_e(\mathbf{x}, t)$ with a phenomenological[1] model for the ionic currents – involving a single gating variable $w = w(\mathbf{x}, t)$ which plays the role of a recovery function thus allowing to model

---

1 Ionic models may be divided into three categories (Sundnes et al. 2006): phenomenological, first generation, and second generation models. Phenomenological models describe the AP without accounting for the underlying physiology. On the contrary, first and second generation models attempt to include a description of the mechanisms of the cell; while the former are based on simplified formulations to approximate the electrical behavior, the latter use instead sophisticated techniques allowing to represent subcellular processes. In the following, we will focus only on phenomenological models.

refractoriness of cells – results in the following nonlinear time-dependent system reproducing the EP phenomena inducing the muscle contraction:

$$
\begin{cases}
\dfrac{\partial u}{\partial t} - \operatorname{div}(\mathbf{D}_i \nabla u) - \operatorname{div}(\mathbf{D}_i \nabla u_e) + I_{\text{ion}}(u, w) = I_{\text{app}}^i & (\mathbf{x}, t) \in \Omega \times (0, T), \\[2mm]
-\operatorname{div}(\mathbf{D}_i \nabla u) - \operatorname{div}((\mathbf{D}_i + \mathbf{D}_e)\nabla u_e) = I_{\text{app}}^i + I_{\text{app}}^e & (\mathbf{x}, t) \in \Omega \times (0, T), \\[2mm]
\dfrac{\partial w}{\partial t} + g(u, w) = 0 & (\mathbf{x}, t) \in \Omega \times (0, T), \\[2mm]
\mathbf{D}_i \nabla(u + u_e) \cdot \mathbf{n} = 0 & (\mathbf{x}, t) \in \partial\Omega \times (0, T), \\[2mm]
(\mathbf{D}_i + \mathbf{D}_e)\nabla u_e \cdot \mathbf{n} + \mathbf{D}_i \nabla u \cdot \mathbf{n} = 0 & (\mathbf{x}, t) \in \partial\Omega \times (0, T), \\[2mm]
u(\mathbf{x}, 0) = u_0, \ w(\mathbf{x}, 0) = w_0 & \mathbf{x} \in \Omega.
\end{cases}
\tag{6.1}
$$

Here, t and $u = u(\mathbf{x}, t)$ denote a rescaled and dimensionless time and transmembrane potential,[2] depending on the ionic model considered, $\mathbf{n}$ denotes the outward directed unit vector normal to the boundary $\partial\Omega$ of the domain Ω, whereas $I_{\text{app}}^i = I_{\text{app}}^i(\mathbf{x}, t)$ and $I_{\text{app}}^e = I_{\text{app}}^e(\mathbf{x}, t)$ are the intra- and the extracellular applied currents representing, e.g. the activation of the tissue. The initial conditions $(6.1)_6$, representing the initial state of the transmembrane potential and the gating variable, are $u_0 = 0$ and $w_0 = 0$, in our case, whereas the homogeneous Neumann boundary conditions $(6.1)_4$ and $(6.1)_5$ are related to the electrical isolation of the portion of the myocardium Ω considered. The parabolic nonlinear diffusion-reaction equation $(6.1)_1$ for u, which must be in principle solved at any point $\mathbf{x} \in \Omega$, is two-way coupled with the ODE system $(6.1)_3$; indeed, the reaction term I_{ion} and the function g depend on both u and w. The most common choices for the two functions I_{ion} and g in order to efficiently reproduce the AP are, e.g. the FitzHugh–Nagumo (FitzHugh 1961; Nagumo et al. 1962), the Aliev–Panfilov (A–P) (Aliev and Panfilov 1996; Nash and Panfilov 2004), the Roger–McCulloch (R–M) (Rogers and McCulloch 1994) or the Mitchell and Schaeffer models (Mitchell and Schaeffer 2003). The diffusivity tensors $\mathbf{D}_i$, $\mathbf{D}_e$ usually depend on the fibers-sheet structure of the tissue, affecting directional conduction velocities and directions. In particular, by assuming an axisymmetric distribution of the fibers, the intra- and extracellular conductivity tensors take the form

$$
\begin{aligned}
\mathbf{D}_i(\mathbf{x}) &= \sigma_t^i\, I + (\sigma_l^i - \sigma_t^i)\, \mathbf{f}_0 \otimes \mathbf{f}_0, \\
\mathbf{D}_e(\mathbf{x}) &= \sigma_t^e\, I + (\sigma_l^e - \sigma_t^e)\, \mathbf{f}_0 \otimes \mathbf{f}_0,
\end{aligned}
\tag{6.2}
$$

where $\otimes$ indicates the tensor product of vectors, i.e. $(\mathbf{x} \otimes \mathbf{y})_{ij} = x_i y_j$, σ_l^i, σ_l^e, and σ_t^i, σ_t^e are the conductivities in the fibers direction $\mathbf{f}_0$ and the transversal one, for the intra- and extracellular conductivity tensors.

A simplified model, compared to the Bidomain model, requiring lower computational efforts, is given by the Monodomain equation (Colli Franzone et al. 2014), written only in terms of the transmembrane potential u. Indeed, by assuming that the intra- and the extracellular conductivity tensors are such that $\mathbf{D}_i = \lambda \mathbf{D}_e$, it is possible to simplify the Bidomain equations (6.1). By setting

$$
\mathbf{D} = \frac{1}{1 + \lambda} \mathbf{D}_i \quad \text{and} \quad I_{\text{app}} = \frac{\lambda}{1 + \lambda} I_{\text{app}}^i + \frac{1}{1 + \lambda} I_{\text{app}}^e,
$$

---

2 Dimensional times and potential (Aliev and Panfilov 1996) are given by $\tilde{t}\,[\text{ms}] = 12.9t$ and $\tilde{u}\,[\text{mV}] = 100u - 80$. The transmembrane potential ranges from the resting state of $-80\,\text{mV}$ to the excited state of $+20\,\text{mV}$.

the resulting coupled Monodomain system reads:

$$\begin{cases} \dfrac{\partial u}{\partial t} - \text{div}(\mathbf{D}\nabla u) + I_{\text{ion}}(u, w) = I_{\text{app}}(\mathbf{x}, t) & (\mathbf{x}, t) \in \Omega \times (0, T), \\[2mm] \dfrac{\partial w}{\partial t} + g(u, w) = 0 & (\mathbf{x}, t) \in \Omega \times (0, T), \\[2mm] \nabla u \cdot \mathbf{n} = 0 & (\mathbf{x}, t) \in \partial\Omega \times (0, T), \\[2mm] u(\mathbf{x}, 0) = u_0, \; w(\mathbf{x}, 0) = w_0 & \mathbf{x} \in \Omega, \end{cases} \tag{6.3}$$

where the conductivity tensor is defined as:

$$\mathbf{D}(\mathbf{x}) = \sigma_t \, I + (\sigma_l - \sigma_t) \, \mathbf{f}_0 \otimes \mathbf{f}_0. \tag{6.4}$$

When a simple phenomenological ionic model is considered, such as the FitzHugh–Nagumo, the A–P (Aliev and Panfilov 1996), or the R–M (Rogers and McCulloch 1994) model, the ionic current takes the form of a cubic nonlinear function of u and a single (dimensionless) gating variable plays the role of a recovery function, allowing to model refractoriness of cells. In this work, we focus on the simple phenomenological A–P and R–M ionic models in order to decrease the computational costs associated to the solution of (6.1) and (6.3). The first consists in taking:

$$\begin{aligned} I_{\text{ion}}(u, w) &= Ku(u - a)(u - 1) + uw, \\[2mm] g(u, w) &= \left(\epsilon_0 + \dfrac{c_1 w}{c_2 + u} \right)(-w - Ku(u - b - 1)), \end{aligned} \tag{6.5}$$

where the parameters K, a, b, ϵ_0, c_1, and c_2 are related to the cell. Here, a represents an oscillation threshold, whereas the weighting factor $\epsilon_0 + \frac{c_1 w}{c_2 + u}$ was introduced in Aliev and Panfilov (1996) to tune the restitution curve to experimental observations by adjusting the parameters c_1 and c_2; see, e.g. Clayton et al. (2011), Quarteroni et al. (2017, 2019), and Colli Franzone et al. (2014).

For the R–M ionic model, we rely on the following variant provided in Rogers and McCulloch (1994)

$$\begin{aligned} I_{\text{ion}}(u, w) &= Gu \left(1 - \dfrac{u}{u_{\text{th}}} \right) \left(1 - \dfrac{u}{u_p} \right) + \eta_1 uw, \\[2mm] g(u, w) &= \eta_2 \left(\dfrac{u}{u_p} - \eta_3 w \right), \end{aligned} \tag{6.6}$$

where G, η_1, η_2, and η_3 are positive coefficients, u_{th} is a threshold potential, and u_p is the peak potential.

The solution of cardiac EP systems entails several mathematical (i.e. nonlinearity and coupling of the equations) and numerical (i.e. high computational costs related to small time-step sizes, otherwise the system might be unstable, and mesh sizes, in order to capture the steep fronts (Sundnes et al. 2007; Colli Franzone and Pavarino 2004; Colli Franzone et al. 2014)) critical issues. Moreover, the coupled systems (6.1) and (6.3) usually depend on several parameters affecting either functional or geometric data such as, e.g. material properties, initial and boundary conditions, or the shape of the domain. For instance, relevant physical situations are those in which input parameters affect the diffusivity matrix

D (through the conduction velocities) and the applied current I_{app}. All these instances can be cast in either *multi-query* and/or *real-time* contexts. In the former case, the equations must be solved for a huge number of parameter instances because the parameter-quantity of interest map is repetitively evaluated in order to perform multi-scenario analysis, to deal with uncertainties and with inter- and intra-subject variability and to consider specific pathological scenarios; in the latter case, outputs of interest must be computed in a very limited amount of time, in view of the integration of computational model in the clinical practice.

6.2 Reduced Order Modeling

The solution of a parametrized system of PDEs by means of a *full order model* (FOM), i.e. the dynamical system arising by the space discretization of the equations by means of numerical methods, such as the Galerkin-finite element (FE) method (Quarteroni and Valli 1994) and isogeometric analysis (IGA) (Cottrell et al. 2009), whenever dealing with real-time or multi-query scenarios, may entail prohibitive computational costs if the FOM is high-dimensional, as anticipated in Section 6.1.2. Cardiac EP problems fit into real-time and multi-query contexts, due to the fact that outputs of interest must be computed in very short times and repetitive solutions of systems (6.1) and (6.3) are required in order to analyze different pathological scenarios (or different patients).

Reduced order modeling techniques aim at replacing the FOM by a *reduced order model* (ROM), featuring a much lower dimension, however, still able to express the physical features of the problem described by the FOM, thus being able to efficiently approximate the global map $(t; \mu) \mapsto \mathbf{u}_h(t; \mu)$, where $t \in (0, T)$ denotes time, $\mu \in \mathcal{P} \subset \mathbb{R}^{n_\mu}$ a vector of input parameters and $\mathbf{u}_h(t; \mu) \in \mathbb{R}^{N_h}$ the solution of a dynamical system arising from the space discretization of time-dependent (non)linear parametrized PDEs, such as the one of systems (6.1) and (6.3). The basic assumption underlying the construction of such a ROM is that the solution of the parametrized PDE, belonging a priori to a high-dimensional (discrete) space, lies on a low-dimensional manifold embedded in this space. The goal of a ROM is then to approximate the *solution manifold* – that is, the set of all PDE solutions when the parameters vary in the parameter space – through a suitable, approximated *trial manifold*.

A widespread family of reduced order modeling techniques relies on the assumption that the reduced order approximation can be expressed by a linear combination of problem-dependent basis functions, built starting from a set of FOM solutions obtained for different values of the parameters, also called snapshots. Among these techniques, proper orthogonal decomposition (POD) – equivalent to principal component analysis in statistics (Hastie et al. 2001), or Karhunen–Loève expansion in stochastic processes – and the greedy algorithm (Prud'homme et al. 2001; Buffa et al. 2012) are the most common strategies to build a reduced basis (RB). The former exploits the singular value decomposition (SVD) of a suitable snapshot matrix (or the eigen-decomposition of the corresponding snapshot correlation matrix); the latter consists in an adaptive sampling of the parameter space to minimize the snapshots to be computed, relying on the evaluation of efficient estimates of the error between the FOM and the ROM, thus yielding *linear* ROMs, in which the ROM approximation is given by the linear superimposition of POD modes. Relying on either POD or greedy algorithms, the solution manifold is approximated through a *linear* trial manifold, i.e. the ROM approximation is sought in a low-dimensional linear trial subspace.

Projection-based methods are linear ROMs in which the ROM approximation of the PDE solution, for any new parameter value, results from the solution of a low-dimensional (non-linear, dynamical) system, whose unknowns are the ROM degrees of freedom (or generalized coordinates). Both for linear and nonlinear PDEs, ROM's operators are obtained by imposing that the projection of the FOM residual evaluated on the ROM trial solution is orthogonal to a low-dimensional, linear test subspace, which might coincide with the trial subspace (Benner et al. 2015, 2017; Quarteroni et al. 2016). This is the core idea of the reduced basis method (Quarteroni et al. 2016), that has been successfully applied in several contexts (Grepl and Patera 2010; Veroy and Patera 2005) and to a broad range of applications, such as structural dynamics and elasticity (Willcox and Peraire 2002; Amsallem et al. 2009; Bonomi et al. 2017), aerodynamics (Carlberg et al. 2013; Bui-Thanh et al. 2004, 2008), cardiovascular fluid-dynamics (Manzoni et al. 2012; Colciago et al. 2014; Ballarin et al. 2016), and many other fields.

However, linear ROMs may experience computational bottlenecks at different extents when dealing with parametrized problems featuring coherent structures (possibly dependent on parameters) that propagate over time, namely, in transport, wave-type phenomena, front propagation processes, such as cardiac EP or convection-dominated flows, as soon as the physical behavior under analysis is strongly affected by parametric dependence. For larger parametric variations or stronger dependence of coherent structures on parameters, the dimension of the linear trial manifold can easily become extremely large (if compared to the intrinsic dimension of the solution manifold for the sake of accuracy) thus compromising the ROM efficiency. The same difficulty may also affect (often expensive) hyper-reduction techniques, such as the (discrete) empirical interpolation (DEIM) (Barrault et al. 2004; Chaturantabut and Sorensen 2010). Such hyper-reduction techniques are essential to assemble the operators appearing in the ROM in order to not rely on expensive N_h-dimensional arrays, see, e.g. Farhat et al. (2020) for further details. Moreover, projections-based methods, such as POD-Galerkin ROMs, are usually intrusive and, in several applications, deriving the reduced equations starting from the FOM entails high computational costs.

Deep learning (DL) (Goodfellow et al. 2016) techniques come as an inspiration to handle the complex reduction process of dynamical systems, unveiling low-dimensional features from black-box data streams (Guo and Hesthaven 2018, 2019). This choice is motivated by their ability of effectively approximating nonlinear maps and by their ability to learn from data and generalize to unseen data. On the other hand, DL models enable us to build non-intrusive, completely data-driven, ROMs, since their construction only requires to access the dataset, the parameter values and the snapshot matrix, but not the FOM arrays (Regazzoni et al. 2019; Salvador et al. 2021). For example, in Kaiser et al. (2018) and Brunton et al. (2016a,2016b) the SINDy method is applied in combination with autoencoder (AE) neural networks (NNs) to discover the underlying model of dynamical systems (Champion et al. 2019). In González and Balajewicz (2018) an autoencoder is used to compress the state and is followed by a recurrent NN, (Carlberg et al. 2019) applies hierarchical dimensionality reduction comprising autoencoders and principal component analysis (PCA) (Jolliffe and Cadima 2016) followed by dynamics learning to recover missing computational fluid dynamics (CFD) data and in Takeishi et al. (2017) and Lusch et al. (2018) autoencoders are applied to learn approximate invariant subspaces of the Koopman operator. NNs have witnessed a dramatic blooming in the past ten years also in CFD (see, e.g. (Brunton et al. 2020; Kutz 2017)).

Our goal is to set up nonintrusive DL-based *nonlinear* ROMs to approximate the solution manifold through a *nonlinear* trial manifold, whose dimension is nearly equal (if not equal) to the intrinsic dimension of the solution manifold, we wish to approximate. In this way, we aim at overcoming the critical issues of projection-based linear ROMs, that arise when addressing problems featuring wave-type phenomena and problems characterized by remarkable variability of the solution (with respect to the problem parameters), such as physiological and pathological cardiac EP.

6.2.1 Problem Formulation

We describe ROMs in algebraic terms, for the sake of generality, starting from the high-fidelity (spatial) approximation of nonlinear, time-dependent, parametrized PDEs; note that cardiac EP problems fall into this class. By introducing suitable space discretizations, techniques, such as the FE method (Quarteroni and Valli 1994) or IGA (Cottrell et al. 2009), the high-fidelity FOM can be expressed as a nonlinear parametrized dynamical system (Patelli et al. 2017; Pegolotti et al. 2019; Bucelli et al. 2021). Given $\mu \in P$, a vector of input parameters suitably sampled over the parameter space, we aim at solving the initial value problem:

$$\begin{cases} \dot{\mathbf{u}}_h(t; \mu) = \mathbf{f}(t, \mathbf{u}_h(t; \mu); \mu), & t \in (0, T), \\ \mathbf{u}_h(0; \mu) = \mathbf{u}_0(\mu), \end{cases} \tag{6.7}$$

where the parameter space $P \subset \mathbb{R}^{n_\mu}$ is a bounded and closed set, $\mathbf{u}_h : [0, T) \times P \to \mathbb{R}^{N_h}$ is the parametrized solution of (6.7), $\mathbf{u}_0 : P \to \mathbb{R}^{N_h}$ is the initial datum and $\mathbf{f} : (0, T) \times \mathbb{R}^{N_h} \times P \to \mathbb{R}^{N_h}$ is a (nonlinear) function, encoding the system dynamics. The FOM dimension N_h is related with the finite-dimensional approximating subspace introduced in the discretization and it can be extremely high whenever the PDE problem shows complex physical behaviors and/or high degrees of accuracy are required to its solution.

Our goal is the efficient numerical approximation of the whole set:

$$S_h = \{\mathbf{u}_h(t; \mu) \mid t \in [0, T) \text{ and } \mu \in P \subset \mathbb{R}^{n_\mu}\} \subset \mathbb{R}^{N_h} \tag{6.8}$$

of solutions to problem (6.7) when $(t; \mu)$ varies in $[0, T) \times P$, also referred to as solution manifold. Assuming that, for any given parameter $\mu \in P$, problem (6.7) admits a unique solution, for each $t \in (0, T)$, the intrinsic dimension of the solution manifold is at most $n_\mu + 1 \ll N_h$, where n_μ is the number of parameters (time plays the role of an additional parameter). This means that each point $\mathbf{u}_h(t; \mu)$ belonging to S_h is completely defined in terms of at most $n_\mu + 1$ intrinsic coordinates, or equivalently, the tangent space to the manifold at any given $\mathbf{u}_h(t; \mu)$ is spanned by $n_\mu + 1$ basis vectors.

6.2.2 Nonlinear Dimensionality Reduction

Motivated by the need of avoiding the drawbacks of linear ROMs and setting a general paradigm for the construction of efficient, low-dimensional ROMs, we resort to nonlinear dimensionality reduction techniques, exploiting DL algorithms (Fresca et al. 2020a).

Therefore, we build a nonlinear ROM to approximate $\tilde{\mathbf{u}}_h(t; \boldsymbol{\mu}) \approx \mathbf{u}_h(t; \boldsymbol{\mu})$ by:

$$\tilde{\mathbf{u}}_h(t; \boldsymbol{\mu}) = \boldsymbol{\Psi}_h(\mathbf{u}_n(t; \boldsymbol{\mu})), \tag{6.9}$$

where $\mathbf{u}_n : [0, T) \times P \to \mathbb{R}^n$ denotes the vector-valued function of two arguments representing the intrinsic coordinates of the ROM approximation and $\boldsymbol{\Psi}_h : \mathbb{R}^n \to \mathbb{R}^{N_h}$, $\boldsymbol{\Psi}_h : \mathbf{s}_n \mapsto \boldsymbol{\Psi}_h(\mathbf{s}_n)$, $n \ll N_h$, is a nonlinear, differentiable function; similar approaches can be found in González and Balajewicz (2018) and Lee and Carlberg (2020). Precisely, the solution manifold S_h is approximated by a *reduced nonlinear trial manifold*:

$$\tilde{S}_n = \{ \boldsymbol{\Psi}_h(\mathbf{u}_n(t; \boldsymbol{\mu})) \mid \mathbf{u}_n(t; \boldsymbol{\mu}) \in \mathbb{R}^n,$$
$$t \in [0, T) \text{ and } \boldsymbol{\mu} \in P \subset \mathbb{R}^{n_\mu} \} \subset \mathbb{R}^{N_h} \tag{6.10}$$

so that $\tilde{\mathbf{u}}_h : [0, T) \times P \to \tilde{S}_n$. Our goal is to build a ROM whose dimension n is as close as possible to the intrinsic dimension $n_\mu + 1$ of the solution manifold S_h, i.e. $n \geq n_\mu + 1$, in order to correctly capture the solution of the dynamical system by containing the size of the approximation spaces (Lee and Carlberg 2020).

To model the relationship between each pair $(t; \boldsymbol{\mu}) \to \mathbf{u}_n(t; \boldsymbol{\mu})$, and to describe the system dynamics on the reduced nonlinear trial manifold $\tilde{S}_n$ in terms of the intrinsic coordinates, we consider a nonlinear map under the form:

$$\mathbf{u}_n(t; \boldsymbol{\mu}) = \boldsymbol{\Phi}_n(t; \boldsymbol{\mu}), \tag{6.11}$$

where $\boldsymbol{\Phi}_n : [0, T) \times \mathbb{R}^{n_\mu} \to \mathbb{R}^n$ is a differentiable, nonlinear function. No additional assumptions such as the (exact or approximate) affine $\boldsymbol{\mu}$-dependence as in the POD-Galerkin ROM, are needed, thus avoiding (intrusive and often expensive) hyper-reduction techniques.

6.3 Decreasing Complexity in Cardiac Electrophysiology

Exploring the parameter space, i.e. solving the equations modeling the propagation of the electrical signal in the heart, for several values of parameters, it is of paramount importance, in order to investigate different scenarios or intra- and inter-subject variability. Solving the equations may quickly become unaffordable if such a coupled system must be solved for several parameters instances. *Multi-query* analysis is relevant in a variety of situations: when analyzing multiple scenarios, when dealing with sensitivity analysis and uncertainty quantification (UQ) problems in order to account for inter-subject variability (Mirams et al. 2016; Johnstone et al. 2016; Hurtado et al. 2017; Clayton et al. 2020), for parameter estimation or data assimilation, in which some unknown (or unaccessible) quantities characterizing the mathematical model must be inferred from a set of measurements (Dhamala et al. 2018; Quaglino et al. 2018; Johnston et al. 2018; Pathmanathan et al. 2019; Levrero-Florencio et al. 2020). In all these cases, to achieve computational efficiency, multi-query analysis in cardiac EP must rely on suitable *surrogate* models see, e.g. Niederer et al. (2020) for a recent review on the topic. Although typically more intrusive to implement, ROMs often yield more accurate approximations than data fitting and usually generate more significant computational gains than lower-fidelity models.

Conventional projection-based ROMs built, e.g. through the reduced basis (RB) method (Quarteroni et al. 2016), yields inefficient ROMs when dealing with nonlinear time-dependent parametrized PDE-ODE system as the one arising from cardiac EP. The three major computational bottlenecks shown by such kind of ROMs for cardiac EP are:

- the linear superimposition of modes would cause the dimension of the ROM to be excessively large if we want to guarantee an acceptable accuracy;
- evaluating the ROM requires the solution of a dynamical system, which might be unstable unless the size of time-step Δt is very small;
- the ROM must also account for the dynamics of the gating variables, even when aiming at computing just the electrical potential. This fact entails an extremely intrusive and costly hyper-reduction stage to reduce the solution of the ODE system to a few, selected mesh nodes (Pagani et al. 2018).

To overcome the limitations of projection-based ROMs, we apply the class of new, non-intrusive ROM techniques based on DL algorithms introduced in Fresca et al. (2020a) and Fresca and Manzoni (2022). By combining in a suitable way a convolutional AE and a deep feedforward neural network (DFNN), DL-based ROMs (DL-ROMs) and POD-enhanced DL-ROMs (POD-DL-ROMs) enable the construction of an efficient ROM, whose dimension is as close as possible to the number of parameters upon which the solution of the differential problem depends. In particular, the numerical assessment of our POD-DL-ROM technique has been performed on a very broad range of examples such as computational fluid dynamics (Fresca and Manzoni 2021) and cardiac EP problems (Fresca et al. 2021b) or the approximation of the nonlinear dynamics of micro-electro-mechanical-systems (MEMS) (Fresca et al. 2021a).

The POD-DL-ROM technique can be effectively used to handle parametrized problems in cardiac EP, accounting for both physiological and pathological conditions, in order to provide fast and accurate solutions. The proposed POD-DL-ROM is extremely efficient during the testing stage, that is for any new scenario unseen during the training stage, after a fast training phase. This is particularly useful in view of the evaluation of patient-specific features to enable the integration of computational methods in current clinical platforms.

6.3.1 POD-Enhanced Deep Learning-Based ROMs

The recently proposed DL-ROM technique (Fresca et al. 2020a) combines data-driven and physics-based models. Indeed, it exploits snapshots taken from a set of FOM solutions (for selected parameter values and time instances) and deep neural network (DNN) architectures to learn, in a nonintrusive way, both (i) the nonlinear trial manifold where the ROM solution is sought, and (ii) the nonlinear reduced dynamics. In a linear ROM built, e.g. through POD, the trial manifold is nothing but a set of basis functions, while the latter task corresponds to the projection stage in the subspace spanned by these basis functions. A first attempt to solve, by means of DL-ROMs, parametrized benchmark test cases in cardiac EP described by the Monodomain equations, has been carried out in Fresca et al. (2020b). Although extremely efficient at testing (i.e. online) time, when evaluating the problem solution for any new testing-parameter instance, DL-ROMs require an expensive training (i.e. offline) stage, because of the extremely large number of network parameters to be estimated. POD-DL-ROMs provide a possible enhancement of DL-ROMs, which avoids expensive training stages, by (i) performing a prior dimensionality reduction through POD, and (ii) using a multi-fidelity pretraining stage, where different physical models can be efficiently combined, as recently shown in Fresca and Manzoni (2022). In particular, through the use of randomized POD (rPOD), the POD-DL-ROM training phase is extremely fast, especially if compared to the training stage of DL-ROMs. For example, in Fresca and Manzoni (2022), where we consider the solution of the parametrized Monodomain equation in a square slab of cardiac tissue on a FOM dimension $N_h = 4096$, the use of the POD-enhanced DL-ROM reduces the GPU training time from 15 hours to 24 minutes, while preserving extremely efficient testing times.

Tailored on the applications at hand, the goal of POD-DL-ROMs is to approximate the map $(t; \mu) \mapsto \mathbf{u}_h(t; \mu)$, where $t \in (0, T)$ denotes time, $\mu \in \mathcal{P} \subset \mathbb{R}^{n_\mu}$ a vector of input parameters and $\mathbf{u}_h(t; \mu) \in \mathbb{R}^{N_h}$ the transmembrane potential solution of (6.1) or (6.3). This may be achieved without taking into account, and then expensively solving, the dynamics of the extracellular potential $\mathbf{u}_{e,h}(t; \mu)$, in the case of the Bidomain equations, and the gating variable $\mathbf{w}_h(t; \mu)$ in the construction of the ROM. More precisely, we build a nonlinear ROM to approximate $V^T\mathbf{u}_h(t; \mu) \approx \tilde{\mathbf{u}}_N(t; \mu)$ by:

$$\tilde{\mathbf{u}}_N(t; \mu) = \Psi_N(\mathbf{u}_n(t; \mu)), \tag{6.12}$$

where $\Psi_N : \mathbb{R}^n \to \mathbb{R}^N$, $\Psi_N : \mathbf{s}_n \mapsto \Psi_N(\mathbf{s}_n)$, $n \ll N$, is a nonlinear, differentiable function and $V \in \mathbb{R}^{N_h \times N}$ is the POD basis matrix of a N-dimensional subspace of $\mathbb{R}^{N_h}$. In particular, the columns of V form an orthonormal basis of dimension N, computed by means of randomized SVD (rSVD) (Halko et al. 2011). In this way, the manifold $S_N = \{V^T\mathbf{u}_h(t; \mu) \mid t \in [0, T)$ and $\mu \in \mathcal{P} \subset \mathbb{R}^{n_\mu}\} \subset \mathbb{R}^N$ is approximated by the n-dimensional reduced nonlinear trial manifold:

$$\tilde{S}_n = \{\Psi_N(\mathbf{u}_n(t; \mu)) \mid \ \mathbf{u}_n(t; \mu) \in \mathbb{R}^n$$
$$t \in [0, T) \text{ and } \mu \in \mathcal{P} \subset \mathbb{R}^{n_\mu}\} \subset \mathbb{R}^N. \tag{6.13}$$

Note that $\tilde{\mathbf{u}}_N : [0, T) \times \mathcal{P} \to \tilde{S}_n$. The function $\mathbf{u}_n : [0, T) \times \mathcal{P} \to \mathbb{R}^n$ denotes the minimal coordinates of $\tilde{\mathbf{u}}_N$ on the nonlinear trial manifold $\tilde{S}_n$. Our goal is to set-up a ROM whose dimension n is as close as possible to the intrinsic dimension $n_\mu + 1$ (time plays the role of an additional coordinate) of the solution manifold S_h, i.e. $n \geq n_\mu + 1$, to correctly capture the degrees of freedom of the set S_N by containing its size (Lee and Carlberg 2020). To model the relationship between each pair $(t; \mu) \mapsto \mathbf{u}_n(t; \mu)$, and to describe the reduced dynamics on the reduced nonlinear trial manifold $\tilde{S}_n$, we consider a nonlinear map under the form:

$$\mathbf{u}_n(t; \mu) = \Phi_n(t; \mu), \tag{6.14}$$

where $\Phi_n : [0, T) \times \mathbb{R}^{n_\mu} \to \mathbb{R}^n$ is a differentiable, nonlinear function. As for DL-ROMs (see, e.g. (Fresca et al. 2020a)), both the reduced dynamics and the reduced nonlinear manifold where the ROM solution is sought (or trial manifold) must be learnt. In particular,

- **Reduced dynamics learning**: We aim at learning the dynamics of the set S_N on the nonlinear trial manifold $\tilde{S}_n$ in terms of minimal coordinates by means of a DFNN. Indeed, we set the function Φ_n in (6.11) equal to:

$$\Phi_n(t; \mu, \theta_{\text{FFNN}}) = \phi_n^{\text{DF}}(t; \mu, \theta_{\text{FFNN}}),$$

where θ_{FFNN} denotes the vector of parameters of the DFNN, collecting all the corresponding weights and biases of each layer of the DFNN;

- **Nonlinear trial manifold learning**: We employ the decoder function of a convolutional autoencoder (AE), that is, we define the function in (6.9) as:

$$\Psi_N(\mathbf{u}_n(t; \mu, \theta_{\mathrm{FFNN}}); \theta_{\mathrm{dec}}) = \mathbf{f}_N^D(\mathbf{u}_n(t; \mu, \theta_{\mathrm{FFNN}}); \theta_{\mathrm{dec}}),$$

where $\mathbf{f}_N^D$ depends on the vector θ_{dec} of parameters of the convolutional/dense layers of the decoder.

By combining the two previous stages, the POD-DL-ROM approximation $\tilde{\mathbf{u}}_N$ finally takes the form:

$$\tilde{\mathbf{u}}_N(t; \mu, \theta_{\mathrm{FFNN}}, \theta_{\mathrm{dec}}) = \mathbf{f}_N^D(\phi_n^{\mathrm{DF}}(t; \mu, \theta_{\mathrm{FFNN}}); \theta_{\mathrm{dec}}). \tag{6.15}$$

The encoder function of the convolutional AE can then be exploited to map the intrinsic coordinates $\mathbf{V}^T\mathbf{u}_h$ associated to $(t; \mu)$ onto a low-dimensional representation:

$$\tilde{\mathbf{u}}_n(t; \mu, \theta_{\mathrm{enc}}) = \mathbf{f}_n^E(\mathbf{V}^T\mathbf{u}_h(t; \mu); \theta_{\mathrm{enc}}),$$

where $\mathbf{f}_n^E$ denotes the encoder function, depending upon a vector θ_{enc} of parameters. The architecture of the POD-DL-ROM neural network, employed at training time, is the one shown in Figure 6.3. At testing time, we can discard the encoder function.

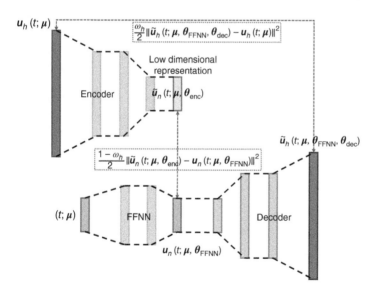

Figure 6.3 Starting from the FOM solution $\mathbf{u}_h(t; \mu)$, the intrinsic coordinates $\mathbf{V}^T\mathbf{u}_h(t; \mu)$ are computed through rSVD; their approximation $\tilde{\mathbf{u}}_N(t; \mu)$ is provided by the NN as output, so that the reconstructed solution $\tilde{\mathbf{u}}_h(t; \mu)$ is recovered through the rPOD basis matrix. In particular, the intrinsic coordinates $\mathbf{V}^T\mathbf{u}_h(t; \mu)$ are provided as input to block (A), which returns as output $\tilde{\mathbf{u}}_n(t; \mu)$. The same parameter instance $(t; \mu)$ enters block (B), which provides as output $\mathbf{u}_n(t; \mu)$, and the error between the low-dimensional vectors is accumulated. The minimal coordinates $\mathbf{u}_n(t; \mu)$ are given as input to block (C), which returns the approximated intrinsic coordinates $\tilde{\mathbf{u}}_N(t; \mu)$. Then, the reconstruction error is computed.

Provided the snapshot matrix $\mathbf{S} \in \mathbb{R}^{N_h \times N_{train} N_t}$, i.e. the matrix collecting FOM solutions (or snapshots) computed for different parameter values, and the parameter matrix $\mathbf{M} \in \mathbb{R}^{(n_\mu+1) \times N_s}$, i.e. the matrix collecting all the parameter instances corresponding to the computed snapshots, computing the POD-DL-ROM approximation (6.15) thus consists of solving the optimization problem:

$$\min_\theta \mathcal{J}(\theta) = \min_\theta \frac{1}{N_s} \sum_{i=1}^{N_{train}} \sum_{k=1}^{N_t} \mathcal{L}(t^k, \mu_i; \theta), \tag{6.16}$$

where the per-example loss function is given by:

$$\mathcal{L}(t^k, \mu_i; \theta) = \frac{\omega_N}{2} \| \mathbf{V}^T \mathbf{u}_h(t^k; \mu_i) - \tilde{\mathbf{u}}_N(t^k; \mu_i, \theta_{FFNN}, \theta_{dec}) \|^2$$
$$+ \frac{1-\omega_N}{2} \| \tilde{\mathbf{u}}_n(t^k; \mu_i, \theta_{enc}) - \mathbf{u}_n(t^k; \mu_i, \theta_{FFNN}) \|^2, \tag{6.17}$$

N_{train} and N_{test} are the number of training- and testing-parameter instances, respectively, N_t is the number of time instances, $N_s = N_{train} N_t$ and $\omega_N \in [0, 1]$. The POD-DL-ROM approximation of the FOM solution $\tilde{\mathbf{u}}_h(t; \mu) \approx \mathbf{u}_h(t; \mu)$ is then recovered by means of the rPOD basis matrix as:

$$\tilde{\mathbf{u}}_h(t; \mu, \theta_{FFNN}, \theta_{dec}) = \mathbf{V} \tilde{\mathbf{u}}_N(t; \mu, \theta_{FFNN}, \theta_{dec}).$$

6.3.1.1 POD-DL-ROM Architecture and Algorithms

The configuration of the POD-DL-ROM neural network used in our test cases is the one given below. We choose a 12-layer DFNN equipped with 50 neurons per hidden layer and n neurons in the output layer, where n represents the dimension of the (nonlinear) reduced trial manifold. The architectures of the encoder and decoder functions are instead reported in Tables 6.1 and 6.2. No activation function is applied at the last convolutional layer of the decoder neural network, as usually done when dealing with AEs.

We detail the algorithms through which the training and the testing of the neural network are performed in Algorithms 6.1 and 6.2. During the training phase, the optimal parameters of the POD-DL-ROM are found by solving the optimization problem (6.16) and (6.17) over the training set through the back-propagation (Rumelhart et al. 1986) and ADAM algorithms (Kingma and Ba 2015) (see Algorithm 6.1). At testing time, the encoder function is instead discarded and the optimal parameters, found during the training phase, are

Table 6.1 Attributes of convolutional and dense layers in the encoder $\mathbf{f}_n^E$.

Layer	Input dimension	Output dimension	Kernel size	# of filters	Stride	Padding
1	$[N, N, 1]$	$[N, N, 8]$	$[5, 5]$	8	1	SAME
2	$[N, N, 8]$	$[N/2, N/2, 16]$	$[5, 5]$	16	2	SAME
3	$[N/2, N/2, 16]$	$[N/4, N4, 32]$	$[5, 5]$	32	2	SAME
4	$[N/4, N/4, 32]$	$[N/8, N/8, 64]$	$[5, 5]$	64	2	SAME
5	N	64				
6	64	n				

Algorithm 6.1 POD-DL-ROM training algorithm

Input: Parameter matrix $\mathbf{M} \in \mathbb{R}^{(n_\mu+1)\times N_s}$, snapshot matrix $\mathbf{S} \in \mathbb{R}^{N_h \times N_s}$, training-validation splitting fraction α, starting learning rate η, batch size N_b, maximum number of epochs N_{epochs}, and number of minibatches $N_{\text{mb}} = (1-\alpha)N_s/N_b$.

Output: Optimal model parameters $\theta^* = (\theta^*_{\text{enc}}, \theta^*_{\text{FFNN}}, \theta^*_{\text{dec}})$.

1: Compute rPOD basis matrix $\mathbf{V}_N$
2: Randomly shuffle $\mathbf{M}$ and $\mathbf{S}$
3: Split data in $\mathbf{M} = [\mathbf{M}^{\text{train}}, \mathbf{M}^{\text{val}}]$ and $\mathbf{S} = [\mathbf{S}^{\text{train}}, \mathbf{S}^{\text{val}}]$ (with $\mathbf{M}^{\text{val}} \in \mathbb{R}^{(n_\mu+1)\times\alpha N_s}$ and $\mathbf{S}^{\text{val}} \in \mathbb{R}^{N_h \times \alpha N_s}$)
4: Compute intrinsic coordinates $\mathbf{S}^{\text{train}}_N = \mathbf{V}_N^T \mathbf{S}^{\text{train}}$
5: Compute intrinsic coordinates $\mathbf{S}^{\text{val}}_N = \mathbf{V}_N^T \mathbf{S}^{\text{val}}$
6: Normalize data in $\mathbf{M}$ and $\mathbf{S}_N = [\mathbf{S}^{\text{train}}_N, \mathbf{S}^{\text{val}}_N]$
7: Randomly initialize $\theta^0 = (\theta^0_{\text{enc}}, \theta^0_{\text{FFNN}}, \theta^0_{\text{dec}})$
8: $n_e = 0$
9: **while** ($\neg$early-stopping **and** $n_e \leq N_{\text{epochs}}$) **do**
10:     **for** $k = 1 : N_{\text{mb}}$ **do**
11:         Sample a minibatch $(\mathbf{M}^{\text{batch}}, \mathbf{S}^{\text{batch}}_N) \subseteq (\mathbf{M}^{\text{train}}, \mathbf{S}^{\text{train}}_N)$
12:         $\mathbf{S}^{\text{batch}}_N = \text{reshape}(\mathbf{S}^{\text{batch}}_N) \in \mathbb{R}^{N_b \times \sqrt{N} \times \sqrt{N} \times d}$
13:         $\widetilde{\mathbf{S}}^{\text{batch}}_n(\theta^{N_{\text{mb}}n_e+k}_{\text{enc}}) = \mathbf{f}^E_n(\mathbf{S}^{\text{batch}}_N; \theta^{N_{\text{mb}}n_e+k}_{\text{enc}})$
14:         $\mathbf{S}^{\text{batch}}_n(\theta^{N_{\text{mb}}n_e+k}_{\text{FFNN}}) = \boldsymbol{\phi}^{DF}_n(\mathbf{M}^{\text{batch}}; \theta^{N_{\text{mb}}n_e+k}_{\text{FFNN}})$
15:         $\widetilde{\mathbf{S}}^{\text{batch}}_N(\theta^{N_{\text{mb}}n_e+k}_{\text{FFNN}}, \theta^{N_{\text{mb}}n_e+k}_{\text{dec}}) = \mathbf{f}^D_N(\mathbf{S}^{\text{batch}}_n(\theta^{N_{\text{mb}}n_e+k}_{\text{FFNN}}); \theta^{N_{\text{mb}}n_e+k}_{\text{dec}})$
16:         $\widetilde{\mathbf{S}}^{\text{batch}}_N = \text{reshape}(\widetilde{\mathbf{S}}^{\text{batch}}_N) \in \mathbb{R}^{N_b \times N \times d}$
17:         Accumulate loss (6.17) on $(\mathbf{M}^{\text{batch}}, \mathbf{S}^{\text{batch}}_N)$ and compute $\widehat{\nabla}_\theta J$
18:         $\theta^{N_{\text{mb}}n_e+k+1} = \text{ADAM}(\eta, \widehat{\nabla}_\theta J, \theta^{N_{\text{mb}}n_e+k})$
19:     **end for**
20:     Repeat instructions 12–16 on $(\mathbf{M}^{\text{val}}, \mathbf{S}^{\text{val}}_N)$ with the updated weights $\theta^{N_{\text{mb}}n_e+k+1}$
21:     Accumulate loss (6.17) on $(\mathbf{M}^{\text{val}}, \mathbf{S}^{\text{val}}_N)$ to evaluate early-stopping criterion
22:     $n_e = n_e + 1$
23: **end while**

Algorithm 6.2 POD-DL-ROM testing algorithm

Input: Testing parameter matrix $\mathbf{M}^{\text{test}} \in \mathbb{R}^{(n_\mu+1)\times(N_{\text{test}}N_t)}$, rPOD basis matrix $\mathbf{V}_N, (\theta^*_{\text{FFNN}}, \theta^*_{\text{dec}})$.

Output: ROM approximation matrix $\widetilde{\mathbf{S}}_h \in \mathbb{R}^{N_h \times (N_{\text{test}}N_t)}$.

1: Load θ^*_{FFNN} and θ^*_{dec}
2: $\mathbf{S}_n(\theta^*_{\text{FFNN}}) = \boldsymbol{\phi}^{DF}_n(\mathbf{M}^{\text{test}}; \theta^*_{\text{FFNN}})$
3: $\widetilde{\mathbf{S}}_N(\theta^*_{\text{FFNN}}, \theta^*_{\text{dec}}) = \mathbf{f}^D_N(\mathbf{S}_n(\theta^*_{\text{FFNN}}); \theta^*_{\text{dec}})$
4: $\widetilde{\mathbf{S}}_N = \text{reshape}(\widetilde{\mathbf{S}}_N)$
5: $\widetilde{\mathbf{S}}_h = \mathbf{V}_N \widetilde{\mathbf{S}}_N$

Table 6.2 Attributes of dense and transposed convolutional layers in the decoder f^D_N.

Layer	Input dimension	Output dimension	Kernel size	# of filters	Stride	Padding
1	n	256				
2	256	N_h				
3	$[N/8, N/8, 64]$	$[N/4, N/4, 64]$	$[5, 5]$	64	2	SAME
4	$[N/4, N/4, 64]$	$[N/2, N/2, 32]$	$[5, 5]$	32	2	SAME
5	$[N/2, N/2, 32]$	$[N, N, 16]$	$[5, 5]$	16	2	SAME
6	$[N, N, 16]$	$[N, N, 1]$	$[5, 5]$	1	1	SAME

employed to predict the ROM solution for new, unseen parameter instances (see Algorithm 6.2). By exploiting an early stopping criterion, we stop the training if the loss function does not decrease over a certain number of epochs over the validation set.

6.4 Numerical Results

In this section, we apply the POD-DL-ROM technique to meaningful problems in cardiac EP, both in physiological and pathological scenarios, solved on a rectangular slab, a LV, and a LA surface geometry. Dealing with realistic geometries, large-scale problems and pathological scenarios, such as reentry and reentry breakup, shows the feasibility of POD-DL-ROM to be integrated in the clinical practice in order to compute outputs of interest, e.g. activation maps (ACs), APD, electrograms, and location of rotors' cores (Fresca et al. 2021b). To evaluate the performance of POD-DL-ROM, we rely on the loss function (6.17) and on:

- the error indicator $\epsilon_{rel} \in \mathbb{R}$ given by

$$\epsilon_{rel} = \frac{1}{N_{test}} \sum_{i=1}^{N_{test}} \left(\frac{\sqrt{\sum_{k=1}^{N_t} ||\mathbf{u}_h^k(\boldsymbol{\mu}_{test,i}) - \tilde{\mathbf{u}}_h^k(\boldsymbol{\mu}_{test,i})||^2}}{\sqrt{\sum_{k=1}^{N_t} ||\mathbf{u}_h^k(\boldsymbol{\mu}_{test,i})||^2}} \right); \tag{6.18}$$

- the relative error $\epsilon_k \in \mathbb{R}^{N_h}$, for $k = 1, \dots, N_t$, defined as:

$$\epsilon_k = \frac{|\mathbf{u}_h^k(\boldsymbol{\mu}_{test}) - \tilde{\mathbf{u}}_h^k(\boldsymbol{\mu}_{test})|}{\sqrt{\frac{1}{N_t} \sum_{k=1}^{N_t} ||\mathbf{u}_h^k(\boldsymbol{\mu}_{test})||^2}}. \tag{6.19}$$

While (6.18) is a synthetic error indicator, the quantity defined in (6.19) is instead a spatially distributed function.

To solve the optimization problem (6.16) and (6.17), we use the ADAM algorithm (Kingma and Ba 2015), which is a stochastic gradient descent method computing an adaptive approximation of the first and second momentum of the gradients of the loss function. In particular, it computes exponentially weighted moving averages of the gradients and of the squared gradients. We set the starting learning rate to $\eta = 10^{-4}$, and perform cross-validation in order to tune the hyperparameters of the POD-DL-ROM, by splitting the data in training and validation sets with a proportion $8:2$. Moreover, we implement an early stopping regularization technique to reduce overfitting (Goodfellow et al. 2016), stopping the training if the loss does not decrease over a certain amount of epochs. As nonlinear activation function, we employ the ELU function (Clevert et al. 2015). The parameters, weights and biases, are initialized through the He uniform initialization (He et al. 2015).

6.4.1 Test 1: Two-Dimensional Slab with Figure of Eight Reentry

The most recognized cellular mechanisms sustaining AT is reentry (Nattel 2002). The particular kind of reentry we deal with in this test case is the so-called figure of eight reentry, and can be obtained by solving Eq. (6.3). To induce the reentry, we apply a classical S1–S2 protocol (Nagaiah et al. 2013; Colli Franzone et al. 2014). In particular, we consider a square slab of cardiac tissue $\Omega = (0, 2 \text{ cm})^2$ and apply an initial stimulus (S1) at the bottom edge of the domain, i.e.:

$$I_{\text{app}}^1(\mathbf{x}, t) = \mathbf{1}_{\Omega_1}(\mathbf{x}) \mathbf{1}_{[t_1^i, t_1^f]}(\tilde{t}), \tag{6.20}$$

where $\mathbf{1}_{\Omega_1}$ is the characteristic function which is equal to 1 for all points in $\Omega_1 = \{\mathbf{x} \in \Omega : y \leq 0.1\}$ and is equal to 0 elsewhere, $t_1^i = 0$ ms and $t_1^f = 5$ ms. A second stimulus (S2) under the form:

$$I_{\text{app}}^2(\mathbf{x}, t; \mu) = \mathbf{1}_{\Omega_2(\mu)}(\mathbf{x}) \mathbf{1}_{[t_2^i, t_2^f]}(\tilde{t}), \tag{6.21}$$

with $\Omega_2(\mu) = \{\mathbf{x} \in \Omega : (x - 1)^2 + (y - \mu)^2 \leq (0.2)^2\}$, $t_2^i = 70$ ms and $t_2^f = 75$ ms, is then applied. Here, the parameter μ is the y-coordinate of the center of the second circular stimulus. The parameter space is given by $\mathcal{P} = [0.8, 1.1]$ cm and this choices have been made to obtain a reentry elicited and sustained until $T = 175$ ms. Moreover, we restrict ourselves to the time interval $[95, 175]$ ms, without considering the time window $[0, 95)$ ms in which the reentry has not arisen yet, and is common to all μ instances. The time-step is $\Delta t = 0.2/12.9$. We consider a FOM dimension $N_h = 256 \times 256 = 65,536$, implying a mesh size $h = 0.0784$ mm; this mesh size is recognized to correctly solve the tiny transition front developing during depolarization of the tissue, see Trayanova (2011) and Plank et al. (2008). The fibers are parallel to the x-axis and the conductivities in the longitudinal and transversal directions to the fibers are $\sigma_l = 2 \times 10^{-3} \text{ cm}^2/\text{ms}$ and $\sigma_t = 3.1 \times 10^{-4} \text{ cm}^2/\text{ms}$, respectively. The parameters appearing in (6.5) are set to $K = 8$, $a = 0.1$, $b = 0.1$, $\varepsilon_0 = 0.01$, $c_1 = 0.14$, and $c_2 = 0.3$, see ten Tusscher (2004).

The snapshot matrix is built by solving problem (6.3), by means of linear finite elements and a one-step, semi-implicit, first order time scheme, completed with the applied currents (6.20) and (6.21) over $N_t = 400$ time instances. Moreover, we consider $N_{\text{train}} = 13$ training-parameter instances uniformly distributed in the parameter space and $N_{\text{test}} = 12$ testing-parameter instances, each of them corresponding to the midpoint of two consecutive training-parameter instances. The maximum number of epochs is set equal to

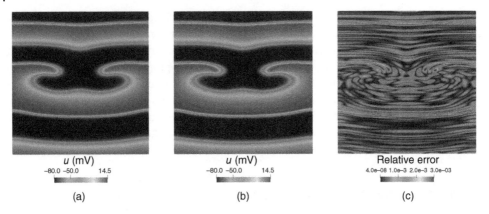

(a) (b) (c)

Figure 6.4 *Test 1*: comparison between FOM and POD-DL-ROM solutions for a testing-parameter instance. FOM (a) and POD-DL-ROM (b) solutions, with $n = 5$ and $N = 1024$, and relative error ϵ_k (c), for the testing-parameter instance $\mu_{\text{test}} = 0.9125$ cm at $\tilde{t} = 147$ ms. The relative error ϵ_k is below 1%.

$N_{\text{epochs}} = 6000$, the batch size is $N_b = 40$. Regarding the early stopping criterion, we stop the training if the loss does not decrease in 1000 epochs.

In Figure 6.4, we report the FOM and the POD-DL-ROM solutions, the latter with $n = 5$ and $N = 1024$, along with the relative error ϵ_k, for the testing-parameter instance $\mu_{\text{test}} = 0.9125$ cm at $\tilde{t} = 147$ ms, corresponding to almost the same level of accuracy ϵ_{rel} achieved by a DL-ROM on this problem in Fresca et al. (2020b).

The comparison among the DL-ROM, the POD-DL-ROM and the POD-Galerkin ROM with $N_c = 4$ clusters training and testing computational times obtained by keeping the same degree of accuracy for the three models, is provided in Table 6.3. The DL-ROM and POD-DL-ROM training and testing phases are carried out on a GTX 1070 8 GB GPU while the POD-Galerkin ROM tests are performed on a full 64 GB node (20 Intel® Xeon® E5-2640 v4 2.4 GHz cores) of our in-house HPC cluster. The use of POD-DL-ROM introduces a first level of dimensionality reduction, by means of the rSVD, equal to $N_h/N = 64$, which reflects in the striking reduction of the total training and validation time with respect to the ones of the DL-ROM and the POD-Galerkin ROM. Finally, we remark that the POD-DL-ROM technique results to be the most efficient both at training and testing time.

Table 6.3 *Test 1*: DL-ROM, POD-DL-ROM and POD-Galerkin ROM computational times.

	# params	# epochs	Total time	Test (s)
DL-ROM (GPU)	33,891,843	5633	64 h	0.6
POD DL-ROM (GPU)	395,907	12,738	138 m	0.4
POD-Galerkin ROM ($N_c = 4$)	—	—	238 m	33

6.4.2 Test 2: Three-Dimensional Left Ventricle Geometry

We consider the solution of the system (6.3) coupled with the A–P ionic model (6.5) in a three-dimensional LV geometry, obtained from the 3D human heart model provided by Zygote Zygote (2014). Here, we consider a single ($n_\mu = 1$) parameter, given by the longitudinal conductivity in the fibers direction.

The conductivity tensor takes the form

$$\mathbf{D}(\mathbf{x}; \mu) = \sigma_t I + (\mu - \sigma_t)\mathbf{f}_0 \otimes \mathbf{f}_0, \tag{6.22}$$

where $\sigma_t = 12.9 \cdot 0.02 \, \text{mm}^2/\text{ms}$; $\mathbf{f}_0$ is determined at each mesh point through a rule-based approach, by solving a suitable Laplace problem (Rossi et al. 2014). The resulting fibers field is reported in Figure 6.5. The applied current is defined as:

$$I_{\text{app}}(\mathbf{x}, t) = \frac{C}{(2\pi)^{3/2}\alpha} \exp\left(-\frac{||\mathbf{x} - \bar{\mathbf{x}}||^2}{2\beta}\right) \mathbf{1}_{[0,\bar{t}]}(t),$$

where $\bar{t} = 2 \, \text{ms}$, $C = 1000 \, \text{mA}$, $\alpha = 50$, $\beta = 50 \, \text{mm}^2$, and $\bar{\mathbf{x}} = (44.02, 1349.61, 63.28)^T \, \text{mm}$. In order to build the snapshot matrix $\mathbf{S}$, we solve problem (6.2) completed with the conductivity tensor (6.22) on a mesh made by $N_h = 65,503$ vertices over the interval $(0, T)$ with $T = 300 \, \text{ms}$ and time-step $\Delta t = 0.1/12.9$. We uniformly sample $N_t = 1000$ time instances in $(0, T)$. The parameter space is provided by $\mathcal{P} = 12.9 \cdot [0.04, 0.4] \, \text{mm}^2/\text{ms}$; here, we consider $N_{\text{train}} = 25$ training-parameter instances and $N_{\text{test}} = 24$ testing-parameter instances computed as in Test 4. In this case, the maximum number of epochs is set to $N_{\text{epochs}} = 30,000$, the batch size is $N_b = 40$ and the training is stopped if the loss does not decrease over 4000 epochs.

In Figure 6.6, we report the FOM and POD-DL-ROM solutions, the latter with $n = 2$ and $N = 256$, and the relative error ϵ_k, at $\tilde{t} = 297.1 \, \text{ms}$, for the testing-parameter instance $\mu_{\text{test}} = 12.9 \cdot 0.3243 \, \text{mm}^2/\text{ms}$. The POD-DL-ROM approximation accurately reconstructs the FOM solution, the maximum values of the error ϵ_k being associated to a very small region in the spatial domain.

Figure 6.5 *Test 2:* fibers field on the Zygote LV geometry.

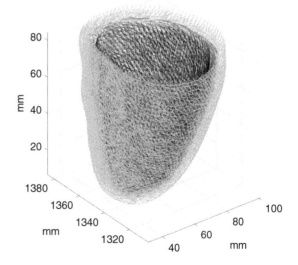

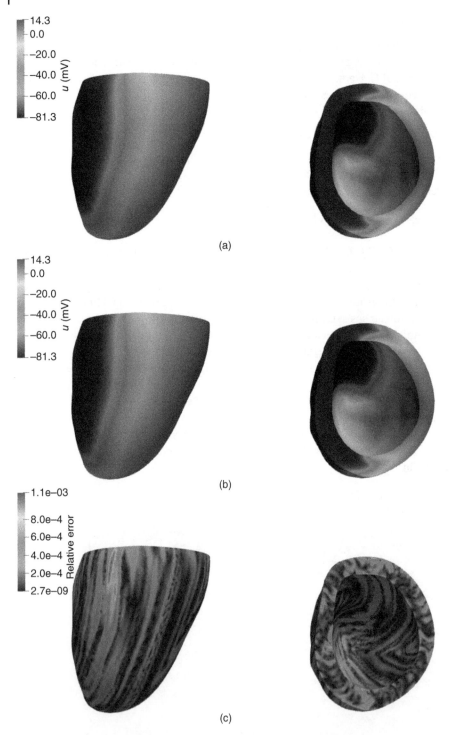

Figure 6.6 *Test 2*: comparison between FOM and POD-DL-ROM solutions for a testing-parameter instance. FOM (a), POD-DL-ROM (b), with $n = 3$ and $N = 256$, solutions and relative error ϵ_k (c), for the testing-parameter instance $\mu_{\text{test}} = 12.9 \cdot 0.3243$ mm^2/ms at $\tilde{t} = 297.1$ ms. The relative error ϵ_k is below 1%.

Table 6.4 *Test 2*: FOM, POD-Galerkin ROM and POD-DL-ROM computational times.

FOM	POD-GalerkinROM: train	POD-GalerkinROM: test	POD-DL-ROM: train	POD-DL-ROM: test
3.5 h	28 h	120 s	49 m	0.25 ms

In Table 6.4, we report the CPU FOM computational time together with the training (offline), and testing (online) times required by the POD-Galerkin ROM with $N_c = 4$ local bases, obtained on a full 64 GB node (20 Intel® Xeon® E5-2640 v4 2.4 GHz cores) of a HPC cluster, and the POD-DL-ROM training (total training and validation time) and testing times obtained on a GTX 1070 8 GB GPU. The POD-DL-ROM allows to achieve a training speed-up equal to 34 and a testing one of 4.8×10^5, if compared to the POD-Galerkin ROM training and testing times, respectively. In particular, a POD-DL-ROM approximation enables extremely efficient testing computational times, even faster than real-time solutions (here, $T = 0.3$ ms).

6.4.3 Test 3: Left Atrium Surface by Varying the Stimuli Location

Here, we focus on the computation of the solution of the Bidomain equations (6.1) coupled with the R–M model (6.6) on an idealized LA surface geometry. The direction of the cardiac fibers is determined as in the previous example. The equations have been discretized in space by means of IGA exploiting P2 Non-Uniform Rational B-Splines (NURBS) basis functions (Cottrell et al. 2009), the majority with a global C1 continuity, with $N_h = 154{,}036$. Time integration is performed over the interval $(0, T)$, with $T = 200$ ms and a time-step $\Delta t = 0.1$ ms.

The parameters $(n_\mu = 3)$ consist in the coordinates of the center of the intracellular applied current, and belong to the two-dimensional subdomain, the dark gray region shown in Figure 6.7, together with the portion of the domain affected by the stimulus, the light gray region. The intracellular applied current is defined as:

$$I_{app}^i(\mathbf{x}, t) = C \mathbf{1}_{\Omega_{app}(\mu)}(\mathbf{x}) \mathbf{1}_{[t^i, t^f]}(t),$$

with $C = 100$ mA, $\Omega_{app}(\mu) = \{\mathbf{x} \in \Omega : (x - \mu_1)^2 + (y - \mu_2)^2 + (z - \mu_3)^2 \leq (0.5)^2\}$, and $t^i = 0$ ms and $t^f = 5$ ms.

For the training phase, we uniformly sample $N_t = 200$ time instances in the interval $(0, T)$ and consider $N_{train} = 18$ training-parameter instances randomly sampled from the parameter space. For the testing phase, $N_{test} = 14$ randomly sampled testing-parameter instances have been considered. The maximum number of epochs is $N_{epochs} = 40{,}000$, the batch size is $N_b = 40$, the starting learning rate is $\eta = 2 \times 10^{-4}$ and, regarding early stopping, we stop the training if the loss function does not decrease along 2000 epochs.

Figure 6.7 *Test 3*: parameter space $\mathcal{P}$ in which the coordinates of the center of the intracellular applied current vary (dark gray region) and portion of domain affected by the stimulus (light gray region).

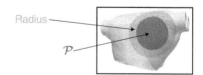

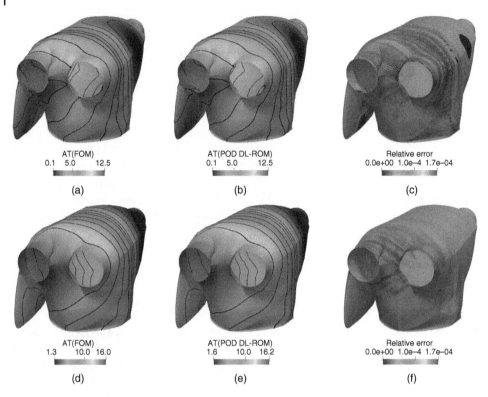

Figure 6.8 *Test 3*: comparison between FOM and POD-DL-ROM activation maps for different testing-parameter instances. FOM (a, d) and POD-DL-ROM (b, e), with $n = 4$ and $N = 256$, ACs and relative error ϵ_k (c, f), for the testing-parameter instances $\mu_{\text{test}} = (1.72, -0.35, -1.70)$ cm (a–c) and $\mu_{\text{test}} = (1.44, -0.80, -1.44)$ cm (d–f). The POD-DL-ROM technique is able to capture the variability of the solution over the parameter space highlighted by the different shape of the contour lines.

In order to point out the ability of the POD-DL-ROM approximation to approach the FOM solution when computing outputs of interest we show, in Figure 6.8, the FOM and POD-DL-ROM activation maps (ACs) or activation times (ATs), together with the associated ϵ_k, for the testing-parameter instances $\mu_{\text{test}} = (1.72, -0.35, -1.70)$ cm and $\mu_{\text{test}} = (1.44, -0.80, -1.44)$ cm. We highlight the strong variability of the solution over the parameter space, shown by the different shape of the contour lines in Figure 6.8a–c and d–f, meaning that the propagation direction of the front remarkably varies over $\mathcal{P}$, and the ability of the POD-DL-ROM solution to capture it accurately.

Finally, in Table 6.5, we report the FOM CPU computational time and the POD-DL-ROM GPU training and testing times; the time needed to assemble the snapshot matrix **S** is not

Table 6.5 *Test 3*: FOM and POD-DL-ROM computational times.

FOM	POD-DL-ROM: training	POD-DL-ROM: testing
10 h	5 h	0.2 s

included. Solving the FOM, for a single testing-parameter instance, requires 10 hours, with respect to the POD-DL-ROM total training and validation time, which is equal to 5 hours. POD-DL-ROM also proves to be extremely efficient at testing time, since it provides, once again, accurate results in almost real-time.

6.4.4 Test 4: Reentry Breakup

Few attempts have been made in order to solve, by means of DL algorithms, problems featuring a chaotic and disorganized solution. In Raissi (2018) the Kuramoto–Sivashinsky equation, in a chaotic regime, is solved by means of physics-informed neural networks (PINNs), but the algorithm leads to not completely satisfactory results. In Pathak et al. (2018a,2018b) a hybrid forecasting scheme based on reservoir computing in conjunction with knowledge-based models are successfully applied to prototype spatiotemporal chaotic systems. In Yeo (2017) a DNN for a model-free prediction of a chaotic dynamical system from noisy observations is presented. In that case, the proposed DL model aims to predict the conditional probability distribution of the state variable. Here, we want to apply the technique presented to the chaotic solution of the reentry breakup problem.

In particular, we focus on the solution of the Monodomain equation (6.3) coupled with the A–P ionic model (6.5) over the domain $\Omega = (0, 4 \text{ cm})^2$ discretized by means of linear finite elements with $N_h = 128 \times 128 = 16,384$ grid points. Time integration is performed over the interval $(0, T)$, with $T = 900$ ms and a time-step $\Delta t = 0.2/12.9$, by means of a one-step, semi-implicit, first order scheme. The fibers are parallel to the x-axis and the conductivities in the longitudinal and transversal directions to the fibers are $\sigma_l = 2 \times 10^{-3} \text{ cm}^2/\text{ms}$ and $\sigma_t = 3.1 \times 10^{-4} \text{ cm}^2/\text{ms}$, respectively. We set the parameters of the A–P model equal to $K = 8$, $a = 0.1$, $\epsilon_0 = 0.01$, $b = 0.1$, $c_2 = 0.3$ and $c_1 = 0.05$ (ten Tusscher 2004) and apply the cross-field stimulation protocol to generate the reentry breakup.

The parameter (here $n_\mu = 1$) consists of the x-coordinate of the location of the S2 stimulus, which takes the form

$$I_{app}^{i,2}(\mathbf{x}, t) = C\mathbf{1}_{\Omega_2(\mu)}(\mathbf{x})\mathbf{1}_{[t_2^i, t_2^f]}(\tilde{t}),$$

where $C = 1$ mA, $\Omega_2(\mu) = \{\mathbf{x} \in \Omega : x \leq \mu\}$, $t_2^i = 125$ ms, $t_2^f = 130$ ms and $\mu \in \mathcal{P} = [0.5, 2.25]$ cm.

In order to investigate the feasibility of applying the POD DL-ROM technique on this challenging problem, we analyze the decay of the eigenvalues of the training snapshot matrix. In particular, we uniformly sample $N_{train} = 8, 15, 25, 35$ training-parameter instances from $\mathcal{P}$, and we compute the respective snapshot matrix. In Figure 6.9, we show the decay of the eigenvalues for $\epsilon_{POD} = 10^{-3}$, which results in a dimension of the linear trial subspace equal to $N = 2247, 3804, 5632, 6678$. The dimension N remarkably increases with respect to N_{train}, meaning that it is not possible to reduce the problem over the parameter space by means of a linear ROM; indeed, a huge number of modes would be required to get an accurate approximation of the dynamics. Motivated by this fact, we decided to apply the DL-ROM technique to the problem under investigation.

We consider $N_t = 1000$ time instances uniformly distributed over the interval $(600, 900)$ ms, $N_{train} = 26$ training- and $N_{test} = 21$ testing-parameter instances, randomly

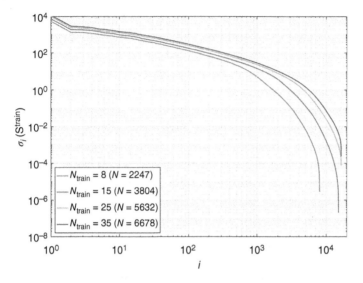

Figure 6.9 *Test 4*: decay of eigenvalues for different values of N_{train}.

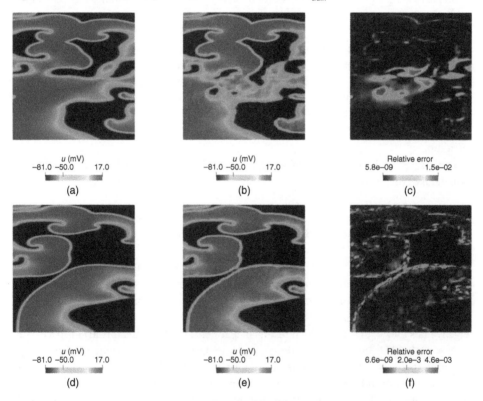

Figure 6.10 *Test 4*: comparison between FOM and DL-ROM solutions for different testing-parameter instances. FOM (a, d) and DL-ROM (b, e), with $n = 10$, solutions, together with ϵ_k (c, f), for the testing-parameter instances $\mu_{\text{test}} = 0.535$ cm (a–c) and $\mu_{\text{test}} = 0.7125$ cm (d–f) at $\bar{t} = 688$ ms. The DL-ROM technique is able to reconstruct the chaotic behavior of the solution.

sampled from the parameter space. The maximum number of epochs is $N_{\text{epochs}} = 30,000$ and the batch size is $N_b = 40$. Regarding early stopping, we stop the training if the loss does not decrease in 3000 epochs.

In Figure 6.10, we show the FOM and DL-ROM solutions, the latter with $n = 20$, along with the relative error ϵ_k, for the testing-parameter instances $\mu_{\text{test}} = 0.535$ cm and $\mu_{\text{test}} = 0.7125$ cm at $\tilde{t} = 688$ ms. In particular, $\mu_{\text{test}} = 0.535$ cm consists in the midpoint among two training-parameter instances whereas $\mu_{\text{test}} = 0.7125$ cm is a testing-parameter instance close to the training-parameter instance $\mu_{\text{train}} = 0.7$ cm; indeed in the last case the relative error ϵ_k is smaller. We highlight the impressive variability shown by the solution for different parameters values, at each single time. Even if the steep fronts of the FOM solution are not sharply reconstructed, the DL-ROM solution is able to capture all the multiple re-entries and the main dynamics, providing useful information like the location of rotors' cores.

In the previous results, we have considered a quite large parameter space, considered the strong variability of the solution of the reentry breakup problem over $\mathcal{P}$, equal to almost half edge of the domain. We expect that, by reducing the dimension of the parameter space, a higher accuracy could be achieved. Finally, the DL-ROM testing computational time, on a GTX 1070 8 GB GPU, is 0.35 seconds, thus generating a speed-up, with respect to the FOM CPU computational time (numerical tests have been performed on a MacBook Pro Intel Core i7 6-core with 16 GB RAM), equal to 1.48×10^3.

At the best of our knowledge, this is the first attempt in which chaotic regimes featuring so many scales and depending on physical parameters are accurately reproduced by reduced order modeling techniques.

6.5 Conclusions

The numerical simulation of cardiac EP problems in real-time and multi-query contexts, by means of traditional FOMs, such as the FE method or NURBS-based IGA, is practically prohibitive because of the huge computational costs associated to the numerical solution of the equations. Indeed, small time-step sizes must be selected to ensure stability and small mesh sizes are required to capture the steep fronts and preserve accuracy.

Leveraged on a recently proposed technique (Fresca and Manzoni 2022) to build low-dimensional ROMs by exploiting DL algorithms. This strategy allows us to overcome typical computational bottlenecks shown by standard, linear projection-based ROM techniques (such as POD-Galerkin ROMs) when dealing with problems featuring coherent structures propagating over time.

Thanks to their data-driven and nonintrusive nature, POD-DL-ROMs might be considered as turn-key reduced order modeling techniques to handle applications of interest and great complexity. In particular, we applied the proposed ROM framework to parametrized physiological and pathological problems in cardiac EP: the results reported in Section 6.4 represent the first attempt for reducing the computational complexity associated to the reentry and the reentry breakup problems, this opening, virtually, a new path toward the model personalization in real-time, even when dealing with extremely challenging, and computationally involved, scenarios. The possibility to perform real-time numerical simulations in cardiac EP can help moving forward the translation of computational methods in the clinical practice, aiming at complementing clinical data, quantifying risks related to cardiac pathologies, and planning therapies.

Author Biographies

- **Stefania Fresca** is Young Researcher in Numerical Analysis at MOX (Laboratory for Modeling and Scientific Computing), Department of Mathematics, Politecnico di Milano, Italy. After carrying out her PhD (awarded cum laude in 2021) in the framework of the ERC Advanced Grant Project iHEART (PI: Prof. Alfio Quarteroni) devoted to cardiac modeling, she spent two years as Post-Doctoral Research Fellow at MOX. Her research interests and expertise include scientific machine learning, reduced order modeling, deep learning, numerical approximation of PDEs, with several applications to engineering problems. She is (co)author of more than 10 peer-reviewed articles on international journals. Her PhD Thesis has been awarded the Runner-up Best PhD Award in Biomedical Engineering in 2022 at the 7th International Conference on Computational & Mathematical Biomedical Engineering (CMBE22).
- **Luca Dedè** is Associate Professor of Numerical Analysis at MOX, Department of Mathematics, Politecnico di Milano. His research activity focuses on the development of mathematical models and numerical methods for the numerical simulation of problems arising from different applications, including the emerging field of Computational Medicine with application to the human heart. His research contributions and expertise include mathematical modelling, numerical methods for partial differential equations, Finite Element and isogeometric methods, methods for High Performance Computing, Scientific Machine Learning. He is (co)author of several publications, including more than 80 peer-reviewed articles on international journals and one book.
- **Andrea Manzoni** is Associate Professor of Numerical Analysis at MOX, Department of Mathematics, Politecnico di Milano. His research interests and expertise include the development of reduced-order modelling techniques for PDEs, PDE-constrained optimization, uncertainty quantification, computational statistics, and machine/deep learning, aiming at the rapid and reliable numerical simulation of problems arising from different applications. He is (co)author of several publications, including more than 80 peer-reviewed articles on international journals and three books. He won the ECCOMAS Award for the best PhD thesis in Europe about computational methods in applied sciences and engineering in 2012, the Biannual SIMAI prize (Italian Society of Applied and Industrial Mathematics) in 2017, and the ECCOMAS Jacques Louis Lions Young-investigator Award in 2022.

References

Aliev, R.R. and Panfilov, A.V. (1996). A simple two-variable model of cardiac excitation. *Chaos, Solitons and Fractals* 7 (3): 293–301. https://doi.org/10.1016/0960-0779(95)00089-5.

Allessie, M. and de Groot, N. (2014). Crosstalk opposing view: rotors have not been demonstrated to be the drivers of atrial fibrillation. *Journal of Physiology* 592 (15): 3167–3170. https://doi.org/10.1113/jphysiol.2014.271809.

Alonso, A. and Bengtson, L.G.S. (2014). A rising tide: the global epidemic of atrial fibrillation. *Circulation* 129 (8): 829–830. https://doi.org/10.1161/circulationaha.113.007482.

Altman, P. and Dittmer, D. (1971). Respiration and Circulation. *Technical Report*. Bethesda, MD: Federation of American Societies for Experimental Biology. https://doi.org/10.1086/406910.

Amsallem, D., Cortial, J., Carlberg, K., and Farhat, C. (2009). A method for interpolating on manifolds structural dynamics reduced-order models. *International Journal for Numerical Methods in Engineering* 80 (9): 1241–1258. https://doi.org/10.1002/nme.2681.

Ballarin, F., Faggiano, E., Ippolito, S. et al. (2016). Fast simulations of patient-specific haemodynamics of coronary artery bypass grafts based on a POD-Galerkin method and a vascular shape parametrization. *Journal of Computational Physics* 315: 609–628. https://doi.org/10.1016/j.jcp.2016.03.065.

Barrault, M., Maday, Y., Nguyen, N.C., and Patera, A.T. (2004). An 'empirical interpolation' method: application to efficient reduced-basis discretization of partial differential equations. *Comptes Rendus Mathématiques des l'Académie des Sciences* 339 (9): 667–672. https://doi.org/10.1016/j.crma.2004.08.006.

Benner, P., Gugercin, S., and Willcox, K. (2015). A survey of projection-based model reduction methods for parametric dynamical systems. *SIAM Review* 57 (4): 483–531. https://doi.org/10.1137/130932715.

Benner, P., Cohen, A., Ohlberger, M., and Willcox, K. (2017). *Model Reduction and Approximation: Theory and Algorithms*. SIAM. https://doi.org/10.1137/1.9781611974829.

Bonomi, D., Manzoni, A., and Quarteroni, A. (2017). A matrix DEIM technique for model reduction of nonlinear parametrized problems in cardiac mechanics. *Computer Methods in Applied Mechanics and Engineering* 324: 300–326. https://doi.org/10.1016/j.cma.2017.06.011.

Boyle, P., Hakim, J.B., Zahid, S. et al. (2018). The fibrotic substrate in persistent atrial fibrillation patients: comparison between predictions from computational modeling and measurements from focal impulse and rotor mapping. *Frontiers in Physiology* 9: https://doi.org/10.3389/fphys.2018.01151.

Brooks, C. and Lu, H. (1972). *The Sinoatrial Pacemaker of the Heart*. Charles C. Thomas Publisher.

Brunton, S.L., Proctor, J.L., and Kutz, J.N. (2016a). Discovering governing equations from data by sparse identification of nonlinear dynamical systems. *Proceedings of the National Academy of Sciences of the United States of America* 113 (15): 3932–3937. https://doi.org/10.1073/pnas.1517384113.

Brunton, S.L., Proctor, J.L., and Kutz, J.N. (2016b). Sparse identification of nonlinear dynamics with control (SINDYc). *IFAC-PapersOnLine* 49 (18): 710–715. https://doi.org/10.1016/j.ifacol.2016.10.249.

Brunton, S.L., Noack, B.R., and Koumoutsakos, P. (2020). Machine learning for fluid mechanics. *Annual Review of Fluid Mechanics* 52: 477–508. https://doi.org/10.1146/annurev-fluid-010719-060214.

Bucelli, M., Salvador, M., Dede', L., and Quarteroni, A. (2021). Multipatch isogeometric analysis for electrophysiology: simulation in a human heart. *Computer Methods in Applied Mechanics and Engineering* 376: 113666. https://doi.org/10.1016/j.cma.2021.113666.

Buffa, A., Maday, Y., Patera, A.T. et al. (2012). A priori convergence of the greedy algorithm for the parametrized reduced basis method. *ESAIM: Mathematical Modelling and Numerical Analysis - Modélisation Mathématique et Analyse Numérique* 46 (3): 595–603. https://doi.org/10.1051/m2an/2011056.

Bui-Thanh, T., Damodaran, M., and Willcox, K. (2004). Aerodynamic data reconstruction and inverse design using proper orthogonal decomposition. *AIAA Journal* 42 (8): 1505–1516. https://doi.org/10.2514/1.2159.

Bui-Thanh, T., Willcox, K., and Ghattas, O. (2008). Parametric reduced-order models for probabilistic analysis of unsteady aerodynamic applications. *AIAA Journal* 46 (10): 2520–2529. https://doi.org/10.2514/1.35850.

Carlberg, K., Farhat, C., Cortial, J., and Amsallem, D. (2013). The GNAT method for nonlinear model reduction: effective implementation and application to computational fluid dynamics and turbulent flows. *Journal of Computational Physics* 242: 623–647. https://doi.org/10.1016/j.jcp.2013.02.028.

Carlberg, K.T., Jameson, A., Kochenderfer, M. et al. (2019). Recovering missing CFD data for high-order discretizations using deep neural networks and dynamics learning. *arXiv preprint arXiv:1812.01177*. https://arxiv.org/abs/1812.01177.

Champion, K., Lusch, B., Kutz, J.N., and Brunton, S.L. (2019). Data-driven discovery of coordinates and governing equations. *Proceedings of the National Academy of Sciences of the United States of America* 116 (45): 22445–22451. https://doi.org/10.1073/pnas.1906995116.

Chaturantabut, S. and Sorensen, D.C. (2010). Nonlinear model reduction via discrete empirical interpolation. *SIAM Journal on Scientific Computing* 32 (5): 2737–2764. https://doi.org/10.1137/090766498.

Clayton, R.H. and Taggart, P. (2005). Regional differences in APD restitution can initiate wavebreak and re-entry in cardiac tissue: a computational study. *Biomedical Engineering Online* 4 (54): https://doi.org/10.1186/1475-925X-4-54.

Clayton, R.H., Bernus, O., Cherry, E.M. et al. (2011). Models of cardiac tissue electrophysiology: progress, challenges and open questions. *Progress in Biophysics and Molecular Biology* 104 (1): 22–48. https://doi.org/10.1016/j.pbiomolbio.2010.05.008. Cardiac physiome project: Mathematical and modelling foundations.

Clayton, R.H., Aboelkassem, Y., Cantwell, C.D. et al. (2020). An audit of uncertainty in multi-scale cardiac electrophysiology models. *Philosophical Transactions of the Royal Society A: Mathematical, Physical and Engineering Sciences* 378 (2173): 20190335. https://doi.org/10.1098/rsta.2019.0335.

Clevert, D., Unterthiner, T., and Hochreiter, S. (2015). Fast and accurate deep network learning by exponential linear units (ELUs). *arXiv preprint arXiv:1511.07289*. https://arxiv.org/abs/1511.07289.

Colciago, C.M., Deparis, S., and Quarteroni, A. (2014). Comparisons between reduced order models and full 3D models for fluid-structure interaction problems in haemodynamics. *Journal of Computational and Applied Mathematics* 265: 120–138. https://doi.org/10.1016/j.cam.2013.09.049. Current Trends and Progresses in Scientific Computation.

Colli Franzone, P. and Pavarino, L.F. (2004). A parallel solver for reaction–diffusion systems in computational electrocardiology. *Mathematical Models and Methods in Applied Sciences* 14 (06): 883–911. https://doi.org/10.1142/S0218202504003489.

Colli Franzone, P., Pavarino, L.F., and Scacchi, S. (2014). *Mathematical Cardiac Electrophysiology, Modeling, Simulation & Applications*, vol. 13. Springer.

Cottrell, J.A., Hughes, T.J.R., and Bazilevs, Y. (2009). *Isogeometric Analysis: Toward Integration of CAD and FEA*, 1e. Wiley Publishing.

Davis, W.T., Montrief, T., Koyfman, A., and Long, B. (2019). Dysrhythmias and heart failure complicating acute myocardial infarction: an emergency medicine review. *The American Journal of Emergency Medicine* 37 (7): https://doi.org/10.1016/j.ajem.2019.04.047.

Dhamala, J., Arevalo, H.J., Sapp, J. et al. (2018). Quantifying the uncertainty in model parameters using Gaussian process-based Markov chain Monte Carlo in cardiac electrophysiology. *Medical Image Analysis* 48: 43–57. https://doi.org/10.1016/j.media.2018.05.007.

Dzialowski, E.M. and Crossley, D.A. (2015). *The Cardiovascular System*, 6e. San Diego, CA: Academic Press https://doi.org/10.1016/B978-0-12-407160-5.00011-7.

Farhat, C., Grimberg, S., Manzoni, A., and Quarteroni, A. (2020). Computational bottlenecks for PROMs: pre-computation and hyperreduction.

FitzHugh, R. (1961). Impulses and physiological states in theoretical models of nerve membrane. *Biophysical Journal* 1 (6): 445–466.

Fresca, S. and Manzoni, A. (2021). Real-time simulation of parameter-dependent fluid flows through deep learning-based reduced order models. *Fluids* 6 (7): https://doi.org/10.3390/fluids6070259.

Fresca, S. and Manzoni, A. (2022). POD-DL-ROM: enhancing deep learning-based reduced order models for nonlinear parametrized PDEs by proper orthogonal decomposition. *Computer Methods in Applied Mechanics and Engineering* 388: 114181. https://doi.org/10.1016/j.cma.2021.114181.

Fresca, S., Dede', L., and Manzoni, A. (2020a). A comprehensive deep learning-based approach to reduced order modeling of nonlinear time-dependent parametrized PDEs. *Journal of Scientific Computing* 87 (2): 67. https://doi.org/10.1007/s10915-021-01462-7.

Fresca, S., Manzoni, A., Dedè, L., and Quarteroni, A. (2020b). Deep learning-based reduced order models in cardiac electrophysiology. *PLoS ONE* 15 (10): 1–32. https://doi.org/10.1371/journal.pone.0239416.

Fresca, S., Gobat, G., Fedeli, P. et al. (2021a). Deep learning-based reduced order models for the real-time simulation of the nonlinear dynamics of microstructures. *International Journal for Numerical Methods in Engineering* 123 (20): 4749–4777. https://doi.org/10.1002/nme.7054.

Fresca, S., Manzoni, A., Dede', L., and Quarteroni, A. (2021b). POD-enhanced deep learning-based reduced order models for the real-time simulation of cardiac electrophysiology in the left atrium. *Frontiers in Physiology* 12: https://doi.org/10.3389/fphys.2021.679076.

García-Cosío, F., Pastor Fuentes, A., and Núñez Angulo, A. (2012). Clinical approach to atrial tachycardia and atrial flutter from an understanding of the mechanisms. Electrophysiology based on anatomy. *Revista Española de Cardiología (English Edition)* 65 (4): 363–375. https://doi.org/10.1016/j.recesp.2011.11.020.

Geselowitz, D.B. and Miller, W.T. III (1983). A bidomain model for anisotropic cardiac muscle. *Annals of Biomedical Engineering* 11 (3–4): 191–206. https://doi.org/10.1007/BF02363286.

González, F.J. and Balajewicz, M. (2018). Deep convolutional recurrent autoencoders for learning low-dimensional feature dynamics of fluid systems. *arXiv preprint arXiv:1808.01346*. https://arxiv.org/abs/1808.01346.

Goodfellow, I., Bengio, Y., and Courville, A. (2016). *Deep Learning*. MIT Press.

Grepl, M.A. and Patera, A.T. (2010). A posteriori error bounds for reduced-basis approximations of parametrized parabolic partial differential equations. *ESAIM: Mathematical Modelling and Numerical Analysis* 39 (1): 157–181. https://doi.org/10.1051/m2an:2005006.

Guo, M. and Hesthaven, J.S. (2018). Reduced order modeling for nonlinear structural analysis using Gaussian process regression. *Computer Methods in Applied Mechanics and Engineering* 341: 807–826. https://doi.org/10.1016/j.cma.2018.07.017.

Guo, M. and Hesthaven, J.S. (2019). Data-driven reduced order modeling for time-dependent problems. *Computer Methods in Applied Mechanics and Engineering* 345: 75–99. https://doi.org/10.1016/j.cma.2018.10.029.

Halko, N., Martinsson, P., and Tropp, J.A. (2011). Finding structure with randomness: probabilistic algorithms for constructing approximate matrix decompositions. *SIAM Review* 53: 217–288. https://doi.org/10.1137/090771806.

Hastie, T., Tibshirani, R., and Friedman, J. (2001). *The Elements of Statistical Learning*, Springer Series in Statistics. New York: Springer New York Inc.

He, K., Zhang, X., Ren, S., and Sun, J. (2015). Delving deep into rectifiers: surpassing human-level performance on ImageNet classification. *Proceedings of the IEEE International Conference on Computer Vision (ICCV)*, 1026–1034.

Hurtado, D.E., Castro, S., and Madrid, P. (2017). Uncertainty quantification of two models of cardiac electromechanics. *International Journal for Numerical Methods in Biomedical Engineering* 33 (12): e2894. https://doi.org/10.1002/cnm.2894.

Jarvik, R. (2004). The total artificial heart. *Scientific American* 244 (1): 74–81.

Johnston, B.M., Coveney, S., Chang, E.T.Y. et al. (2018). Quantifying the effect of uncertainty in input parameters in a simplified bidomain model of partial thickness ischaemia. *Medical & Biological Engineering & Computing* 56 (5): 761–780. https://doi.org/10.1007/s11517-017-1714-y.

Johnstone, R.H., Chang, E.T.Y., Bardenet, R. et al. (2016). Uncertainty and variability in models of the cardiac action potential: can we build trustworthy models? *Journal of Molecular and Cellular Cardiology* 96: 49–62. https://doi.org/10.1016/j.yjmcc.2015.11.018. Special Issue: Computational Modelling of the Heart.

Jolliffe, I.T. and Cadima, J. (2016). Principal component analysis: a review and recent developments. *Philosophical Transactions of the Royal Society A: Mathematical, Physical and Engineering Sciences* 374 (2065): 20150202. https://doi.org/10.1098/rsta.2015.0202.

Kaiser, E., Kutz, J.N., and Brunton, S.L. (2018). Sparse identification of nonlinear dynamics for model predictive control in the low-data limit. *Proceedings of the Royal Society A* 474 (2219): 20180335. https://doi.org/10.1098/rspa.2018.0335.

Kingma, D.P. and Ba, J. (2015). Adam: a method for stochastic optimization. *International Conference on Learning Representations (ICLR)*.

Klabunde, R. (2011). *Cardiovascular Physiology Concepts*. Wolters Kluwer Health/Lippincott Williams & Wilkins.

Kutz, J.N. (2017). Deep learning in fluid dynamics. *Journal of Fluid Mechanics* 814: 1–4. https://doi.org/10.1017/jfm.2016.803.

Lee, K. and Carlberg, K. (2020). Model reduction of dynamical systems on nonlinear manifolds using deep convolutional autoencoders. *Journal of Computational Physics* 404: 108973. https://doi.org/10.1016/j.jcp.2019.108973.

Levrero-Florencio, F., Margara, F., Zacur, E. et al. (2020). Sensitivity analysis of a strongly-coupled human-based electromechanical cardiac model: effect of mechanical parameters on physiologically relevant biomarkers. *Computer Methods in Applied Mechanics and Engineering* 361: 112762. https://doi.org/10.1016/j.cma.2019.112762.

Lusch, B., Kutz, J.N., and Brunton, S. (2018). Deep learning for universal linear embeddings of nonlinear dynamics. *Nature Communications* 9: https://doi.org/10.1038/s41467-018-07210-0.

Manzoni, A., Quarteroni, A., and Rozza, G. (2012). Model reduction techniques for fast blood flow simulation in parametrized geometries. *International Journal for Numerical Methods in Biomedical Engineering* 28 (6-7): 604–625. https://doi.org/10.1002/cnm.1465.

Mirams, G.R., Pathmanathan, P., Gray, R.A. et al. (2016). Uncertainty and variability in computational and mathematical models of cardiac physiology. *The Journal of Physiology* 594 (23): 6833–6847. https://doi.org/10.1113/JP271671.

Mitchell, C.C. and Schaeffer, D.G. (2003). A two-current model for the dynamics of cardiac membrane. *Bulletin of Mathematical Biology* 65 (5): 767–793. https://doi.org/10.1016/S0092-8240(03)00041-7.

Morillo, C., Banerjee, A., Perel, P. et al. (2017). Atrial fibrillation: the current epidemic. *Journal of Geriatric Cardiology* 14: 195–203. https://doi.org/10.11909/j.issn.1671-5411.2017.03.011.

Nagaiah, C., Kunisch, K., and Plank, G. (2013). Optimal control approach to termination of re-entry waves in cardiac electrophysiology. *Journal of Mathematical Biology* 67 (2): 359–388. https://doi.org/10.1007/s00285-012-0557-2.

Nagumo, J., Arimoto, S., and Yoshizawa, S. (1962). An active pulse transmission line simulating nerve axon. *Proceedings of the IRE* 50 (10): 2061–2070.

Narayan, S.M. and Jalife, J. (2014). Crosstalk proposal: rotors have been demonstrated to drive human atrial fibrillation. *The Journal of Physiology* 592 (15): 3163–3166. https://doi.org/10.1113/jphysiol.2014.271031.

Narayan, S.M., Krummen, D.E., Shivkumar, K. et al. (2012a). Treatment of atrial fibrillation by the ablation of localized sources CONFIRM (conventional ablation for atrial fibrillation with or without focal impulse and rotor modulation) trial. *Journal of the American College of Cardiology* 60 (7): 628–636. https://doi.org/10.1016/j.jacc.2012.05.022.

Narayan, S.M., Patel, J., Mulpuru, S., and Krummen, D.E. (2012b). Focal impulse and rotor modulation ablation of sustaining rotors abruptly terminates persistent atrial fibrillation to sinus rhythm with elimination on follow-up: a video case study. *Heart Rythym* 9 (9): 1436–1439. https://doi.org/10.1016/j.hrthm.2012.03.055.

Nash, M.P. and Panfilov, A.V. (2004). Electromechanical model of excitable tissue to study reentrant cardiac arrhythmias. *Progress in Biophysics and Molecular Biology* 85: 501–522. https://doi.org/10.1016/j.pbiomolbio.2004.01.016.

Nattel, S. (2002). New ideas about atrial fibrillation 50 years on. *Nature* 415: 219–226. https://doi.org/10.1038/415219a.

Niederer, S.A., Aboelkassem, Y., Cantwell, C.D. et al. (2020). Creation and application of virtual patient cohorts of heart models. *Philosophical Transactions of the Royal Society A: Mathematical, Physical and Engineering Sciences* 378 (2173): 20190558. https://doi.org/10.1098/rsta.2019.0558.

Nishida, K. and Nattel, S. (2014). Atrial fibrillation compendium. *Circulation Research* 114 (9): 1447–1452. https://doi.org/10.1161/CIRCRESAHA.114.303466.

Opie, L. (2004). *Heart Physiology: From Cell to Circulation*. Lippincott Williams & Wilkins.

Pagani, S., Manzoni, A., and Quarteroni, A. (2018). Numerical approximation of parametrized problems in cardiac electrophysiology by a local reduced basis method. *Computer Methods in Applied Mechanics and Engineering* 340: 530–558. https://doi.org/10.1016/j.cma.2018.06.003.

Patelli, A.S., Dede', L., Lassila, T. et al. (2017). Isogeometric approximation of cardiac electrophysiology models on surfaces: an accuracy study with application to the human left atrium. *Computer Methods in Applied Mechanics and Engineering* 317: 248–273. https://doi.org/10.1016/j.cma.2016.12.022.

Pathak, J., Hunt, B., Girvan, M. et al. (2018a). Model-free prediction of large spatiotemporally chaotic systems from data: a reservoir computing approach. *Physical Review Letters* 120: 024102. https://doi.org/10.1103/PhysRevLett.120.024102.

Pathak, J., Wikner, A., Fussell, R. et al. (2018b). Hybrid forecasting of chaotic processes: using machine learning in conjunction with a knowledge-based model. *Chaos* 28 (4): 041101. https://doi.org/10.1063/1.5028373.

Pathmanathan, P., Cordeiro, J.M., and Gray, R.A. (2019). Comprehensive uncertainty quantification and sensitivity analysis for cardiac action potential models. *Frontiers in Physiology* 10: https://doi.org/10.3389/fphys.2019.00721.

Pegolotti, L., Dede', L., and Quarteroni, A. (2019). Isogeometric analysis of the electrophysiology in the human heart: numerical simulation of the bidomain equations on the atria. *Computer Methods in Applied Mechanics and Engineering* 343: 52–73. https://doi.org/10.1016/j.cma.2018.08.032.

Plank, G., Zhou, L., Greenstein, J. et al. (2008). From mitochondrial ion channels to arrhythmias in the heart: computational techniques to bridge the spatio-temporal scales. *Philosophical Transactions. Series A, Mathematical, Physical, and Engineering Sciences* 366: 3381–3409. https://doi.org/10.1098/rsta.2008.0112.

Prud'homme, C., Rovas, D.V., Veroy, K. et al. (2001). Reliable real-time solution of parametrized partial differential equations: reduced-basis output bound methods. *Journal of Fluids Engineering* 124 (1): 70–80. https://doi.org/10.1115/1.1448332.

Quaglino, A., Pezzuto, S., Koutsourelakis, P. et al. (2018). Fast uncertainty quantification of activation sequences in patient-specific cardiac electrophysiology meeting clinical time constraints. *International Journal for Numerical Methods in Biomedical Engineering* 34 (7): e2985. https://doi.org/10.1002/cnm.2985.

Quarteroni, A. and Valli, A. (1994). *Numerical Approximation of Partial Differential Equations*, vol. 23. Springer-Verlag.

Quarteroni, A., Manzoni, A., and Negri, F. (2016). *Reduced Basis Methods for Partial Differential Equations: An Introduction*, vol. 92. Springer.

Quarteroni, A., Manzoni, A., and Vergara, C. (2017). The cardiovascular system: mathematical modeling, numerical algorithms, clinical applications. *Acta Numerica* 26: 365–590.

Quarteroni, A., Dede', L., Manzoni, A., and Vergara, C. (2019). *Mathematical modelling of the human cardiovascular system: data, numerical approximation, clinical applications*. In: *Cambridge Monographs on Applied and Computational Mathematics*. Cambridge University Press. https://doi.org/10.1017/9781108616096.

Raissi, M. (2018). Deep hidden physics models: deep learning of nonlinear partial differential equations. *Journal of Machine Learning Research* 19: 1–24.

Regazzoni, F., Dede', L., and Quarteroni, A. (2019). Machine learning for fast and reliable solution of time-dependent differential equations. *Journal of Computational Physics* 397: https://doi.org/10.1016/j.jcp.2019.07.050.

Rogers, J.M. and McCulloch, A.D. (1994). A collocation-Galerkin finite element model of cardiac action potential propagation. *IEEE Transactions on Biomedical Engineering* 41 (8): 743–757. https://doi.org/10.1109/10.310090.

Rossi, S., Lassila, T., Ruiz Baier, R. et al. (2014). Thermodynamically consistent orthotropic activation model capturing ventricular systolic wall thickening in cardiac electromechanics. *European Journal of Mechanics - A/Solids* 48: 129–142. https://doi.org/10.1016/j.euromechsol.2013.10.009.

Rumelhart, D., Hinton, G., and Williams, R. (1986). Learning representations by back-propagating errors. *Nature* 323: 533–536. https://doi.org/10.1038/323533a0.

Saha, M., Roney, C.H., Bayer, J.D. et al. (2018). Wavelength and fibrosis affect phase singularity locations during atrial fibrillation. *Frontiers in Physiology* 9: 1207. https://doi.org/10.3389/fphys.2018.01207.

Sakamoto, S., Nitta, T., Ishii, Y. et al. (2005). Interatrial electrical connections: the precise location and preferential conduction. *Journal of Cardiovascular Electrophysiology* 16 (10): 1077–1086. https://doi.org/10.1111/j.1540-8167.2005.40659.x.

Salvador, M., Dede', L., and Manzoni, A. (2021). Non intrusive reduced order modeling of parametrized pdes by kernel pod and neural networks. *Computers & Mathematics with Applications* 104: 1–13. https://doi.org/10.1016/j.camwa.2021.11.001.

Sundnes, J., Lines, G.T., Cai, X. et al. (2006). *Computing the Electrical Activity in the Heart*. Berlin, Heidelberg: Springer-Verlag https://doi.org/10.1007/3-540-33437-8.

Sundnes, J., Lines, G.T., Cai, X. et al. (2007). *Computing the Electrical Activity in the Heart*, vol. 1. Springer Science & Business Media.

Takeishi, N., Kawahara, Y., and Yairi, T. (2017). Learning Koopman invariant subspaces for dynamic mode decomposition. *Proceedings of the 31st International Conference on Neural Information Processing Systems (NIPS'2017)*, 1130–1140.

Trayanova, N.A. (2011). Whole-heart modeling applications to cardiac electrophysiology and electromechanics. *Circulation Research* 108: 113–128. https://doi.org/10.1161/CIRCRESAHA.110.223610.

ten Tusscher, K. (2004). Spiral wave dynamics and ventricular arrhythmias. PhD thesis. Universiteit Utrecht, the Netherlands.

Veroy, K. and Patera, A.T. (2005). Certified real-time solution of the parametrized steady incompressible Navier–Stokes equations: rigorous reduced-basis a posteriori error bounds. *International Journal for Numerical Methods in Fluids* 47: 773–788. https://doi.org/10.1002/fld.867.

Willcox, K. and Peraire, J. (2002). Balanced model reduction via the proper orthogonal decomposition. *American Institute of Aeronautics and Astronautics Journal* 40 (11): 2323–2330. https://doi.org/10.2514/2.1570.

Yeo, K. (2017). Model-free prediction of noisy chaotic time series by deep learning. *arXiv preprint arXiv:1710.01693*.

Zygote Media Group Inc. (2014). Zygote Solid 3D Heart Generation II Developement Report. *Technical report*. Zygote Media Group Inc.

7

The Potential of Microbiome Big Data in Precision Medicine: Predicting Outcomes Through Machine Learning

Silvia Turroni and Simone Rampelli

Unit of Microbiome Science and Biotechnology, Department of Pharmacy and Biotechnology, University of Bologna, 40126, Bologna, Italy

7.1 The Gut Microbiome: A Major Player in Human Physiology and Pathophysiology

The gut microbiome, i.e. the 10-trillion microbial community that inhabits our gut, is undoubtedly a leading player in human physiology. Countless studies have in fact shown that this microbial counterpart is essential for the extraction of energy from the diet (i.e. from fibers), the synthesis of vitamins (mainly of group B), the barrier effect against potential enteropathogens, the development, and regulation of the immune system (involving both innate and adaptive arms), as well as the modulation of the central nervous system (the so-called "gut-brain axis"), just to name a few (Candela et al. 2015; de Vos et al. 2022). These actions are due to the large and diversified pool of small bioactive molecules produced or contributed by the microbiome, which enter the bloodstream and reach extraintestinal organs (Turroni et al., 2018). Among these, it is certainly worth mentioning the short-chain fatty acids (SCFAs), i.e. the end-products of the fermentation of polysaccharides, which act as signaling molecules and exert decisive roles in the maintenance of metabolic and immunological homeostasis (Koh et al. 2016). Indeed, SCFAs have generally been attributed to anti-inflammatory and immunomodulatory activities and overall beneficial metabolic effects, e.g. by affecting satiety, intestinal gluconeogenesis, adipose tissue, and liver function. In contrast, it is known that other microbial metabolites have a harmful impact on the host health, as is the case of (i) phenolic compounds from amino acid metabolism; (ii) trimethylamine from dietary choline and carnitine conversion, which is then oxidized by host enzymes to trimethylamine-N-oxide (TMAO), a risk factor for cardiovascular disease; and (iii) bile acids, whose deconjugation and further metabolism by the gut microbiome interfere with their downstream signaling (Barone et al. 2021).

Although the gut microbiome includes all the domains of life, bacteria are certainly the predominant and most studied component (to which the vast majority of the statements made here basically refer). Alongside them, archaea and micro-eukaryotes (i.e. fungi and protists) are frequently encountered, as well as viruses, which are attributed crosstalk with the host and have potential implications for health as well (Iliev and Leonardi 2017;

Big Data Analysis and Artificial Intelligence for Medical Sciences, First Edition.
Edited by Bruno Carpentieri and Paola Lecca.
© 2024 John Wiley & Sons Ltd. Published 2024 by John Wiley & Sons Ltd.

Shkoporov et al. 2019). From an ecological standpoint, such a microbial community shows a certain degree of diversity, which is index of functioning, stability, and productivity of the population (Fassarella et al. 2021). With specific regard to stability, it should be remembered that the gut microbiome actually oscillates in a dynamic equilibrium, which allows it to change in the face of a perturbation and then return to the same or to a new but stable ecological state in a landscape of healthy configurations (resilience phenomenon). The main drivers of microbiome variation are recognized to be of an exogenous nature and include diet, lifestyle, host location (or geographical effect) (He et al. 2018), or, more generally, the exposome, i.e. the totality of the exposures that accompany us during life (Vujkovic-Cvijin et al. 2020). Interestingly, age and body mass index (BMI) have also been identified among the microbiome-associated confounding factors, further stressing the correlation between the gut microbiome and our metabolic health across lifespan.

Likewise, it is a fact that the dynamic equilibrium of the gut microbiome can be severely disturbed by certain stressors, leading to significant reductions in microbial diversity and functional richness, and possibly resulting in recalcitrant unhealthy states associated with disease (Fassarella et al. 2021). Again, countless studies have reported imbalances in the compositional and functional structure of the gut microbiome in the context of disparate disorders, including intestinal (e.g. inflammatory bowel disease, irritable bowel syndrome, etc.) but also hepatic, metabolic, respiratory, cardiovascular, neurological, and oncological (Lynch and Pedersen 2016). As anticipated, a reduction in diversity is typically observed, together with a decrease in health-associated taxa (mainly SCFA producers) and an increase in pathogens or so-called pathobionts (microorganisms with pathogenic potential) (Jochum and Stecher 2020), even if the magnitude and direction of the changes as well as the specific actors involved are clearly context-dependent (Duvallet et al. 2017). In general, it can be argued that certain microbiome profiles are reasonably supposed to predict the onset and progression of such disorders, including response to treatment (Helmink et al. 2019, Integrative HMP (iHMP) Research Network Consortium 2019). It is, therefore, not surprising that their inclusion in current models of disease prediction, diagnosis, and prognosis is strongly recommended. Once the microbiome signatures have been precisely identified, they can be used as targets in personalized, precision, integrated preventive, and therapeutic strategies, also aimed at correcting the gut microbiome (e.g. by increasing the resilience of healthy states or decreasing and overcoming that of unhealthy states) to promote long-term health. Such strategies may be based on diet, as well as on pre-biotics, (traditional and/or next-generation) probiotics (or live biotherapeutics) (O'Toole et al. 2017), synbiotics or postbiotics, or, ultimately, on fecal microbiota transplantation for the *ex novo* establishment of a healthy community, eradicating the dysbiotic one. In this scenario, the need to manage and integrate multidimensional big data, such as those of the gut microbiome obtained through high-throughput technologies, e.g. 16S rRNA gene sequencing (for alpha diversity and compositional profiling) (Goodrich et al. 2014), shotgun metagenomics (for species-level and functional insights) (Quince et al. 2017), metatranscriptomics (for the determination of the active fraction of the microbiome and actively transcribed genes) (Zhang et al. 2021), metaproteomics (for proteome profiling) (Salvato et al. 2021), and metabolomics (for metabolite analysis) (Vernocchi et al. 2016), is extremely evident. As described below, machine learning represents a great opportunity and solution for data integration and mining to discover clinically translatable knowledge, thus enabling concrete applications in precision medicine, from the development of predictive biomarkers to tailored modulation of the gut microbiome (Cammarota et al. 2020).

7.2 Machine Learning Applied to Microbiome Research

In this section, we will discuss previous research that has applied machine learning approaches to the human microbiome in health and disease settings, along with current projects and future prospects for concrete opportunities to harness microbiome big data in medical sciences. Specifically, two case studies will be dealt with:

i. obesity, for which extensive microbiome datasets are now available and exploited precisely to predict the development of this condition;
ii. cancer (with a focus on colorectal cancer (CRC)), where research is certainly more backward, but the prospects are equally valid.

Next, we will briefly explore the potential of microbiomes in personalized nutrition, i.e. in assisting the design of precision dietary interventions for successful prophylactic and treatment purposes. Finally, we will discuss the possibility of using microbiome data from other body niches to predict the gut microbiome in a meta-community framework, with a view to integrating the numerous large-scale retrospective studies that did not include fecal sampling and also helping paleomicrobiologists in reconstructing the microbiome–host coevolutionary history.

7.2.1 Case Study 1: Obesity

Obesity and related comorbidities are one of the conditions for which the contribution of the gut microbiome is best known (Barone et al. 2021). Mechanistic studies in animal models have even suggested a causal role for the microbiome, particularly with regard to blood glucose levels and insulin resistance, although demonstration of causality in humans has yet to be performed (Cani and Van Hul 2020). In any case, researchers have consistently reported an obesity-associated dysbiotic profile, poor in fiber-degrading SCFA-producing taxa while rich in pathobionts, which can trigger intestinal barrier dysfunction, leading to translocation of microbial metabolites (or even microbes) and pathogen-associated molecular patterns (e.g. lipopolysaccharide), thus driving metabolic inflammation and dysregulation (Tilg and Moschen 2014; Tilg et al. 2020). It is, therefore, not surprising that much work has been done over the years to harness the potential of the gut microbiome for predictive purposes. One of the first noteworthy attempts dates back to 2018, when, in a cohort-based study involving around 1000 Israeli individuals, Rothschild et al. (2018) demonstrated that microbiome data significantly improved prediction accuracy for many human traits, especially glucose and obesity measures. They also defined a term, "microbiome-association index," to quantify overall association between the microbiome and host phenotypes (including anthropometric and blood measurements), and found significant values (i.e. the gut microbiome allowed a significant fraction of the phenotypic variance to be inferred) for a number of obesity-related variables, such as BMI, glycemic status and fasting glucose, cholesterol, and waist and hip circumference (and their ratio). Although the authors were aware of the correlative nature of this measure and the possible confounding effect of host metadata, they strongly suggested the inclusion of microbiome data in current prediction models that use only genetic and environmental data.

In a recent longitudinal work, Rampelli et al. (2018) have taken a step forward in this direction by investigating the impact of the microbiome-diet axis in the development of childhood obesity in Europe. According to their findings, the individual gut microbiome layout (in terms of diversity, taxa represented, and interactions between them) together with long-term dietary habits strongly influence the host metabolic and immunological home-ostasis and, in the context of other lifestyle variables (e.g. physical activity), may help predict the development of obesity. It must be said that such results were not based on machine learning algorithms, but the authors nevertheless hypothesized the development of a pre-dictive model of obesity, also based on microbiome features, to be implemented in the near future with more subjects, sampling times, and possibly other omics data. Interestingly, their findings formed the basis for the EIT Food project CLiMB-Out (child microbes pre-dict how to stay away from obesity – https://www.eitfood.eu/projects/climb-out), aimed at developing microbiome-informed predictive tools that help detect obesity-associated risks and facilitate the implementation of timely interventions based on lifestyle and dietary changes for the well-being of the child and subsequently of the adult. Microbiome data (i.e. the relative abundance of microbial taxa) are just one of several covariates to be included within such new predictors, which can be termed as "One Health tools," as data from multi-ple fields are collected and linked together with the ultimate goal of improving public health (i.e. preventing obesity). Other covariates include dietary data (e.g. those obtained from food frequency questionnaires or dietary recalls) and lifestyle data (e.g. physical activity, socioe-conomic status, environmental exposure, etc.), as well as medical history, anthropometry, and measures of physiological, immunological, and psychological parameters. No results are available yet, but they are expected to contribute to the design of innovative educa-tional and communication programs to engage families and healthcare professionals in the adoption of healthy diets and lifestyles across different socioeconomic environments.

In previous years, other attempts to develop microbiome-based predictive tools for obe-sity have been done without much success, perhaps because they were mostly based on a small variety of data. In particular, in the first study, Pasolli et al. (2016) implemented a Random Forest-based tool that used only microbiome data (i.e. relative abundance tables from 16S rRNA amplicon sequencing) and performed poorly in predicting obesity and type 2 diabetes. Another work led by Fernández-Navarro et al. (2019) focused on developing several machine learning approaches, including decision tree, ensemble, and support vec-tor machine methods (Namkung 2020), to identify the best predictors for obesity. Notably, their approach found that serum levels of eicosapentaenoic acid and the relative abun-dance of *Bacteroides* in feces were directly associated with a nonobese phenotype. Very recently, Liu et al. (2021) combined the linear discriminant analysis effect size (LEfSe) anal-ysis (Segata et al. 2011) and Random Forest classifier (Breiman 2001) feature importance calculation to obtain the compositional and functional characteristics of the gut micro-biome that correlated with obesity in a cohort of 2263 Chinese individuals. Specifically, they used gut metagenomic compositional (including 751 species) and functional (covering 506 metabolic pathways) data to find associations with BMI categories (underweight, normal weight, slightly overweight, and overweight). Three species were identified as biomarkers of nonobesity: *Bacteroides caccae*, *Odoribacter splanchnicus*, and *Roseburia hominis* (i.e. their proportions were significantly higher in normal-weight individuals than in obese individuals). As for functionality, the obesity-related gut microbiome showed higher potential for metabolic pathways involved in lipid and ubiquinol biosynthesis.

Overall, this body of literature demonstrates that implementing a microbiome-based machine learning tool to predict obesity and suggest dietary and lifestyle changes based on outcomes is potentially feasible, but there is a need for a larger volume of data to build a robust approach.

7.2.2 Case Study 2: Cancer

Several studies on the human microbiome in different types of cancer, such as colorectal, gastric, oral, lung, and pancreatic cancer, have highlighted distinct microbial profiles and suggested potential protective or vice versa oncogenic signatures, with immense clinical implications (Vivarelli et al. 2019). What is emerging is the possibility of using data from the microbiome (mainly the intestinal one but not only) to predict the onset of cancer, its progression, and response to therapies (therefore, to better stratify patients), but also to design integrated treatment strategies aimed at achieving long-term disease-free survival (D'Amico et al. 2022). Although the research field is relatively new, large datasets are accumulating that are now available for machine learning applications. As mentioned above, we will provide and discuss some examples in the field of CRC, along with more general perspectives in precision oncology.

By applying a Random Forest classifier to metagenomic data (i.e. the relative abundance table of taxa at the species level) from CRC patients, six key gut microbes have been identified (including *Porphyromonas asaccharolytica*, *Peptostreptococcus stomatis*, *Fusobacterium* sp., *Parvimonas* sp., *Streptococcus vestibularis,* and *Flavonifractor plautii*), which discriminated patients from healthy controls (Ai et al. 2019). Another work based on a Random Forest classifier sought to link the presence of *F. plautii* (a flavonoid-degrading gut bacterium) with the progression of CRC in Indian patients using both metagenomics and metabolomics data (i.e. relative abundance tables of microbial taxa, functions, and metabolites). Interestingly, *F. plautii* was the most important species in driving the separation of CRC samples from healthy controls (Gupta et al. 2019). Flemer et al. (2018) also found changes in gut microbiome structure closely related to CRC, using relative abundance tables from 16S rRNA amplicon sequencing as input, but have the particular merit of using Random Forest to look for associations between gut and oral microbiome configurations. According to the authors, combining data from both ecosystems dramatically increased (over 76%) the sensitivity of their classification model to distinguish individuals with CRC or polyps from controls. As will be discussed later, research in this direction could open new perspectives in cancer diagnosis and prognosis, where oral microbiome profiling can be configured as an alternative approach to detect disease and assess its progression. More recently, Jang et al. (2020) used a Bayesian network model to identify bacterial species related to a positive outcome after CRC chemotherapy treatment. In another study, Kharrat et al. (2019) applied an ensemble method in order to identify CRC-related species. A similar approach using Random Forest and logistic regression was also employed in two other studies (Koohi-Mugadham et al. 2019; Wirbel et al. 2019). As for tumors developing outside the gastrointestinal tract, it is worth mentioning the recently established ONCOBIOME project, which aims to find out the gut microbiome signatures associated with cancer onset, prognosis, and response to therapy (https://www.oncobiome.eu/). All these applications are making it possible to define marker microbial species that could be adopted/targeted by tailored treatments (e.g. based on pre/probiotics). In this scenario, machine learning could also help to identify not only new potential targets but also probiotic candidates to be validated experimentally.

Despite the tantalizing promises, it must be said that the challenges can be multifaceted. First, the results from the different studies available show different (and sometimes conflicting) microbiome–cancer associations, and extracting a consolidated list of microbes that are unique to patients with particular cancers or unique to healthy humans is still an open challenge. Second, and more generally, establishing a correlation between a microbiome component and the disease obviously does not imply causation but simple associations that can be direct or indirect, i.e. microbes can directly contribute to the development of the disease by secreting products such as peptides and small molecules that alter the cellular microenvironment and interfere with the cell cycle or could thrive in the diseased environment without a direct connection. Researchers who ignore such dichotomies may end up compromising the accuracy of their predictions. With specific regard to cancer, one solution could be to check the sequences of oncogenes for possible mutations, deletions, or insertions, and to include such data in machine learning approaches to look for direct connections with microbes.

7.2.3 Case Study 3: Personalized Nutrition

As easily understood, machine learning also has enormous potential in the near future of microbiome-based personalized nutrition (Kolodziejczyk et al. 2019). Artificial intelligence pipelines may in fact find use in the design of precision diets for prophylactic (for diseases for which an individual is at high risk due to genetics and/or lifestyle), therapeutic (for a plethora of diseases), or lifestyle optimization (e.g. in sport) purposes. The prerequisite is to have datasets of gut microbiome, clinical features, and physiological responses to diet to train models capable of learning the effect of a specific food on physiology. The ultimate goal is to identify personalized dietary combinations to impact microbiome composition and function, as well as host physiology. In this regard, it should be mentioned the milestone work by Zeevi et al. (2015), who accurately predicted interpersonal variability in postprandial glycemic response to identical foods in a cohort of 800 healthy and prediabetic Israeli subjects. The authors implemented a machine learning approach that integrated comprehensive multidimensional data, including the compositional and functional structure of the gut microbiome, blood parameters, anthropometrics, physical activity, and lifestyle. Strikingly, based on these predictions, they designed tailored dietary interventions that had the expected impact on the postprandial glycemic response and gut microbiome. Specifically, they applied their algorithm in a leave-one-out scheme to rank each participant's meal and design two short-term (one-week) diets, one "good" and one "bad" consisting of meals that were predicted to have low and high postprandial glycemic responses, respectively. Despite some real-life noise, their prediction turned out to be very accurate. As correctly concluded by the authors, the predictor-based approach has wider applicability, being potentially valuable in the rational design of nutritional interventions in a variety of multifactorial inflammatory, metabolic, and oncological disorders.

7.2.4 Case Study 4: Exploiting the Meta-Community Theory for New Machine Learning Approaches

In the field of the human microbiome, a new frontier is represented by the meta-community theory, according to which the host and the surrounding microbiomes are in an intimate relationship, showing reciprocal exchanges and influences (Koskella et al. 2017; Miller et al. 2018). Precisely, the meta-community theory views "the world as a collection of patches – spatially distinct areas of suitable habitat surrounded by a matrix of unsuitable habitat" (Costello et al. 2012), each of which contains a community of organisms. Such communities are linked together to form a meta-community by the dispersal of organisms from patch to patch. This is also true for human-associated microbial communities, where meta-community theory may be particularly useful for understanding ecological dynamics, including the assembly of various microbiomes in the human body. In this framework, a close association between oral and gut microbiomes has recently been advanced, with the former reflecting changes in the latter, in both healthy and diseased individuals (Bajaj et al. 2015; Iwauchi et al. 2019; Prodan et al. 2019; Schmidt et al. 2019).

Based on this meta-community vision, Rampelli et al. (2021) recently implemented a deep learning tool (G2S), which exploits this close link between oral and gut microbial ecosystems to predict the configurations of the latter from the data of the former. The tool relies specifically on a convolutional neural network (Alzubaidi et al. 2021), trained on paired oral and fecal samples from modern populations across the globe. Again, the accuracy of the inference (in this case, the family-level configuration of the gut microbiome) was superior to other approaches, including Random Forest and a stochastic method developed for this comparison, which generated mock profiles in the range of the training datasets. According to the authors, this superiority is most likely attributable to the predictive power of deep learning that automatically detects patterns in data by also embedding the computation of variables to yield end-to-end models. This type of approach could be of practical clinical relevance in retrospective studies, where gut microbiome analyses were not performed due to lack of funds or simply were not foreseen, but also in the area of paleomicrobiology to infer microbiome changes across the evolutionary timeline. In particular, G2S can help characterize the gut microbiome–human host coevolutionary trajectories by retrieving more information from ancient specimens, such as dental calculi that are far more common and better preserved than coprolites. Machine learning tools based on meta-community theory could therefore represent a unique opportunity to recover data on modern or ancient samples that, for various reasons, have not been collected.

7.3 Conclusions and Perspectives

Machine learning is increasingly being used to make inferences about microbiome big data in an attempt to optimize patient stratification for diagnostic and prognostic purposes and to guide the design of personalized precision intervention strategies. Since the first applications, many efforts have been made, but more time is needed to develop more powerful and reliable approaches that can actually be used by researchers and physicians in their daily practice. In particular, a large amount of data is required to implement robust machine learning-based algorithms. In this regard, the new technologies of massive sequencing, with their lower cost of analysis, are significantly increasing our capacity to generate data, but this has at the same time increased the challenges of bioinformatic analysis. For instance, there is a high need to simplify information by reducing dimensionality to handle data of hundreds of thousands of functional genes from metagenomics analysis. The same is also true when we use a gene-marker sequencing approach, such as 16S rRNA gene sequencing, where we deal with thousands of operational taxonomic units (OTUs – groups of sequences sharing at least 97% identity) or amplicon sequence variants (ASVs – exact unique sequences). What is certain is that machine learning is showing its great potential in the microbiome field. We expect top-notch machine learning-based approaches to be implemented in the coming years, and this might be an important step forward for many disciplines related to microbiome science, such as precision medicine.

Author Biographies

Silvia Turroni is an Associate Professor in Chemistry and Biotechnology of Fermentation, Department of Pharmacy and Biotechnology, University of Bologna (Bologna, Italy). Her research activity, documented by >180 publications in international peer-reviewed journals and >140 participations in national and international congresses (>60 as invited speaker), is mainly focused on the compositional and functional profiling of the human microbiome and the exploration of its impact on health. She has strong expertise in next-generation sequencing technologies, including 16S rRNA amplicon sequencing and omics approaches, i.e. metagenomics, metatranscriptomics, and, more recently, culturomics, as well as microbiome–host interaction studies in *ex vivo* models.

Simone Rampelli is Assistant Professor in Chemistry and Biotechnology of Fermentation, Department of Pharmacy and Biotechnology, University of Bologna (Bologna, Italy). His research activity, documented by >85 publications in international peer-reviewed journals and >30 participations in national and international conferences (>10 as invited speakers), is mainly focused on the compositional and functional profiling of microbiome and the development of bioinformatic approaches for microbiome data. He has strong expertise in bioinformatics and biostatistics on metagenomics and metatranscriptomics, including evolutionary approaches for tracking adaptation and evolution of microbial genomes.

References

Ai, D., Pan, H., Han, R. et al. (2019). Using decision tree aggregation with random forest model to identify gut microbes associated with colorectal cancer. *Genes (Basel)* 10 (2): 112. https://doi.org/10.3390/genes10020112.

Alzubaidi, L., Zhang, J., Humaidi, A.J. et al. (2021). Review of deep learning: concepts, CNN architectures, challenges, applications, future directions. *Journal of Big Data* 8 (53): 1–74. https://doi.org/10.1186/s40537-021-00444-8.

Bajaj, J.S., Betrapally, N.S., Hylemon, P.B. et al. (2015). Salivary microbiota reflects changes in gut microbiota in cirrhosis with hepatic encephalopathy. *Hepatology* 62: 1260–1271. https://doi.org/10.1002/hep.27819.

Barone, M., D'Amico, F., Fabbrini, M. et al. (2021). Over-feeding the gut microbiome: a scoping review on health implications and therapeutic perspectives. *World Journal of Gastroenterology* 27 (41): 7041–7064. https://doi.org/10.3748/wjg.v27.i41.7041.

Breiman, L. (2001). Random forests. *Machine Learning* 45: 5–32. https://doi.org/10.1023/A:1010933404324.

Cammarota, G., Ianiro, G., Ahern, A. et al. (2020). Gut microbiome, big data and machine learning to promote precision medicine for cancer. *Nature Reviews Gastroenterology & Hepatology* 17 (10): 635–648. https://doi.org/10.1038/s41575-020-0327-3.

Candela, M., Biagi, E., Turroni, S. et al. (2015). Dynamic efficiency of the human intestinal microbiota. *Critical Reviews in Microbiology* 41 (2): 165–171.

Cani, P.D. and Van Hul, M. (2020). Gut microbiota and obesity: causally linked? *Expert Review of Gastroenterology & Hepatology* 14 (6): 401–403. https://doi.org/10.1080/17474124.2020.1758064.

Costello, E.K., Stagaman, K., Dethlefsen, L. et al. (2012). The application of ecological theory toward an understanding of the human microbiome. *Science* 336 (6086): 1255–1262. https://doi.org/10.1126/science.1224203.

D'Amico, F., Barone, M., Tavella, T. et al. (2022). Host microbiomes in tumor precision medicine: how far are we? *Current Medicinal Chemistry* https://doi.org/10.2174/0929867329666220105121754.

Duvallet, C., Gibbons, S.M., Gurry, T. et al. (2017). Meta-analysis of gut microbiome studies identifies disease-specific and shared responses. *Nature Communications* 8 (1): 1784. https://doi.org/10.1038/s41467-017-01973-8.

Fassarella, M., Blaak, E.E., Penders, J. et al. (2021). Gut microbiome stability and resilience: elucidating the response to perturbations in order to modulate gut health. *Gut* 70 (3): 595–605. https://doi.org/10.1136/gutjnl-2020-321747.

Fernández-Navarro, T., Díaz, I., Gutiérrez-Díaz, I. et al. (2019). Exploring the interactions between serum free fatty acids and fecal microbiota in obesity through a machine learning algorithm. *Food Research International* 121: 533–541. https://doi.org/10.1016/j.foodres.2018.12.009.

Flemer, B., Warren, R.D., Barrett, M.P. et al. (2018). The oral microbiota in colorectal cancer is distinctive and predictive. *Gut* 67 (8): 1454–1463. https://doi.org/10.1136/gutjnl-2017-314814.

Goodrich, J.K., Di Rienzi, S.C., Poole, A.C. et al. (2014). Conducting a microbiome study. *Cell* 158 (2): 250–262. https://doi.org/10.1016/j.cell.2014.06.037.

Gupta, A., Dhakan, D.B., Maji, A. et al. (2019). Association of *Flavonifractor plautii*, a Flavonoid-1422 Degrading Bacterium, with the gut microbiome of colorectal cancer patients in India. *mSystems* 4 (6): e00438–e00419. https://doi.org/10.1128/mSystems.00438-19.

He, Y., Wu, W., Zheng, H.M. et al. (2018). Regional variation limits applications of healthy gut microbiome reference ranges and disease models. *Nature Medicine* 24 (10): 1532–1535. https://doi.org/10.1038/s41591-018-0164-x.

Helmink, B.A., Khan, M.A.W., Hermann, A. et al. (2019). The microbiome, cancer, and cancer therapy. *Nature Medicine* 25 (3): 377–388. https://doi.org/10.1038/s41591-019-0377-7.

Iliev, I.D. and Leonardi, I. (2017). Fungal dysbiosis: immunity and interactions at mucosal barriers. *Nature Reviews Immunology* 17 (10): 635–646. https://doi.org/10.1038/nri.2017.55.

Integrative, H.M.P. (2019). (iHMP) research network consortium. The integrative human microbiome project. *Nature* 569 (7758): 641–648. https://doi.org/10.1038/s41586-019-1238-8.

Iwauchi, M., Horigome, A., Ishikawa, K. et al. (2019). Relationship between oral and gut microbiota in elderly people. *Immunity, Inflammation and Disease* 7 (3): 229–236. https://doi.org/10.1002/iid3.266.

Jang, B.S., Chang, J.H., Chie, E.K. et al. (2020). Gut microbiome composition is associated with a pathologic response after preoperative chemoradiation in patients with rectal cancer. *International Journal of Radiation Oncology, Biology, Physics* 107 (4): 736–746. https://doi.org/10.1016/j.ijrobp.2020.04.015.

Jochum, L. and Stecher, B. (2020). Label or concept – what is a pathobiont? *Trends in Microbiology* 28 (10): 789–792. https://doi.org/10.1016/j.tim.2020.04.011.

Kharrat, N., Assidi, M., Abu-Elmagd, M. et al. (2019). Data mining analysis of human gut microbiota links *Fusobacterium* spp. with colorectal cancer onset. *Bioinformation* 15 (6): 372–379. https://doi.org/10.6026/97320630015372.

Koh, A., De Vadder, F., Kovatcheva-Datchary, P., and Bäckhed, F. (2016). From dietary fiber to host physiology: short-chain fatty acids as key bacterial metabolites. *Cell* 165 (6): 1332–1345. https://doi.org/10.1016/j.cell.2016.05.041.

Kolodziejczyk, A.A., Zheng, D., and Elinav, E. (2019). Diet-microbiota interactions and personalized nutrition. *Nature Reviews Microbiology* 17 (12): 742–753. https://doi.org/10.1038/s41579-019-0256-8.

Koohi-Moghadam, M., Borad, M.J., Tran, N.L. et al. (2019). MetaMarker: a pipeline for de novo discovery of novel metagenomic biomarkers. *Bioinformatics* 35 (19): 3812–3814. https://doi.org/10.1093/bioinformatics/btz123.

Koskella, B., Hall, L.J., and Metcalf, C.J.E. (2017). The microbiome beyond the horizon of ecological and evolutionary theory. *Nature Ecology & Evolution* 1 (11): 1606–1615. https://doi.org/10.1038/s41559-017-0340-2.

Liu, W., Fang, X., Zhou, Y. et al. (2021). Machine learning-based investigation of the relationship between gut microbiome and obesity status. *Microbes and Infection* 24 (2): 104892. https://doi.org/10.1016/j.micinf.2021.104892.

Lynch, S.V. and Pedersen, O. (2016). The human intestinal microbiome in health and disease. *New England Journal of Medicine* 375 (24): 2369–2379. https://doi.org/10.1056/NEJMra1600266.

Miller, E.T., Svanbäck, R., and Bohannan, B.J.M. (2018). Microbiomes as metacommunities: understanding host-associated microbes through metacommunity ecology. *Trends in Ecology & Evolution* 33 (12): 926–935. https://doi.org/10.1016/j.tree.2018.09.002.

Namkung, J. (2020). Machine learning methods for microbiome studies. *Journal of Microbiology* 58 (3): 206–216. https://doi.org/10.1007/s12275-020-0066-8.

O'Toole, P.W., Marchesi, J.R., and Hill, C. (2017). Next-generation probiotics: the spectrum from probiotics to live biotherapeutics. *Nature Microbiology* 2: 17057. https://doi.org/10.1038/nmicrobiol.2017.57.

Pasolli, E., Truong, D.T., Malik, F. et al. (2016). Machine learning meta-analysis of large metagenomic datasets: tools and biological insights. *PLoS Computational Biology* 12 (7): e1004977. https://doi.org/10.1371/journal.pcbi.1004977.

Prodan, A., Levin, E., and Nieuwdorp, M. (2019). Does disease start in the mouth, the gut or both? *eLife* 8: e45931. https://doi.org/10.7554/eLife.45931.

Quince, C., Walker, A.W., Simpson, J.T. et al. (2017). Shotgun metagenomics, from sampling to analysis. *Nature Biotechnology* 35 (9): 833–844. https://doi.org/10.1038/nbt.3935.

Rampelli, S., Guenther, K., Turroni, S. et al. (2018). Pre-obese children's dysbiotic gut microbiome and unhealthy diets may predict the development of obesity. *Communications Biology* 1: 222. https://doi.org/10.1038/s42003-018-0221-5.

Rampelli, S., Fabbrini, M., Candela, M. et al. (2021). G2S: a new deep learning tool for predicting stool microbiome structure from oral microbiome data. *Frontiers in Genetics* 12: 644516. https://doi.org/10.3389/fgene.2021.644516.

Rothschild, D., Weissbrod, O., Barkan, E. et al. (2018). Environment dominates over host genetics in shaping human gut microbiota. *Nature* 555 (7695): 210–215. https://doi.org/10.1038/nature25973.

Salvato, F., Hettich, R.L., and Kleiner, M. (2021). Five key aspects of metaproteomics as a tool to understand functional interactions in host-associated microbiomes. *PLoS Pathogens* 17 (2): e1009245. https://doi.org/10.1371/journal.ppat.1009245.

Schmidt, T.S., Hayward, M.R., Coelho, L.P. et al. (2019). Extensive transmission of microbes along the gastrointestinal tract. *eLife* 8: e42693. https://doi.org/10.7554/eLife.42693.

Segata, N., Izard, J., Waldron, L. et al. (2011). Metagenomic biomarker discovery and explanation. *Genome Biology* 12 (6): R60. https://doi.org/10.1186/gb-2011-12-6-r60.

Shkoporov, A.N., Clooney, A.G., Sutton, T.D.S. et al. (2019). The human gut virome is highly diverse, stable, and individual specific. *Cell Host & Microbe* 26 (4): 527–541.e5. https://doi.org/10.1016/j.chom.2019.09.009.

Tilg, H. and Moschen, A.R. (2014). Microbiota and diabetes: an evolving relationship. *Gut* 63 (9): 1513–1521. https://doi.org/10.1136/gutjnl-2014-306928.

Tilg, H., Zmora, N., Adolph, T.E., and Elinav, E. (2020). The intestinal microbiota fuelling metabolic inflammation. *Nature Reviews Immunology* 20 (1): 40–54. https://doi.org/10.1038/s41577-019-0198-4.

Turroni, S., Brigidi, P., Cavalli, A., and Candela, M. (2018). Microbiota-host transgenomic metabolism, bioactive molecules from the inside. *Journal of Medicinal Chemistry* 61 (1): 47–61. https://doi.org/10.1021/acs.jmedchem.7b00244.

Vernocchi, P., Del Chierico, F., and Putignani, L. (2016). Gut microbiota profiling: metabolomics based approach to unravel compounds affecting human health. *Frontiers in Microbiology* 7: 1144. https://doi.org/10.3389/fmicb.2016.01144.

Vivarelli, S., Salemi, R., Candido, S. et al. (2019). Gut microbiota and cancer: from pathogenesis to therapy. *Cancers (Basel)* 11 (1): 38. https://doi.org/10.3390/cancers11010038.

de Vos, W.M., Tilg, H., Van Hul, M., and Cani, P.D. (2022). Gut microbiome and health: mechanistic insights. *Gut* https://doi.org/10.1136/gutjnl-2021-326789.

Vujkovic-Cvijin, I., Sklar, J., Jiang, L. et al. (2020). Host variables confound gut microbiota studies of human disease. *Nature* 587 (7834): 448–454. https://doi.org/10.1038/s41586-020-2881-9.

Wirbel, J., Pyl, P.T., Kartal, E. et al. (2019). Meta-analysis of fecal metagenomes reveals global microbial signatures that are specific for colorectal cancer. *Nature Medicine* 25 (4): 679–689, 2019679-689. https://doi.org/10.1038/s41591-019-0406-6.

Zeevi, D., Korem, T., Zmora, N. et al. (2015). Personalized nutrition by prediction of glycemic responses. *Cell* 163 (5): 1079–1094. https://doi.org/10.1016/j.cell.2015.11.001.

Zhang, Y., Thompson, K.N., Branck, T. et al. (2021). Metatranscriptomics for the human microbiome and microbial community functional profiling. *Annual Review of Biomedical Data Science* 4: 279–311. https://doi.org/10.1146/annurev-biodatasci-031121-103035.

8

Predictive Patient Stratification Using Artificial Intelligence and Machine Learning

Thanh-Phuong Nguyen[1], Thanh T. Giang[2], Quang T. Pham[2] and Dang H. Tran[3]

[1] Innovation Business Unit, Dennemeyer TechSys, Luxembourg, Luxembourg
[2] Faculty of Natural Science and Technology, Tay Bac University, Sonla, Vietnam
[3] Faculty of Computer Science, Hanoi National University of Education, Hanoi, Vietnam

8.1 Overview of Artificial Intelligence for Patient Stratification

Patient stratification is the division of a patient population into disease subgroups, also referred to as "strata" or "blocks." Each sub-group has different disease characteristics and disease causes. For example, patients could be divided up according to age, gender, ethnicity, social background, medical history, or any other relevant factor. Disease signatures, known as a combination of genomic and non-genomic features, exhibit highly diverse factors depending on the specific diseases.

Nowadays, thanks to the availability of huge patient data sets, the research on patient stratification is blooming and brings a lot of challenges. To deal with Big Data, there is a crucial need of artificial intelligence (AI), especially high-performed machine learning solutions. By using the full potential of the novel AI applications in biomedicine, an enormous patient population can be accurately stratified into distinguishable sub-groups of patients based on high dimensional and multivariate patient data. These sub-groups can be studied to find novel targets for drug discovery or repurposing, and for personalizing the most suitable treatments available for an individual patient based on their personal genetic makeup, phenotype, and comorbidities/co-prescriptions (Suri et al. 2022; Schutte et al. 2022; Shao et al. 2022).

Multiple factors, ranging from genetics to lifestyle and the environment, contribute to the development of complex diseases such as cancers, diabetes, and neurodegenerative disorders. For the complex disease, patients stratification is much more challenging because of the multifactorial characteristics and their interactions (Suri et al. 2022; Schutte et al. 2022; Shao et al. 2022). Among those complex diseases, cancers and Alzheimer disease (AD) have been attracted a lot of research due to the severity, the complication, and the high prevalence as emerging. Computational methods in general, the AI-based method in particular, have significantly contributed to cancer and AD diagnosis, prognosis, and treatment (Patel et al. 2020; Fabrizio et al. 2021).

There are a number of significant research projects that have been carried out to offer insights into different aspects of cancers. Early cancer diagnosis using AI was reviewed in Hunter et al. (2022). Classification and determination of cancer types or severity levels were studied in Soh et al. (2017) and Couture et al. (2018). Patients clustering and a potential treatment regimen was proposed for cancer patients (Pekic et al. 2019; Hussain et al. 2019). Identification of disease genes were inferred to assist cancer diagnosis and treatment in Gkountela et al. (2019) and Speicher and Pfeifer (2015). A predictive model for cancer therapeutic drugs was presented in Li et al. (2020). Approaching temporal factors of cancer, Azadeh et al. studied the prognosis of ability, survival time of cancer patients (Bashiri et al. 2017). Cancer patients stratification is one of most crucial steps making sure right medication at the right time for cancer patients (Sorbye et al. 2007; Chand et al. 2018; Kalinin et al. 2018; Fröhlich et al. 2018; Jang et al. 2019; Giang et al. 2020). De Meulder et al. proposed a computational framework to cluster potential patient groups having complex diseases (De Meulder et al. 2018). They applied their framework for ovarian cancer by combining multiple-omics large-scale datasets and spectral clustering with a consensus clustering step. Fröhlich et al. worked on predicting high or low risk for premenopausal breast cancer patients based on several multi-omics analysis (Fröhlich et al. 2018). Jang et al. developed a predictive model using gene markers to stratify cancer patients and later analyzed survivals (Jang et al. 2019). Giang et al. proposed a novel stratification model using fast multiple kernel learning (fMKL) and dimensionality reduction to classify survival/non-survival patients for various cancers (Giang et al. 2020).

Cancer datasets used in patient stratification are often large, high dimensional (possibly up to millions dimensions). Consequently, conventional methods are unable to cope with the significant computational costs and intricacies associated with these conditions (Fan and Li 2006; Pavlopoulou et al. 2015). Second, the patient datasets are various in types, gene expression, DNA methylation, and miRNA expression, each of which brings particularly cancers' insightful characteristics. Integrative approaches excel in handling data consistently and robustly by incorporating multiple sources of information and considering various aspects of the problem at hand. By leveraging the collective power of different data modalities, such as genomics, proteomics, and clinical data, integrative approaches enable a deeper understanding of the underlying disease mechanisms. Wang et al. proposed a similarity network method to synthesize data from three types, including gene expression, DNA methylation, and miRNA expression (Wang et al. 2014). Taking advantage of deep learning, a data integration model was built for classifying cancer patients more robustly (Liang et al. 2014).

To improve the computational performance, there have been many studies on dimensionality reduction (Hira and Gillies 2015; Alshamlan et al. 2015; Taguchi 2016; Giang et al. 2018). Alshamlan et al. utilized a combination of the minimum redundancy maximum relevance (mRMR) and artificial bee colony (ABC) methods to identify significant genes in cancer classification. This hybrid approach aims to select a set of genes that exhibit both high relevance to the cancer classification task and minimal redundancy among themselves (Alshamlan et al. 2015). Taguchi et al. employed the principal component analysis (PCA) method to predict miRNA/mRNA interactions across six different types of cancers

(Taguchi 2016). By applying PCA, they aimed to reduce the dimensionality of the data and extract the most informative features for predicting the interactions between miRNAs and mRNAs in cancer (Taguchi 2016). This approach provides insights into the regulatory mechanisms underlying cancer development and progression. Similarly, Giang et al. developed a fast framework for dimensionality reduction and data integration by integrating MKL with dimensionality reduction techniques (Giang et al. 2018). This framework enables the efficient integration of diverse data sources and the simultaneous reduction of high-dimensional data. By combining MKL and dimensionality reduction, the proposed method achieved improved computational efficiency and enhanced performance in data integration tasks. While the aforementioned methods successfully addressed the challenges of data heterogeneity and high dimensionality to a certain extent, they did not provide efficient solutions for learning models from molecular biology datasets that often contain noise, outliers, and missing data. Dealing with these issues is crucial for accurate and reliable analysis in the field of molecular biology.

AD patient stratification has been approached in a different way. Thanks to magnetic resonance imaging (MRI)s high-quality three-dimensional images of brain, most of work on the AD stratification were based on MRI data. Regions of interest (ROI) which affect disease development could be revealed and this factor contributes to AD diagnosis and treatment notably. There are two main approaches based on ROIs, the single-ROI-based approach and the multiple-ROI-based approach (Chupin et al. 2009; Liu et al. 2017a,2017b, 2018; Dai et al. 2013; Suk et al. 2014; Ben Ahmed et al. 2015; Khedher et al. 2015). Chupin et al. (2009) modeled probabilistic and anatomical priors for hippocampus segmentation to determine three subgroups AD, normal controls (NC), and mild cognitive impairment (MCI). Ahmed et al. selected visual features from the most involved regions in AD to construct an automatic classification framework for AD, NC, and MCI (Ben Ahmed et al. 2015).

Several multivariate approaches, such as partial least squares and PCA, were developed to build a discrimination model (Khedher et al. 2015). Liu et al. took the network-based approach using ROIs, modeled individual networks, and applied them as inputs of a classification model (Liu et al. 2017b). The support vector machine (SVM) was applied to train a classification model based on multiple ROIs and control-group feature normalization. The method enhanced the performance of AD diagnosis (Linn et al. 2016). In Liu et al. (2017a, 2018), Liu et al. showed that both of ROIs and the correlations between them were strongly relevant to AD diagnosis results. Hazarika et al. used brain magnetic resonance scans to implement some commonly used deep neural network models for classifying AD patients (Hazarika et al. 2023). Although previous methods have achieved notable results, they have not fully resolved the challenges of high-dimensional data in terms of accuracy and computational performance. Further advancements are needed in efficient algorithms for dimensionality reduction and feature selection, as well as the utilization of advanced machine learning models tailored for high-dimensional data.

In Section 8.2, we introduce a patient stratification model that combines robust principal component analysis (RPCA) and MKL. We begin by presenting RPCA and its application in dimensionality reduction and feature extraction in Sections 8.2.1 and 8.2.2, respectively. Section 8.2.3 outlines the construction of the predictive model using MKL. The experimental datasets are described in Section 8.2.4, followed by two experiments conducted on cancer and Alzheimer disease patients in Section 8.2.5. Section 8.2.6 presents the results of comparative evaluation and discusses the key findings. Finally, in Section 8.3, we conclude the chapter.

8.2 A RPCA and MKL Combination Model for Patient Stratification

In this section, we present the patient stratification model, combining the data dimensionality reduction based on RPCA and MKL classification model based on MKBoost-S2 (Xia and Hoi 2012) and weighted multiple kernel learning (wMKL) (Cai et al. 2012). MKL is a machine learning technique that combines information from multiple kernels or similarity measures to improve the performance of a learning algorithm. Kernels define the similarity or distance between data points and are fundamental in many machine learning algorithms, such as SVMs. MKL has been successfully applied in various domains, including bioinformatics, computer vision, and natural language processing, where multiple sources of information or diverse feature representations need to be effectively integrated for improved learning and prediction performance (Cortes et al. 2009). Meanwhile, wMKL is an extension of MKL that assigns different weights to individual kernels during the learning process. In wMKL, each kernel is assigned a weight that determines its contribution to the final decision or prediction. MKBoost-S2 (multiple kernel boosting with second-order information) is a machine learning algorithm that combines the principles of MKL and boosting. By considering second-order information, MKBoost-S2 aims to capture complex relationships and dependencies in the data that may not be fully captured by first-order information alone. This can lead to improved discrimination and generalization ability, especially in scenarios where the data exhibits nonlinear or complex patterns.

The model extracted the most relevant features to classify patient subgroups. Figure 8.1 shows the illustration of our two-step stratification model which are:

1. Apply RPCA to reduce dimensions and to extract relevant features from the patient datasets.
2. Build classifiers based on MKBoost-S2 from each preprocessed datasets by RPCA and integrate them based on MKBoost-S2 and wMKL algorithms.

The inputs of the model were the patient datasets. In our two case studies, we used gene expression, DNA methylation, and miRNA expression for cancer patients and twelve data types of the MRI data for Alzheimer disease patients. The outputs of the model were the different subgroups of the cancer patients in the first application, and Alzheimer disease patients in the second one. The details of the two steps are presented in Sections 8.2.2 and 8.2.3.

8.2.1 Robust Principal Component Analysis

The RPCA method is derived from the key idea of PCA method which is to reduce the dimension of a dataset with large number of interrelated variables while retaining the variation in the dataset. The reduction is achieved by transforming feature representation from the old feature space to a new one. The new feature space includes a new set of variables (the

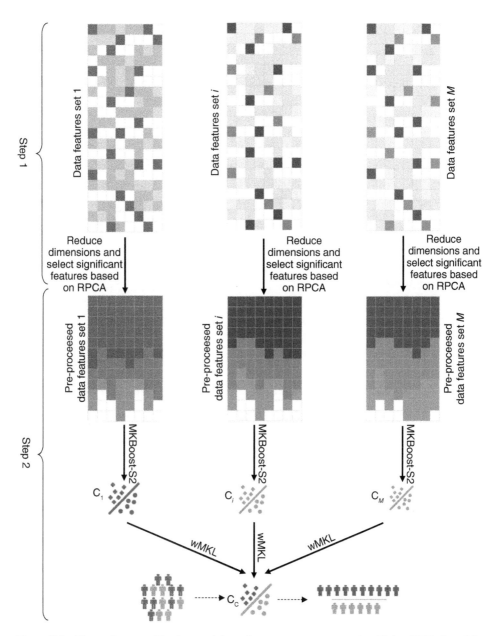

Figure 8.1 The patient stratification model employs a two-step approach utilizing RPCA. Step 1 is to reduce dimensions and to identify important features based on RPCA. Step 2 is to execute the MKBoost2-based models and combine the results to form the final model.

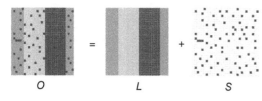

Figure 8.2 Robust principal component analysis illustration. O is the original data matrix, L is the low-rank matrix, and S is the sparse matrix.

$O \qquad L \qquad S$

principal components), which are uncorrelated and ordered, therefore, the first few retain most of the variation present in all of the original variables (Jolliffe 2005). PCA decomposes the original data matrix $O \in R^{m \times n}$ into the sum of two $O = L + N$ matrices, given a low-rank matrix L (containing most of the information called principal components) and a noise matrix N. N can be eliminated with minimal loss of information.

The PCA method represents data in a new space by finding an orthogonal coordinate system. The PCA problem can simply be solved by using singular value decomposition (SVD). However, SVD is very sensitive to outlier data, hence, PCA is not robust on datasets containing corrupted, missing, or outlier data. While PCA reduces N small to minimize information loss, RPCA defines S as a sparse matrix with the elements having arbitrary large values. Thus, RPCA is very suitable for the noisy datasets (Candès et al. 2011). The RPCA solves the problem of finding the low-rank matrix L and the sparse matrix S, then $O = L + S$ (see more in Figure 8.2).

The RPCA problem is transferred to the optimization problem based on l_0-norm (l_0-norm is pseudo-norm, and l_0-norm of a vector is the number of its nonzero components. l_0-norm is used in sparse constraint problems.) as follows:

$$\text{minimize rank}(L) + \lambda ||S||_0$$
$$\text{subject to } O = L + S \tag{8.1}$$

with $\lambda > 0$ is the Lagrange multiplier. The problem (8.1) is a NP-hard (non-deterministic polynomial-time hard) problem (Candès et al. 2011).

The problem of low-rank and sparse matrices decomposition is transformed based on the principal component pursuit method (Candès et al. 2011). Accelerated proximal gradient (Xia and Hoi 2012) or the augmented Lagrange multipliers (Bishop 2006) methods are later used to solve the RPCA optimization problem.

RPCA overcomes the limitation of PCA and has been successfully applied in many areas such as machine vision (Candès et al. 2011), image alignment (Peng et al. 2012), subspace recovery (Peng et al. 2012), and clustering problems (Candès et al. 2011). We applied RPCA to pre-process several patient datasets and to extract relevant features (see more in Section 8.2.2).

8.2.2 Dimensionality Reduction and Features Extraction Based on RPCA

Most RPCA studies have been based on $O = L + S$ matrix decompressing. The matrix keeps the low-rank matrix L that contains highly similar features with low dimension and the remove matrix S. In many datasets, the sparse matrix S containing outlier data are often more useful for classifying data than the low-rank matrix. This is because the sparse matrix captures differential features that can be crucial for accurate classification, while the low-rank matrix may not adequately represent the distinct characteristics of the data (Lin et al. 2009). In the cancers' datasets, although the expression levels of thousands of genes are measured simultaneously, only small numbers of genes are essential in the cancer diagnosis and treatment. From this hypothesis, we applied RPCA in the data pre-processing step to obtain two matrices, the low-rank matrix L (containing genes similarly expressed) and the sparse matrix S (containing genes differentially expressed). We used the processed data in the sparse matrix by rearranging and removing nonrelevant features. This rearranged matrix was used as the input data matrix for the next processing steps.

The RPCA-based data decomposition model for gene expression data type is described as follows. The same models were similarly developed for DNA methylation, miRNA expression in the cancer patient datasets, and the other data types in the AD patient datasets.

- **Step 1. Decompose the original data matrix**: Figure 8.3 illustrates the decompressing model for gene expression data based on RPCA. O is the original observation data matrix that presents the gene expression dataset, L is the low-rank matrix representing the similar genes, and S is the sparse matrix representing the differential genes. Each row of matrix corresponds to a transcription level of a gene, and each column is a sample. White and light gray blocks denote 0 and near-zero values, dark gray blocks refer differential values of genes. As shown in Figure 8.3, the matrix S of the differential expressed genes (the red blocks) can be recovered from the matrix O of gene expression data by RPCA.
- **Step 2. Sort genes based on their values**: Each line of the matrix S represents a transcriptional response of an observed sample's gene, each column of S represents expression levels of m genes in a sample. The matrix S is presented as follows:

$$S = \begin{bmatrix} s_{11} & s_{12} & \cdots & s_{1n} \\ s_{21} & s_{22} & \cdots & s_{2n} \\ \vdots & \vdots & \ddots & \vdots \\ s_{m1} & s_{m2} & \cdots & s_{mn} \end{bmatrix}. \tag{8.2}$$

The values of elements of S can be positive or negative because the gene expressions are adjusted. To discover the differential expressed genes, only the absolute values of entries in S will be taken into account. First, we calculated the absolute values of the element in the sparse matrix S. Second, we summed the values by a row of the matrix to get the evaluating vector E as shown in the following formula:

$$E = \begin{bmatrix} \sum_{i=1}^{n} |s_{1i}| & \cdots & \sum_{i=1}^{n} |s_{mi}| \end{bmatrix}^{T}. \tag{8.3}$$

Third, the vector E was arranged in a descending order of elements to obtain a new evaluation vector $\hat{E}$. Without loss of generality, we assumed that the first c_1 elements in $\hat{E}$ were nonzero:

$$\hat{E} = \begin{bmatrix} \hat{e}_1, \cdots, \hat{e}_{c_1}, \underbrace{0, \cdots, 0}_{m-c_1} \end{bmatrix}^{T}. \tag{8.4}$$

- **Step 3. Extract relevant genes**: One important principle states that if the value of an element in a vector is evaluated as 0, removing that element does not impact the optimality of the remaining variables. Even deleting a nonzero element (with a small value) will not affect too much associations with the remaining variables. Based on this principle, we see

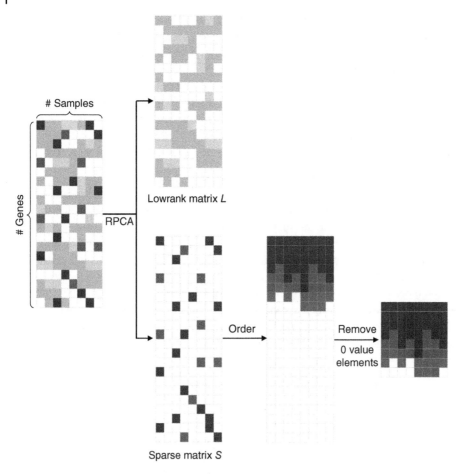

Figure 8.3 Gene expression preprocessing model based on RPCA. The gene expression data are processed to generate two matrices, denoted as *L* and *S*. The resulting matrix *S* are sorted, and any values equal to zero are removed.

that, in $\hat{E}$, the larger the values are, the greater the differences in gene expression are and more important that genes are. Therefore, we only selected $\text{num}_1 (\text{num}_1 < c_1)$ genes as the ordered in $\hat{E}$ as the input for the classification model in the next step.

8.2.3 Predictive Model Construction Based on Multiple Kernel Learning

Recent studies have demonstrated that models that integrate multiple data sources outperform those that rely solely on a single data source. Additionally, MKL with different kernel functions have been proven their efficiency in data analysis (Gönen and Alpaydın 2011). We propose a MKL-based model to stratify cancer patients and AD patients from multiple data sources (illustrated in Step 2 of Figure 8.1).

The three data types in cancer datasets, and the twelve data types in Alzheimer datasets were preprocessed to extract relevant features based on the proposed model in Section 8.2.2.

The preprocessed datasets were the input of the MKL model at the later step. In the model, MKL is implemented in two steps as described below.

First, for each dataset, MKBoost-S2 was used to create a hybrid kernel corresponding to a classifier achieving the best accuracy from a dataset and a set of kernel functions (see details in Xia and Hoi (2012)). Because the polynomial kernel function achieves good global optimal performance and the Gaussian kernel function obtains good local optimal performance, in our study, we used 13 base kernels as follows:

- **Polynomial kernel function**:

$$k_{\text{Polynomial}}(x, y) = (x^\top y + 1)^d$$

with $x^\top$ is transformation matrix of x and d is degree of polynomial. In this paper, we use three values of d, including $d = \{1, 2, 3\}$ to build three kernel functions for MKBoost-S2.
- **Gaussian kernel function**:

$$k_{\text{Gaussian}}(x, y) = \exp\left(\frac{||x - y||^2}{2\sigma^2}\right).$$

We built 10 Gaussian kernel functions with $\sigma = \{2^{-4}, 2^{-3}, \ldots, 2^4, 2^5\}$ for MKBoost-S2.

MKBoost-S2 uses 13 kernel functions to build a classifier. From M data types, and we have M classifiers, namely C_1, C_i, and C_M.

Second, we used wMKL to combine M classifiers C_1, C_i, and C_M into a unified classifier (notation as C_C) as follows:

$$C_C = \sum_{i=1}^{M} \lambda_i C_i$$

with C_i is the classifier corresponding to each data type, λ_i is the corresponding weight of these classifiers. Especially, the combination classifier was built based on the summation of the M classifiers with corresponding weights. In this study, we used the classifier's accuracy as weight for each component.

8.2.4 Materials

8.2.4.1 Cancer Patient Datasets

We investigated the cancer datasets from The Cancer Genome Atlas (TCGA) 2020.[1] The classifier attribute was *Dead* state of patients. The datasets were Lung Squamous Cell Carcinoma (LUNG), Glioblastoma Multiforme (GBM), Breast Invasive Carcinoma (BREAST), Ovarian Serous Cystadenocarcinoma (OV). The LUNG dataset includes 106 patients (42 dead). The GBM dataset includes 275 patients (73 dead). The BREAST dataset includes 435 patients (75 dead), and the OV dataset includes 541 patients (258 dead).

For each cancer patient dataset, we used three related data types, including gene expression, DNA methylation, and miRNA expression. Details of the data are shown in Table 8.1.

---

1 www.cancer.gov.

Table 8.1 The cancer dataset statistics.

			# features		
Cancer	# samples	Alive/dead	Gene expression	DNA methylation	miRNA expression
LUNG	106	42/64	12,042	23,074	352
GBM	275	202/73	12,042	22,896	534
BREAST	435	360/75	12,042	24,978	354
OV	541	283/258	12,042	21,825	799

Table 8.2 The Alzheimer disease MRI image dataset statistics.

Type	# samples	Age	Gender	MMSE
NC	230	73.13 ± 6.24	116/84	29.16 ± 0.82
MCInc	160	76.26 ± 5.35	89/71	27.56 ± 1.18
MCIc	120	75.95 ± 6.27	53/67	26.38 ± 1.52
MCI	280	76.11 ± 5.98	142/138	26.97 ± 1.34
AD	200	76.63 ± 5.91	122/108	23.54 ± 2.07

8.2.4.2 Alzheimer Disease Patient Datasets

MRI images of Alzheimer disease patients were extracted from Alzheimer disease neuroimaging initiative (ADNI).[2] The dataset consists of 710 T1-weighted subjects (data samples), including 200 subjects diagnosed with AD (the patient of Alzheimer disease), 280 subjects with MCI, and 230 NC subjects. Among 280 subjects with MCI, there are 120 subjects who have MCI and convert to AD within 18 months (MCIc) and 160 subjects who have MCI and do not convert to AD (MCInc). Details of the data (type, number of samples, age statistics, gender (number of males/number of females) and Minimum mean square error (MMSE)) are shown in Table 8.2. To analyze the MRI images, we applied the six measures for cortical and subcortical regions proposed by Liu et al. (2017b). More specifically, those six measures are cortical gray matter volume (CGMV), cortical thickness (CT), cortical surface area (CSA), cortical curvature (CC), cortical folding index (CFI) and subcortical volume (SV). We performed a complete procedure of image pre-processing, including spatial normalization, intensity normalization, skull stripping, and segmentation and fill for obtaining the higher quality images. As a result, all images were registered with Automated Anatomical Labelling Atlas (AAL atlas) (Tzourio-Mazoyer et al. 2002) before the anatomic reconstruction by FreeSurfer software.[3]

First, the six measures for cortical and subcortical regions were calculated. Later, we represented the obtained data in terms of graphs. We generated six graphs G_k corresponding

---

2 http://adni.loni.usc.edu.
3 https://surfer.nmr.mgh.harvard.edu.

to six measures, denoted by G_{CGMV}, G_{CT}, G_{CSA}, G_{CC}, G_{CFI}, G_{SV}. In a graph G_k, the set V_k denotes set of vertices (v_i), representing the regions. We denote E_k as the set of edges (e_{ii}), that comprise the weighted connections between two regions. The pre-processing step were described in Giang et al. (2018). After pre-processing MRI images step, we got twelve data types including V_{CGMV}, V_{CT}, V_{CSA}, V_{CC}, V_{CFI}, V_{SV}, E_{CGMV}, E_{CT}, E_{CSA}, E_{CC}, E_{CFI}, and E_{SV}.

8.2.5 Experiment Design

8.2.5.1 Experiment of Stratifying Cancer Patients

Each dataset in the gene expression, DNA methylation, miRNA expression was represented as O matrix. Each row corresponds to a feature, and each column is an observed sample (a patient). We obtained the feature extracting model based on the RPCA to each dataset and the output were three preprocessed data matrices.

MKBoost-S2 was applied to model the three classifier C_{GE}, C_{DNA}, and C_{RNA} from the corresponding datasets. We run 13 base kernel functions for each dataset to obtain the best performance of the MKBoost-S2 method. wMKL was later employed to combine three classifiers into an unified C_C classifier, denoted as *3-combination classifier*. To evaluate the performance of the integrative model, we also carried out additional experiments running on different combinations of two classifiers, specifically C_{GE-DNA}, C_{GE-RNA}, and $C_{DNA-RNA}$ classifiers, denoted as *2-combination classifiers*.

Accuracy and receiver operating characteristic (ROC) curve were calculated for the comparative evaluation. We compared the computational performance of our RPCA-based model with the performance of the models running on original dataset (without any dimensionality reduction) and fMKL-DR method results (Giang et al. 2020). The classifiers' accuracy and AUC (the area under the ROC curve) of the proposed model on the 2 of 3 datasets was compared with the ones obtained on all of the 3 datasets. We ran the experiment 20 times to ensure the unbiased results. At each run, we randomly took 2/3 of the dataset to train the model and the remaining dataset to test. The average accuracy of 20 runs is the final accuracy of the classification model.

8.2.5.2 Experiment of Stratifying Alzheimer Disease Patients

The experiment based on Alzheimer disease patient datasets is designed similar to the experiments for cancers, but with other inputs. Twelve data types were input to the Alzheimer disease patient stratification model. Those data types are described in Section 8.2.4.2. We used RPCA to extract relevant features from each data type, and we obtained twelve preprocessed data matrices accordingly.

MKBoost-S2 was used to build C_i classifiers, respectively. At the later step, we combined those classifiers by performing the wMKL algorithm. The outputs were the four predictive models to classify AD/NC (the AD patient and NC), AD/MCI (the AD patient and MCI), NC/MCI (the NC and MCI), and MCIc/MCInc (MCI converted and MCI not converted).

The evaluation process are done similarly to the cancer patient stratification model. We compared accuracy and ROC curve with other previously proposed methods.

8.2.6 Results and Discussions

In this section, we show the key results and discussions for the two applications of cancer patient stratification and AD patient stratification.

Table 8.3 Accuracy of classifier based on the original dataset and the pre-processing dataset by RPCA (the highest values are in bold).

Cancer	# samples	Accuracy (%)					
		Original dataset			Pre-processing dataset by RPCA		
		$GE^{a)}$	$DNA^{a)}$	$RNA^{a)}$	C_{GE}	C_{DNA}	C_{RNA}
LUNG	106	61.88	64.85	70.94	**64.68**	**67.81**	**71.41**
GBM	275	74.22	75.28	76.39	**80.83**	**76.39**	**80.88**
BREAST	435	88.10	88.03	91.48	**90.14**	**90.1**	**91.51**
OV	541	59.22	58.22	54.92	**68.72**	**67.61**	**66.50**

a) GE: gene expression, DNA: DNA methylation, RNA: miRNA expression.

8.2.6.1 Application of Stratifying Cancer Patients

Table 8.3 shows accuracy of the classifiers on the original datasets and the datasets obtained by the RPCA method. The results shows that, on most of cancer patient datasets, accuracy of our method was significantly higher than the one on the original datasets. Especially, for GBM and OV diseases, accuracy of all three data types was considerably outperformed. The biggest accuracy difference increased from 54.92% to 66.5% with the miRNA expression dataset for the OV disease. It shows that our dimensionality reduction and features extraction model based on RPCA improved the cancer patients stratification.

Table 8.4 illustrates accuracy of the classifiers on two or three data types based on wMKL. The results have shown that *2-combination classifiers* achieved better accuracy than the ones on a single data type (in Table 8.3). For each type of cancers, the combination of the classifiers has a different impact, for example, in LUNG disease, the combination of C_{GE} and C_{RNA} or C_{DNA} and C_{RNA} has better accuracy (with 72.66%) compared with the accuracy of combination between C_{GE} and C_{DNA} is 69.22%. For OV cancer, the combination of C_{GE} and C_{DNA} produced the best accuracy with 69.25%. Although the *2-combination classifiers*

Table 8.4 The classifiers' accuracy was assessed using various combinations of two or three data types (the highest values are in bold).

Cancer	# samples	Accuracy (%)				
		C_{GE-DNA}	C_{GE-RNA}	$C_{DNA-RNA}$	C_C	C_C^*
LUNG	106	69.22	72.66	72.35	**77.35**	*76.65*
GBM	275	81.67	82.72	81.61	**85.23**	*84.80*
BREAST	435	91.44	91.43	92.17	**92.92**	*92.73*
OV	541	69.25	68.70	67.64	**69.80**	*69.56*

The highest accuracy was observed when utilizing *3-combination classifiers* for all cancer types, as indicated in the sixth column denoted as C_C.

Table 8.5 The AUC was calculated for classifiers based on combinations of two or three data types.

Cancer	# samples	Accuracy (%)			
		C_{GE-DNA}	C_{GE-RNA}	$C_{DNA-RNA}$	C_C
LUNG	106	0.7324	0.7093	0.7225	**0.8135**
GBM	275	0.7383	0.7066	0.7251	**0.7683**
BREAST	435	0.7241	0.7624	0.7498	**0.7925**
OV	541	0.6217	0.6255	0.6132	**0.6746**

The best result is obtained by *3-combination classifiers* across all types of cancers, as indicated in the sixth column denoted as C_C.

are better than the single one, the best results are obtained by *3-combination classifiers* in all type of cancers. Noticeably, in GBM and BREAST diseases, accuracy increased to 85.23% and 84.80%, respectively. These results are much better than the results of fMKL-DR (Giang et al. 2020) on GBM (81.11%) and OV (62.22%) datasets. The C_C^* column in Table 8.4 presents the statistical hypothesis tested with confident value at 95%. The findings shows that our classification model is statistically significant.

Table 8.5 shows AUC of the classification models, and Figure 8.4 illustrates the ROC curves. The results show that the *3-combination classifiers* C_C returned better AUC than *2-combination classifiers*. Especially, for LUNG disease, AUC of the C_C is 0.8135, that is much higher than the other classifiers, while the largest value of *2-combination classifiers* is 0.7324. Similar to other cancers, the largest AUC is achieved when combining three data types. Comparing to fMKL-DR (Giang et al. 2020), on all four datasets, our model achieved

Table 8.6 The accuracy of the previous methods and the proposed method was evaluated across different AD patient groups (the highest values are in bold).

Method	Accuracy %			
	AD/NC	AD/MCI	NC/MCI	MCIc/MCInc
Chupin et al. (2009)	80.51	73.48	71.94	64.21
Ben Ahmed et al. (2015)	86.40	74.51	76.29	68.72
Khedher et al. (2015)	88.96	84.59	82.41	70.11
Dai et al. (2013)	90.81	85.92	81.92	71.04
Suk et al. (2014)	93.05	88.98	83.67	72.86
Liu et al. (2017b)	95.24	90.85	86.35	74.28
Giang et al. (2020)	96.50	91.25	87.65	78.49
Proposed method	96.25	90.75	87.5	**82.55**
Proposed method (at 90% confidence level of *t-test*)	*95.95*	*89.5*	*87.1*	**82.15**

Our proposed method, as shown in the last two rows, achieved the highest level of accuracy among all the methods.

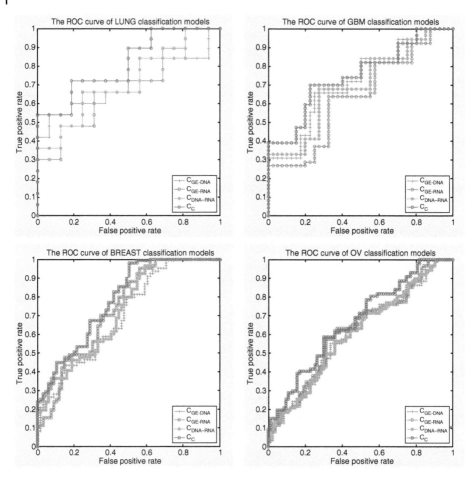

Figure 8.4 The ROC curves of the classifiers for four types of cancer are displayed: (a) for Lung cancer, (b) for GBM, (c) for Breast cancer, and (d) for Ovarian cancer. The most optimal outcome is achieved when all three types of data are combined, represented by the dark gray curves.

significantly better results of AUC values. This result confirmed that all of three data type are important, and the integrative analysis produced better results.

8.2.7 Application of Stratifying Alzheimer Disease Patients

Table 8.6 shows accuracy of the classifiers built by the previous proposed method and our proposed method. The results showed that accuracy of our proposed method was mostly less than previous methods, except MCIc/MCInc classifier. Accuracy of our proposed method is 82.55%, which is significantly higher than the one of previous methods. As a result, our method is useful in the case of high similarity between patient subgroups, but not for all cases of the AD patients.

Table 8.7 shows AUCs of the classifiers. Similarly, the AUC of MCIc/MCInc classifier was remarkably higher than other methods. The results showed that all of the classifiers are reliable thanks to high AUCs.

Table 8.7 AUC of the previous methods and the proposed method for different AD patient groups (the highest values are in bold).

Method	AUC			
	AD/NC	AD/MCI	NC/MCI	MCIc/MCInc
Chupin et al. (2009)	0.7851	0.7328	0.7155	0.6638
Ben Ahmed et al. (2015)	0.8487	0.7562	0.7677	0.6814
Khedher et al. (2015)	0.9256	0.8859	0.8134	0.7076
Dai et al. (2013)	0.9429	0.8743	0.8118	0.7086
Suk et al. (2014)	0.9475	0.9007	0.8203	0.7123
Liu et al. (2017b)	0.9754	0.9355	0.9107	0.7885
Giang et al. (2020)	0.9786	0.9412	0.9151	0.8024
Proposed method	0.9724	0.9386	0.9091	**0.8538**
Proposed method (at 90% confidence level of *t-test*)	*0.9702*	*0.9350*	*0.9015*	***0.8452***

8.3 Conclusion

In this chapter, we have reviewed state-of-the-art methods using AI in patient stratification for complex diseases. We then presented our AI-based method for stratifying cancer patients and AD patients. The model applied dimensionality reduction and feature extraction based on RPCA, and MKL using a combination of MKBoost-S2 and wMKL. Experiment results showed that our proposed model was efficiently preprocessed the cancer patient and Alzheimer disease patient data. Integrating multiple classifiers returned higher accuracy and AUC. The BREAST data set accuracy was 92.92% and 97.24% with AD/NC classifying. Moreover, our method can be easily reproduced for other diseases. In the future, the use of AI will be more and more popular and play a crucial role in clinical practices for the prediction of individual disease risk as well as patient stratification in order to finally develop effective and personalized therapies.

Author Biographies

Thanh-Phuong Nguyen received her BS (2003) and MS (2005) in Information Technology from Hanoi University of Technology (HUT), Vietnam. In September 2008, she received a PhD in Bioinformatics and Machine Learning from the School of Knowledge Science at the Japan Institute of Science and Technology (JAIST). With experience spanning both public institutions and private corporations, she has recently taken up a position at Dennemeyer Group as the Lead of the Data Science and AI team. Her primary areas of focus include data science, machine learning, AI, and the application of large language models to analyze Big Data.

Thanh Trung Giang received the BS from Tay Bac University in 2008, MS in Computer Science from Hanoi University of Education in 2012, and his PhD degree in System Information from University of Engineering and Technology, VNU in 2023. Presently, he holds the position of the head of the IT department at GCL Invest. Leveraging his extensive expertise in bioinformatics, data mining, and financial analysis, he spearheads innovative initiatives and improves business operations.

Quang Trung Pham received his B.S. from the University of Information and Communication Technology, Thai Nguyen University in 2005, and his M.S. in Computer Science from Hanoi University of Education in 2010. Currently, he is a lecturer at Tay Bac University, where he applies his expertise in bioinformatics and data mining to teaching and research.

Dang Hung Tran received the BS from Faculty of Mathematic and Informatics, Hanoi National University of Education in 2001, MS in Computer Science from University of Engineering and Technology, VNU in 2006, and PhD degree in Knowledge Science from Japan Advance Institute of Science and Technology (JAIST) in 2009. He currently holds the positions of associate professor and dean at the Faculty of Information Technology, Hanoi National University of Education (HNUE). His extensive research focuses on the fields of bioinformatics, data mining, and machine learning.

References

Alshamlan, H., Badr, G., and Alohali, Y. (2015). mRMR-ABC: a hybrid gene selection algorithm for cancer classification using microarray gene expression profiling. *BioMed Research International* 2015: 604910.

Bashiri, A., Ghazisaeedi, M., Safdari, R. et al. (2017). Improving the prediction of survival in cancer patients by using machine learning techniques: experience of gene expression data: a narrative review. *Iranian Journal of Public Health* 46 (2): 165.

Ben Ahmed, O., Benois-Pineau, J., Allard, M. et al. (2015). Classification of Alzheimer's disease subjects from MRI using hippocampal visual features. *Multimedia Tools and Applications* 74 (4): 1249–1266.

Bishop, C.M. (2006). Pattern recognition. *Machine Learning* 128 (9).

Cai, D., He, X., and Han, J. (2012). Speed up kernel discriminant analysis via approximating kernel matrices. *IEEE Transactions on Knowledge and Data Engineering* 24 (6): 1079–1091.

Candès, E.J., Li, X., Ma, Y., and Wright, J. (2011). Robust principal component analysis? *Journal of the ACM (JACM)* 58 (3): 1–37.

Chand, M., Keller, D.S., Mirnezami, R. et al. (2018). Novel biomarkers for patient stratification in colorectal cancer: a review of definitions, emerging concepts, and data. *World Journal of Gastrointestinal Oncology* 10 (7): 145.

Chupin, M., Gérardin, E., Cuingnet, R. et al. (2009). Fully automatic hippocampus segmentation and classification in Alzheimer's disease and mild cognitive impairment applied on data from ADNI. *Hippocampus* 19 (6): 579–587.

Cortes, C., Mohri, M., and Rostamizadeh, A. (2009). Learning non-linear combinations of kernels. *Advances in Neural Information Processing Systems* 22 (NIPS 2009), 396–404.

Couture, H.D., Williams, L.A., Geradts, J. et al. (2018). Image analysis with deep learning to predict breast cancer grade, ER status, histologic subtype, and intrinsic subtype. *npj Breast Cancer* 4 (1): 1–8.

Dai, D., He, H., Vogelstein, J.T., and Hou, Z. (2013). Accurate prediction of ad patients using cortical thickness networks. *Machine Vision and Applications* 24 (7): 1445–1457.

De Meulder, B., Lefaudeux, D., Bansal, A.T. et al., the U-BIOPRED Study Group, and the eTRIKS Consortium (2018). A computational framework for complex disease stratification from multiple large-scale datasets. *BMC Systems Biology* 12 (1): 60. https://doi.org/10.1186/s12918-018-0556-z.

Fabrizio, C., Termine, A., Caltagirone, C., and Sancesario, G. (2021). Artificial intelligence for Alzheimer's disease: promise or challenge? *Diagnostics* 11 (8): https://doi.org/10.3390/diagnostics11081473.

Fan, J. and Li, R. (2006). Statistical challenges with high dimensionality: feature selection in knowledge discovery. *arXiv preprint math/0602133*.

Fröhlich, H., Patjoshi, S., Yeghiazaryan, K. et al. (2018). Premenopausal breast cancer: potential clinical utility of a multi-omics based machine learning approach for patient stratification. *EPMA Journal* 9 (2): 175–186.

Giang, T.T., Nguyen, T.P., Nguyen, T.Q.V., and Tran, D.H. (2018). fmKL-DR: a fast multiple kernel learning framework with dimensionality reduction. *International Symposium on Integrated Uncertainty in Knowledge Modelling and Decision Making*, 153–165. Springer.

Giang, T.-T., Nguyen, T.-P., and Tran, D.-H. (2020). Stratifying patients using fast multiple kernel learning framework: case studies of Alzheimer's disease and cancers. *BMC Medical Informatics and Decision Making* 20 (1): 1–15.

Gkountela, S., Castro-Giner, F., Szczerba, B.M. et al. (2019). Circulating tumor cell clustering shapes DNA methylation to enable metastasis seeding. *Cell* 176 (1–2): 98–112.

Gönen, M. and Alpaydın, E. (2011). Multiple kernel learning algorithms. *The Journal of Machine Learning Research* 12: 2211–2268.

Hazarika, R.A., Maji, A.K., Kandar, D. et al. (2023). An approach for classification of Alzheimer's disease using deep neural network and brain magnetic resonance imaging (MRI). *Electronics* 12 (3): https://doi.org/10.3390/electronics12030676.

Hira, Z.M. and Gillies, D.F. (2015). A review of feature selection and feature extraction methods applied on microarray data. *Advances in Bioinformatics* 2015: 198363.

Hunter, B., Hindocha, S., and Lee, R.W. (2022). The role of artificial intelligence in early cancer diagnosis. *Cancers* 14 (6): https://doi.org/10.3390/cancers14061524.

Hussain, F., Saeed, U., Muhammad, G. et al. (2019). Classifying cancer patients based on DNA sequences using machine learning. *Journal of Medical Imaging and Health Informatics* 9 (3): 436–443.

Jang, Y., Seo, J., Jang, I. et al. (2019). CaPSSA: visual evaluation of cancer biomarker genes for patient stratification and survival analysis using mutation and expression data. *Bioinformatics* 35 (24): 5341–5343.

Jolliffe, I. (2005). Principal component analysis. In: *Encyclopedia of Statistics in Behavioral Science*. John Wiley.

Kalinin, A.A., Higgins, G.A., Reamaroon, N. et al. (2018). Deep learning in pharmacogenomics: from gene regulation to patient stratification. *Pharmacogenomics* 19 (7): 629–650.

Khedher, L., Ramírez, J., Górriz, J.M. et al., Alzheime's Disease Neuroimaging Initiative (2015). Early diagnosis of Alzheime's disease based on partial least squares, principal component analysis and support vector machine using segmented MRI images. *Neurocomputing* 151: 139–150.

Li, K., Du, Y., Li, L., and Wei, D.-Q. (2020). Bioinformatics approaches for anti-cancer drug discovery. *Current Drug Targets* 21 (1): 3–17.

Liang, M., Li, Z., Chen, T., and Zeng, J. (2014). Integrative data analysis of multi-platform cancer data with a multimodal deep learning approach. *IEEE/ACM Transactions on Computational Biology and Bioinformatics* 12 (4): 928–937.

Lin, Z., Ganesh, A., Wright, J. et al. (2009). Fast convex optimization algorithms for exact recovery of a corrupted low-rank matrix. *Coordinated Science Laboratory Report no. UILU-ENG-09-2214, DC-246.*

Linn, K.A., Gaonkar, B., Satterthwaite, T.D. et al. (2016). Control-group feature normalization for multivariate pattern analysis of structural MRI data using the support vector machine. *NeuroImage* 132: 157–166. https://doi.org/10.1016/j.neuroimage.2016.02.044.

Liu, J., Li, M., Pan, Y. et al. (2017a). Classification of schizophrenia based on individual hierarchical brain networks constructed from structural MRI images. *IEEE Transactions on Nanobioscience* 16 (7): 600–608. https://doi.org/10.1109/TNB.2017.2751074.

Liu, J., Wang, J., Tang, Z. et al. (2017b). Improving Alzheimer's disease classification by combining multiple measures. *IEEE/ACM Transactions on Computational Biology and Bioinformatics* 15 (5): 1649–1659.

Liu, J., Li, M., Lan, W. et al. (2018). Classification of Alzheimer's disease using whole brain hierarchical network. *IEEE/ACM Transactions on Computational Biology and Bioinformatics* 15: 624–632.

Patel, S.K., George, B., and Rai, V. (2020). Artificial intelligence to decode cancer mechanism: beyond patient stratification for precision oncology. *Frontiers in Pharmacology* 11: https://doi.org/10.3389/fphar.2020.01177.

Pavlopoulou, A., Spandidos, D.A., and Michalopoulos, I. (2015). Human cancer databases. *Oncology Reports* 33 (1): 3–18.

Pekic, S., Soldatovic, I., Miljic, D. et al. (2019). Familial cancer clustering in patients with prolactinoma. *Hormones and Cancer* 10 (1): 45–50.

Peng, Y., Ganesh, A., Wright, J. et al. (2012). RASL: Robust alignment by sparse and low-rank decomposition for linearly correlated images. *IEEE Transactions on Pattern Analysis and Machine Intelligence* 34 (11): 2233–2246.

Schutte, K., Brulport, F., Harguem-Zayani, S. et al. (2022). An artificial intelligence model predicts the survival of solid tumour patients from imaging and clinical data. *European Journal of Cancer* 174: 90–98. https://doi.org/10.1016/j.ejca.2022.06.055.

Shao, H., Shi, L., Lin, Y., and Fonseca, V. (2022). Using modern risk engines and machine learning/artificial intelligence to predict diabetes complications: a focus on the bravo model. *Journal of Diabetes and its Complications* 36 (11): 108316. https://doi.org/10.1016/j.jdiacomp.2022.108316.

Soh, K.P., Szczurek, E., Sakoparnig, T., and Beerenwinkel, N. (2017). Predicting cancer type from tumour DNA signatures. *Genome Medicine* 9 (1): 1–11.

Sorbye, H., Köhne, C.-H., Sargent, D.J., and Glimelius, B. (2007). Patient characteristics and stratification in medical treatment studies for metastatic colorectal cancer: a proposal for standardization of patient characteristic reporting and stratification. *Annals of Oncology* 18 (10): 1666–1672.

Speicher, N.K. and Pfeifer, N. (2015). Integrating different data types by regularized unsupervised multiple kernel learning with application to cancer subtype discovery. *Bioinformatics* 31 (12): i268–i275.

Suk, H.-I., Lee, S.-W., and Shen, D., Alzheimer's Disease Neuroimaging Initiative (2014). Hierarchical feature representation and multimodal fusion with deep learning for AD/MCI diagnosis. *NeuroImage* 101: 569–582.

Suri, J.S., Paul, S., Maindarkar, M.A. et al. (2022). Cardiovascular/stroke risk stratification in Parkinson's disease patients using atherosclerosis pathway and artificial intelligence paradigm: a systematic review. *Metabolites* 12 (4): https://doi.org/10.3390/metabo12040312.

Taguchi, Y.H. (2016). Identification of more feasible microRNA–mRNA interactions within multiple cancers using principal component analysis based unsupervised feature extraction. *International Journal of Molecular Sciences* 17 (5): 696.

Tzourio-Mazoyer, N., Landeau, B., Papathanassiou, D. et al. (2002). Automated anatomical labeling of activations in SPM using a macroscopic anatomical parcellation of the MNI MRI single-subject brain. *NeuroImage* 15 (1): 273–289.

Wang, B., Mezlini, A.M., Demir, F. et al. (2014). Similarity network fusion for aggregating data types on a genomic scale. *Nature Methods* 11 (3): 333–337.

Xia, H. and Hoi, S.C.H. (2012). MKBoost: a framework of multiple kernel boosting. *IEEE Transactions on Knowledge and Data Engineering* 25 (7): 1574–1586.

9

Hybrid Data-Driven and Numerical Modeling of Articular Cartilage

Seyed Shayan Sajjadinia[1], Bruno Carpentieri[1] and Gerhard A. Holzapfel[2,3]

[1] *Faculty of Engineering, Free University of Bozen-Bolzano, Bozen-Bolzano, Italy*
[2] *Institute of Biomechanics, Graz University of Technology, Graz, Austria*
[3] *Department of Structural Engineering, Norwegian University of Science and Technology, Trondheim, Norway*

9.1 Introduction

Articular cartilage (AC) is a load-bearing and lubricating soft tissue between articulating bony ends, which under healthy conditions exhibits excellent resistance and shock-absorbing abilities (Lu and Mow 2008). Nevertheless, the damage to this tissue, especially, due to biomechanical factors, causes significant health care costs (Salmon et al. 2016). Therefore, the analysis of cartilage is a very active area in the biomedical sciences, hopefully, to prevent or detect damage in its early stages, which requires a good understanding of the biomechanics involved (Martínez-Moreno et al. 2019).

Artificial intelligence (AI), particularly using machine learning (ML), has made significant strides in biomechanical cartilage studies. These advancements are evident in recent investigations on the heterogeneous material characterization of knee cartilage (Niasar and Li 2023), damage classification through unique biomechanical markers (Alunni Cardinali et al. 2023), and fiber orientation prediction in tissue (Mirmojarabian et al. 2023). However, the acquisition of clinical data for training these models is still a considerable challenge. This limitation has led to a predominant preference for physics-based models, especially using numerical methods.

Numerical modeling, notably using finite element (FE) methods, is crucial in solving (and approximating) cartilage-related physics problems (Freutel et al. 2014). Such methods find application in many scenarios: simulating crack propagation under cyclic loading (Orozco et al. 2022), analyzing fibrillar components (Sajjadinia and Haghpanahi 2021), and comparing healthy and damaged tissues (Vulović et al. 2021), to name a few. Despite their functionality, these techniques are highly iterative algorithms with significant computation time, varying from minutes to days based on the hardware settings and simulation definitions (Haut Donahue et al. 2002; Kazemi et al. 2011; Beidokhti et al. 2016; Wang and Yang 2018; Lostado Lorza et al. 2021).

One method to overcome the high computational costs of numerical simulations, including cartilage analysis, is to use ML to create similar data-driven models. These models that learn the behavior of numerical models by samples extracted from them are usually far

Big Data Analysis and Artificial Intelligence for Medical Sciences, First Edition.
Edited by Bruno Carpentieri and Paola Lecca.
© 2024 John Wiley & Sons Ltd. Published 2024 by John Wiley & Sons Ltd.

faster than the main numerical models that can be used instead of them; hence, they are called surrogates. Surrogates of biomechanical cartilage models receive special attention, see, e.g. Paiva et al. (2012), Arbabi et al. (2016a,2016b), Egli et al. (2021), and Sajjadinia et al. (2022). One goal of this chapter is to revisit these models and relevant issues, with a focus on hybrid paradigms that use both physics-based and data-driven approaches.

This study is organized as follows: Section 9.2 first summarizes the role of cartilage in joint biomechanics and next the cartilage components in load-bearing. Section 9.3 first gives a general picture of numerical modeling, followed by a brief explanation of an example of advanced constitutive (material) equations to get a better understanding of their application and complexity. Section 9.4 gives an overview of the most important methods of ML with regular and hybrid algorithms, whereas Section 9.5 concludes this work.

9.2 Knee and Cartilage

9.2.1 Main Joint Substructures

A tibiofemoral joint is the largest joint within the knee and entire body (as shown in Figure 9.1), consisting of the touching long ends of bones (namely femur and tibia), cartilaginous tissue (including femoral cartilage, tibial cartilage, and menisci), and ligaments. The shape of the bones allows condyloid joints, while the cam shape of the femoral condyles allows rotation in all axes (Goldblatt and Richmond 2003). The asymmetry within this joint was created over the course of evolution to accommodate the joint to the complex asymmetrical dynamics of the knee caused by various musculoskeletal movements of the body, e.g. with the regular gait (Dye 1987).

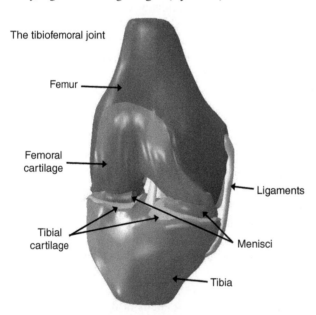

Figure 9.1 Main substructures in a knee model. Source: Image is extracted from Cooper et al. (2019) under its CC BY 4.0 license, permitting reuse with a proper citation.

Soft tissues play a key role in protecting the knee capsule from pathological motion and conditions. Ligaments stabilize it and avoid unphysiological positions and movements. Meniscus substructures, with their wedge-like cross-sections, allow the distribution of the axial force on articulating surfaces; this reduces the peak contact pressure (Walker and Erkman 1975; Mameri et al. 2022). In addition, AC absorbs this compressive distributed force and enables a low-friction sliding motion (Forster and Fisher 1996). Although meniscal tissue has a cartilage-like composition with different but similar biomechanical roles (Danso et al. 2014; Chen et al. 2017), we particularly focus on AC due to its high importance in osteoarthritis studies (Buckwalter 1995; Pearle et al. 2005; Goldring 2012; Brody 2015).

Osteoarthritis, a degenerative joint disease, predominantly impairs cartilage by gradually deteriorating its structure, leading to joint pain, discomfort, and eventual loss of joint function (Lespasio et al. 2017). It affects roughly a third of individuals aged 65 and above, with a notable predominance in women, thereby incurring significant socioeconomic costs on healthcare systems (Chen et al. 2012; Hawker 2019). Despite an incomplete understanding of the precise mechanism, recent review studies highlight potential correlations, including lifestyle elements such as poor diet, some comorbidities like diabetes, biomechanical factors (e.g. traumatic injuries), and hereditary aspects such as genetic risk loci (Loeser et al. 2016; Mobasheri et al. 2017; Astephen Wilson and Kobsar 2021).

In light of these correlations, biomechanical studies have proven essential in shaping strategies for rehabilitation and exercise (Kong et al. 2022). On the other hand, AC, much like other connective tissues, gains its functional properties largely from extracellular components, specifically collagen fibrils and proteoglycan proteins (Culav et al. 1999; Brody 2015). Consequently, a large focus of biomechanical research involves simulating the interaction of these components or phases (Klika et al. 2016; Ebrahimi et al. 2019; Sajjadinia et al. 2019; Lin et al. 2021; Paz et al. 2022), which is outlined in Section 9.2.2.

9.2.2 Load-Bearing Cartilage Phases

Aggrecans, the most common proteoglycan molecules in AC, are connected to the chains of hyaluronic acid to form large aggregates that are trapped in the collagen network. Because of their constituent glycosaminoglycan (GAG), which are negatively charged compounds, they have a fixed negative charge, resulting in a chemical potential gradient that attracts water to achieve chemical equilibrium, i.e. the mechanism of osmosis (Kiani et al. 2002; Gómez-Florit et al. 2020; Johnson et al. 2021). The aggregates are then responsible for the vital osmotic pressure that contributes to the load-bearing of the tissue by counteracting the applied loads. Moreover, this internal pressure swells the tissue, which is compensated by stretching of the collagen network, which increases the reversible deformation of the tissue (Dudhia 2005).

Thanks to the osmotic pressure of AC and the porous structure of the tissue, water makes up about 60–80% of the tissue (Cederlund and Aspden 2022). This not only maintains perfect lubrication on the surface of AC but also resists external loads as the hydrostatic fluid pressure, usually more than the other load-bearing components (Quiroga et al. 2017; Sajjadinia et al. 2019). Together with the solid constituents, the tissue can then be viewed as a biphasic mixture with a fluid phase and an effective solid phase (considering the overall effect of solid components such as aggregates and collagen networks). In addition, the water flow in the small solid pores at the beginning of cartilage deformation creates a considerable drag force between the two phases, which balance out over time (Mow et al. 1980). This results in a greater resistance to tissue deformation, which is regularly determined by the level of permeability (Eschweiler et al. 2021).

Besides, collagen fibrillar networks reinforce AC against tensile forces, like structural wire ropes (Bozec et al. 2007; Bielajew et al. 2020). It is observed that the fibrils can be classified into primary anisotropic (direction-dependent) and secondary isotropic (direction-independent) bundles (Clark 1985; Wilson et al. 2004). The isotropic bundles of the healthy tissue tend to be oriented roughly parallel to and between all axes of Euclidean (geometrical) space, while the anisotropic bundles are oriented in an arcade-like fashion: they extend perpendicularly from the calcified regions in the deep zone of AC and gradually rotate in the middle zone to become parallel to the AC surface (Wilson et al. 2004). While the fibrils are anchored to the bones in this way, they protect the surface from shear-induced damage (Shirazi and Shirazi-Adl 2008; Motavalli et al. 2014).

For further clarification, Figure 9.2 is extracted from an osteoarthritis study, which represents one of the possible scenarios in this condition, assuming that AC is viscoelastic, while elasticity describes the reversible deformation of the tissue; viscosity is the energy loss during this deformation (e.g. due to drag force). In this particular case, the main measurable material properties, including the storage and loss moduli, correspond to the ability to store elastic energy and the ability to dissipate energy, respectively (Banks et al. 2011). However, in a more general formulation of AC biomechanics, calculating the precise long-term and short-term local responses requires multi-physics constitutive equations (which simultaneously account for at least some of the abovementioned constituents). Because of their complexity, they are implemented by some numerical approximation methods, e.g. the FE method (Freutel et al. 2014).

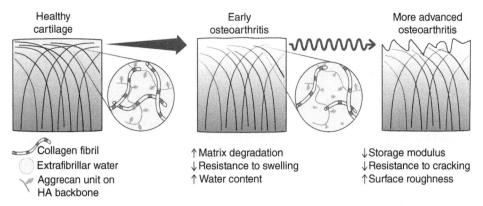

Figure 9.2 A possible scenario for osteoarthritis in articular cartilage is as follows: in the early stages, the tissue matrix undergoes degradation, resulting in an increase in water content. However, in more advanced conditions, it manifests itself through wear and tear on the tissue surface. Source: The image has been modified from Cooke et al. (2018) under its CC BY 4.0 license, allowing for reuse with correct citation. Abbreviation: HA = hyaluronic acid.

9.3 Physics-Based Modeling

9.3.1 Numerical Modeling

In cartilage modeling, the effects of weight and inertia are usually ignored, given the low density of the tissue (Pearle et al. 2005). By applying Newton's second law, we can argue that any force exerted on the tissue boundary, i.e. surface traction, should be balanced (although it can deform the model to reach equilibrium). This balance can be illustrated by the following simplified equilibrium equation in 3D Euclidean space, i.e.

$$\int_S \mathbf{t} dS = \mathbf{0}, \tag{9.1}$$

where S is the surface area of the deformed solid material, and $\mathbf{t}$ is the surface traction, which is correlated with the total Cauchy stress tensor σ_T as:

$$\mathbf{t} = \sigma_T \cdot \mathbf{n}, \tag{9.2}$$

where $\mathbf{n}$ is the outward normal to the surface and the stress tensor can be roughly interpreted as the distribution of force effects at each point. Now, we use the divergence theorem on the surface integral, which relates the flux of a field (stress in this case) on a closed surface to the spatial divergence of that field within the volume, such that

$$\int_S \sigma_T \cdot \mathbf{n} dS = \int_V \nabla_\mathbf{x} \sigma_T dV, \tag{9.3}$$

where $\nabla_\mathbf{x}(\bullet)$ is the gradient operator of $\bullet$ with respect to the deformed position vector $\mathbf{x}$. We can eliminate the integration to get the following differential equation:

$$\nabla_\mathbf{x} \sigma_T = \mathbf{0}. \tag{9.4}$$

FE software packages commonly use the weak form of differential equations. For example, using the principle of virtual work (Antman and Osborn 1979), Eq. (9.4) can be rewritten as follows:

$$\int_V \nabla_\mathbf{x} \sigma_T \cdot \delta \mathbf{u} dV = 0, \tag{9.5}$$

where $\delta \mathbf{u}$ denotes the virtual (nonzero) displacement field, which generates the virtual work. In practice, this variation simplifies the equation, as the result of the integral is now a scalar value. Furthermore, using the integration by parts of this equation, the divergence theorem, and Eq. (9.2), we can now directly impose the traction on the boundaries and remove the derivative term from the stress parameter (Holzapfel 2000; Belytschko et al. 2014):

$$\int_V \sigma_T : \nabla_\mathbf{x} \delta \mathbf{u} dV - \int_S \mathbf{t} \cdot \delta \mathbf{u} dS = 0. \tag{9.6}$$

Next, to account for the fluid contribution in cartilage load-bearing, we can use the continuity equation with the assumption that AC is a porous medium fully saturated with water. Thus,

$$\frac{d}{dt}\left(\int_V \rho \phi^F dV\right) + \int_S \rho \phi^F \mathbf{n} \cdot \mathbf{v}_r dS = 0, \tag{9.7}$$

where ρ is the mass density of the fluid, $\mathbf{v}_r$ is the relative velocity of the fluid with respect to the solid structure, and ϕ^F is the local volume fraction of the fluid. Conceptually, the first term models the rate of fluid change inside the tissue, whereas the second term reflects the amount crossing the boundary. Introducing the volume ratio J into the first term (to include the deformation of the solid structure) and applying the divergence theorem to the second term, the following partial differential equation is achieved:

$$\frac{1}{J}\frac{d}{dt}\left(J\rho\phi^F\right) + \nabla \cdot \left(\rho\phi^F\mathbf{v}_r\right) = 0. \tag{9.8}$$

The finite difference method can be used to approximate the temporal derivative by discretizing the time domain into time step Δt. In particular, the backward Euler formula is used to approximate the temporal derivative of a function y by shifting the current time step one step forward and then applying the backward difference approximation according to:

$$\left[\frac{dy}{dt}\right]_{t+\Delta t} \approx \frac{y_{t+\Delta t} - y_t}{\Delta t}. \tag{9.9}$$

Now, similar to the equilibrium equation, a weak form can be derived from Eq. (9.8), and then the divergence theorem can be applied, yielding:

$$\int_V \left([\delta P]_{t+\Delta t}\left(\left[J\rho\phi^F\right]_{t+\Delta t} - \left[J\rho\phi^F\right]_t\right) - \Delta t\left[\rho\phi^F\nabla_x\delta P \cdot \mathbf{v}_r\right]_{t+\Delta t}\right)dV$$
$$+ \Delta t \int_S \left[\delta P\rho\phi^F\mathbf{n} \cdot \mathbf{v}_r\right]_{t+\Delta t}dS = 0, \tag{9.10}$$

where δP is the virtual fluid pressure.

Next, FE methods are used to discretize the continuous spatial domain. For example, given a nonlinear 1D function $f(x)$, it can be approximated by $\overline{f}(x)$ as follow:

$$\overline{f}(x) = \sum_{i=1}^n \sum_{j=1}^2 \mathcal{N}_j^i(x)f(x_i). \tag{9.11}$$

Here, the geometrical domain is discretized into 1D FEs, where x_i is the nodal input value of the element i corresponding to the nodal result $f(x_i)$ with domain $[x_{i-1}, x_i]$, and $\mathcal{N}(x)$ is the shape function that can be defined by:

$$\mathcal{N}_1^i(x) = \frac{x_i - x}{x_i - x_{i-1}} \quad \text{and} \quad \mathcal{N}_2^i(x) = \frac{x - x_{i-1}}{x_i - x_{i-1}}. \tag{9.12}$$

Conceptually, these particular shape functions approximate $f(x)$ as a group of simpler linear functions connected with each other at their nodes. Likewise, by generalizing this to the 3D space with displacement and fluid pressure nodal values, the shape functions $\mathcal{N}^P$ and $\mathcal{N}^u$ are defined to spatially discretize, respectively, P and $\mathbf{u}$ (and their virtual variations). Substituting them into Eqs. (9.10) and (9.6) results in:

$$\mathcal{F} = 0, \tag{9.13}$$

where, $\mathcal{F} = [\mathcal{F}_1, \mathcal{F}_2]^T$ with

$$\mathcal{F}_1 = \int_V \left[\sigma : \nabla_x\mathcal{N}^u\right]_{t+\Delta t}dV - \int_S \left[\mathbf{t} \cdot \mathcal{N}^u\right]_{t+\Delta t}dS, \tag{9.14}$$

$$\mathscr{F}_2 = \int_V \left(\mathscr{N}^P_{t+\Delta t} \left(\left[J \rho \phi^F \right]_{t+\Delta t} - \left[J \rho \phi^F \right]_t \right) - \Delta t \left[\rho \phi^F \nabla_{\mathbf{x}} \mathscr{N}^P \cdot \mathbf{v}_r \right]_{t+\Delta t} \right) dV$$

$$+ \Delta t \int_S \left[\mathscr{N}^P \rho \phi^F \mathbf{n} \cdot \mathbf{v}_r \right]_{t+\Delta t} dS. \tag{9.15}$$

This discretization technique is referred to as implicit FE modeling because it provides a set of equations between the unknown parameters at the end of time step $t + \Delta t$ and the known parameters at step t (obviously once the discretized constitutive equations and additional conditions have been applied). Due to the high stability of this method, well-established software packages such as (Abaqus 2021) use similar formulations. However, the existence of a nonlinear system of equations requires the use of a root-finding technique such as the Newton's method (Almeida and Spilker 1997; Belytschko et al. 2014).

We denote $\mathscr{U}$ as the vector of system variables, such as $\{u_1, u_2, u_3, P\}$, where u_1, u_2, and u_3 correspond to the components of $\mathbf{u}$ in the 3D Cartesian coordinate system. To linearize Eq. (9.13), the Newton's method uses the Jacobian matrix $\mathfrak{J}^{(i)}$ at each iteration i, i.e.

$$\mathfrak{J}^{(i)} = \begin{bmatrix} \frac{\partial \mathcal{F}_1^{(i)}}{\partial u_1^{(i)}} & \cdots & \frac{\partial \mathcal{F}_1^{(i)}}{\partial P^{(i)}} \\ \frac{\partial \mathcal{F}_2^{(i)}}{\partial u_1^{(i)}} & \cdots & \frac{\partial \mathcal{F}_2^{(i)}}{\partial P^{(i)}} \end{bmatrix}, \tag{9.16}$$

where

$$\mathcal{F}^{(i)} = \mathcal{F} \big|_{\mathscr{U}^t = \mathscr{U}^{(i-1)}, \ \mathscr{U}^{t+\Delta t} = \mathscr{U}^{(i)}}, \tag{9.17}$$

assuming that $i \in \mathbb{N}$ and $\mathscr{U}^{(0)}$ is the previously known value of $\mathscr{U}$ at the beginning of the increment (i.e. the values that have been computed from the previous increment or the initial state). In this manner, it linearizes the nonlinear equations iteratively with an initial guess $\mathscr{U}^{(1)}$, i.e.

$$\mathcal{F}^{(i+1)} = \mathcal{F}^{(i)} + \left(\mathscr{U}^{(i+1)} - \mathscr{U}^{(i)} \right) \cdot \mathfrak{J}^{(i)}. \tag{9.18}$$

To solve this problem, at each step the integrations in the discretized equations for each FE are calculated (typically with numerical approximation), resulting in a set of linear equations. These equations can then be solved either directly or iteratively using well-established techniques in linear algebra, thereby determining $\mathscr{U}^{(i+1)}$. This process is assumed converged once $\left(\mathcal{F}^{(i+1)} \right)^2$ becomes sufficiently small, indicating that Eq. (9.13) is approximately solved and the unknown parameters are estimated at step $t + \Delta t$. This is an extremely simplified representation of the numerical modeling, which can give an overall understanding of the solution procedure and its highly iterative nature (Belytschko et al. 2014). Furthermore, the exact definition of the shape functions may vary depending on the specific physics problem, e.g. the existence of contact mechanics and geometric complexity (Figure 9.3). Some implementations may use more advanced linearization techniques or apply an explicit FE method (Almeida and Spilker 1997; Korsawe et al. 2006; Nakahara et al. 2016). But regardless of these differences, they are still developed based on similar iterative algorithms, which explains why they can be expensive to run.

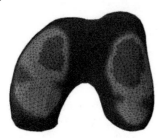
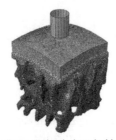
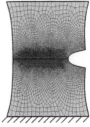

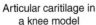
Articular caritilage in
a knee model

Cartilage and subchondral bone
interaction under indenter compression

Tear simulation in
articular cartilage

Figure 9.3 Examples of finite element studies, showing that element shapes depend on the geometric complexity and physics problems. Source: Orava et al. (2022), Orozco et al. (2022)/Elsevier/CC BY 4.0, and Ardatov et al. (2023).

9.3.2 Constitutive Modeling

We first introduce the tensors that are often used in constitutive modeling of nonlinear materials (Holzapfel 2000). Suppose $\nabla_X(\bullet)$ is the gradient operator of $\bullet$ with respect to the vector of undeformed position $\mathbf{X}$ and $\mathbf{I}$ is the identity tensor, the deformation gradient $\mathbf{F}$ is calculated as:

$$\mathbf{F} = \mathbf{I} + \nabla_X \mathbf{u}. \tag{9.19}$$

This is a measure of the relative deformation, formulated by a second-order tensor, which can be decomposed into an orthogonal tensor (i.e. the rotation tensor $\mathbf{R}$) and a positive definite symmetric tensor (i.e. the left stretch tensor $\mathbf{V}$), i.e.

$$\mathbf{F} = \mathbf{VR}. \tag{9.20}$$

This equation allows us to focus only on the stretch in the tissue (which is responsible for the stress response of the tissue in AC analyses), since $\mathbf{R}^T\mathbf{R} = \mathbf{I}$. The left Cauchy–Green tensor $\mathbf{B}$ is thus defined in such a way to exclude the effect of rigid body rotation. For this reason,

$$\mathbf{B} = \mathbf{FF}^T = \mathbf{V}^2. \tag{9.21}$$

These tensors can be associated with the volume ratio by

$$J = \sqrt{\det \mathbf{B}} = \det \mathbf{F} > 0. \tag{9.22}$$

With anisotropic materials, it is imperative to include the direction dependency in their equations. For example, the direction of the fibril bundle I is given by the unit direction vector $\mathbf{N}^I$, which can change to its new unit direction $\mathbf{n}^I$ after deformation. It can be calculated by first deforming the initial direction vector (using the deformation gradient) and then scaling it to its unit size, i.e.

$$\mathbf{n}^I = \frac{\mathbf{FN}^I}{\|\mathbf{FN}^I\|_2}, \tag{9.23}$$

where $\|\bullet\|_2$ denotes the l^2 norm of $\bullet$. Instead of considering the entire deformation, we can now focus on the deformation in the specific direction of the fibrils using the logarithmic strain ϵ^I in the direction of the deformed bundles (as a measure of the large deformation). Thus,

$$\epsilon^I = \log(\lambda^I), \tag{9.24}$$

where λ^I is the fibrillar stretch, which can be correlated with the total deformation using finite strain theory, i.e.

$$\lambda^I = \sqrt{\mathbf{n}^I \cdot \mathbf{B} \cdot \mathbf{n}^I}. \tag{9.25}$$

Now, the solid–fluid interaction is modeled using the classical porous media theory and Darcy's law, stating that the fluid flows from a region of higher pressure to lower pressure, and the rate of that depends on the material properties (Terzaghi 1943; Dullien 1979). Thus,

$$\phi^F \mathbf{v}_r = -\frac{1}{\mu} \mathbf{K} \cdot \nabla_x P, \tag{9.26}$$

where μ is the dynamic viscosity (the internal flow resistance of the fluid) and $\mathbf{K}$ is the permeability tensor (the ability to transmit fluids through the porous structure). In addition, the stress caused by this pressure together with the effective stress tensor σ^{EFF} (that transmits to the solid structure) determines the total stress σ_T as:

$$\sigma_T = \sigma^{EFF} - P\mathbf{I}. \tag{9.27}$$

By defining the constitutive behavior of the solid structure and its relationship with tissue deformation, Eq. (9.27) is fully determined. Once this equation and Eq. (9.26) are discretized (as explained in Section 9.3.1), they can be introduced into the governing equation, Eq. (9.13), to replace the relative velocity and stress tensor. Regardless of this, the inclusion of advanced multi-physics constitutive models of AC might make this process even more iterative. This is explained here by exemplifying one of the most up-to-date multiphasic cartilage models (Sajjadinia et al. 2021a).

The constrained mixture theory is used (Klisch 1999), which is arguably the most popular constitutive multi-physics model to define the effective stress in AC. It assumes the non-fluid phases are confined together and have a similar deformation, yielding

$$\sigma^{EFF} = \sigma^{COL} + \sigma^{MAT} - \sigma^{GAG}. \tag{9.28}$$

Here, the superscripts COL, MAT, and GAG denote the contributions of the fibrillar collagen network, the non-fibrillar extracellular matrix, and the osmotic pressure, respectively (Mow et al. 1980; Wilson et al. 2005; Sajjadinia et al. 2019).

Regarding the collagen fibrils, it is experimentally observed that they bear loads nonlinearly correlated with their strains (Charlebois et al. 2004), e.g. by $(E_1 + E_2\epsilon^I)\epsilon^I$, where E_1 and E_2 signify the degree of nonlinearity. This response, before application to its constitutive equation, needs two modifications: (i) multiplication by λ^I/J, the inverse of the fibril bundle surface area, to account for surface area effects; and (ii) multiplication by the components' volume fractions, reflecting each component's contribution according to the mixture theory. Thus, the tensile stress in each fibril bundle σ^I can be evaluated as follows (Wilson et al. 2007; Sajjadinia et al. 2019):

$$\sigma^I = \phi_0^S \rho_C^I \frac{\lambda^I}{J}(E_1 + E_2\epsilon^I)\epsilon^I, \tag{9.29}$$

where ρ_C^I is the volume fraction of the relevant fibrils and ϕ_0^S is the initial value of the solid volume fraction. Then the stress in the collagen fibril network σ^{COL} can be defined considering the contributions of all fibrils (Wilson et al. 2004), i.e.

$$\sigma^{COL} = \sum_{I=1}^{9} \sigma^I \mathbf{n}^I \otimes \mathbf{n}^I, \tag{9.30}$$

where $\otimes$ denotes the dyadic product. This summation takes into account the orientations of all bundles (as explained in Section 9.2.2) and their stress contributions.

Next, the osmotic pressure can be defined by first deriving a model for glycosaminoglycan-related electrostatic force and then simplifying it by relating this force only to the deformation in the solid matrix (Ateshian et al. 2004). This can lead to an exponential form of the osmotic stress contribution via two positive material constants, i.e. α_1 and α_2 (Buschmann and Grodzinsky 1995; Stender et al. 2013), i.e.

$$\sigma^{GAG} = \alpha_1 J^{-\alpha_2} \mathbf{I}. \tag{9.31}$$

The other components of the solid phase are usually represented by an isotropic nonlinear elastic model, e.g. using one of the popular neo-Hookean equations, formulated on the basis of the thermodynamics of rubber-like materials, see, e.g. Kim et al. (2012). This model is modified to consider the effects of the volume fractions of the material (Wilson et al. 2007; Sajjadinia et al. 2021a), i.e.

$$\sigma^{MAT} = \phi_0^S G_m \frac{1 - \rho_0^{COL}}{J} \left[-\frac{\ln J}{6} \left(3\phi_0^S \frac{J \ln J}{(J - \phi_0^S)^2} - 1 - 3\frac{J + \phi_0^S}{J - \phi_0^S} \right) \mathbf{I} + (\mathbf{B} - J^{2/3}\mathbf{I}) \right], \tag{9.32}$$

where G_m is an additional material constant and ρ_0^{COL} is the initial value of the total collagen volume fraction ρ^{COL}. The volume fractions are updated by the continuity equation of the solid phases as:

$$\varphi = \frac{\varphi_0}{J} \quad \varphi \in \{\phi^S, \rho^{COL}\}. \tag{9.33}$$

While the above-mentioned equations formulate the constitute behavior for FE analysis of cartilage, due to the fixed charges in this tissue, the *in vivo* data recorded in the literature mostly consider the prestressed state as the initial condition. This is in contrast to mathematical models, which typically consider the stress-free state as the initial state, resulting in a large discrepancy between the initial numerical conditions and the *in vivo* conditions. The pre-stress σ_0 can be verified by setting $\mathbf{F} = \mathbf{I}$ (which only applies the initial boundary conditions), i.e.

$$\sigma_0 = -\alpha \mathbf{I}. \tag{9.34}$$

This causes the tissue to swell until it reaches equilibrium (as mentioned in Section 9.2.2). This can then change the initial geometrical properties and material fractions, e.g. according to Eq. (9.33). Therefore, the numerical solvers should first find the pre-stressed state (observable as *in vivo*) by starting from the unknown stress-free state. The initial state can be approximated using a pre-stressing algorithm, which is essentially an optimization algorithm that employs multiple FE analyses to test various stress-free states and identify the approximate stress-free states (Wang et al. 2018; Sajjadinia et al. 2021a). The application of this algorithm makes the numerical simulation more iterative, which may be alleviated by ML, as briefly discussed in Section 9.4.

9.4 Al-Enhanced Modeling

9.4.1 Deep Learning

Assuming $\mathcal{X}$ and $\mathcal{Y}$ are the sets of corresponding measurable spaces, supervised ML is the task of constructing a model function f that can ideally map each element of input data $\mathcal{X}$ to its corresponding member in the output set $\mathcal{Y}$ according to

$$f : \mathcal{X} \longrightarrow \mathcal{Y}. \tag{9.35}$$

The output examples, used for generation and evaluation of the model, known as labels, are typically obtained by human or systemic supervision. Each input–output pair of samples can be characterized by multidimensional quantitative properties (or features). For example, in a pre-stressing simulation, the known pre-stressed geometry, physical constraints, and constitutive parameters can be used as input features, while the labels can be the observed or numerically calculated stress-free states.

Given a subset of labeled data $\mathcal{Z} \subset \mathcal{X} \times \mathcal{Y}$, a learning algorithm, especially in the context of deep learning, finds the best function f, using the errors measured by a loss function $\mathcal{L}$, i.e.

$$\mathcal{L} : \mathcal{M}(\mathcal{X}, \mathcal{Y}) \times \mathcal{Z} \longrightarrow \mathbb{R}, \tag{9.36}$$

where $\mathcal{M}(\mathcal{X}, \mathcal{Y})$ is the set of possible measurable and learnable functions with different hypothetical architectures, such as artificial neural networks (Abiodun et al. 2019). In the basic multilayer feed-forward neural network (FFNN) with fully connected or dense layers (Rumelhart et al. 1986), the sequence of input features (i.e. the input layer) is connected to its subsequent layer. The data derived from the previous layers provide the input signals of the next layer up to the very last output layer (generating the output data). Assuming such an FFNN model represented by $\Psi \in \mathcal{M}(\mathcal{X}, \mathcal{Y})$, then

$$\Psi(x; \cdot, \Theta) = \psi^{(L)}\left(\psi^{(L-1)}\left(\cdots\left(\psi^{(1)}\left(\psi^{(0)}(x)\right)\right)\right)\right). \tag{9.37}$$

Here, $\psi^{(i)}$ is a transformation through the layer $i \in [0, L]$, with the assumption that layer 0 is the input layer, i.e. $\psi^{(0)}(x) = x$. Also, Θ (the set of trainable parameters) and hyperparameters (like the number of layers) define the exact definition of each layer $\psi^{(i)}$. For most regression problems, the basic definition of $\psi^{(i)}$ is as follows:

$$\psi^{(i)}(x) = \begin{cases} W^{(i)}\psi^{(i-1)}(x) + b^{(i)} & \text{if } i = L, \\ a\left(W^{(i)}\psi^{(i-1)}(x) + b^{(i)}\right) & \text{others,} \end{cases} \tag{9.38}$$

where W and b are the trainable weight and bias parameters, respectively (finding the best linear combination), and a is the activation function, which nonlinearly amplifies or attenuates the effects of the input signals to help capture nonlinear patterns (Berner et al. 2022). An efficient activation function is the rectified linear unit function, which is basically a ramp function that ignores the negative signals (Fukushima 1980; Nair and Hinton 2010), i.e.

$$a(x) = \max(0, x). \tag{9.39}$$

During training, an initial guess of the trainable parameters is first made, which may result in some errors in the generated output data compared to the labels. This error can then be minimized by using an optimization algorithm that iteratively changes the trainable parameters until the most accurate and generalizable model is achieved.

The algorithm has undergone significant enhancements, most notably the integration of normalization layers, which stabilize the training of models by normalizing different distributions of input signals (Bianchi et al. 2012; Salimans and Kingma 2016; Bjorck et al. 2018; Xu et al. 2019). This allows implementation of neural networks with many hidden layers to tackle complex problems. In addition, specialized variations have been developed to cater to distinct data structures: recurrent neural networks (Yu et al. 2019) and transformers (Lin et al. 2022) for temporal information, and convolutional neural networks (Ajit et al. 2020) for spatial information. A challenge, however, is the lack of permutation invariance in these algorithms. This means the order of features is relevant, which becomes problematic with FE nodal data, where the order of nodal features to be considered is usually of no importance (Géron 2019).

In this regard, message-passing graph neural networks (MPGNNs) have two key benefits: their ability to maintain permutation invariance and to efficiently process varying numbers of nodes. The salient feature of MPGNNs is their focus on individual nodes and their connections to neighboring nodes rather than the entire mesh. Given a node n with a feature vector denoted by $\mathfrak{v}_n$, the set $\Gamma(n)$ of its neighboring nodes is derived from the mesh topology, i.e. the nodal connections. Subsequently, information about the neighbors is aggregated using an aggregation function, such as a sum function, to be further processed by an FFNN, i.e.

$$\mathfrak{v}'_n = \text{FFNN}\left(\sum_{i \in \Gamma(n)} \mathfrak{v}_i, \mathfrak{v}_n \right), \tag{9.40}$$

where $\mathfrak{v}'_n$ is the updated nodal representation. An enrichment of global information is possible by increasing the number of sequentially message-passing layers connected to one another. Despite the versatility of this method, it can be enhanced further through variations, e.g. by assigning features to each connection, i.e. edge features defined by different distance metrics to account for the nodal geometrical information. This approach eliminates the need to directly encode nodal positions as nodal features and allows spatial equivariance in the surrogate (Cai et al. 2018; Zhou et al. 2020; Wu et al. 2021).

Incorporating edge features or other types of features may alter the aggregation functions applied to each entity, such as the node and the edge, thus potentially changing Eq. (9.40). However, the underlying concepts remain the same: the mesh data is initially converted into a graph, and two FFNNs update each node or edge feature after aggregating the neighboring features. Consequently, a transformed graph representation is generated that facilitates learning by isolating highly local data. This process can be reiterated with further message passing until it reaches the output layer, yielding nodal outputs (Sperduti and Starita 1997; Battaglia et al. 2018; Riba et al. 2018).

9.4.2 Surrogate Modeling

Training the surrogates of cartilage models by supervised ML requires a set of data samples generated from a high-fidelity numerical model, as discussed in Section 9.3, which may become prohibitively expensive. Therefore, typical FFNNs were trained on the data generated from simplified FE models, e.g. Paiva et al. (2012) used a surrogate for their multiscale cartilage simulation but using a very simplified elastic model (ignoring the nonlinear multi-physics). Arbabi et al. (2016a) included the biphasic equations in their surrogate of a 2D cartilage model, but ignored the vital osmotic pressure. Arbabi et al. (2016b) then managed to use a multi-physics model to train the surrogate, but with 10,000 samples.

Under specific conditions, such as reducing the scale of the simulation, a surrogate may be generated with only a few samples; see, e.g. (Faisal et al. 2023). However, for complex multi-physics equations, particularly in large-scale and high-dimensional data, having a large training dataset becomes unavoidable. If the primary purpose of applying ML is to enhance efficiency, the models should ideally be trained on a limited number of samples, especially when the numerical generation of these samples is costly (Forrester et al. 2008). This factor often leads to the underutilization of AI-enhanced modeling techniques.

Our research group recently developed a specialized hybrid ML algorithm (Sajjadinia et al. 2022) that can be trained on very small datasets of the multi-physics models of soft tissues, especially cartilage-like materials. The key idea is to insert a simplified version of the numerical model into the surrogate model by ignoring some of the physical behaviors of the high-fidelity model, e.g. some of the constitutive equations, to create a dataset with low-fidelity but inexpensive samples. The ML model then finds a mapping between the low-fidelity and high-fidelity data, and therefore, the high-fidelity model is only used for training. The low-fidelity numerical model used in the surrogate transforms the input features into more informative features, i.e. an approximation of the high-fidelity results that can significantly improve the training performance with small datasets. This has been shown experimentally by 2D and 3D simulations.

The 2D simulations, shown in Figure 9.4, chose a multi-physics model with and without pre-stressing optimizers for the low-fidelity and high-fidelity models, respectively, on two sets of in-distribution validation samples and out-of-distribution test samples (to also

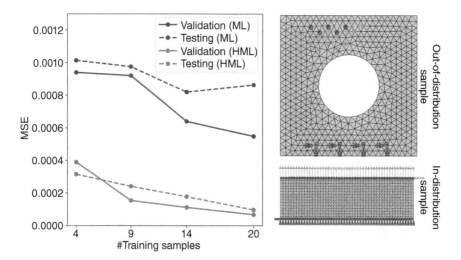

Figure 9.4 Examples of 2D in-distribution and out-of-distribution models used in the validation and test sets (right) and the corresponding plot of the trained surrogate errors in these sets versus the number of training samples (left). Source: Sajjadinia et al. (2022). Abbreviation: MSE = mean squared error; ML = machine learning; HML = hybrid machine learning.

assess the generalizability of the surrogates). The results indicate that the hybrid ML model can outperform the ML surrogates with only four samples (using the MPGNNs that allow generalizable inference). Likewise, through pointwise evaluation (Sajjadinia et al. 2021b), we observed similar performance improvements in another 3D model in that study. The latency (run-time after training) of this model was relatively 2 to 14 times smaller, even though the numerical model had been simplified for fast data generation.

While specialized surrogate models are not commonly applied in AC modeling, likely due to the complexity of implementing numerical models, previous studies have successfully used multi-fidelity approaches with different hybrid or full ML surrogates. These approaches have yielded comparable performance improvements in other application domains. Traditional ML techniques, such as Gaussian processes, have predominantly been used (Cheng et al. 2021; Zhang et al. 2022), while advanced physics problems are often implemented using different neural network architectures (Yang and Perdikaris 2019; Ahn et al. 2022). With these promising results, multi-fidelity, and hybrid surrogates are expected to further advance in the biomechanical modeling of AC.

9.5 Discussion and Conclusion

This chapter has provided an overview of biomechanical modeling methods enhanced with AI that perform advanced numerical simulations using ML surrogates. Focusing on the biomechanical constitutive modeling of cartilage, we first reviewed the main load-bearing components of AC (to be included in the high-fidelity simulations) and then we elaborated on the constitutive equations to demonstrate the complexity of such models. In particular, it was pointed out that these models are commonly implemented through advanced multi-physics equations and iterative numerical algorithms, making their data generation too time-consuming. We have tried to clarify that ML surrogates may solve this problem, especially when implemented by the multi-fidelity and hybrid ML algorithms.

The hybrid ML implementations showed encouraging results as they could be trained with fewer samples compared to the regular ML counterparts. However, they were only tested on simplified numerical models, and the important collagen fibrils were neglected. Therefore, an interesting research direction for future studies is to evaluate such hybrid methods using all major biomechanical components of cartilage. This raises further questions regarding the exact learning and numerical methods that can find the best compromise between the performance and computational efforts for different simulation tasks.

In summary, the contribution of hybrid surrogates to AC modeling can be seen as an example of the meaningful application of AI in biomechanical simulation or more generally in the field of *in silico* biomedicine.

Author Biographies

Seyed Shayan Sajjadinia is currently a PhD student in Computer Science at the Faculty of Engineering, University of Bozen-Bolzano with also an educational background in biomechanical engineering. His research interest is application of deep learning and finite element analysis in computer simulation, especially in advanced biomechanical analysis, which is the focus of his PhD research dissertation.

Bruno Carpentieri earned a Laurea degree in Applied Mathematics from Bari University in 1997 and then pursued his PhD studies in Computer Science at Toulouse, France. He has gained professional experience as a postdoctoral researcher at the University of Graz, as an Assistant Professor at the University of Groningen, and as a Reader at Nottingham Trent University. Since May 2017, he holds the position of Associate Professor in Applied Mathematics at the Faculty of Engineering, University of Bozen-Bolzano. His scientific interests include numerical linear algebra and high-performance computing.

Gerhard A. Holzapfel is a Professor and head of the Institute of Biomechanics at Graz University of Technology, an Adjunct Professor at the Norwegian University of Science and Technology, and a Visiting Professor at the University of Glasgow. He has made significant contributions in the field of experimental and computational biomechanics, with a particular interest in soft biological tissues. He has received numerous awards and honors for his work and is listed in "The World's Most Influential Scientific Minds: 2014" by Thomas Reuters. Professor Holzapfel is also the cofounder and coeditor-in-chief of the journal of Biomechanics and Modeling in Mechanobiology.

References

Abaqus (2021). Dassault Systèmes Simulia Corp. Providence, RI. http://www.simulia.com.

Abiodun, O.I., Jantan, A., Omolara, A.E. et al. (2019). Comprehensive review of artificial neural network applications to pattern recognition. *IEEE Access* 7: 158820–158846. https://doi.org/10.1109/ACCESS.2019.2945545.

Ahn, J.G., Yang, H.I., and Kim, J.G. (2022). Multi-fidelity meta modeling using composite neural network with online adaptive basis technique. *Computer Methods in Applied Mechanics and Engineering* 388: 114258. https://doi.org/10.1016/j.cma.2021.114258.

Ajit, A., Acharya, K., and Samanta, A. (2020). A review of convolutional neural networks. *2020 International Conference on Emerging Trends in Information Technology and Engineering (ic-ETITE)*, 1–5. https://doi.org/10.1109/ic-ETITE47903.2020.049.

Almeida, E.S. and Spilker, R.L. (1997). Mixed and penalty finite element models for the nonlinear behavior of biphasic soft tissues in finite deformation: Part I – alternate formulations. *Computer Methods in Biomechanics and Biomedical Engineering* 1(1): 25–46. https://doi.org/10.1080/01495739708936693.

Alunni Cardinali, M., Govoni, M., Tschon, M. et al. (2023). Brillouin–Raman micro-spectroscopy and machine learning techniques to classify osteoarthritic lesions in the human articular cartilage. *Scientific Reports* 13(1): 1690. https://doi.org/10.1038/s41598-023-28735-5.

Antman, S.S. and Osborn, J.E. (1979). The principle of virtual work and integral laws of motion. *Archive for Rational Mechanics and Analysis* 69(3): 231–262. https://doi.org/10.1007/BF00248135.

Arbabi, V., Pouran, B., Campoli, G. et al. (2016a). Determination of the mechanical and physical properties of cartilage by coupling poroelastic-based finite element models of indentation with artificial neural networks. *Journal of Biomechanics* 49(5): 631–637. https://doi.org/10.1016/j.jbiomech.2015.12.014.

Arbabi, V., Pouran, B., Weinans, H., and Zadpoor, A.A. (2016b). Combined inverse-forward artificial neural networks for fast and accurate estimation of the diffusion coefficients of cartilage based on multi-physics models. *Journal of Biomechanics* 49(13): 2799–2805. https://doi.org/10.1016/j.jbiomech.2016.06.019.

Ardatov, O., Aleksiuk, V., Macknickas, A. et al. (2023). Modeling the impact of meniscal tears on von Mises stress of knee cartilage tissue. *Bioengineering* 10(3): https://doi.org/10.3390/bioengineering10030314.

Astephen Wilson, J.L. and Kobsar, D. (2021). Osteoarthritis year in review 2020: mechanics. *Osteoarthritis and Cartilage* 29(2): 161–169. https://doi.org/10.1016/j.joca.2020.12.009.

Ateshian, G.A., Chahine, N.O., Basalo, I.M., and Hung, C.T. (2004). The correspondence between equilibrium biphasic and triphasic material properties in mixture models of articular cartilage. *Journal of Biomechanics* 37(3): 391–400. https://doi.org/10.1016/S0021-9290(03)00252-5.

Banks, H.T., Hu, S., and Kenz, Z.R. (2011). A brief review of elasticity and viscoelasticity for solids. *Advances in Applied Mathematics and Mechanics* 3(1): 1–51. https://doi.org/10.4208/aamm.10-m1030.

Battaglia, P.W., Hamrick, J.B., Bapst, V., et al. (2018). Relational inductive biases, deep learning, and graph networks. https://doi.org/10.48550/arxiv.1806.01261.

Beidokhti, H.N., Janssen, D., Khoshgoftar, M. et al. (2016). A comparison between dynamic implicit and explicit finite element simulations of the native knee joint. *Medical Engineering & Physics* 38(10): 1123–1130. https://doi.org/10.1016/j.medengphy.2016.06.001.

Belytschko, T., Liu, W.K., Moran, B., and Elkhodary, K. (2014). *Nonlinear Finite Elements for Continua and Structures*. Wiley.

Berner, J., Grohs, P., Kutyniok, G., and Petersen, P. (2022). The modern mathematics of deep learning. In: *Mathematical Aspects of Deep Learning* (ed. P. Grohs and G. Kutyniok), 1–111. Cambridge University Press. https://doi.org/10.1017/9781009025096.002.

Bianchi, M., Kassay, G., and Pini, R. (2012). Conditioning for optimization problems under general perturbations. *Nonlinear Analysis: Theory, Methods & Applications* 75(1): 37–45. https://doi.org/10.1016/j.na.2011.07.061.

Bielajew, B.J., Hu, J.C., and Athanasiou, K.A. (2020). Collagen: quantification, biomechanics and role of minor subtypes in cartilage. *Nature Reviews Materials* 5(10): 730–747. https://doi.org/10.1038/s41578-020-0213-1.

Bjorck, N., Gomes, C.P., Selman, B., and Weinberger, K.Q. (2018). Understanding batch normalization. In: *Advances in Neural Information Processing Systems*, vol. 31 (ed. S. Bengio, H. Wallach, H. Larochelle, et al.). Curran Associates, Inc. https://proceedings.neurips.cc/paper/2018/file/36072923bfc3cf47745d704feb489480-Paper.pdf.

Bozec, L., van der Heijden, G., and Horton, M. (2007). Collagen fibrils: nanoscale ropes. *Biophysical Journal* 92(1): 70–75. https://doi.org/10.1529/biophysj.106.085704.

Brody, L.T. (2015). Knee osteoarthritis: clinical connections to articular cartilage structure and function. *Physical Therapy in Sport* 16(4): 301–316. https://doi.org/10.1016/j.ptsp.2014.12.001.

Buckwalter, J.A. (1995). Osteoarthritis and articular cartilage use, disuse, and abuse: experimental studies. *The Journal of Rheumatology. Supplement* 43: 13–15. http://europepmc.org/abstract/MED/7752117.

Buschmann, M.D. and Grodzinsky, A.J. (1995). A molecular model of proteoglycan-associated electrostatic forces in cartilage mechanics. *Journal of Biomechanical Engineering* 117(2): 179–192. https://doi.org/10.1115/1.2796000.

Cai, H., Zheng, V.W., and Chang, K.C. (2018). A comprehensive survey of graph embedding: problems, techniques, and applications. *IEEE Transactions on Knowledge and Data Engineering* 30(9): 1616–1637. https://doi.org/10.1109/TKDE.2018.2807452.

Cederlund, A.A. and Aspden, R.M. (2022). Walking on water: revisiting the role of water in articular cartilage biomechanics in relation to tissue engineering and regenerative medicine. *Journal of The Royal Society Interface* 19(193): 20220364. https://doi.org/10.1098/rsif.2022.0364.

Charlebois, M., McKee, M.D., and Buschmann, M.D. (2004). Nonlinear tensile properties of bovine articular cartilage and their variation with age and depth. *Journal of Biomechanical Engineering* 126(2): 129–137. https://doi.org/10.1115/1.1688771.

Chen, A., Gupte, C., and Akhtar, K. (2012). The global economic cost of osteoarthritis: how the UK compares. *Arthritis* 2012: 698709. https://doi.org/10.1155/2012/698709.

Chen, S., Fu, P., Wu, H., and Pei, M. (2017). Meniscus, articular cartilage and nucleus pulposus: a comparative review of cartilage-like tissues in anatomy, development and function. *Cell and Tissue Research* 370(1): 53–70. https://doi.org/10.1007/s00441-017-2613-0.

Cheng, M., Jiang, P., Hu, J. et al. (2021). A multi-fidelity surrogate modeling method based on variance-weighted sum for the fusion of multiple non-hierarchical low-fidelity data. *Structural and Multidisciplinary Optimization* 64(6): 3797–3818. https://doi.org/10.1007/s00158-021-03055-2.

Clark, J.M. (1985). The organization of collagen in cryofractured rabbit articular cartilage: a scanning electron microscopic study. *Journal of Orthopaedic Research* 3(1): 17–29. https://doi.org/10.1002/jor.1100030102.

Cooke, M.E., Lawless, B.M., Jones, S.W., and Grover, L.M. (2018). Matrix degradation in osteoarthritis primes the superficial region of cartilage for mechanical damage. *Acta Biomaterialia* 78: 320–328. https://doi.org/10.1016/j.actbio.2018.07.037.

Cooper, R.J., Wilcox, R.K., and Jones, A.C. (2019). Finite element models of the tibiofemoral joint: a review of validation approaches and modelling challenges. *Medical Engineering & Physics* 74: 1–12. https://doi.org/10.1016/j.medengphy.2019.08.002.

Culav, E.M., Clark, C.H., and Merrilees, M.J. (1999). Connective tissues: matrix composition and its relevance to physical therapy. *Physical Therapy* 79(3): 308–319. https://doi.org/10.1093/ptj/79.3.308.

Danso, E.K., Honkanen, J.T.J., Saarakkala, S., and Korhonen, R.K. (2014). Comparison of nonlinear mechanical properties of bovine articular cartilage and meniscus. *Journal of Biomechanics* 47(1): 200–206. https://doi.org/10.1016/j.jbiomech.2013.09.015.

Dudhia, J. (2005). Aggrecan, aging and assembly in articular cartilage. *Cellular and Molecular Life Sciences CMLS* 62(19): 2241–2256. https://doi.org/10.1007/s00018-005-5217-x.

Dullien, F.A.L. (1979). *Porous Media: Fluid Transport and Pore Structure*. Elsevier Science.

Dye, S.F. (1987). An evolutionary perspective of the knee. *The Journal of Bone and Joint Surgery. American Volume* 69(7): 976–983. http://europepmc.org/abstract/MED/3654710.

Ebrahimi, M., Ojanen, S., Mohammadi, A. et al. (2019). Elastic, viscoelastic and fibril-reinforced poroelastic material properties of healthy and osteoarthritic human tibial cartilage. *Annals of Biomedical Engineering* 47(4): 953–966. https://doi.org/10.1007/s10439-019-02213-4.

Egli, F.S., Straube, R.C., Mielke, A., and Ricken, T. (2021). Surrogate modeling of a nonlinear, biphasic model of articular cartilage with artificial neural networks. *PAMM* 21(1): e202100188. https://doi.org/10.1002/pamm.202100188.

Eschweiler, J., Horn, N., Rath, B. et al. (2021). The biomechanics of cartilage – an overview. *Life* 11(4): https://doi.org/10.3390/life11040302.

Faisal, T.R., Adouni, M., and Dhaher, Y.Y. (2023). Surrogate modeling of articular cartilage degradation to understand the synergistic role of MMP-1 and MMP-9: a case study. *Biomechanics and Modeling in Mechanobiology* 22(1): 43–56. https://doi.org/10.1007/s10237-022-01630-0.

Forrester, A.I.J., Sóbester, A., and Keane, A.J. (2008). *Engineering Design via Surrogate Modelling*. Wiley. https://doi.org/10.1002/9780470770801.

Forster, H. and Fisher, J. (1996). The influence of loading time and lubricant on the friction of articular cartilage. *Proceedings of the Institution of Mechanical Engineers, Part H: Journal of Engineering in Medicine* 210(2): 109–119. https://doi.org/10.1243/PIME_PROC_1996_210_399_02.

Freutel, M., Schmidt, H., Dürselen, L. et al. (2014). Finite element modeling of soft tissues: material models, tissue interaction and challenges. *Clinical Biomechanics* 29(4): 363–372. https://doi.org/10.1016/j.clinbiomech.2014.01.006.

Fukushima, K. (1980). Neocognitron: a self-organizing neural network model for a mechanism of pattern recognition unaffected by shift in position. *Biological Cybernetics* 36(4): 193–202. https://doi.org/10.1007/BF00344251.

Géron, A. (2019). *Hands-On Machine Learning with Scikit-Learn, Keras, and TensorFlow: Concepts, Tools, and Techniques to Build Intelligent Systems*, 2e. O'Reilly Media, Inc. ISBN: 9781492032649.

Goldblatt, J.P. and Richmond, J.C. (2003). Anatomy and biomechanics of the knee. *Operative Techniques in Sports Medicine* 11(3): 172–186. https://doi.org/10.1053/otsm.2003.35911. The Multiple Ligament Injured Knee, Part I.

Goldring, M.B. (2012). Articular cartilage degradation in osteoarthritis. *HSS Journal®* 8(1): 7–9. https://doi.org/10.1007/s11420-011-9250-z.

Gómez-Florit, M., Domingues, R.M.A., Bakht, S.M. et al. (2020). 1.3.6 –natural materials. In: *Biomaterials Science*, 4e (ed. W.R. Wagner, S.E. Sakiyama-Elbert, G. Zhang, et al.), 361–375. Academic Press. ISBN: 978-0-12-816137-1. https://doi.org/10.1016/B978-0-12-816137-1.00026-X.

Haut Donahue, T.L., Hull, M.L., Rashid, M.M. et al. (2002). A finite element model of the human knee joint for the study of tibio-femoral contact. *Journal of Biomechanical Engineering* 124(3): 273–280. https://doi.org/10.1115/1.1470171.

Hawker, G.A. (2019). Osteoarthritis is a serious disease. *Clinical and Experimental Rheumatology* 37(5 Suppl 120): 3–6. http://europepmc.org/abstract/med/31621562.

Holzapfel, G.A. (2000). *Nonlinear Solid Mechanics: A Continuum Approach for Engineering*. Chichester: Wiley.

Johnson, D., Hashaikeh, R., and Hilal, N. (2021). 1 - basic principles of osmosis and osmotic pressure. In: *Osmosis Engineering* (ed. N. Hilal, A.F. Ismail, M. Khayet, et al.), 1–15. Elsevier. ISBN: 978-0-12-821016-1. https://doi.org/10.1016/B978-0-12-821016-1.00011-5.

Kazemi, M., Li, L.P., Savard, P., and Buschmann, M.D. (2011). Creep behavior of the intact and meniscectomy knee joints. *Journal of the Mechanical Behavior of Biomedical Materials* 4(7): 1351–1358. https://doi.org/10.1016/j.jmbbm.2011.05.004.

Kiani, C., Chen, L., Wu, Y.J. et al. (2002). Structure and function of aggrecan. *Cell Research* 12(1): 19–32. https://doi.org/10.1038/sj.cr.7290106.

Kim, B., Lee, S.B., Lee, J. et al. (2012). A comparison among neo-Hookean model, Mooney-Rivlin model, and Ogden model for chloroprene rubber. *International Journal of Precision Engineering and Manufacturing* 13(5): 759–764. https://doi.org/10.1007/s12541-012-0099-y.

Klika, V., Gaffney, E.A., Chen, Y.C., and Brown, C.P. (2016). An overview of multiphase cartilage mechanical modelling and its role in understanding function and pathology. *Journal of the Mechanical Behavior of Biomedical Materials* 62: 139–157. https://doi.org/10.1016/j.jmbbm.2016.04.032.

Klisch, S.M. (1999). Internally constrained mixtures of elastic continua. *Mathematics and Mechanics of Solids* 4(4): 481–498. https://doi.org/10.1177/108128659900400405.

Kong, H., Wang, X.Q., and Zhang, X.A. (2022). Exercise for osteoarthritis: a literature review of pathology and mechanism. *Frontiers in Aging Neuroscience* 14: https://doi.org/10.3389/fnagi.2022.854026.

Korsawe, J., Starke, G., Wang, W., and Kolditz, O. (2006). Finite element analysis of poro-elastic consolidation in porous media: standard and mixed approaches. *Computer Methods in Applied Mechanics and Engineering* 195(9): 1096–1115. https://doi.org/10.1016/j.cma.2005.04.011.

Lespasio, M.J., Piuzzi, N.S., Husni, M.E. et al. (2017). Knee osteoarthritis: a primer. *The Permanente Journal* 21: 16–183. https://doi.org/10.7812/tpp/16-183.

Lin, W., Meng, Q., Li, J. et al. (2021). The effect of highly inhomogeneous biphasic properties on mechanical behaviour of articular cartilage. *Computer Methods and Programs in Biomedicine* 206: 106122. https://doi.org/10.1016/j.cmpb.2021.106122.

Lin, T., Wang, Y., Liu, X., and Qiu, X. (2022). A survey of transformers. *AI Open* 3: 111–132. https://doi.org/10.1016/j.aiopen.2022.10.001.

Loeser, R.F., Collins, J.A., and Diekman, B.O. (2016). Ageing and the pathogenesis of osteoarthritis. *Nature Reviews Rheumatology* 12(7): 412–420. https://doi.org/10.1038/nrrheum.2016.65.

Lostado Lorza, R., Somovilla Gomez, F., Corral Bobadilla, M. et al. (2021). Comparative analysis of healthy and cam-type femoroacetabular impingement (FAI) human hip joints using the finite element method. *Applied Sciences* 11(23): https://doi.org/10.3390/app112311101.

Lu, X.L. and Mow, V.C. (2008). Biomechanics of articular cartilage and determination of material properties. *Medicine & Science in Sports & Exercise* 40(2): https://doi.org/10.1249/mss.0b013e31815cb1fc.

Mameri, E.S., Dasari, S.P., Fortier, L.M. et al. (2022). Review of meniscus anatomy and biomechanics. *Current Reviews in Musculoskeletal Medicine* 15(5): 323–335. https://doi.org/10.1007/s12178-022-09768-1.

Martínez-Moreno, D., Jiménez, G., Gálvez-Martín, P. et al. (2019). Cartilage biomechanics: a key factor for osteoarthritis regenerative medicine. *Biochimica et Biophysica Acta (BBA) - Molecular Basis of Disease* 1865(6): 1067–1075. https://doi.org/10.1016/j.bbadis.2019.03.011.

Mirmojarabian, S.A., Kajabi, A.W., Ketola, J.H.J. et al. (2023). Machine learning prediction of collagen fiber orientation and proteoglycan content from multiparametric quantitative MRI in articular cartilage. *Journal of Magnetic Resonance Imaging* 57(4): 1056–1068. https://doi.org/10.1002/jmri.28353.

Mobasheri, A., Rayman, M.P., Gualillo, O. et al. (2017). The role of metabolism in the pathogenesis of osteoarthritis. *Nature Reviews Rheumatology* 13(5): 302–311. https://doi.org/10.1038/nrrheum.2017.50.

Motavalli, M., Akkus, O., and Mansour, J.M. (2014). Depth-dependent shear behavior of bovine articular cartilage: relationship to structure. *Journal of Anatomy* 225(5): 519–526. https://doi.org/10.1111/joa.12230.

Mow, V.C., Kuei, S.C., Lai, W.M., and Armstrong, C.G. (1980). Biphasic creep and stress relaxation of articular cartilage in compression: theory and experiments. *Journal of Biomechanical Engineering* 102(1): 73–84. https://doi.org/10.1115/1.3138202.

Nair, V. and Hinton, G.E. (2010). Rectified linear units improve restricted Boltzmann machines. *Proceedings of the 27th International Conference on International Conference on Machine Learning, ICML'10*, 807–814. ISBN 9781605589077. https://icml.cc/Conferences/2010/papers/432.pdf.

Nakahara, K., Morita, Y., Tomita, Y., and Nakamachi, E. (2016). Stress evaluation of articular cartilage chondrocyte cell by using multi-scale finite element method and smoothed particle hydrodynamics method. *Biomedical and Biotechnology Engineering of ASME International Mechanical Engineering Congress and Exposition*, Volume 3. https://doi.org/10.1115/IMECE2016-66416.

Niasar, E.H.A. and Li, L.P. (2023). Characterizing site-specific mechanical properties of knee cartilage with indentation-relaxation maps and machine learning. *Journal of the Mechanical Behavior of Biomedical Materials* 142: 105826. https://doi.org/10.1016/j.jmbbm.2023.105826.

Orava, H., Huang, L., Ojanen, S.P. et al. (2022). Changes in subchondral bone structure and mechanical properties do not substantially affect cartilage mechanical responses –a finite element study. *Journal of the Mechanical Behavior of Biomedical Materials* 128: 105129. https://doi.org/10.1016/j.jmbbm.2022.105129.

Orozco, G.A., Tanska, P., Gustafsson, A. et al. (2022). Crack propagation in articular cartilage under cyclic loading using cohesive finite element modeling. *Journal of the Mechanical Behavior of Biomedical Materials* 131: 105227. https://doi.org/10.1016/j.jmbbm.2022.105227.

Paiva, G., Bhashyam, S., Thiagarajan, G., et al. (2012). A data-driven surrogate model to connect scales between multi-domain biomechanics simulations. *Annual International Conference of the IEEE Engineering in Medicine and Biology Society*, 3077–3080. https://doi.org/10.1109/EMBC.2012.6346614.

Paz, A., Orozco, G.A., Tanska, P. et al. (2022). A novel knee joint model in FEBio with inhomogeneous fibril-reinforced biphasic cartilage simulating tissue mechanical responses during gait: data from the osteoarthritis initiative. *Computer Methods in Biomechanics and Biomedical Engineering* 26(11): 1353–1367. https://doi.org/10.1080/10255842.2022.2117548.

Pearle, A.D., Warren, R.F., and Rodeo, S.A. (2005). Basic science of articular cartilage and osteoarthritis. *Clinics in Sports Medicine* 24(1): 1–12. https://doi.org/10.1016/j.csm.2004.08.007.

Quiroga, J.M.P., Wilson, W., Ito, K., and van Donkelaar, C.C. (2017). Relative contribution of articular cartilage's constitutive components to load support depending on strain rate. *Biomechanics and Modeling in Mechanobiology* 16(1): 151–158. https://doi.org/10.1007/s10237-016-0807-0.

Riba, P., Fischer, A., Lladós, J., Fornés, A. (2018). Learning graph distances with message passing neural networks. *24th International Conference on Pattern Recognition (ICPR)*, 2239–2244. https://doi.org/10.1109/ICPR.2018.8545310.

Rumelhart, D.E., Hinton, G.E., and Williams, R.J. (1986). Learning representations by back-propagating errors. *Nature* 323(6088): 533–536. https://doi.org/10.1038/323533a0.

Sajjadinia, S.S. and Haghpanahi, M. (2021). A parametric study on the mechanical role of fibrillar rotations in an articular cartilage finite element model. *Scientia Iranica* 28(2): 830–836. https://doi.org/10.24200/sci.2020.51785.2362.

Sajjadinia, S.S., Haghpanahi, M., and Razi, M. (2019). Computational simulation of the multiphasic degeneration of the bone-cartilage unit during osteoarthritis via indentation and unconfined compression tests. *Proceedings of the Institution of Mechanical Engineers, Part H: Journal of Engineering in Medicine* 233(9): 871–882. https://doi.org/10.1177/0954411919854011.

Sajjadinia, S.S., Carpentieri, B., and Holzapfel, G.A. (2021a). A backward pre-stressing algorithm for efficient finite element implementation of in vivo material and geometrical parameters into fibril-reinforced mixture models of articular cartilage. *Journal of the Mechanical Behavior of Biomedical Materials* 114: 104203. https://doi.org/10.1016/j.jmbbm.2020.104203.

Sajjadinia, S.S., Carpentieri, B., and Holzapfel, G.A. (2021b). A pointwise evaluation metric to visualize errors in machine learning surrogate models. In: *Proceedings of CECNet 2021, Frontiers in Artificial Intelligence and Applications*, vol. 345 (ed. A.J. Tallón-Ballesteros), 26–34. IOS Press https://doi.org/10.3233/FAIA210386.

Sajjadinia, S.S., Carpentieri, B., Shriram, D., and Holzapfel, G.A. (2022). Multi-fidelity surrogate modeling through hybrid machine learning for biomechanical and finite element analysis of soft tissues. *Computers in Biology and Medicine* 148: 105699. https://doi.org/10.1016/j.compbiomed.2022.105699.

Salimans, T. and Kingma, D.P. (2016). Weight normalization: a simple reparameterization to accelerate training of deep neural networks. In: *Advances in Neural Information Processing Systems*, vol. 29 (ed. D. Lee, M. Sugiyama, U. Luxburg, et al.). Curran Associates, Inc. https://proceedings.neurips.cc/paper/2016/file/ed265bc903a5a097f61d3ec064d96d2e-Paper.pdf.

Salmon, J.H., Rat, A.C., Sellam, J. et al. (2016). Economic impact of lower-limb osteoarthritis worldwide: a systematic review of cost-of-illness studies. *Osteoarthritis and Cartilage* 24(9): 1500–1508. https://doi.org/10.1016/j.joca.2016.03.012.

Shirazi, R. and Shirazi-Adl, A. (2008). Deep vertical collagen fibrils play a significant role in mechanics of articular cartilage. *Journal of Orthopaedic Research* 26(5): 608–615. https://doi.org/10.1002/jor.20537.

Sperduti, A. and Starita, A. (1997). Supervised neural networks for the classification of structures. *IEEE Transactions on Neural Networks* 8(3): 714–735. https://doi.org/10.1109/72 .572108.

Stender, M.E., Raub, C.B., Yamauchi, K.A. et al. (2013). Integrating qPLM and biomechanical test data with an anisotropic fiber distribution model and predictions of TGF-β1 and IGF-1 regulation of articular cartilage fiber modulus. *Biomechanics and Modeling in Mechanobiology* 12(6): 1073–1088. https://doi.org/10.1007/s10237-012-0463-y.

Terzaghi, K. (1943). *Theoretical Soil Mechanics*. Hoboken, NJ: Wiley.

Vulović, A., Filardo, G., and Filipović, N. (2021). Comparison of mechanical response of knee joint with healthy and damaged femoral cartilage. *IEEE 21st International Conference on Bioinformatics and Bioengineering (BIBE)*, 1–4. https://doi.org/10.1109/BIBE52308.2021 .9635319.

Walker, P.S. and Erkman, M.J. (1975). The role of the menisci in force transmission across the knee. *Clinical Orthopaedics and Related Research* 109: 184–192. https://doi.org/10.1097/ 00003086-197506000-00027.

Wang, M. and Yang, N. (2018). Three-dimensional computational model simulating the fracture healing process with both biphasic poroelastic finite element analysis and fuzzy logic control. *Scientific Reports* 8(1): 6744. https://doi.org/10.1038/s41598-018-25229-7.

Wang, X., Eriksson, T.S.E., Ricken, T., and Pierce, D.M. (2018). On incorporating osmotic prestretch/prestress in image-driven finite element simulations of cartilage. *Journal of the Mechanical Behavior of Biomedical Materials* 86: 409–422. https://doi.org/10.1016/j.jmbbm .2018.06.014.

Wilson, W., van Donkelaar, C.C., van Rietbergen, B. et al. (2004). Stresses in the local collagen network of articular cartilage: a poroviscoelastic fibril-reinforced finite element study. *Journal of Biomechanics* 37(3): 357–366. https://doi.org/10.1016/S0021-9290(03)00267-7.

Wilson, W., van Donkelaar, C.C., van Rietbergen, B., and Huiskes, R. (2005). A fibril-reinforced poroviscoelastic swelling model for articular cartilage. *Journal of Biomechanics* 38(6): 1195–1204. https://doi.org/10.1016/j.jbiomech.2004.07.003.

Wilson, W., Huyghe, J.M., and van Donkelaar, C.C. (2007). Depth-dependent compressive equilibrium properties of articular cartilage explained by its composition. *Biomechanics and Modeling in Mechanobiology* 6(1): 43–53. https://doi.org/10.1007/s10237-006-0044-z.

Wu, Z., Pan, S., Chen, F. et al. (2021). A comprehensive survey on graph neural networks. *IEEE Transactions on Neural Networks and Learning Systems* 32(1): 4–24. https://doi.org/10.1109/ tnnls.2020.2978386.

Xu, J., Sun, X., Zhang, Z. et al. (2019). Understanding and improving layer normalization. In: *Advances in Neural Information Processing Systems*, vol. 32 (ed. H. Wallach, H. Larochelle, A. Beygelzimer, et al.). Curran Associates, Inc. https://proceedings.neurips.cc/paper/2019/ file/2f4fe03d77724a7217006e5d16728874-Paper.pdf.

Yang, Y. and Perdikaris, P. (2019). Conditional deep surrogate models for stochastic, high-dimensional, and multi-fidelity systems. *Computational Mechanics* 64(2): 417–434. https://doi.org/10.1007/s00466-019-01718-y.

Yu, Y., Si, X., Hu, C., and Zhang, J. (2019). A review of recurrent neural networks: LSTM cells and network architectures. *Neural Computation* 31(7): 1235–1270. https://doi.org/10.1162/ neco_a_01199.

Zhang, L., Wu, Y., Jiang, P. et al. (2022). A multi-fidelity surrogate modeling approach for incorporating multiple non-hierarchical low-fidelity data. *Advanced Engineering Informatics* 51: 101430. https://doi.org/10.1016/j.aei.2021.101430.

Zhou, J., Cui, G., Hu, S. et al. (2020). Graph neural networks: a review of methods and applications. *AI Open* 1: 57–81. https://doi.org/10.1016/j.aiopen.2021.01.001.

10

A Hybrid of Differential Evolution and Minimization of Metabolic Adjustment for Succinic and Ethanol Production

Zhang N. Hor[1], Mohd S. Mohamad[2,3], Yee W. Choon[4,5], Muhammad A. Remli[4,5] and Hairudin A. Majid[1]

[1] *Faculty of Computing, Universiti Teknologi Malaysia, 81310 UTM Johor Bahru, Johor, Malaysia*
[2] *Health Data Science Lab, Department of Genetics and Genomics, College of Medical and Health Sciences, United Arab Emirates University, Al Ain, Abu Dhabi, United Arab Emirates*
[3] *Big Data Analytics Center, United Arab Emirates University, Al Ain, Abu Dhabi, United Arab Emirates*
[4] *Artificial Intelligence Lab, Institute for Artificial Intelligence and Big Data, Universiti Malaysia Kelantan, Kota Bharu 16100, Kelantan, Malaysia*
[5] *Faculty of Data Science and Computing, Universiti Malaysia Kelantan, Kota Bharu 16100, Kelantan, Malaysia*

10.1 Introduction

Succinic acid is commonly used for flavor improvement in nutritional products and pharmaceutical supplements, while ethanol is widely used in the automobile, pharmaceutical, antiseptic, and good solvent sectors. Previous research has demonstrated some available approaches to overcome the problem of metabolic engineering. Several approaches have been used in previous experiments for gene knockouts in microorganisms such as genetic algorithm (GA) (Alter et al. 2018), OptKnock (Burgard et al. 2003), and MOMAKnock (Ren et al. 2013). OptKnock is one of the programming frameworks to suggest gene knockout strategies of metabolites. The framework is categorized as a bi-level optimization method to propose gene knockout techniques for biochemical overproduction. OptKnock is used to obtain the potential gene to be eliminated to increase metabolic production while retaining the distribution of the flux. In addition to gene deletion, other internal flux distributions, such as growth or other biological targets, are often configured. MOMAKnock is a bi-level architecture originating from OptKnock and MOMA. The architecture used formulation of bi-level programming problem for maximum targeted production with maximum growth rate. It should be noted that bi-level programming problem is one optimization method where one problem is embedded within another. Optimal genetic manipulations may be identified under the MOMA assumption. OptReg (Pharkya and Maranas 2006) is an algorithmic extension of OptKnock to allow up- and/or downregulation in addition to gene knockouts to achieve the target of bio-production. It uses the formulation of OptKnock as a starting point. OptReg's goal is to calculate which reactions can be modulated or eliminated in such a way that the biochemical of interest is overproduced. However, the breadth and complexity of the recently considered genetic manipulations present several new variables

Big Data Analysis and Artificial Intelligence for Medical Sciences, First Edition.
Edited by Bruno Carpentieri and Paola Lecca.
© 2024 John Wiley & Sons Ltd. Published 2024 by John Wiley & Sons Ltd.

and nonlinearities requiring new and nontrivial theoretical treatment for the generation of single-level optimization problems.

These approaches have, however, faced some challenges, such as poor performance in local and global optimization processes, not taking into account the minimal shift in flux between mutant and wild-type, high computational time, and low capacity to run a whole genome that is a large-scale model (Tang et al. 2015). Nor does the conventional approach allow for a single run with different trade-offs between the two objectives of optimizing biomass and ethanol and succinic acid production. While GA has been explored and used in the development of succinic acid, there is a certain drawback where it fails to maximize the production of succinic acid and causes premature convergence. Differential Evolution (DE) (Storn and Price 1997) is a stochastic and population-based optimization approach with an objective function that can model the objective of the problem while integrating constraints. Recent works also focus on several methods and algorithms targeting the optimization of succinic and ethanol production (Dzulkalnine et al. 2022; Tan et al. 2023).

10.2 Method

10.2.1 Differential Evolution (DE)

DE is a stochastic and population-based optimization approach with an objective function that can be used to formulate the objective of the problem while integrating constraints. DE is one of the evolutionary algorithms (EAs) that evolves from improved GA. One of the benefits of DE is the ability to accommodate non-differentiable, nonlinear, and multi-modal cost functions. In addition, DE has few control parameters to make the algorithm function with fast convergence and easier to control (Storn and Price 1997). Operators in DE algorithm are similar to GA, where mutation, crossover, and selection are used. The mutation uses random number to generate new solution from children, while crossover produces new solution from parents. The selection operator chooses potential candidate solutions to become parents for the next generation. Although the operators used are similar, DE depends on a mutation operation, as opposed to GA on a crossover operation. The core activity of DE is based on variations in the population of randomly selected pairs of solutions. The mutation operation in DE is used in the search process, and the potential area in the search space is specifically searched by the selection operation. The child vector parameters are then taken more frequently than others by a nonuniform crossover from one parent. The components of the current population representatives are used to create a trivial vector to allow the crossover operator to shuffle information about effective combinations. As a consequence, the search for better solution space is allowed. Figure 10.1 displays the flowchart for the DE algorithm.

10.2.2 Mutation

A mutant vector (G) is generated for each target vector x_i, by:

$$v_{i,} G + 1 = x_{r1,} G + K \cdot (x_{r2,} G - xi, G) + F \cdot (x_{r2,} G - x_{r3,} G) \tag{10.1}$$

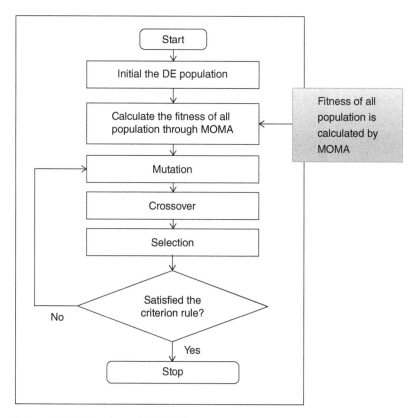

Figure 10.1 Flow chart of DEMOMA.

with i, r_1, r_2, $r_3 \in \{1, 2, \dots, NP\}$ is selected randomly and independently from each other. The r_1, r_2, and r_3 are the random integers with different values from running index i. In Eq. (10.1), K is the combination factor, while F is the scaling factor that has an impact on the difference vector $(x_{r2}, G - x_{r3}, G)$. In this operator, DE initializes new solution vectors randomly by adding the weight between two other solution vectors to a third vector. More details of how it is derived can be referred to Storn and Price (1997).

10.2.3 Crossover

Crossover as a second process is intended to enhance the diversity of the population. In a crossover process, the jth gene of the ith individual of the next generation is created from the disrupted individuals, v_{ji}, $G+1$ and x_{ji}, G. The trial individual is formed by:

$$u_{ji}, G+1 = \begin{cases} v_{ji}, G+1 \text{ if } (\text{rnd}_j \le CR) \text{ or } j = rn_i, \\ x_{ji}, G \text{ if } (\text{rnd}_j > CR) \text{ or } j \ne rn_i, \end{cases} \tag{10.2}$$

where $\text{rnd}_j \in [0;1]$ is random number and $rn_i \in (1, 2, \dots, D)$ is randomly chosen index. The crossover operator is purposely increasing the diversity of the solution vectors (exploration). The predetermined solution vectors and trial vectors from mutation process are evaluated with the objective function. The best value will then replace the target vector.

10.2.4 Selection

Trial individual $u_{i,} G+1$ is compared to the target vector x_i, G by using a greedy criterion to determine whether to become a generation member, $G+1$. If the fitness of the trial individual is equal to or less than the fitness of the target vector, the target vector will be replaced by the trial individual. Otherwise, the old target vector will still be maintained. The operation can be expressed as follows:

$$x_{i,} G+1 = \begin{cases} u_i, G+1 \text{ if } u_{i,} G+1 \le x_i, G, \\ x_i, G \text{ if } u_{i,} G+1 > x_i, G, \end{cases} \tag{10.3}$$

Equation (10.3), $x_{i,} G+1$ is the new target vector.

10.2.5 Minimization of Metabolic Adjustment

Minimization of Metabolic Adjustment (MOMA) is an extension of the flux balance analysis (FBA) that has the same stoichiometric restrictions as the FBA. MOMA provides a mathematically compact approximation for the intermediate suboptimal condition. It is based on the conjecture that, initially, the mutant stays as near as possible to the wild-type maximum in terms of flux values (Segrè et al. 2002). In addition, MOMA is ideal for simulating the behavior of disrupted metabolic networks, as it calculates a minimal distance solution or a solution with a minimum number of changes. The internal problem of constraining the dispersion of the metabolic flux distribution is formulated with steady-state phenotypes of wild-type strains. In other words, metabolic flux distribution problem is depicted as constrain problem of steady-state phenotypes. The formulation is represented using quadratic programming (QP). Feasible space ϕ^j has been determined and has a minimum distance from the current vector w. In MOMA, the aim is to find the vector $x \in \phi^j$ in such a way that the Euclidean distance is reduced. Equation (10.4) indicates the Euclidean distance from w to v.

$$D(w, v) = \sqrt{\sum_{i=1}^{N}(w_i - v_i)^2} \tag{10.4}$$

In Eq. (10.4), v is fluxes in the "reference" state (wild-type), while w is fluxes of interest (mutant). Equation (10.5) is used to minimize the linear constraint. By noting that minimizing function D is equal to minimizing its square and that avoids constant terms from the objective function, one may select Q to be an $N \times N$ unit matrix and set $L = -w$, and then minimize the minimization of D to the minimization of $f(x)$.

$$f(x) = L \cdot x + \frac{1}{2}x^T Q x \tag{10.5}$$

In Eq. (10.5), L is a vector of length N, Q is $N \times N$ matrix (linear and quadratic components of the objective function), and x^T is a transposal of x. In conclusion, FBA is used to create maximal wild-type FBA predictions. MOMA is used at the point nearest to the optimum wild-type FBA (Chong et al. 2014), and it helps to identify a better list of genes to knock out with optimization capability.

10.2.6 A Hybrid of Differential Evolution and Minimization of Metabolic Adjustment

The proposed method of this chapter is to hybridize Differential Evolution and Minimization of Metabolic Adjustment (DEMOMA). DE is an effective heuristic algorithm and stochastic optimization to minimize the objective function that can form the goals of the problem when incorporating constraints. Figure 10.1 illustrates the DEMOMA flow chart, and MOMA is used to measure population fitness based on the distribution of wild-type metabolic flux. There are four main steps used in this process. The phases include; generating initial population using random numbers (candidate solutions), evaluating fitness of the population, and following DE operations which are mutation, crossover, and selection. The criterion rule then will be tested before it repeats or stops. In this method, the fitness of the population is evaluated using MOMA equation (10.5). That is, the MOMA acts as objective function which can improve the list of knockout genes which can give more accurate result. The candidates' solutions generated from random number generator in DE will be mutated, and crossover using DE operators in Eqs. (10.1)–(10.3) until the solutions are near to optimal. The list of genes that are produced from DEMOMA will help predict better production of succinate and ethanol.

10.3 Experiments and Discussion

10.3.1 Dataset

The dataset used in this chapter is *E. coli* K-12 MG1655 and can be freely downloaded from the Systems Biology Research Group (https://systemsbiology.ucsd.edu/Downloads/EcoliCore). Various models of *E. coli* K-12 MG1655 are available for download, and the core *E. coli* metabolic network model has been chosen to determine the optimal set of gene knockouts that produced succinic acid and ethanol using DEMOMA. The core *E. coli* metabolic network model is the *i*AF1260 genome-scale metabolic reconstruction subset with 137 genes, 95 reactions, and 72 metabolites.

10.3.2 Parameter Setting

In order to maximize efficiency, experimental setting and control parameters are involved. One of the aims of this chapter is to review and analyze the method used for gene knockout in the production of succinic acid and ethanol in *E. coli*. The target reactions are thus succinic acid, succinate (*EX_succ(e)*) and ethanol (*EX_etoh(e)*). The maximum number of iterations for experiment is set to 50. In other words, each population runs 50 times. Population number, D is set at 50, and F as the weight applied to the random differential (scaling factor) is set at 1. The strategy is set at 7 (DE/rand/1/bin) because it is the most effective and commonly used (Babu and Jehan 2003). By using the seventh technique, the disruption can be either in the best vector of the previous generation or in any randomly picked vector. For disruptions of a single vector variance, the weighted vector differential of any two vectors is applied to the third vector out of the three distinctly selected vectors. Then, the disruption of two vector variations, five separate vectors, rather than the target vector, are selected randomly from the current population. As a consequence, the weighted vector difference of each pair of any four vectors is applied to the fifth vector for perturbation. In addition to the crossover probability, CR is set to 0.5 to execute on each of the D variables if a randomly chosen number is between 0 and 1 (Choon et al. 2014). Next, DEMOMA is conducted for a total of 50 runs in order to obtain the optimum solution with the maximum growth rate of *E. coli*, succinic acid, and ethanol production. DEMOMA is evaluated by setting the number of knockouts from 2 to 5. In addition, the minimum growth rate for each population is set at 0.01 h^{-1} to guarantee that the cell is alive and that any population with a growth rate of less than 0.01 h^{-1} is discarded.

10.3.3 Experimental Results

The growth rate of *E. coli* after gene knockout is measured in unit one per hour (h^{-1}) and the production rate of succinic acid and ethanol is measured in unit millimole per gram of dry cell weight per hour (mmol gDW^{-1} h^{-1}). The findings obtained from DEMOMA to produce succinic acid and ethanol are summarized. Table 10.1 shows the results to produce succinic acid, while Table 10.2 shows the results to produce ethanol. In Tables 10.1 and 10.2, there are four knockout strategies identified which are resulted from DEMOMA. That knockout contains their respective reaction, number of genes, and the gene names. The best result with the highest production rate is selected for each reaction knockout number. Both tables are the near-optimal solution (knockout strategies) to produce succinate and ethanol.

Table 10.1 Result for succinic acid production.

Reaction knockout number	Knockout list		Succinic acid production (mmol gDW^{-1} h^{-1})	Growth rate (h^{-1})
	Reaction	Gene		
2	RPE	*sgcE, rpe*	6.693	0.4352
	ACONTb	*acnA, acnB*		
3	Plt2r	*pitA, pitB*	6.7172	0.4320
	PPCK	*pck*		
	ATPM	—		
4	ACONTa	*acnA, acnB*	7.7987	0.2863
	GND	*gnd*		
	ME1	*maeA*		
	PPS	*ppsA*		
5	ACONTa	*acnA, acnB*	10.6676	0.1707
	ATPS4r	*ATP*		
	PYK	*pykF, pykA*		
	O2t	—		
	EX_nh4e(e)	—		

Table 10.2 Result for ethanol production.

Reaction knockout number	Knockout list		Ethanol production (mmol gDW^{-1} h^{-1})	Growth rate (h^{-1})
	Reaction	Gene		
2	NH4t	amtB	11.8488	0.0822
	G6PDH2r	zwf		
3	FBP	glpX, fbp	11.8488	0.0822
	ICDHyr	icd		
	PDH	lpd, aceE, aceF		
4	CS	gltA	11.8488	0.0822
	GLUt2r	gltP		
	TKT1	tktA, tktB		
	EX_akg(e)	—		
5	D-LACt2	glcA, lldP	11.8488	0.0822
	ICDHyr	icd		
	ICL	aceA		
	EX_gln-L(e)	—		
	FRD7	frdD, frdA, frdC, frdB		

For the two reactions of succinic acid production, *RPE* and *ACONTb* are chosen by DEMOMA and knocked out from the reaction list. *RPE* is the abbreviation of 5-phosphate 3-epimerase, whereas *ACONTb* is aconitase (half-reaction B, isocitrate hydro-lyase). The *RPE* reaction is made up of *sgcE* and *rpe* genes. It is the oxidative pentose phosphate pathway and is responsible for the interconversion of ribulose-5-phosphate and xylulose-5-phosphate (Caldwell et al. 2007). Knockout of the *sgcE* and *rpe* genes causes the *TKT2* reaction to operate in reverse direction so that pentose phosphate pathways cannot produce *NADPH* and more flux is guided by glycolysis (Ip et al. 2014). *ACONTb* consists of *acnA* and *acnB*. Reaction in the citric acid cycle is responsible for the reaction of aconitate to isocitrate.

ATPM, *Plt2r*, and *PPCK* are chosen for the three reactions knockout of succinic acid production. *ATPM* is an *ATP* maintenance requirement that involves retaining the *ADP* before folding into *ATP*. *Plt2r* is a reversible phosphate transport that brings phosphate to *E. coli*. The small amount of available phosphate limits the formation of *ATP* (Marzan and Shimizu 2011). *PPCK* is a reaction within anaplerotic reaction and consists of a *pck* gene. The function of the *pck* gene is to preserve the ratio of phosphoenolpyruvate to oxaloacetate and to stabilize the pool of intermediate products of the citric acid cycle (de Mey et al. 2007). Knockout of the *pck* gene induces an increase in oxaloacetate, and more oxaloacetate can be used to produce succinic acid.

ACONTa, *GND*, *ME1*, and *PPS* are chosen for the four reactions knockout of succinic acid production. *ACONTa* is aconitase (half-reaction A, citrate hydro-lyase) composed of the *acnA* and *acnB* genes. Reaction in the citric acid cycle is responsible for the reaction of citrate to aconitate. *GND* is phosphogluconate dehydrogenase and consists of the *gnd* gene. It is a reaction within the pentose phosphate pathway which catalyzes the reaction of 6-Phospho-D-gluconate to D-Ribulose 5-phosphate. The knockout of the *gnd* gene block 6-Phospho-D-gluconate transforms to D-Ribulose 5-phosphate and decreases the flux to the pentose phosphate pathway (Wendisch et al. 2006). *ME1* is a malic enzyme composed of the *maeA* gene. It is responsible for the pyruvate reaction of L-malate. Knockout of *ME1* decreases the concentration of pyruvate, and pyruvate is more condensed in acetyl-CoA, then converted into acetate, and creates ethanol as a byproduct. In order to increase the production of succinic acid, it is important to remove all byproducts (Chong et al. 2014). On the other hand, *ME1* knockout allows nicotinamide adenine dinucleotide to be completely used in the citric acid cycle, thereby increasing the production of succinic acid. Next, *PPS* is phosphoenolpyruvate synthase, a reaction within glycolysis. It consists of the *ppsA* gene and is responsible for producing pyruvate phosphoenolpyruvate.

ACONTa, ATPS4r, O2t, PYK, and EX_nh4e(e) are chosen for the five reactions knockout of succinic acid production. *ACONTa* is aconitase (half-reaction A, citrate hydro-lyase) which is a reaction in the citric acid cycle. It consists of the *acnA* and *acnB* genes and is responsible for the reaction of citrate to aconitate. *ATPS4r* is an *ATP* synthase that transforms *ADP* to *ATP*. *ATPS4r* deletion allows low energy to be produced. *O2t* is the diffusion of travel. *O2t* deletion means that E. coli grows in an anaerobic environment. *PYK* is a pyruvate kinase composed of the *pykF* and *pykA* genes. It includes the formation of pyruvate from phospho-enolpyruvate. As described above the reduction in pyruvate would increase the production of succinic acid, as byproducts such as acetate and ethanol have been reduced. EX_nh4e(e) is an exchange of ammonia. *EX_nh4e(e)* deletion shows that no ammonia is used in the reaction.

NH4t and G6PDH2r are identified by DEMOMA and knockout from the reaction list for the two reactions deletion for the production of ethanol. NH4t is a reversible transport of ammonia, while G6PDH2r is Glucose 6-phosphate dehydrogenase. NH4t consists of the amtB gene and is a response to the production of ammonium. Deletion of NH4t is the absence of ammonium in the reaction. G6PDH2r is a reaction under the pentose phosphate pathway. It consists of the zwf gene and is responsible for the reaction of glucose 6-phosphate to 6-phospho-D-glucono-1, 5-lactone. Knockout of the zwf gene drives glucose 6-phosphate into glycolysis and transforms 6-phosphate fructose to improve the production of ethanol.

FBP, ICDHyr, and PDH are identified for the three reactions knockout in ethanol production. FBP is a fructose-bisphosphatase composed of the genes glpX and fbp. It is a reaction within glycolysis which is responsible for the reaction of fructose 1, 6-bisphosphate to fructose 6-phosphate. Since conversion is a reversible reaction, the conversion of the genes glpX and fbp is rendered nonfunctional. This in turn raises the amount of fructose 1, 6-bisphosphate, driving the glycolysis process to produce more acetyl-CoA, thus maximizing the production of ethanol. Next, ICDHyr isocitrate dehydrogenase, a reaction within the citric acid cycle. It consists of the icd gene and is responsible for the transformation of isocitrate into oxoglutarate. Knockout of the icd gene would cause the citric acid cycle to be interrupted (Wendisch et al. 2006). PDH is pyruvate dehydrogenase, which consists of lpd, acee, and acef genes. It is responsible for the pyruvate reaction to acetyl-CoA.

CS, EX_akg(e), GLUt2r, and TKT1 are identified for the four reactions knockout of ethanol production. CS is a citrate synthase. It consists of the gltA gene and the gltA gene block reaction of acetyl-Coa converted to citrate, which ensures that acetyl-Coa can be completely used for the production of ethanol. Then, EX_akg(e) is a 2-oxoglutarate exchange and EX_akg(e) indicates no 2-oxoglutarate exists in the reaction. GLUt2r is a transport of glutamate transporting glutamate. It consists of gltP genes and the deletion of gltP genes means that glutamate cannot be transferred to *E. coli*. TKT1 is a transketolase that reacts within the pentose phosphate pathway. TKT1 consists of tktA and tktB genes. Deletion of tktA and tktB genes decreases the efficiency of gluconeogenesis resulting in an enhanced concentration of phosphoenolpyruvate. Phosphoenolpyruvate is then converted to pyruvate and to be used for ethanol production, specifically for biofuel.

For the five reactions knockout of ethanol production, D-LACt2, EX_gln-L(e), FRD7, ICDHyr, and ICL are identified. D-LACt2 is a D-lactate transport composed of the genes glcA and lldP. It is responsible for the reversible transport of D-lactate to *E. coli*. Next, EX_gln-L(e) is an exchange of L-Glutamine. Knockout of EX_gln-L(e) means that there is no L-Glutamine in the reaction. In addition, FRD7 is fumarate reductase which is the reaction inside oxidative phosphorylation and which is responsible for the reaction of fumarate to succinate. FRD7 consists of the frdA, frdB, frdC, and frdD genes. Knockout of the frdA, frdB, frdC, and frdD genes inhibits the conversion of fumarate to succinate. ICDHyr is an isocitrate dehydrogenase composed of an icd gene. As described above, it is responsible for the reaction of transforming isocitrate to oxoglutarate, and the deletion of the icd gene breaks the citric acid cycle. Next, ICL is an isocitrate lyase that is made up of the aceA gene. It is a reaction under anaplerotic reaction that is responsible for succinate isocitrate reactions. The deletion of the aceA gene would restrict the process of isocitrate conversion to succinate (Wendisch et al. 2006).

Table 10.3 Comparison between different methods for production rate and growth rate of succinic acid.

Method	Reaction knockout number	Knockout list	Production rate (mmol gDW^{-1} h^{-1})	Growth rate (h^{-1})
DEMOMA	2	RPE, ACONTb	6.693	0.4352
	3	Plt2r, PPCK, ATPM	6.7172	0.4320
	4	ACONTa, GND, ME1, PPS	7.7987	0.2863
	5	ACONTa, ATPS4r, PYK, O2t, EX_nh4e(e)	10.6676	0.1707
OptKnock	2	PFL, LDH_D	1.65	0.31
	3	PFL, LDH_D, ACALD	4.79	0.31
	4	PYK, ACKr, PTAr, GLCpts	6.21	0.16
MOMA-Knock	3	SUCDi, PGL, URIC	5.02	—
	4	SUCDi, ACKr, MTHFD, TKT1	5.02	—
	5	SUCDi, GLUDC, PGCD, PSERT, GND	5.02	—
ACO-MOMA	3	G6PDH2r, PDH, SUCDi	7.9015	0.2761
		FUM, G6PDH2r, PDH	7.9015	0.2761

Table 10.4 Comparison between different methods for production rate and growth rate of ethanol.

Method	Reaction knockout number	Knockout list	Production rate (mmol gDW^{-1} h^{-1})	Growth rate (h^{-1})
DEMOMA	2	NH4t, G6PDH2r	11.8488	0.0822
	3	FBP, ICDHyr, PDH	11.8488	0.0822
	4	CS, GLUt2r, TKT1, EX_akg(e)	11.8488	0.0822
	5	D-LACt2, ICDHyr, ICL , EX_gln-L(e) , FRD7	11.8488	0.0822
OptReg	3	PGI, PFL, O2t	18.7400	0.08
Wet laboratory	2	MG1655 (pZSKLMgldA) dhaKLM, gldA	8.70	—

10.3.4 Comparative Analysis

The findings obtained from DEMOMA are compared with previous approaches. The Opt-Knock, MOMAKnock, and ACOMOMA results are used to compare with the DEMOMA results. However, the findings of the OptReg and Wet laboratory are used to compare *E. coli* with DEMOMA with the results of ethanol production as well as the growth rate of *E. coli*. Table 10.3 shows the comparison between the different methods for the production rate and the growth rate of succinic acid, while Table 10.4 shows the comparison between the different methods for the production rate and the growth rate of ethanol. The highest rate of production and growth of *E. coli* is highlighted in the table.

In Table 10.3, DEMOMA is capable of producing highest production rate and growth rate (highlighted in gray). The production rate and growth rate values are 10.6676 and 0.4352. The maximum production involves five genes which are ACONTa, ATPS4r, PYK, O2t, and EX_nh4e(e). The maximum growth involves two genes which are RPE and ACONTb. In Table 10.4, the highest production rate involves three genes (PGI, PFL, and O2t) that produced 18.7400. On the other hand, the growth rate produced the same number with different list of knockout genes. In summary, the proposed DEMOMA is capable of producing the highest rate of production and growth that are beneficial in succinate and ethanol production.

10.4 Conclusion

This chapter focuses on the use of the knockout genes to increase the production of succinic acid and ethanol in *E. coli*. In this chapter, a DEMOMA hybrid algorithm was implemented to predict optimal sets of gene knockouts to optimize the production of succinic acid and ethanol. As a result, succinic acid and ethanol production with four distinct numbers of knockout reactions were produced. For succinic acid production with five knockout reactions, the selected reactions were *ACONTa, ATPS4r, PYK, O2t*, and *EX_nh4e(e)*, while the selected genes were *acnA, acnB, ATP, pykF*, and *pykA*. Production and growth contributed to 10.6676 mmol gDW^{-1} h^{-1} and 0.1707 h^{-1}, respectively. For ethanol production with five knockout reactions, the selected reactions were *D-LACt2, ICDHyr, ICL, FRD7*, and *EX_gln-L(e)*, while the selected genes were *glcA, lldP, icd, aceA, frdD, frdA, frdC*, and *frdB*. Production and growth were 11.8488 mmol gDW^{-1} h^{-1} and 0,0822 h^{-1}, respectively.

The results of the hybrid algorithm were then compared to the previous approaches. The result of succinic acid production is compared with OptKnock, MOMAKnock, and ACOMOMA, while the result of ethanol production is compared with OptReg and the wet laboratory results. The results obtained from DEMOMA were better than other approaches in terms of the rate of production or growth. In conclusion, DEMOMA successfully predicted the deletion of genes to increase the production of succinic acid and ethanol in *E. coli*.

However, the population formed in DEMOMA is random due to the stochastic characteristics of DE. Thus, it may not be possible to foresee any gene knockouts that may greatly affect the outcome of succinic acid and ethanol production. In comparison, DEMOMA was only tested on the core *E. coli* metabolic network model. For future work, the DEMOMA algorithm may be extended to various datasets to assess its robustness. Study the DEMOMA algorithm for a gene or reaction number greater than five and enhance the MOMA technique by adding kinetic and regulatory knowledge to help measure the flux balance in the cell.

Acknowledgment

We would like to thank the Skim Geran Penyelidikan Fundamental (no grant: R.J130000.7828.4F720) from the Ministry of Education Malaysia for their support in making this research a success. Also, thank to Universiti Malaysia Kelantan for supporting this research via Post-Doctoral (Research) Scheme and UMK Fund (R/FUND/A0100/01850A/001/2020/00816).

Author Bibliographies

Zhang Neng Hor received his Master's Degree and Bachelor's Degree in Computer Science from Universiti Malaya and Universiti Teknologi Malaysia in year 2016 and 2022, respectively. His research interests are artificial intelligence, bioinformatics, and machine learning.

Dr. Saberi is a Professor of Artificial Intelligence and Health Data Science. He is now the Director of the Health Data Science Lab in the Department of Genetics and Genomics (CMSH-UAEU). His research interests include AI, Data Science, and Bioinformatics. Before joining CMHS-UAEU, he served at several universities in Malaysia as the Director of the Institute for AI and Big Data, Head of the AI and Bioinformatics Research Group, founder of the Department of Data Science, Manager of IT, and Deputy Director (academic) for Center of Computing and Informatics.

Dr. Yee Wen Choon received her Doctorate and Bachelor's Degree in Computer Science from Universiti Teknologi Malaysia in 2010 and 2014, respectively. Her research interests are artificial intelligence, bioinformatics, machine learning, and algorithms.

Dr. Muhammad Akmal Remli is a director at Institute for Artificial Intelligence and Big Data (AIBIG), Universiti Malaysia Kelantan (UMK). He is also a senior lecturer at Faculty of Data Science and Computing UMK. He received a Master's and a PhD degree in Computer Science from Universiti Teknologi Malaysia in 2014 and 2018. In 2016, he worked at The Bioinformatics, Intelligent Systems and Educational Technology (BISITE) Research Group at University of Salamanca, Spain, and was working in cancer bioinformatics. His main research interests are artificial intelligence, data science, business intelligence, and computational systems biology.

Mr. Hairudin Abdul Majid is a Senior Lecturer at Faculty of Computing, Universiti Teknologi Malaysia, since 1998 until now. He is a member of Artificial Intelligence and Bioinformatics Lab (AIBIG). His research interests are pattern recognition, soft computing, maintenance modeling, operational research, and image processing. Currently, more than 40 papers are published on the website, and also get involved in many research projects under the Ministry of Education (KPT) grants like Fundamental Research Grant Scheme (FRGS) and e-science under the Ministry of Science, Technology, and Innovation (MOSTI) or internal grants under University of Technology Malaysia Grant for University Publication (GUP UTM). The most achievement project was under knowledge transfer grant (KTP) collaborate with the Ministry of Health to predict the number of dentistry in 2030.

References

Alter, T., Blank, L., and Ebert, B. (2018). Genetic optimization algorithm for metabolic engineering revisited. *Metabolites* 8: 33. https://doi.org/10.3390/metabo8020033.

Babu, B.V. and Jehan, M.M.L. (2003. CEC '03). Differential evolution for multi-objective optimizatior. In: *Proceedings of the 2003 Congress on Evolutionary Computation*, 2696–2703. IEEE.

Burgard, A.P., Pharkya, P., and Maranas, C.D. (2003). Optknock: a bilevel programming framework for identifying gene knockout strategies for microbial strain optimization. *Biotechnology and Bioengineering* 84: 647–657. https://doi.org/10.1002/bit.10803.

Caldwell, P.E., MacLean, M.R., and Norris, P.R. (2007). Ribulose bisphosphate carboxylase activity and a calvin cycle gene cluster in sulfobacillus species. *Microbiology (NY)* 153: 2231–2240. https://doi.org/10.1099/mic.0.2007/006262-0.

Chong, S.K., Mohamad, M.S., Mohamed Salleh, A.H. et al. (2014). A hybrid of ant colony optimization and minimization of metabolic adjustment to improve the production of succinic acid in *Escherichia coli*. *Computers in Biology and Medicine* 49: 74–82. https://doi .org/10.1016/j.compbiomed.2014.03.011.

Choon, Y.W., Mohamad, M.S., Deris, S. et al. (2014). Differential bees flux balance analysis with OptKnock for in silico microbial strains optimization. *PLoS One* 9: e102744. https://doi.org/10.1371/journal.pone.0102744.

Dzulkalnine, M.F., Mohamad, M.S., Choon, Y.W. et al. (2022). Optimizing ethanol production in *Escherichia coli* using a hybrid of particle swarm optimization and artificial bee colony. In: *Proceedings of the 2022 The 6th International Conference on Advances in Artificial Intelligence*, 140–146. New York, NY, USA: ACM.

Ip, K., Donoghue, N., Kim, M.K., and Lun, D.S. (2014). Constraint-based modeling of heterologous pathways: application and experimental demonstration for overproduction of fatty acids in *Escherichia coli*. *Biotechnology and Bioengineering* 111: 2056–2066. https://doi .org/10.1002/bit.25261.

Marzan, L. and Shimizu, K. (2011). Metabolic regulation of *Escherichia coli* and its PhoB and PhoR genes knockout mutants under phosphate and nitrogen limitations as well as at acidic condition. *Microbial Cell Factories* 10: 39. https://doi.org/10.1186/1475-2859-10-39.

de Mey, M., de Maeseneire, S., Soetaert, W., and Vandamme, E. (2007). Minimizing acetate formation in *E. Coli* fermentations. *Journal of Industrial Microbiology & Biotechnology* 34: 689–700. https://doi.org/10.1007/s10295-007-0244-2.

Pharkya, P. and Maranas, C.D. (2006). An optimization framework for identifying reaction activation/inhibition or elimination candidates for overproduction in microbial systems. *Metabolic Engineering* 8: 1–13. https://doi.org/10.1016/j.ymben.2005.08.003.

Ren, S., Zeng, B., and Qian, X. (2013). Adaptive bi-level programming for optimal gene knockouts for targeted overproduction under phenotypic constraints. *BMC Bioinformatics* 14: S17. https://doi.org/10.1186/1471-2105-14-S2-S17.

Segrè, D., Vitkup, D., and Church, G.M. (2002). Analysis of optimality in natural and perturbed metabolic networks. *Proceedings of the National Academy of Sciences* 99: 15112–15117. https://doi.org/10.1073/pnas.232349399.

Storn, R. and Price, K. (1997). Differential evolution – a simple and efficient heuristic for global optimization over continuous spaces. *Journal of Global Optimization* 11: 341–359. https://doi .org/10.1023/A:1008202821328.

Tan, J.B., Mohamad, M.S., Moorthy, K. et al. (2023). A hybrid of ant colony optimization, genetic algorithm and flux balance analysis for optimization of succinic acid production in *Escherichia Coli*. *International Journal of Modeling, Simulation, and Scientific Computing* https://doi.org/10.1142/S179396232350040X.

Tang, P.W., Choon, Y.W., Mohamad, M.S. et al. (2015). Optimising the production of succinate and lactate in escherichia coli using a hybrid of artificial bee colony algorithm and minimisation of metabolic adjustment. *Journal of Bioscience and Bioengineering* 119: 363–368. https://doi.org/10.1016/j.jbiosc.2014.08.004.

Wendisch, V.F., Bott, M., and Eikmanns, B.J. (2006). Metabolic engineering of *Escherichia Coli* and *Corynebacterium Glutamicum* for biotechnological production of organic acids and amino acids. *Current Opinion in Microbiology* 9: 268–274. https://doi.org/10.1016/j.mib.2006 .03.001.

11

Analysis Pipelines and a Platform Solution for Next-Generation Sequencing Data

Víctor Duarte[1,2], Alesandro Gómez[1,2] and Juan M. Corchado[1,2,3]

[1]*BISITE Research Group, University of Salamanca, 37007 Salamanca, Spain*
[2]*Air Institute, IoT Digital Innovation Hub, 37188 Salamanca, Spain*
[3]*Department of Electronics, Information and Communication, Faculty of Engineering, Osaka Institute of Technology, Osaka 535-8585, Japan*

11.1 Introduction

Following the completion of the Human Genome Project there have been considerable advances in high-throughput sequencing, converting this technology into a routine tool in many research laboratories and genetic centers which use it in varying areas of work, and in both large and small projects. It has been discovered that our genomes contain the answers to the countless questions that humanity has continually asked itself. Genomes can give us information about the root cause of all types of medical problems and they can even help us understand the source of human intelligence. However, the new paradigm generates an enormous amount of data that classical computational approaches are not able to handle. This has led to the emergence of multiple tools and algorithms for the analysis and management of all the data collected by different sequencing platforms. The set of next-generation sequencing (NGS) data processing tools has been classified according to the stage in which the tools intervene. There are numerous applications that fully exploit the potential of high-performance sequencing: genomic DNA sequencing makes it possible to discover new, unknown genomes, to study genetic variants in the population, or to clinically diagnose Mendelian diseases and more complex syndromes such as cancer; RNA sequencing, also known as RNA-seq, makes it possible to analyze a complete transcriptome as a complement to the use of classical microarrays.

This chapter analyzes and compares the multiple algorithms and software tools needed to run a pipeline of massive genomic sequencing data analysis in clinical settings, with the aim of finding causal relationships between genetic variants and a phenotypic set corresponding to a disease. The stages involved in this type of analysis include evaluation of the quality of the reads, alignment against a reference genome, identification of the variants, and, finally, their annotation to give biological significance to the data. It is normally necessary to add some intermediate steps to the main workflow, such as data filtering and preprocessing. To solve this problem, DeepNGS has been developed a technological solution in the form of a web platform that assists in and facilitates the process of analyzing data from human

Big Data Analysis and Artificial Intelligence for Medical Sciences, First Edition.
Edited by Bruno Carpentieri and Paola Lecca.
© 2024 John Wiley & Sons Ltd. Published 2024 by John Wiley & Sons Ltd.

genomic samples to detect and interpret their potential pathogenicity, and therefore, their possible association with a clinical phenotype. In a single click, this platform automates the tedious process of data analysis and leaves it in the hands of expert workflow management systems deployed both in the cloud and on-premises to optimize computational loads and parallelization, in a reliable and secure environment for working with genomic data of relevance. The use of novel artificial intelligence (AI) algorithms enables optimal clinical detection and interpretation, with machine learning (ML)-based pattern extraction methods that leverage information from multiple resources to create a model tailored to each phenotype, all supported by the American College of Medical Genetics (ACMG) classification rules.

First, the pipeline of massive sequencing data analysis for both short-read (Illumina) and long-read (Oxford Nanopore Technologies [ONT]) technologies will be described, reviewing the state of the art of the main tools used at each point of the workflow. The application of AI and ML in genomic data analysis, and its importance in certain processes, is then briefly described. Next, architectures for describing and executing genomic workflows are reviewed. Finally, the characteristics and functionalities, which capacitate the DeepNGS platform to perform integral analyses of genomic data in clinical practice, are detailed.

11.2 NGS Data Analysis Pipeline and State of the Art Tools

11.2.1 Quality Assessment

The files resulting from any of the sequencing technologies described above contain all the reads detected by the sequencer in a standardized format known as FASTQ (FASTQ Files Explained n.d.). This format presents an input for each sequenced read, where each nucleotide (N) has a quality score assigned by the sequencer. The reason for estimating the quality of the bases is that each sequencing technology identifies true positives according to its own precision value. Sequencing errors are inherent to all techniques, even more so if we consider the human factor and failures related to the employed instrumentation or chemical reagents. To ensure the quality of input sequence analyses, error probability values, estimated as Q scores in the FASTQ files, are routinely used as thresholds for dataset filtering. At this stage, software tools evaluate the quality of the sequences and perform trimming based on different parameters (see Figure 11.1).

A number of state-of-the-art tools have been developed to perform basic read quality analysis and sequence trimming, such as NGSQC Toolkit (Patel and Jain 2012), PRINSEQ (Schmieder and Edwards 2011), or the Galaxy environment (Goecks et al. 2010), which produce general reports of the reads and can filter them. However, most of today's pipelines for sequencing analysis commonly include FASTQC ("Babraham Bioinformatics - FastQC A Quality Control Tool for High Throughput Sequence Data" n.d.) to evaluate the reads and subsequently filter them with Trimmomatic (Bolger et al. 2014). FASTQC and Trimmomatic are two totally independent tools, but both have a wide range of very useful modules. FASTQC is a software that provides many graphs and statistics showing the average quality of the reads, the average quality per base, the distribution of indeterminate Ns or guanine and cytosine content (GC content), etc. Trimmomatic is a very powerful tool for filtering sequences using multiple parameters, it works optimally with the data from the Illumina

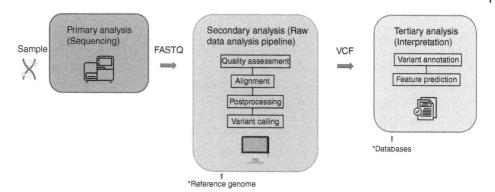

Figure 11.1 General workflow in variant calling NGS data analysis. Three main modules are distinguished: primary analysis, where the biological sample is treated and sequenced; secondary analysis, or the raw data analysis to obtain a set of variants; and tertiary analysis, where interesting features are collected and predicted to obtain an interpretation.

sequencing platform. In addition, it allows for the systematic elimination of adapters which are sequences of no real biological value, that may be generated during the preparation of the libraries of sequencing platforms. Adapters are eliminated to prevent noise in subsequent stages (Pabinger et al. 2014). Albeit it is not the most critical stage of the whole pipeline, it is necessary to clean the reads and facilitate the work of the tools that follow. Despite its importance, there are currently no exhaustive reviews that would compare the performance of different quality control software. Even so, different tools have been developed that might have better performance than Trimmomatic, such as PathoQC (Hong et al. 2014), AfterQC (Chen et al. 2017), or newer ones such as fastp (Chen et al. 2018) and its optimized re-implementation in C++, and FastProNGS (Liu et al. 2019). The latter has better computational cost per run, and this is crucial when analyzing several samples at the same time because hardware requirements increase considerably. One of the recently developed tools is FQStat (Chanumolu et al. 2019), which stands out for offering a parallel programming architecture to optimize the use of resources and the ability to provide quality statistics per lane.

11.2.2 Alignment

Once the reads have been properly processed, it is necessary to perform a mapping or alignment against an existing reference genome, for which there are two main sources, the University of Santa Cruz (UCSC) and the Genome Reference Consortium ("UCSC Genome Browser Home" n.d.; "Human Genome Overview - Genome Reference Consortium" n.d.). Both institutions provide the scientific community with an assembly of references for the human genome, which they continuously improve and optimize to precisely specify the genomic position of millions of reads from a sequencer. As for the alignment process, it is necessary to highlight the enormous computational complexity involved in placing the reads in their correct position within the genome. It is not as simple as it might seem; the human genome is highly complex and has odd regions which it has not been possible to characterize yet, such as repetitions of one or several Ns in the intergenic regions or duplications of the same gene in different chromosomes. Thus, the process carried out by aligning software is incredibly costly.

The different alignment software has been classified according to the type of algorithm they use to map the reads (Mielczarek and Szyda 2016). First, there are hashing-based algorithms – the result of a hash function are keys that unequivocally represent a set of data – which can rapidly elaborate an index to find the position of each read, but unfortunately, they are very prone to errors. RMAP (Smith et al. 2009), SOAP (Li et al. 2008), Novoalign ("Novocraft" n.d.), or SHRiMP (Rumble et al. 2009) fit in this category. Second, there is alignment software that is based on the Smith–Waterman algorithm. This algorithm applies dynamic programming methods to ensure that local alignment is optimal with respect to a given scoring system, for this reason it is more precise but also more time-consuming. An example of this type of software is BFAST (Homer et al. 2009), whose peculiarity is that it implements this algorithm exclusively. Finally, the algorithms based on the Burrows–Wheeler Transform (Manzini 1999) optimize the use of memory, they work optimally with short reads, offering a balance between efficiency, sensitivity, and specificity; currently, there are many tools that implement this algorithm, such as BWA (Li and Durbin 2009), Bowtie (Langmead et al. 2009), SOAP2 (Li et al. 2009b), and SOAP3 (Liu et al. 2012). Numerous studies have evaluated the performance of different aligners for variant identification. According to those studies, the aligners that offer the best performance are BWA, Bowtie, Novoalign, and SOAP. These are also the most used aligners. A characteristic of a good aligner is that it can map reads correctly, even when they contain sequencing errors or genetic polymorphisms that diminish their coincidence with the reference genome. Generally, NGS data analysis projects use BWA or its newer version, Bowtie2. Although some reviews have affirmed that BWA delivers slightly better results (Hwang et al. 2015) at a significantly faster speed (Thankaswamy-Kosalai et al. 2017), other studies have demonstrated the contrary. BWA software is not accurate even when the error rate in the reads is low, generating many incorrectly mapped reads (Ruffalo et al. 2011). Other tools, such as Novoalign, perform optimally in cases where Genome Analysis Toolkit (GATK) is used to identify variants (Cornish and Guda 2015). In addition, it has a greater proportion of true positives when the reads are very short (Thankaswamy-Kosalai et al. 2017). Finally, SOAP and its improved versions have a high accuracy even when there are high error rates in the mapping, so it seems to be the best choice for the identification of single-nucleotide polymorphisms (SNPs) in later stages (Ruffalo et al. 2011).

11.2.3 Post-alignment and pre-variant Calling Processing

The output of the mapping algorithms contains the reads aligned against the reference genome in a quasi-standard format known as Sequence Alignment/Map (SAM) format (Li et al. 2009a). This format gives a lot of information about each of the aligned reads, such as its specific position in the reference, its orientation (the DNA molecule is bicatenary, so it is said to have a positive chain and a negative chain, called forward and reverse, respectively), or its quality. This information is stored in labels known as flags, whose value is the result of the sum of all the individual labels, each one of them represents a type of information that will serve later to manage and filter each read. Once these SAM files have been obtained, it is almost always necessary to carry out a series of preprocesses before the variants can be identified. These preprocesses are usually carried out to facilitate the work of the tools that are used afterward. Most NGS data analysis projects use three main tools for preprocessing: SAMtools (Danecek et al. 2021), GATK (McKenna et al. 2010) – a suite of analysis tools that are fundamental in variant identification – and Picard ("GitHub - Broadinstitute/Picard: A Set of Command Line Tools (in Java) for Manipulating High-Throughput Sequencing (HTS) Data and Formats Such as SAM/BAM/CRAM and VCF." n.d.). Below, a description is provided of the workflow of these tools in most variant identification studies, given that they follow standardized and revised pipelines within the bioinformatics community (Altmann et al. 2012).

First, most variant calling algorithms require the mapped reads to be ordered and indexed according to their genomic position, i.e. an index file is created to facilitate the search for information in the aligned reads. In addition, it is also common to transform the SAM file into its binary version, binary aligned mapped (BAM), which contains the same information but in a compressed format, making the management of the data easier. This can be done through the SAMtools package, which provides functions to offer summaries of the main alignment statistics, such as the percentage of correctly mapped reads or the proportion of correctly aligned pairs. These statistics make it possible to eliminate certain biases from the alignment software, keeping only the reads that have been mapped correctly or uniquely in the reference genome (Altmann et al. 2012). Subsequently, it is common to follow the protocol or best practices pipeline designed by the creators of this software (van der Auwera et al. 2013) because their use for the identification of variants is highly standardized. The protocol consists in a series of stages in which the aligned reads are processed, then it identifies the variants using GATK and Picard tools. Therefore, using the files from SAMtools as input, the following processes are carried out: creation of a reference sequence dictionary and preparation of information in the reads to update the information in the files; marking or labeling of duplicate sequences using Picard given that multiple sequenced DNA fragments do not provide any type of information and may falsify the coverage values of certain regions of the genome; local realignment around the indels – insertions and deletions – since this type of structural variations leads to the incorrect mapping of the adjacent zones, a typical problem in the majority of today's aligners. Finally, a specific GATK process is executed, it is known as Base Quality Score Recalibration (BQSR) and its aim is to determine the real value of error probability associated with each of the sequenced bases ("Base Quality Score Recalibration (BQSR) – GATK" n.d.). The results of the variant detection process may sometimes not be completely precise. However, obtaining a large portion of true positives is essential because, at a later stage, variant identification algorithms use quality values to calculate the degree of reliability of each of the identified variants (Altmann et al. 2012).

11.2.4 Variant Calling

Until recently, the identification of variants and SNPs was typically done in microarrays, but their density limited the detection of genetic polymorphisms to a certain degree. However, a new mass-sequencing approach has emerged for exhaustive variant identification. This approach covers all the possible points of a genome where there may be a variation with respect to the reference genome. It has also become possible to obtain what we call rare variants, so-called because of their low proportion in the population. The relationship between rare variants and complex diseases has recently been demonstrated (Mielczarek and Szyda 2016; Handel et al. 2014). Therefore, thanks to the development of numerous tools in recent years, we may be able to obtain a complete and much more precise map of the genomic variants of any individual, although it is necessary to run complex algorithms to mitigate the enormous computational cost involved in the new paradigm of mass sequencing.

Genomic variants can be classified into several groups, depending on both their genetic nature and the type of algorithm needed to identify them. The first group is constituted by small-length variants, ranging between a single nucleotide, known as SNP or single-nucleotide variation (SNV); and several pairs of bases – called indels – which are a conjunction of insertions and deletions. SNPs are the most common, and therefore, best-known genomic variants, their variation is simple, it lies in the substitution of one nucleotide base for another. Cellular machinery transforms this nucleotide sequence into a sequence of another type of molecule; amino acids, which constitute what is known as proteins. Thus, the change from one N to another causes a variation in the sequence of amino acids, which can have negative, neutral, or positive effects:

- **Negative**: the protein is truncated and ceases to perform its function, giving way to a disease.
- **Neutral**: the change in the amino acid does not affect the protein as a whole, and it can continue to perform its function.
- **Positive**: the new amino acid enhances the existing protein, either by adding a new function or optimizing the one it already had, which ultimately causes the new sequence to continue to evolve by the basic principle of natural selection.

In addition, the so-called indels are small insertions or deletions of several Ns in a particular position, which commonly alter the sequential reading of the DNA chain. The copy-number variants (CNVs) are repeated fragments of relative size that are distributed along the genome, the number of CNVs on a genome causes the differences between individuals. It has been shown that these types of variants represent up to 9.5% of our entire genome (Zarrei et al. 2015), and like the rest of variants can be the cause of certain diseases (Esteki et al. 2015) or have no visible effect on the body, simply representing genetic variation between individuals. These variants can be flagged and identified thanks to the resources that have been obtained in the 1000 Genomes Project (Auton et al. 2015), which has provided a complete map of structural variation in the human genome.

Finally, structural variants (SV) are based on genetic rearrangements over large areas of our genome, typically more than 50 basepairs, which may move from one chromosome to another or are eliminated, leading to serious genetic problems. CNVs also fit under the category of SVs, however, the tools for detecting CNVs employ different algorithms. The concept of balanced variation is also closely related to genomic rearrangement events. If the total number of nucleotides remains the same after the rearrangement, it is said to be balanced. If, on the contrary, there is a net change in the number of nucleotides in the genome; the variation is said to be imbalanced.

Both types of variants are divided into two groups for technical reasons since the algorithms used for their detection are different. Germline variants are those that occur in the germ cells of an organism (ova and sperm); they are inherited by the offspring and are, therefore, present in all the cells of the offspring's body. Somatic variants, on the other hand, arise in the somatic cells during adult life but are not passed on to the offspring. The latter variants are key to understanding the emergence and development of complex diseases such as cancer. Cancer is considered complex because the same type of cancer may vary considerably from one patient to another. It is, therefore, crucial to establish a framework of precision medicine at all stages of cancer treatment, including its diagnosis or prognosis. Each type of cancer has key genes and specific mutations responsible for its development and/or progress. Nevertheless, minimal generalizations are possible when we differentiate between germline and somatic variations. Hereditary or family cancer syndromes are caused by germline cancer-associated variants which are present in certain genes, increasing the predisposition of an individual to develop a specific tumor. These mutations are known relatively well and have been studied in depth, so their detection does not pose a major challenge. Somatic variants, in turn, are much more difficult to detect because of their heterogeneity. This type of variant arises in specific cells and tissues and at a specific moment in the life of an individual. There are two types of mutations: driver mutations, which are the main cause of tumor development; and passenger mutations, which play a secondary role in the development of a tumor; they arise in the majority of tumors and can aggravate their symptoms. Finally, the more advanced a tumor, the greater the probability of new mutations, so a patient with tumor subpopulations may have sets of cells with different genetic signatures. Thus, the key to a precise diagnosis is the correct detection and identification of somatic variants in tumor processes, which make it possible to precisely predict the progression of the disease and to establish treatments that are specially targeted at mutational signatures (Gao et al. 2019).

Variant calling tools are typically designed to detect a particular type of variant, although others have a modular design that allows for the identification of different types of variants in the same sample. SNPs and indels are more frequent and more known than SVs, for this reason, numerous tools are targeted at this group of variants. SNP and indel variant calling tools follow either heuristic or probabilistic approaches:

- Heuristic methods use multiple sources of information on data quality to assign variants. VarScan2 (Koboldt et al. 2012), for example, also implements statistical methods such as Fisher's test to compare variants with theoretical distributions (Mielczarek and Szyda 2016).
- Probabilistic methods, in turn, are based on Bayesian approaches that optimize the probability of identifying genotypes. Currently, the most widely used probabilistic variant calling tools are SAMtools or GATK.

Germline callers, specifically, have the most standardized detection process among all variant calling tools. The aforementioned GATK, SAMtools or VarScan2, fit under this group, as well as others, such as SNVer (Wei et al. 2011) or FreeBayes (Garrison and Marth 2012). However, out of all of them, the GATK algorithm normally offers the most reliable and accurate results (Cornish and Guda 2015). In addition, GATK has a modular design for the detection of other variants and has several functions for the filtering and recalibrating of results, so it seems to be the best option in most studies. However, other reviews have pointed to the ability of FreeBayes to detect a significant number of high-quality variants, so it may be a good option in cases where greater precision is needed to determine the number of obtained variants (Hwang et al. 2015).

As discussed previously, it is more difficult to detect somatic variants than germline variants. It is assumed that the allelic frequency of germline variants must range between 50% and 100%, which is why the process simply involves determining genotype probabilities. However, the high frequency of germline variants may complicate the detection of somatic variants, especially if the frequency of the somatic variants is low. In addition, the high heterogeneity of the subclones of somatic variants or the possible impurities present in the sample, further complicate the detection of real somatic variants. Most tools follow a strategy known as matched tumor-normal variant calling, in which two samples from the same patient are sequenced, one of the tumor tissue and the other of normal tissue. The results are compared to distinguish somatic variants from the germlines, which are present in both samples. The tools that follow this approach can be divided into groups according to the algorithm they use (Xu et al. 2014). Heuristic algorithms are employed by tools such as VarScan2 (Koboldt et al. 2012), qSNP (Kassahn et al. 2013), Shimmer (Hansen et al. 2013), or VarDict (Lai et al. 2016), which use certain thresholds to detect variants and then apply ad hoc statistical methods, such as Fisher's exact test, to filter the results and obtain only somatic variants. The joint genotype analysis, adopted by tools such as SomaticSniper (Larson et al. 2012), SAMtools (Danecek et al. 2021), JointSNVMix2 (Roth et al. 2012), or Seurat (Christoforides et al. 2013), assumes diploidy in both samples and attempts to infer the joint genotypes by means of Bayes' theorem. However, there may be more heterogeneous subclones in a tumor sample, which means that the diploidy assumption oversimplifies the process. Thus, tools such as Strelka (Saunders et al. 2012), MuTect (Cibulskis et al. 2013), or deepSNV (Gerstung et al. 2012) are based on allelic frequency analysis and attempts to move away from the classical joint genotypes approach. The haplotype-based strategy is used by tools such as Platypus (Rimmer et al. 2014), FreeBayes (Garrison and Marth 2012), or MuTect2 (Ruffalo et al. 2011), and consists in assembling reads locally, in concrete regions, and in generating haplotypes with an associated probability. Finally, algorithms based on ML, such as SomaticSeq (Fang et al. 2015) or SnooPer (Spinella et al. 2016), have gained popularity in recent years. These tools train various classifiers based on a real set of variants; some of those tools are even considered ensemble variant callers because they require the union of variants detected by different tools. As a whole, the choice of one tool over another, within the matched tumor-normal strategy, depends on the type and characteristics of the variant that is being searched for. There are tools that only detect SNVs, while others are more flexible and are also able to obtain indels and SVs. The expected allelic frequency of the variants may be one of the key factors that determines the choice of a tool. The use of joint genotype tools is optimal in cases where variant frequency is high; these tools offer good results in the presence of low-coverage data. However, as suggested by several reports (Xu et al. 2014), when searching for new variants or for variants with a low frequency, it is preferable to make use of the allelic frequency approach, adapted by tools such as Strelka or deepSNV.

The matched tumor-normal variant calling strategy is not the only existing strategy for the detection of somatic variants. In practice, it is not always possible to obtain a normal sample from the same patient, either for economic reasons or because it may no longer be feasible to retrieve a germline sample. This is one of today's major challenges in clinical bioinformatics. It is necessary to develop accurate and effective algorithms that can identify somatic variants in the absence of a normal sample. Some tools have already been developed to this end. They can be divided into two large groups according to their core algorithm. Tools like SNVMix2 (Goya et al. 2010), Shearwater (Gerstung et al. 2014), SPLINTER (Vallania et al. 2012), or SNVer (Wei et al. 2011) firstly report all variants without distinguishing between somatic or germline variants, and then they each use a different method to filter as many germline variants as possible. Other tools, such as ISOWN (Kalatskaya et al. 2017) or SomVarIUS (Smith et al. 2016), clearly distinguish between somatic and germline variants because they use ML algorithms to train classifiers with data on the mutation, its clinical impact, frequency and genomic context, etc. (Xu et al. 2014). All this information comes from somatic variant databases such as COSMIC (Tate et al. 2019), or germline variant databases such as Exome Aggregation Consortium (ExAC), repository that contains the exome data of 60 706 individuals, (Karczewski et al. 2017) or dbSNP (Sherry et al. 1999). Furthermore, certain tools, such as the MuTect2 tool, are capable of carrying out a tumor-only sequencing strategy using a panel of normals, created on the basis of the sequenced data of a tumor sample. It has been demonstrated that MuTect2 can in some cases obtain true somatic variants with an accuracy similar to that of matched tumor-normal calling algorithms. However, the MuTect2 strategy is not as effective given that it can only detect already known variants. In the case of variants with a lower frequency, it is necessary to resort to using a normal sample for comparison (Teer et al. 2017).

The tools designed for short-read sequencing projects can be used for SV detection while long-read sequencing platforms can help minimize some of the difficulties that emerge during the detection of SVs. Today, these projects are not yet fully implemented in clinical practice and there are not many tools focused on this type of reads so that almost all analysis pipelines of SVs focus on methods based on short reads. It should be noted that, due to the great complexity and variety of SVs, there are currently no tools that could efficiently detect all the variants. As we shall see below, different platforms can detect a different type of variant (Kosugi et al. 2019). Each tool employs a different algorithm, though it is possible to draw some parallels between them. Some software, such as Breakdancer (Chen et al. 2009), classifies each read into normal or variant-associated, according to its distance and orientation on the map. The regions with a greater proportion of reads are more likely to overlap a SV, that is why Breakdancer labels those regions. Other tools can be applied to slightly increase the resolution of the algorithm and to detect a wider range of variants. DELLY (Rausch et al. 2012) integrates split-read analysis. LUMPY (Layer et al. 2014) adds information on the depth of coverage between regions; Manta (Chen et al. 2016) implements a parallel analysis with a graph-based approach (Mahmoud et al. 2019). To make the right choice, it is necessary to consider the results of recent benchmarking studies that evaluated the performance of numerous tools (Kosugi et al. 2019). Manta, DELLY, and LUMPY generally have good precision and recall values for all types of SVs. Nevertheless, if the best possible results are to be obtained, the choice of the algorithm depends on the type of variant one is searching for. For example, GRIDSS (Cameron et al. 2017) is the best option for deletions; the Wham tool has the best recall and precision in the case of duplications (Kronenberg et al. 2015); MELT (Gardner et al. 2017) or DELLY can be used for inversions (Rausch et al. 2012). Given that there is no universal software that would detect the whole range of SVs, many projects have focused their efforts on the ensemble approach. This approach focuses on detecting different types of variants by means of different tools so that a merged variant call set is obtained.

The ensemble approach is more robust and reliable because it combines the advantages of different methods and overcomes their limitations. Recently, a number of packages have been developed that implement this approach, instead of having to do it manually, they adjust the parameters and variant callers chosen by the user, such as MetaSV (Mohiyuddin et al. 2015), Parliament2 (Zarate et al. 2021), or SURVIVOR (Jeffares et al. 2017).

11.2.5 Variant Annotation

The NGS data analysis pipeline concludes with the process of variant annotation, during which biological significance is given to the obtained results. Thanks to certain applications and tools, it is possible to perform what is known as the biological or functional annotation of variants. It involves the search for a large amount of information on variants, according to multiple parameters, such as the variant's genomic region, the gene and the protein it affects, etc. All this is possible thanks to all the information available in different databases and online resources, such as dbSNP or the 1000 Genomes Project. Those resources provide a series of metrics for the evaluation of the potential clinical impact of a variant in question. These metrics are essential in clinical research, whose objective is to discover the potential relationship between the disease of a patient and its genomic variants. Metrics based on predictive algorithms have been developed over the last two decades to classify variants according to their pathogenicity, or potential protein damage (Gunning et al. 2020). Prediction is based on annotation features, such as the amino acid change, the evolutionary pressure of the gene where it is found, its consequence on the protein or the variant population frequency, and many of these metrics even have AI to boost their accuracy. Among these metrics, we can highlight Condel (González-Pérez and López-Bigas 2011), PolyPhen (Adzhubei et al. 2010), or sorting intolerant from tolerant (SIFT) (Kumar et al. 2009). There are variants whose pathogenicity is certain, while others are neutral or possibly benign. The function of some of the variants is unknown, these are classified as variant of uncertain significance (VUS). This classification is currently standardized and there are consensus guidelines for its evaluation and application in different NGS data analysis pipelines (Roy et al. 2018). In addition to this classification, variants can also be defined according to the effect they have on the protein chain. Synonymous variants are the ones that do not result in a net change in the sequence of amino acids due to the degeneration of the genetic code. Non-synonymous variants cause a real change in the protein, which can have functional consequences. Likewise, the gain or loss of Ns must be considered in the case of insertions or deletions. Given that the sequence of Ns is read in multiples of three, a structural mutation can cause a change in the normal reading of the sequence, resulting in a totally different chain of amino acids; this type of mutation is called frameshift mutation. In the case of an in-frame mutation, the DNA sequence may be read normally. Although in the past it had been assumed that both punctual and SVs result in a deleterious protein that causes a change in the sequence of amino acids; recent studies have demonstrated that this is not certainly true (Mair et al. 2016). Thus, the functional prediction of the detected variants is more complex than expected.

Most types of NGS analysis software incorporate graphical interfaces or web platforms so that their use does not require a very high level of computational knowledge and it makes functional annotation more intuitive. However, this is not the case with the tools that have been developed to determine whether a variant is synonymous or non-synonymous. This is because sequencing projects offer such a large amount of data and variants that this type of platform cannot support it. Thus, when high parallelization or computation is required, command line tools are employed. Many tools have been developed for this purpose, such as ANNOVAR (Wang et al. 2010), NGS-SNP (Grant et al. 2011), snpEff (Cingolani et al. 2012), or Variant Effect Predictor (VEP) (McLaren et al. 2016), where ANNOVAR and VEP are the most revised and commonly used tools today. This is because they offer a high degree of comprehensiveness and make it possible to annotate in command line or through a graphical interface (Pabinger et al. 2014).

The countless resources and/or databases available today are an important source of information when prioritizing or filtering variants, making it possible to avoid the use of countless variant callers. An earlier section has described two of the largest databases; the dbSNP and the resources made available by the 1000 Genomes Project. However, it is necessary to highlight other resources that can offer valuable information on variants. In 2014, the ExAC created a repository that served as a resource for coding variants and obtaining allelic frequencies. However, in 2016 the ExAC was replaced by the improved Genome Aggregation Database (gnomAD) (Karczewski et al. 2020), which introduced new data sets, resulting in 123 136 exomes and 15 496 complete genomes of unrelated individuals. In addition to this repository, the 100 000 Genomes Project of Genomics England (Robbe et al. 2018) is probably the most ambitious genomic sequencing project to date. The project obtained the complete genome of 100,000 people in the United Kingdom. It is now possible to obtain these data for use in research, which provides valuable information to the variant annotation pipeline. These resources offer general information about the genomes and exomes of individuals. However, in the case of a tumor sample analysis, it is necessary to search for data in specific repositories that characterize this type of disease. Among those, COSMIC, a repository that stores information on somatic mutations related to cancer, or The Cancer Genome Atlas (TCGA) project ("The Cancer Genome Atlas Program - National Cancer Institute" n.d.), which has generated exhaustive and multidimensional maps on key genomic changes in numerous types of cancer. Thanks to those resources it is possible to filter the search for variants according to functional annotation, allelic frequency, or role in certain types of cancers. Thus, the robustness and reliability of the variants and the annotated functional characteristics increase significantly, making it possible to reduce the number of variant callers used in the pipeline (Gao et al. 2019). Studies published in recent years have greatly contributed to improving the process of characterization and functional validation of cancer variants, making it possible to gain valuable insights into cancer driver genes (Bailey et al. 2018). Moreover, it has been possible to learn more about functional mutations thanks to protein structure analysis tools (Niu et al. 2016).

11.3 Nanopore Sequencing Data Analysis

Long-read sequencing technology has expanded the scope of applications and possibilities of mass sequencing in clinical settings to become a method with the potential to be routine practice (Goenka et al. 2022). Third-generation technologies are more recent than short-read sequencing methods, so their characteristics clearly differentiate them from each other. The main difference is that they are based on sequencing long reads and do not depend on the amplification of fragments to be sequenced by polymerase chain reaction (PCR). Their capabilities have made it possible to solve new genomic challenges, such as the detection of SVs (Weischenfeldt et al. 2013) or the assembly of novel genomes, although they have not yet managed to reach the precision ratios obtained by second-generation technologies such as Illumina. Among third-generation sequencing technologies is Pacific Biosciences' method called single molecule real time (SMART) sequencing, as well as the innovative and promising technology developed by Oxford Nanopore (Amarasinghe et al. 2020).

The analysis of data from long read sequencing experiments also requires the management and execution of a pipeline or workflow with several processing steps, as for the analysis of short-read data which has already been reviewed above. Therefore, without going into minute detail, this section describes the main aspects of the pipeline, its differences with respect to technologies such as Illumina, and a review of the state-of-the-art tools used by the community. The analysis of long-read data involves the following stages: base-calling, quality control, error correction and, depending on the specific approach or application, DNA or RNA modification detection, de novo genome assembly, transcriptome analysis, variant calling, and haplotyping/phasing. In this case, the work focuses, as for short reads, on the detection of different types of variants of clinical interest for nanopore sequencing experiments, as it is the technology with the largest presence in clinical settings.

11.3.1 Base-Calling

The DNA or RNA strand passing through the nanopore causes a change in voltage and ionic current within a polymer membrane, specific to each of the bases being translocated. These raw current change measurements need to be further transformed into the sequence itself, in a process known as base-calling, making it a fundamental step in the nanopore data analysis pipeline. For this purpose, both in-house commercial tools and open-source software have been developed by ONT using different algorithmic methods. Undoubtedly, the most widely used software package is part of the set of tools provided by ONT called Guppy, with algorithms such as Scrappie or Bonito (Xu et al. 2021), which together with the MinKNOW service offer a complete experience in terms of managing the sequencing process and obtaining sequenced reads (Wang et al. 2021). Other widely used third-party tools are Causalcall (temporal convolutional network) (Zeng et al. 2020), DeepNano (recurrent neural network) (Boža et al. 2017), or fast-bonito (reimplementation of bonito using neural architecture search technique to speed up execution) (Xu et al. 2021).

11.3.2 Quality Control and Preprocessing

As for the analysis of short-read data, a quality control and preprocessing stage of the data generated in the base-calling phase is necessary to ensure the correct execution of downstream analyses and to evaluate the quality of the generated fragments. For this purpose, many tools have been developed in different languages, such as LongQC (Fukasawa et al. 2020), Poretools (Loman and Quinlan 2014), pore (Watson et al. 2015), NanoOK (Leggett et al. 2016), HPG pore (Tarraga et al. 2016), Nanopack (de Coster et al. 2018), or Filtlong

("GitHub - Rrwick/Filtlong: Quality Filtering Tool for Long Reads" n.d.). Most of them are very useful to assess the quality and general state of the generated data by means of metrics, visualizations, and statistical analysis, as well as to carry out the trimming needed to ensure the quality of a large part of the fragments.

11.3.3 Error Correction

The nanopore-based read generation process, although considerably improved in recent years, carries an inherent error rate of almost 15%, resulting in a good proportion of incorrectly sequenced bases. Despite the advantage of generating very long fragments that can cover large genomic regions with multiple applications, the error rate prevents it from being used to a large extent for detection of point changes or de novo genome assembly. For this reason, there is a next step for error correction using two types of methods: on the one hand, self-correction methods, which use graphs to generate consensus sequences, such as Canu (Koren et al. 2017) or LoRMA (Salmela et al. 2017), and hybrid methods, which take advantage of short reads to correct long reads by means of alignments, such as Nanocorr (Goodwin et al. 2015), Ratatosk (Holley et al. 2021), or FMLRC (Wang et al. 2018). These hybrid methods have been shown to lower the error rate to 1–4%, an equivalent measure to that of short reads (Fu et al. 2019).

11.3.4 Alignment

The advantage of long reads is that, as they cover larger genomic regions, their positioning is more likely to be unique, unlike short reads that often have several possible alignments or secondary mappings, especially in repetitive regions. Therefore, the emergence of this technology has been a relief for general-purpose mappers, although they fail to take full advantage of the characteristics of these long fragments as they are not specifically designed for them. In recent years, several interesting alignment tools have been developed and used, such as LAST (Kiełbasa et al. 2011), GraphMap (Sović et al. 2016), minimap2 (Li 2018), NGLMR (Sedlazeck et al. 2018), or GraphMap2 (Marić et al. 2019). The reference tool which has been demonstrated to obtain good results in terms of both performance and accuracy in call sets is minimap2 with its seed-chain-align algorithm (Zhou et al. 2019). This tool also allows the mapping of short reads. Moreover, the GraphMap2 algorithm – a reimplementation of GraphMap – capable of mapping in splice-aware mode to correctly detect the end of exons and is also useful.

11.3.5 Variant Calling

The goal of this nanopore sequencing data analysis pipeline is the detection of variants that are ultimately of clinical interest, be they SNVs or SVs. One of the main applications of this technology is the detection of large structural genomic changes, thanks to the length of the reads that can span these changes and accurately detect breakpoints. For this purpose, tools specifically designed for this purpose are used, such as NanoSV (Cretu Stancu et al. 2017), Sniffles (Sedlazeck et al. 2018), Picky (Gong et al. 2018), Nanovar (Tham et al. 2020), or dysgu (Cleal and Baird 2022); recent studies have shown that the best results, in general, are obtained with Sniffles (Zhou et al. 2019) and dysgu, the latter incorporating ML algorithms to create consensus call sets from both short read and long read approaches. In the case of SNVs, the high error rate of the readings makes the process of accurate point change detection more complex than in short reads. In this case, it is necessary to include a preliminary error correction step and haplotype-aware variant calling algorithms, such as the PEPPER-Margin-DeepVariant pipeline (Shafin et al. 2021), which are capable of accurately detecting these changes using the tool developed by Google.

11.4 Machine Learning Approaches in Variant Calling

In recent years, numerous tools have been developed to apply AI methods in genomic variant analysis pipelines (Zou et al. 2019). ML algorithms search for patterns in datasets; they are traditionally grouped into two categories: supervised learning and unsupervised learning. The objective of supervised learning is to predict the output value of an input variable on the basis of a training dataset that already has labeled values. Classification methods are used for categorical prediction, while regression methods are used for quantitative prediction. Unsupervised learning aims to discover hidden patterns in the dataset without any real prior label; to this end, clustering or association rule learning is employed. In short, the principal goal of a ML algorithm is to optimize a model by predicting a real value in a problem data set on the basis of previous training data. Hence, the model must behave well on training data and be able to generalize when working with other datasets.

ML algorithms can be included in a pipeline for the analysis of sequencing data, as they can contribute to most of the stages described above. However, this work focuses only on ML in variant calling and annotation, specifically on the use of ML algorithms to identify variants associated with diseases. The reason for focusing on this aspect only is because it is a critical point in most pipelines, where less precision has been achieved to date. Most ML algorithms for the analysis of NGS data employ deep learning methods and neural networks, which fall under regression algorithms in supervised learning (Zou et al. 2019). Algorithms of this type offer better performance than other methods such as classifiers or clustering techniques, as the reader can see below with the numerous studies and methods developed in recent years which improve on the more classical techniques (Schmidt and Hildebrandt 2021). Several general ML tools have been developed for the detection of variants, and their results are quite promising. For example, Scotch and Metal (Curnin et al. 2019) obtain new, previously undetected indels, while DeepVariant (Poplin et al. 2018) is a versatile tool based on a deep convolutional neural network whose main characteristic is that it is able to generalize across different genomic constructions, platforms, and experimental designs. Furthermore, many efforts have been made toward developing ML for the detection of somatic variants in projects related to cancer (Wu et al. 2020). NeuSomatic (Sahraeian et al. 2019), the first algorithm based on a convolutional neural network, has been developed for the precise detection of somatic variants. It incorporates more than 100 parameters, according to which it characterizes each training mutation. DeepSVR (Ainscough et al. 2018), a deep learning model that includes three different algorithms – logistic regression, random forest, and deep learning – which are run to refine a set of already detected variants and obtain a good set of true somatic variants. Finally, some ML tools are specific to long-read sequencing projects, such as Oxford Nanopore and Pacific Biosciences. For example, DeepNano (Boža et al. 2017), a recurrent neural network for reads from the MinION sequencer or Clairvoyant (Luo et al. 2019), a convolutional deep neural network specially designed for the SMRT sequencing platform, although it is also valid for other platforms.

Finally, algorithms focused on improving the functional annotation process of detected variants have also been developed. These algorithms are key for the analysis of unknown somatic variants related to cancer or mutations in noncoding regions. One of these tools is DeepSEA (Zhou and Troyanskaya 2015), a deep learning-based algorithm that identifies functional characteristics of noncoding variants through information from regulatory sequences, chromatin profiles, etc. BadMut (Korvigo et al. 2018) is a meta-estimator that employs deep learning algorithms to integrate several deleteriousness prediction scores, obtaining a valuable prediction of the pathogenic potential of a variant. DeepGene (Yuan et al. 2016) software is a classifier based on a deep neural network that correctly classifies different types of cancer according to the profile of specific somatic mutations; this contributes to a better diagnosis and prognosis of the disease. The DANN tool (Quang et al. 2015) can detect the pathogenicity of variants. It is based on the widely used Combined Annotation Dependent Depletion (CADD) algorithm, which uses ML with support vector machines (Rentzsch et al. 2019). However, given that SVM algorithms are not able to detect non-linear relationships, the tool has been developed based on a deep neural network, which is able to detect all the patterns.

11.5 Next-Generation Sequencing Data Analysis Frameworks

The analysis of NGS data involves numerous stages in which the output generally becomes the input of the next step, giving rise to what is known as a pipeline. Given the complexity of NGS data analysis, a certain level of IT expertise is required to correctly manage the generated files, implement third-party software needed at each stage, and, in most cases, build a script that can be executed in command line. Therefore, over the last few years, the bioinformatics community has been developing analytical pipelines to face this problem. Different tools have been designed to import the raw reads of the sequencer and facilitate the process of obtaining variants that contain relevant biological information. Those tools have made it possible for researchers with no computational background to use and apply analytical pipelines. Software often includes a graphical interface that enables the user to modify parameters; moreover, the interpretation of results is much more intuitive, avoiding what is known in computing as black box; a system in which only the inputs and outputs can be studied but not their internal functioning.

The need for the development of these pipelines and workflows also arises from the large number of challenges posed by the new paradigm of genomic data analysis and the era of mass sequencing. The development of numerous applications and tools has contributed to the evolution and optimization of existing platforms and development of new algorithms capable of addressing complex problems. It has become difficult to choose from such a wide range of sophisticated tools and algorithms for all stages of NGS data analysis. By 2017, there were already more than 11 000 tools for the analysis of omics data cataloged in the OMICtools platform (Henry et al. 2014). This statistic demonstrates that assembling pipelines and choosing the right tool at each step is a complex and time-consuming process for researchers with little IT knowledge. This points to the urgency of standardizing analyses and increasing reproducibility in computational biology (Sandve et al. 2013). Moreover, it is necessary to develop advanced but not technically complex tools so that a much larger group of users can perform this type of analysis (Lam et al. 2012). For example, such tools should not require intricate command-line instructions.

Some analytical pipelines offer a predefined order of steps and processes; thus, they allow little flexibility in modifying or replacing certain modules. HugeSeq (Lam et al. 2012), SIMPLEX (Fischer et al. 2012), TREAT (Asmann et al. 2012), bcbio-nextgen ("Bcbio/Bcbio-Nextgen: Validated, Scalable, Community Developed Variant Calling, RNA-Seq and Small RNA Analysis" n.d.), or Sam2bam (Ogasawara et al. 2016) are some of the examples of such pipelines. They implement an automatic and complete analysis of NGS data, from the reception of reads to the identification of different types of variants. These pipelines can receive different formats, be used on cloud platforms, carry out specific sections of the entire pipeline, and offer researchers comprehensive results in the form of summary reports. However, they are usually not very flexible when inserting new modules or modifying certain stages, making it difficult to adapt them to the specific needs of a given project, so they may lag behind due to their rigidity, especially for the bioinformatics community. As a solution to this problem, new platforms have emerged; they are known as workflow management systems or pipeline frameworks (Wratten et al. 2021). These platforms offer greater openness and flexibility to accommodate different pipelines. In addition, their features are more advanced, processes can be visualized in real time, and it is possible to work in the cloud, use a graphical interface, or containerize various tools (Leipzig 2017). There are a large amount of workflow management systems at present; some of them are more standardized, while others are newer and more innovative. Galaxy (Goecks et al. 2010) is a widely used web platform in bioinformatic analysis; it has more than 100 tools available for the different stages of NGS analysis, with the possibility of creating custom pipelines, reproducing them, and sharing them later with the community. Thanks to its graphical interface, Galaxy's web platform is simple and intuitive to use, even in the creation and customization of scripts. Due to its wide use among the scientific community, Galaxy has become a benchmark system for the rest of the workflow frameworks. SEQprocess (Joo et al. 2019) is a framework for carrying out NGS data analysis; it offers several preinstalled pipelines as well as personalized pipeline-generation features. The main characteristic of the R package is that it implements specific analyses for new oncological applications based on the TGCA. However, to generate a personalized pipeline, the user must have some computational background; they must be able to install the specific software and modify the parameters in configuration files. Closha (Ko et al. 2018), another recently developed workflow framework, is a system optimized for use in the cloud through high-performance computing clusters; it also has a graphical interface and makes it possible to run both ready-made and user-customized pipelines. It has certain technical advantages, such as the implementation of a new system known as KoDS for fast file transfer or the scalability of resources; it increases its performance as computational requirements increase, which makes its execution speed slightly higher than that of Galaxy. NGS-pipe (Singer et al. 2018) is another user-friendly analysis framework for the automated design of custom pipelines, ensuring reproducibility in clinical applications and allowing for parallelization in clusters. However, it also requires the manual installation of software and the modification of a configuration file to adjust the parameters. Regarding this aspect, Bio-Docklet (Kim et al. 2017) is a tool for the management of pipelines from other systems, such as Galaxy, in Docker containers, encapsulating all the necessary preconfigured software. This is a very useful approach, as it prevents researchers from having to install software manually. Furthermore, tools have been developed to vastly improve the processing speed of pipelines. The Sentieon software suite (Freed et al. 2017) offers an optimized reimplantation of tools that are routinely used in variant calling analysis, such as BWA or GATK. Sentieon provides consistent results and improves the overall performance of the whole pipeline. The Parabricks tool comprises numerous genomic pipelines, and it has a very promising graphics processing unit (GPU)-accelerated strategy, capable of transforming, within a matter of hours, the FASTQ data from an entire genome project into a variant call format (VCF) output (Franke and Crowgey 2020).

11.6 DeepNGS

DeepNGS is a rapid and automated platform for clinicians and researchers. It processes human-sequenced DNA samples and obtains a set of genetic variants that are key to the clinical diagnosis of any patient. The platform incorporates all the patient's genetic data in a highly secure cloud environment and achieves a higher level of accuracy. It is capable of digesting information to ensure the accuracy of the final diagnosis and the adequacy of treatment recommendations. ML algorithms are being progressively incorporated to optimize the analysis process and achieve even better and more reliable results (Corchado et al. 2021).

The result is a set of detected variants, which may be SNVs, INDELs, or SVs. The platform also distinguishes germinal variants from somatic variants, which are characteristic of tumor cells and whose correct detection is essential in the diagnosis and treatment of this type of disease. Once the alignment, variant detection, and annotation stages have been completed, the intuitive DeepNGS interface offers a general overview and a wealth of visualizations from which conclusions can be drawn immediately.

11.6.1 Pipeline

This section describes the main tools used in the DeepNGS pipeline, managed by the workflow management system Nextflow, which allows for task and job parallelization, reproducibility, and deployment in different computational environments. Below are the algorithms used for Illumina sequencing data in Table 11.1 and for Oxford Nanopore sequencing data in Table 11.2.

Table 11.1 Illumina sequencing data (short-read technology).

Pipeline stage	Tools
Quality control and preprocessing	fastp
Alignment	bwa-mem
Postprocessing	Samtools, GATK MarkDuplicates, GATK BaseRecalibrator, GATK ApplyBQSR
Germline variant calling (SNVs)	GATK HaplotypeCaller, GATK CNNScoreVariants, DeepVariant, octopus
Somatic variant calling (SNVs)	GATK Mutect2, vardictjava, strelka2, scalpel, lofreq, octopus, somaticseq
Structural variant calling	dysgu
Annotation (SNVs)	Ensembl VEP, tapes, OpenCRAVAT
Annotation (SVs)	AnnotSV

Table 11.2 Oxford Nanopore sequencing data (long-reads technology).

Pipeline stage	Tools
Quality control and preprocessing	NanoPack, filtlong
Alignment	minimap2
Postprocessing	samtools
SNVs calling	PEPPER-Margin-DeepVariant
SVs calling	Sniffles, dysgu
Annotation (SNVs)	Ensembl VEP, tapes, OpenCRAVAT
Annotation (SVs)	AnnotSV

11.6.2 DeepNGS Main Features

11.6.2.1 Power and Speed

Cloud computing enables the tool to process FASTQ files from mass sequencing experiments on Illumina platforms, regardless of whether they are gene panels, exomes, or complete genomes. The platform leverages resources provided by Amazon Web Services to launch jobs in an optimized way, using AWS Batch, EC2 instances, S3 storage, or Elastic Container Registry for containerization.

The platform's capabilities will be extended with the release of a new product specifically designed to be deployed in local on-premises environments. This platform can be customized at the installation level according to the computational requirements of each user and the characteristics of their servers, with continuous technical assistance from experts.

11.6.2.2 Optimized Workflow

The tool uses advanced scripts in a continuous process of optimization, with workflow management systems that enable reproducibility, re-entrancy checkpoints, scalability, and system packaging. We have analyzed and incorporated the latest advances in genomics and adapted them to the specific needs of each type of analysis, with the best reference databases worldwide.

11.6.2.3 Intuitive Design and Interactive Charts

- Visualizations and charts make it easier to interpret and present the results.
- Advanced visualization techniques
- Fully optimized and adapted to the needs of genetic data
- Simple and intuitive display of useful information
- Comfortable and user-friendly interface

11.6.2.4 Extended Information

One of the features that makes DeepNGS stand out is the large amount of biological information associated with each of the detected variants, making it possible to prioritize those that are key to the development of the disease.

Information is provided on a classified basis with different annotation sources: basic properties of variants (genomic location, resulting change in the protein, etc.), pathogenicity predictors, allele frequencies in multiple populations, or clinical information. DeepNGS uses multiple data sources to provide the information, such as ClinVar (Landrum et al. 2018), Ensembl (Cunningham et al. 2022), dbNSFP (Xiaoming Liu et al. 2020), 1000 Genomes, or the platform's own data (see Figure 11.2).

Pathogenicity is predicted by means of various computational methods of great clinical utility, such as SIFT, MetaSVM (Dong et al. 2015), DANN, or BayesDel (Feng 2017). These algorithms allow for the automatic prediction of the potential deleterious effect of a specific genetic variant in the protein (see Figure 11.3).

In addition, the platform has modules for the analysis of the variants' associations with drugs, epigenetics, and transcriptomics. PanDrugs (Piñeiro-Yáñez et al. 2018) is used as a tool to calculate association scores between genes and antitumor drugs, which is of vital importance in the analysis of somatic mutations. Epigenetic analysis allows for the analysis of chemical modifications attached to the DNA structure and its regulated three-dimensional folding, which allows the cell to control transcriptional processes and direct the expression of specific genes in specific situations, giving an extra layer of personalization to the DNA-based phenotype. On the other hand, transcriptomics is one of the most widely used omics in research today to study all kinds of cellular processes and how certain genes are regulated, although it has not yet been fully implemented in clinical practice. Both blocks take clinical genomic analysis to another level, integrating much more information to have a more global vision of the clinical phenotype.

11.6.2.5 Artificial Intelligence and Machine Learning

DeepNGS takes full advantage of AI. The development of specific and optimized ML models and algorithms at multiple points in the pipeline enables continuous improvement and allows for the optimization of the complete analysis pipeline (see Table 11.3).

⬇ EXPORT OPTIONS ▾

Table filters configuration

Category Annotation field

Basic annotation - ›

▼ APPLY NEW FILTER

Showing 1-10 of 43459 items

Chromosome (hg19)	Position (hg19)	Reference allele	Alternative allele	Gene (HUGO)	HGVSc	HGVSp	HGVSg	Probability Path	Prediction ACMG	Start Position (hg19)	End Position (hg19)	Chromosome (hg38)	Pos (hg:
12	103234252	T	C	PAH	ENST00000553106.1:c-1241A>G	ENSP00000448059.1:p-Tyr414Cys	chr12:g-103234252T>C	0.9998	Pathogenic	103234252	103234252	12	102:
1	216424437	C	A	USH2A	ENST00000307340.3:c-1975G>T	ENSP00000305941.3:p-Gly659Ter	chr1:g-216424437C>A	0.9971	Pathogenic	216424437	216424437	1	216:
X	153420052	C	A	OPN1LW	ENST00000369951.4:c-582C>A	ENSP00000358967.4:p-Tyr194Ter	chrX:g-153420052C>A	0.9971	Pathogenic	153420052	153420052	X	154:
6	64431415	C	A	EYS	ENST00000503681.1:c-8512G>T	ENSP00000424243.1:p-Glu2830Ter	chr6:g-64431415C>A	0.9941	Likely Pathogenic	64431415	64431415	6	637:
9	2096706	A	T	SMARCA2	ENST00000382203.1:c-2933A>T	ENSP00000371638.1:p-Tyr978Phe	chr9:g-2096706A>T	0.8999	Likely Pathogenic	2096706	2096706	9	209:
6	161127501	A	G	PLG	ENST00000308192.9:c-112A>G	ENSP00000308938.9:p-Lys38Glu	chr6:g-161127501A>G	0.8121	Likely Pathogenic	161127501	161127501	6	160:
1	9796038	C	T	CLSTN1	ENST00000377298.4:c-1639G>A	ENSP00000377298.4:p-Gly547Arg	chr1:g-9796038C>T	0.8121	VUS	9796038	9796038	1	973:
12	53452525	T	C	TNS2	ENST00000314276.3:c-1349T>C	ENSP00000319756.3:p-Val450Ala	chr12:g-53452525T>C	0.8121	VUS	53452525	53452525	12	530:
15	78572759	A	G	DNAJA4	ENST00000394855.3:c-1238A>G	ENSP00000378324.3:p-Asp413Gly	chr15:g-78572759A>G	0.8121	VUS	78572759	78572759	15	782:
7	150932567	C	T	CHPF2	ENST00000035307.2:c-697C>T	ENSP00000035307.2:p-Arg233Trp	chr7:g-150932567C>T	0.8121	VUS	150932567	150932567	7	151:

Figure 11.2 Overview of final annotation table with information tabs. Annotation categories are displayed at the top, followed by the advanced filter module, and finally, the table with the detected variants sorted according to their pathogenicity.

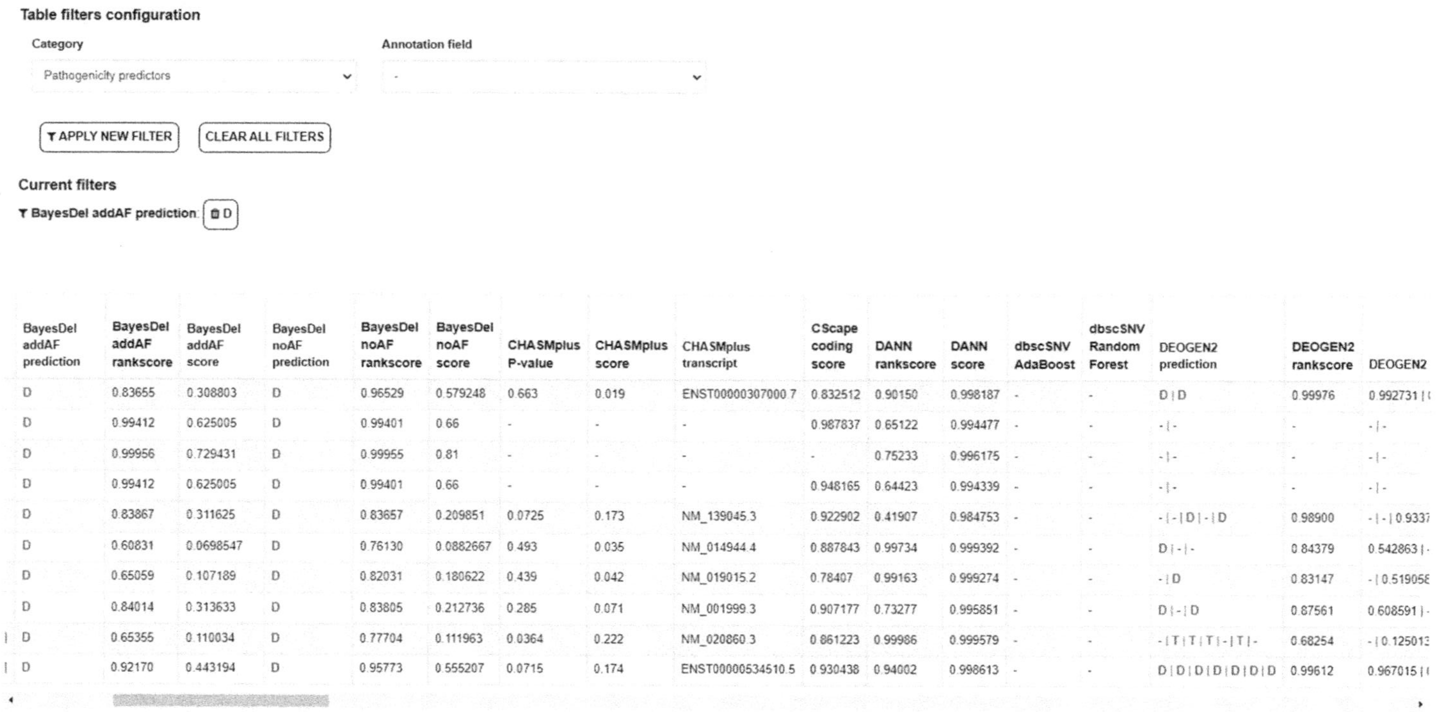

Table filters configuration

Category	Annotation field
Pathogenicity predictors >	- >

APPLY NEW FILTER CLEAR ALL FILTERS

Current filters

▼ BayesDel addAF prediction: ⊗ D

BayesDel addAF prediction	BayesDel addAF rankscore	BayesDel addAF score	BayesDel noAF prediction	BayesDel noAF rankscore	BayesDel noAF score	CHASMplus P-value	CHASMplus score	CHASMplus transcript	CScape coding score	DANN rankscore	DANN score	dbscSNV AdaBoost	dbscSNV Random Forest	DEOGEN2 prediction	DEOGEN2 rankscore	DEOGEN2
D	0.83655	0.308803	D	0.96529	0.579248	0.663	0.019	ENST00000307000 7	0.832512	0.50150	0.998187	-	-	D ¦ D	0.99976	0.992731 ¦ ¦
D	0.99412	0.625005	D	0.99401	0.66	-	-	-	0.987837	0.65122	0.994477	-	-	- ¦ -	-	- ¦ -
D	0.99956	0.729431	D	0.99955	0.81	-	-	-		0.75233	0.996175	-	-	- ¦ -	-	- ¦ -
D	0.99412	0.625005	D	0.99401	0.66	-	-	-	0.948165	0.64423	0.994339	-	-	- ¦ -	-	- ¦ -
D	0.83867	0.311625	D	0.83657	0.209851	0.0725	0.173	NM_139045 3	0.922902	0.41907	0.984753	-	-	- ¦ - ¦ D ¦ - ¦ D	0.98900	- ¦ - ¦ 0.9337
D	0.60831	0.0698547	D	0.76130	0.0882667	0.493	0.035	NM_014944 4	0.887843	0.99734	0.999392	-	-	D ¦ - ¦ -	0.84379	0.542863 ¦ -
D	0.65059	0.107189	D	0.82031	0.180622	0.439	0.042	NM_019015 2	0.78407	0.99163	0.999274	-	-	- ¦ D	0.83147	- ¦ 0.519056
D	0.84014	0.313633	D	0.83805	0.212736	0.285	0.071	NM_001999 3	0.907177	0.73277	0.995851	-	-	D ¦ - ¦ D	0.87561	0.608691 ¦ -
¦ D	0.66365	0.110034	D	0.77704	0.111963	0.0364	0.222	NM_020860 3	0.861223	0.99986	0.999579	-	-	- ¦ T ¦ T ¦ - ¦ T ¦ -	0.68254	- ¦ 0.125012
¦ D	0.92170	0.443194	D	0.95773	0.555207	0.0715	0.174	ENST00000534510 5	0.930438	0.94002	0.998613	-	-	D ¦ D ¦ D ¦ D ¦ D ¦ D	0.99612	0.967015 ¦ ¦

Figure 11.3 Overview of pathogenicity tab with multiple in silico predictors.

Table 11.3 AI algorithms included in the pipeline.

Pipeline stage	Algorithms
Somatic variant calling	Bayesian methods, pattern growth, convolutional, and recurrent neural networks
Pathogenicity prediction	Deep neural networks, random forests, logistic regression
Treatment recommender	Expert system

11.7 Conclusions

As we have seen, there are multiple tools and platforms available today which facilitate the arduous task of analyzing data in a mass sequencing project. Every new tool is more sophisticated than the previous one; this demonstrates how rapidly the field of computational research is evolving and how this leads to a lack of standardization and reproducibility. Therefore, it is necessary to carry out exhaustive studies of the applications in the field of NGS. The elaboration of guidelines and pipelines for each of the applications would be a great step toward improving the transparency and reproducibility of sequencing projects. Second, it has been observed that numerous framework systems have the potential to become standard instruments in any biomedical laboratory; this potential is marked by their characteristics, such as a graphical interface, ease of use, or the possibility of running in parallel in the cloud. Nevertheless, user interfaces are only present in systems that perform the analysis process or customize pipelines, while the final information is not delivered in such a graphical and intuitive way. In cases such as clinical research, where the conclusions of an experiment or even the health of a patient depend on the final information, the interpretation of the results is essential.

This goal has been achieved with the development of DeepNGS, a robust and optimized platform for clinicians in which one of the basic pillars is the biological annotation of the variants and their optimal interpretation, generating graphical and intuitive reports that feature the patient's clinical information. Finally, including ML algorithms in NGS data analysis pipelines implemented in DeepNGS is a novel approach, as it is quite rare in today's standard frameworks. AI has, in recent years, made its way into the field of genomics, which continues to grow and generate an enormous amount of data. Thus, the inclusion of intelligent models and algorithms improves the results obtained by the classical pipeline. In addition to the functionalities already implemented in DeepNGS, the development of a premium version is planned for the near future. The premium version will take variant interpretation and genomic analysis functions to another level. Some of these extra functional modules will offer: cancer-specific databases (COSMIC), the smart prediction of pathogenicity in relation to a set of symptoms or phenotypes, the analysis of duos and trios for complex familial cases, or the analysis of complex genomic samples such as cfDNA, liquid biopsies, or FFPEs. It is also intended to deploy an alternative product for architectures on local servers on-premises, with continuous technical assistance for incident management or execution optimization in subnetworks, all handled by a workflow management system such as Nextflow.

Author Biographies

Víctor Duarte, Graduated in Biotechnology from the University Pablo de Olavide in Seville in 2017. Master's degree in Advanced Bioinformatic Analysis from the same university in 2019 and Master's degree in Bioinformatics and Biostatistics from the Universitat Oberta de Catalunya in 2020. Expert in the development and management of mass sequencing genomic data analysis pipelines. Researcher in bioinformatics in the BISITE research group since September 2019, with interests in the application of computational technologies and artificial intelligence in the analysis of biological data, with special emphasis on the management of clinical genomic data.

Alesandro Gómez, Graduated in Computer Engineering from the University of Salamanca. Master's degree in Computer Engineering from the same university. Course SMART AGRO IT based on disruptive technology for efficient agriculture and livestock of 300 hours of duration by the same university. Team Leader, senior Full Stack developer, with extensive knowledge of back-end languages (PHP, NodeJS, Python, Java, ...) and front-end (VueJS, AngularJS, ...), structured within standard development frameworks (Yii2, Laravel, ...) that handle the OOP paradigm, experience with relational and nonrelational databases, as well as using NLU techniques for the development of chatbots.

Juan Manuel Corchado, Full Professor with Chair at the University of Salamanca. He was Vice President for Research from 2013 to 2017 and the Director of the Science Park of the University of Salamanca. Chosen twice as the Dean of the Faculty of Science, he holds a Ph.D. in Computer Sciences from the University of Salamanca and a Ph.D. in Artificial Intelligence from the University of the West of Scotland. He is the director of a renowned research group called BISITE (Bioinformatics, Intelligent Systems, and Educational Technology), which was created in the year 2000.

References

Adzhubei, I.A., Schmidt, S., Peshkin, L. et al. (2010). A method and server for predicting damaging missense mutations. *Nature Methods* https://doi.org/10.1038/nmeth0410-248.

Ainscough, B.J., Barnell, E.K., Ronning, P. et al. (2018). A deep learning approach to automate refinement of somatic variant calling from cancer sequencing data. *Nature Genetics* 50 (12): 1735–1743. https://doi.org/10.1038/s41588-018-0257-y.

Altmann, A., Weber, P., Bader, D. et al. (2012). A beginners guide to SNP calling from high-throughput DNA-sequencing data. *Human Genetics* https://doi.org/10.1007/s00439-012-1213-z.

Amarasinghe, S.L., Shian, S., Dong, X. et al. (2020). Opportunities and challenges in long-read sequencing data analysis. *Genome Biology* 21 (1): 1–16. https://doi.org/10.1186/S13059-020-1935-5.

Asmann, Y.W., Middha, S., Hossain, A. et al. (2012). TREAT: a bioinformatics tool for variant annotations and visualizations in targeted and exome sequencing data. *Bioinformatics* 28 (2): 277–278. https://doi.org/10.1093/bioinformatics/btr612.

Auton, Adam, Gonçalo R. Abecasis, David M. Altshuler, Richard M. Durbin, David R. Bentley, Aravinda Chakravarti, Andrew G. Clark, et al. 2015. A global reference for human genetic variation. *Nature*. 526(7571), 68–74. https://doi.org/10.1038/nature15393.

van der Auwera, A., Carneiro, M.O., Hartl, C. et al. (2013). From FastQ data to high-confidence variant calls: the Genome Analysis Toolkit best practices pipeline. *Current Protocols in Bioinformatics* 43 (1): 11–10. https://doi.org/10.1002/0471250953.bi1110s43.

Babraham Bioinformatics - FastQC A Quality Control Tool for High Throughput Sequence Data. (n.d.). https://www.bioinformatics.babraham.ac.uk/projects/fastqc/.

Bailey, M.H., Tokheim, C., Porta-Pardo, E. et al. (2018). Comprehensive characterization of cancer driver genes and mutations. *Cell* 173 (2): 371–385.e18. https://doi.org/10.1016/J .CELL.2018.02.060.

Base Quality Score Recalibration (BQSR) – GATK. (n.d.). https://gatk.broadinstitute.org/hc/en-us/articles/360035890531-Base-Quality-Score-Recalibration-BQSR-.

Bcbio/Bcbio-Nextgen: Validated, Scalable, Community Developed Variant Calling, RNA-Seq and Small RNA Analysis. (n.d.). https://github.com/bcbio/bcbio-nextgen.

Bolger, A.M., Lohse, M., and Usadel, B. (2014). Trimmomatic: a flexible trimmer for Illumina sequence data. *Bioinformatics* 30 (15): 2114–2120. https://doi.org/10.1093/bioinformatics/ btu170.

Boža, V., Brejová, B., and Vinař, T. (2017). DeepNano: deep recurrent neural networks for base calling in MinION nanopore reads. *PLoS One* 12 (6): e0178751. https://doi.org/10.1371/ journal.pone.0178751.

Cameron, D.L., Schröder, J., Penington, J.S. et al. (2017). GRIDSS: sensitive and specific genomic rearrangement detection using positional de Bruijn graph assembly. *Genome Research* 27 (12): 2050–2060. https://doi.org/10.1101/gr.222109.117. Epub 2017 Nov 2.

Chanumolu, S.K., Albahrani, M., and Otu, H.H. (2019). FQStat: a parallel architecture for very high-speed assessment of sequencing quality metrics. *BMC Bioinformatics* 20 (1): 424. https://doi.org/10.1186/s12859-019-3015-y.

Chen, K., Wallis, J.W., McLellan, M.D. et al. (2009). BreakDancer: an algorithm for high-resolution mapping of genomic structural variation. *Nature Methods* 6 (9): 677–681. https://doi.org/10.1038/nmeth.1363.

Chen, X., Schulz-Trieglaff, O., Shaw, R. et al. (2016). Manta: rapid detection of structural variants and indels for germline and cancer sequencing applications. *Bioinformatics* 32 (8): 1220–1222. https://doi.org/10.1093/bioinformatics/btv710.

Chen, S., Huang, T., Zhou, Y. et al. (2017). AfterQC: automatic filtering, trimming, error removing and quality control for FASTQ data. *BMC Bioinformatics* 18 (3): 91–100. https://doi .org/10.1186/s12859-017-1469-3.

Chen, S., Zhou, Y., Chen, Y., and Jia, G. (2018). Fastp: an ultra-fast all-in-one FASTQ preprocessor. *Bioinformatics* 34 (17): i884–i890. https://doi.org/10.1093/ BIOINFORMATICS/BTY560.

Christoforides, A., Carpten, J.D., Weiss, G.J. et al. (2013). Identification of somatic mutations in cancer through Bayesian-based analysis of sequenced genome pairs. *BMC Genomics* 14 (1): 302. https://doi.org/10.1186/1471-2164-14-302.

Cibulskis, K., Lawrence, M.S., Carter, S.L. et al. (2013). Sensitive detection of somatic point mutations in impure and heterogeneous cancer samples. *Nature Biotechnology* 31 (3): 213–219. https://doi.org/10.1038/nbt.2514.

Cingolani, P., Platts, A., Wang, L.L. et al. (2012). A program for annotating and predicting the effects of single nucleotide polymorphisms, SnpEff: SNPs in the genome of drosophila melanogaster strain W1118; Iso-2; Iso-3. *Fly* 6 (2): 80–92. https://doi.org/10.4161/fly.19695.

Cleal, K. and Baird, D.M. (2022). Dysgu: efficient structural variant calling using short or long reads. *Nucleic Acids Research* 50 (9): e53. https://doi.org/10.1093/NAR/GKAC039.

Corchado, J.M., Chamoso, P., Hernández, G. et al. (2021). Deepint.net: a rapid deployment platform for smart territories. *Sensors* 21 (1): 236. https://doi.org/10.3390/S21010236.

Cornish, A. and Guda, C. (2015, 2015). A comparison of variant calling pipelines using genome in a bottle as a reference. *BioMed Research International* https://doi.org/10.1155/2015/456479.

de Coster, W., D'Hert, S., Schultz, D.T. et al. (2018). NanoPack: visualizing and processing long-read sequencing data. *Bioinformatics* 34 (15): 2666–2669. https://doi.org/10.1093/BIOINFORMATICS/BTY149.

Cretu Stancu, M., van Roosmalen, M.J., Renkens, I. et al. (2017). Mapping and phasing of structural variation in patient genomes using nanopore sequencing. *Nature Communications* 8 (1): 1–13. https://doi.org/10.1038/s41467-017-01343-4.

Cunningham, F., Allen, J.E., Allen, J. et al. (2022). Ensembl 2022. *Nucleic Acids Research* 50 (D1): D988–D995. https://doi.org/10.1093/NAR/GKAB1049.

Curnin, C., Goldfeder, R.L., Marwaha, S. et al. (2019). Machine learning-based detection of insertions and deletions in the human genome. *BioRxiv* 628222. https://doi.org/10.1101/628222.

Danecek, P., Bonfield, J.K., Liddle, J. et al. (2021). Twelve years of SAMtools and BCFtools. *GigaScience* 10 (2): https://doi.org/10.1093/gigascience/giab008.

Dong, C., Wei, P., Jian, X. et al. (2015). Comparison and integration of deleteriousness prediction methods for nonsynonymous SNVs in whole exome sequencing studies. *Human Molecular Genetics* 24 (8): 2125–2137. https://doi.org/10.1093/hmg/ddu733.

Esteki, Z., Masoud, E.D., Mateiu, L. et al. (2015). Concurrent whole-genome haplotyping and copy-number profiling of single cells. *American Journal of Human Genetics* 96 (6): 894–912. https://doi.org/10.1016/j.ajhg.2015.04.011.

Fang, L.T., Afshar, P.T., Chhibber, A. et al. (2015). An ensemble approach to accurately detect somatic mutations using SomaticSeq. *Genome Biology* 16 (1): 197. https://doi.org/10.1186/s13059-015-0758-2.

FASTQ Files Explained. (n.d.). https://emea.support.illumina.com/bulletins/2016/04/fastq-files-explained.html.

Feng, B.J. (2017). PERCH: a unified framework for disease gene prioritization. *Human Mutation* 38 (3): 243–251. https://doi.org/10.1002/humu.23158.

Fischer, M., Snajder, R., Pabinger, S. et al. (2012). SIMPLEX: cloud-enabled pipeline for the comprehensive analysis of exome sequencing data. Edited by Gajendra P. S. Raghava. *PLoS One* 7 (8): e41948. https://doi.org/10.1371/journal.pone.0041948.

Franke, K.R. and Crowgey, E.L. (2020). Accelerating next generation sequencing data analysis: an evaluation of optimized best practices for Genome Analysis Toolkit algorithms. *Genomics & Informatics* 18 (1): https://doi.org/10.5808/GI.2020.18.1.E10.

Freed, D., Aldana, R., Weber, J.A., and Edwards, J.S. (2017). The Sentieon Genomics Tools - a fast and accurate solution to variant calling from next-generation sequence data. *BioRxiv* 115717. https://doi.org/10.1101/115717.

Fu, S., Wang, A., and Kin Fai, A. (2019). A comparative evaluation of hybrid error correction methods for error-prone long reads. *Genome Biology* 20 (1): 1–17. https://doi.org/10.1186/s13059-018-1605-z.

Fukasawa, Y., Ermini, L., Wang, H. et al. (2020). LongQC: a quality control tool for third generation sequencing long read data. *G3 Genes|Genomes|Genetics* 10 (4): 1193–1196. https://doi.org/10.1534/G3.119.400864.

Gao, P., Zhang, R., and Li, J. (2019). Comprehensive elaboration of database resources utilized in next-generation sequencing-based tumor somatic mutation detection. In: *Biochimica et Biophysica Acta - Reviews on Cancer*. Elsevier B.V. https://doi.org/10.1016/j.bbcan.2019.06 .004.

Gardner, E.J., Lam, V.K., Harris, D.N. et al. (2017). The mobile element locator tool (MELT): population-scale mobile element discovery and biology. *Genome Research* 27 (11): 1916–1929. https://doi.org/10.1101/gr.218032.116.

Garrison, E. and Marth, G. (2012). Haplotype-based variant detection from short-read sequencing. http://arxiv.org/abs/1207.3907.

Gerstung, M., Beisel, C., Rechsteiner, M. et al. (2012). Reliable detection of subclonal single-nucleotide variants in tumour cell populations. *Nature Communications* 3 (1): 1–8. https://doi.org/10.1038/ncomms1814.

Gerstung, M., Papaemmanuil, E., and Campbell, P.J. (2014). Subclonal variant calling with multiple samples and prior knowledge. *Bioinformatics* 30 (9): 1198–1204. https://doi.org/10 .1093/BIOINFORMATICS/BTT750.

GitHub - Broadinstitute/Picard: A Set of Command Line Tools (in Java) for Manipulating High-Throughput Sequencing (HTS) Data and Formats Such as SAM/BAM/CRAM and VCF. (n.d.). https://github.com/broadinstitute/picard.

GitHub - Rrwick/Filtlong: Quality Filtering Tool for Long Reads. (n.d.). https://github.com/ rrwick/Filtlong.

Goecks, J., Nekrutenko, A., Taylor, J. et al. (2010). Galaxy: a comprehensive approach for supporting accessible, reproducible, and transparent computational research in the life sciences. *Genome Biology* 11 (8): https://doi.org/10.1186/gb-2010-11-8-r86.

Goenka, S.D., Gorzynski, J.E., Shafin, K. et al. (2022). Accelerated identification of disease-causing variants with ultra-rapid nanopore genome sequencing. *Nature Biotechnology* 2022 (March): 1–7. https://doi.org/10.1038/s41587-022-01221-5.

Gong, L., Wong, C.H., Cheng, W.C. et al. (2018). Picky comprehensively detects high-resolution structural variants in nanopore long reads. *Nature Methods* 15 (6): 455–460. https://doi.org/ 10.1038/s41592-018-0002-6.

González-Pérez, A. and López-Bigas, N. (2011). Improving the assessment of the outcome of nonsynonymous SNVs with a consensus deleteriousness score, Condel. *American Journal of Human Genetics* 88 (4): 440–449. https://doi.org/10.1016/j.ajhg.2011.03.004.

Goodwin, S., Gurtowski, J., Ethe-Sayers, S. et al. (2015). Oxford nanopore sequencing, hybrid error correction, and de novo assembly of a eukaryotic genome. *Genome Research* 25 (11): 1750–1756. https://doi.org/10.1101/GR.191395.115.

Goya, R., Sun, M.G.F., Morin, R.D. et al. (2010). SNVMix: predicting single nucleotide variants from next-generation sequencing of tumors. *Bioinformatics* 26 (6): 730–736. https://doi.org/ 10.1093/BIOINFORMATICS/BTQ040.

Grant, J.R., Arantes, A.S., Liao, X., and Stothard, P. (2011). In-depth annotation of SNPs arising from resequencing projects using NGS-SNP. *Bioinformatics* 27 (16): 2300–2301. https://doi .org/10.1093/bioinformatics/btr372.

Gunning, A.C., Fryer, V., Fasham, J. et al. (2020). Assessing performance of pathogenicity predictors using clinically relevant variant datasets. *Journal of Medical Genetics* 2020: 107003. https://doi.org/10.1136/jmedgenet-2020-107003.

Handel, A.E., Disanto, G., and Ramagopalan, S.V. (2014). Next-generation sequencing in understanding complex neurological disease. 13 (2): 215–227. https://doi.org/10.1586/ERN .12.165.

Hansen, N.F., Gartner, J.J., Mei, L. et al. (2013). Shimmer: detection of genetic alterations in tumors using next-generation sequence data. *Bioinformatics* 29 (12): 1498–1503. https://doi .org/10.1093/bioinformatics/btt183.

Henry, V.J., Bandrowski, A.E., Pepin, A.S. et al. (2014). OMICtools: an informative directory for multi-omic data analysis. *Database* 2014 (January): https://doi.org/10.1093/DATABASE/ BAU069.

Holley, G., Beyter, D., Ingimundardottir, H. et al. (2021). Ratatosk: hybrid error correction of long reads enables accurate variant calling and assembly. *Genome Biology* 22 (1): 28. https:// doi.org/10.1186/s13059-020-02244-4.

Homer, N., Merriman, B., and Nelson, S.F. (2009). BFAST: an alignment tool for large scale genome resequencing. *PLoS One* 4 (11): e7767. https://doi.org/10.1371/JOURNAL.PONE .0007767.

Hong, C., Manimaran, S., and Johnson, W.E. (2014). PathoQC: computationally efficient read preprocessing and quality control for high-throughput sequencing data sets. *Cancer Informatics* 13 (Suppl 1): 167–176. https://doi.org/10.4137/CIN.S13890.

Human Genome Overview - Genome Reference Consortium (n.d.). https://www.ncbi.nlm.nih .gov/grc/human.

Hwang, S., Kim, E., Lee, I., and Marcotte, E.M. (2015). Systematic comparison of variant calling pipelines using gold standard personal exome variants. *Scientific Reports* 5 (1): 17875. https:// doi.org/10.1038/srep17875.

Jeffares, D.C., Jolly, C., Hoti, M. et al. (2017). Transient structural variations have strong effects on quantitative traits and reproductive isolation in fission yeast. *Nature Communications* 8 (1): 1–11. https://doi.org/10.1038/ncomms14061.

Joo, T., Choi, J.H., Lee, J.H. et al. (2019). SEQprocess: a modularized and customizable pipeline framework for NGS processing in R package. *BMC Bioinformatics* 20 (1): 1–7. https://doi .org/10.1186/s12859-019-2676-x.

Kalatskaya, I., Trinh, Q.M., Spears, M. et al. (2017). ISOWN: accurate somatic mutation identification in the absence of normal tissue controls. *Genome Medicine* 9 (1): 1–18. https:// doi.org/10.1186/s13073-017-0446-9.

Karczewski, K.J., Weisburd, B., Thomas, B. et al. (2017). The ExAC browser: displaying reference data information from over 60 000 exomes. *Nucleic Acids Research* 45 (D1): D840–D845. https://doi.org/10.1093/NAR/GKW971.

Karczewski, K.J., Francioli, L.C., Tiao, G. et al. (2020). The mutational constraint spectrum quantified from variation in 141,456 humans. *Nature* 581 (7809): 434–443. https://doi.org/10 .1038/s41586-020-2308-7.

Kassahn, K.S., Holmes, O., Nones, K. et al. (2013). Somatic point mutation calling in low cellularity tumors. *PLoS One* 8 (11): e74380. https://doi.org/10.1371/journal.pone.0074380.

Kiełbasa, S.M., Wan, R., Sato, K. et al. (2011). Adaptive seeds tame genomic sequence comparison. *Genome Research* 21 (3): 487–493. https://doi.org/10.1101/GR.113985.110.

Kim, B., Ali, T., Lijeron, C. et al. (2017). Bio-Docklets: virtualization containers for single-step execution of NGS pipelines. *GigaScience* 6 (8): gix048. https://doi.org/10.1093/gigascience/gix048.

Ko, G.H., Kim, P.G., Yoon, J. et al. (2018). Closha: bioinformatics workflow system for the analysis of massive sequencing data. *BMC Bioinformatics* 19 (Suppl 1): 43. https://doi.org/10.1186/s12859-018-2019-3.

Koboldt, D.C., Zhang, Q., Larson, D.E. et al. (2012). VarScan 2: somatic mutation and copy number alteration discovery in cancer by exome sequencing. *Genome Research* 22 (3): 568–576. https://doi.org/10.1101/gr.129684.111.

Koren, S., Walenz, B.P., Berlin, K. et al. (2017). Canu: scalable and accurate long-read assembly via adaptive k-mer weighting and repeat separation. *Genome Research* 27 (5): 722–736. https://doi.org/10.1101/GR.215087.116.

Korvigo, I., Afanasyev, A., Romashchenko, N., and Skoblov, M. (2018). Generalising better: applying deep learning to integrate deleteriousness prediction scores for whole-exome SNV studies. *PLoS One* 13 (3): e0192829. https://doi.org/10.1371/journal.pone.0192829.

Kosugi, S., Momozawa, Y., Liu, X. et al. (2019). Comprehensive evaluation of structural variation detection algorithms for whole genome sequencing. *Genome Biology* 20 (1): 1–18. https://doi.org/10.1186/s13059-019-1720-5.

Kronenberg, Z.N., Osborne, E.J., Cone, K.R. et al. (2015). Wham: identifying structural variants of biological consequence. *PLoS Computational Biology* 11 (12): e1004572. https://doi.org/10.1371/JOURNAL.PCBI.1004572.

Kumar, P., Henikoff, S., and Pauline, C.N. (2009). Predicting the effects of coding non-synonymous variants on protein function using the SIFT algorithm. *Nature Protocols* 4 (7): 1073–1082. https://doi.org/10.1038/nprot.2009.86.

Lai, Z., Markovets, A., Ahdesmaki, M. et al. (2016). VarDict: a novel and versatile variant caller for next-generation sequencing in cancer research. *Nucleic Acids Research* 44 (11): 108. https://doi.org/10.1093/nar/gkw227.

Lam, H.Y.K., Pan, C., Clark, M.J. et al. (2012). Detecting and annotating genetic variations using the HugeSeq pipeline. *Nature Biotechnology* 30 (3): 226–229. https://doi.org/10.1038/nbt.2134.

Landrum, M.J., Lee, J.M., Benson, M. et al. (2018). ClinVar: improving access to variant interpretations and supporting evidence. *Nucleic Acids Research* 46 (D1): D1062–D1067. https://doi.org/10.1093/NAR/GKX1153.

Langmead, B., Trapnell, C., Pop, M., and Salzberg, S.L. (2009). Ultrafast and memory-efficient alignment of short DNA sequences to the human genome. *Genome Biology* 10 (3): 1–10. https://doi.org/10.1186/gb-2009-10-3-r25.

Larson, D.E., Harris, C.C., Chen, K. et al. (2012). SomaticSniper: identification of somatic point mutations in whole genome sequencing data. *Bioinformatics* 28 (3): 311–317. https://doi.org/10.1093/bioinformatics/btr665.

Layer, R.M., Chiang, C., Quinlan, A.R., and Hall, I.M. (2014). LUMPY: a probabilistic framework for structural variant discovery. *Genome Biology* 15 (6): 1–19. https://doi.org/10.1186/gb-2014-15-6-r84.

Leggett, R.M., Heavens, D., Caccamo, M. et al. (2016). NanoOK: multi-reference alignment analysis of nanopore sequencing data, quality and error profiles. *Bioinformatics (Oxford, England)* 32 (1): 142–144. https://doi.org/10.1093/BIOINFORMATICS/BTV540.

Leipzig, J. (2017). A review of bioinformatic pipeline frameworks. *Briefings in Bioinformatics* 18 (3): 530–536. https://doi.org/10.1093/bib/bbw020.

Li, H. (2018). Minimap2: pairwise alignment for nucleotide sequences. *Bioinformatics* 34 (18): 3094–3100. https://doi.org/10.1093/BIOINFORMATICS/BTY191.

Li, H. and Durbin, R. (2009). Fast and accurate short read alignment with Burrows–Wheeler Transform. *Bioinformatics* 25 (14): 1754–1760. https://doi.org/10.1093/BIOINFORMATICS/BTP324.

Li, R., Li, Y., Kristiansen, K., and Wang, J. (2008). SOAP: short oligonucleotide alignment program. *Bioinformatics* 24 (5): 713–714. https://doi.org/10.1093/BIOINFORMATICS/BTN025.

Li, H., Handsaker, B., Wysoker, A. et al. (2009a). The sequence alignment/map format and SAMtools. *Bioinformatics* 25 (16): 2078–2079. https://doi.org/10.1093/BIOINFORMATICS/BTP352.

Li, R., Yu, C., Li, Y. et al. (2009b). SOAP2: an improved ultrafast tool for short read alignment. *Bioinformatics* 25 (15): 1966–1967. https://doi.org/10.1093/BIOINFORMATICS/BTP336.

Liu, C.M., Wong, T., Wu, E. et al. (2012). SOAP3: ultra-fast GPU-based parallel alignment tool for short reads. *Bioinformatics* 28 (6): 878–879. https://doi.org/10.1093/BIOINFORMATICS/BTS061.

Liu, X., Yan, Z., Wu, C. et al. (2019). FastProNGS: fast preprocessing of next-generation sequencing reads. *BMC Bioinformatics* 20 (1): 345. https://doi.org/10.1186/s12859-019-2936-9.

Liu, X., Li, C., Mou, C. et al. (2020). DbNSFP v4: a comprehensive database of transcript-specific functional predictions and annotations for human nonsynonymous and splice-site SNVs. *Genome Medicine* 12 (1): 1–8. https://doi.org/10.1186/s13073-020-00803-9.

Loman, N.J. and Quinlan, A.R. (2014). Poretools: a toolkit for analyzing nanopore sequence data. *Bioinformatics* 30 (23): 3399–3401. https://doi.org/10.1093/BIOINFORMATICS/BTU555.

Luo, R., Sedlazeck, F.J., Lam, T.W., and Schatz, M.C. (2019). A multi-task convolutional deep neural network for variant calling in single molecule sequencing. *Nature Communications* 10 (1): 998. https://doi.org/10.1038/s41467-019-09025-z.

Mahmoud, M., Gobet, N., Cruz-Dávalos, D.I. et al. (2019). Structural variant calling: the long and the short of it. *Genome Biology* 20 (1): 1–14. https://doi.org/10.1186/s13059-019-1828-7.

Mair, B., Konopka, T., Kerzendorfer, C. et al. (2016). Gain- and loss-of-function mutations in the breast cancer gene GATA3 result in differential drug sensitivity. *PLoS Genetics* 12 (9): e1006279. https://doi.org/10.1371/JOURNAL.PGEN.1006279.

Manzini, G. (1999). The Burrows-Wheeler Transform: theory and practice. In: *Lecture Notes in Computer Science (Including Subseries Lecture Notes in Artificial Intelligence and Lecture Notes in Bioinformatics)*, vol. 1672, 34–47. https://doi.org/10.1007/3-540-48340-3_4.

Marić, J., Sović, I., Križanović, K. et al. (2019). Graphmap2 – splice-aware RNA-seq mapper for long reads. *BioRxiv* 720458. https://doi.org/10.1101/720458.

McKenna, A., Hanna, M., Eric Banks et al. (2010). The Genome Analysis Toolkit: a MapReduce framework for analyzing next-generation DNA sequencing data. *Genome Research* 20 (9): 1297–1303. https://doi.org/10.1101/GR.107524.110.

McLaren, W., Gil, L., Hunt, S.E. et al. (2016). The ensembl variant effect predictor. *Genome Biology* 17 (1): 1–14. https://doi.org/10.1186/s13059-016-0974-4.

Mielczarek, M. and Szyda, J. (2016). Review of alignment and SNP calling algorithms for next-generation sequencing data. *Journal of Applied Genetics* 57 (1): 71–79. https://doi.org/10.1007/s13353-015-0292-7.

Mohiyuddin, M., Mu, J.C., Li, J. et al. (2015). MetaSV: an accurate and integrative structural-variant caller for next generation sequencing. *Bioinformatics* 31 (16): 2741–2744. https://doi.org/10.1093/bioinformatics/btv204.

Niu, B., Scott, A.D., Sengupta, S. et al. (2016). Protein-structure-guided discovery of functional mutations across 19 cancer types. *Nature Genetics* 48 (8): 827–837. https://doi.org/10.1038/ng.3586.

Novocraft (n.d.). http://www.novocraft.com/.

Ogasawara, T., Cheng, Y., and Tzeng, T.H.K. (2016). Sam2bam: high-performance framework for NGS data preprocessing tools. *PLoS One* 11 (11): e0167100. https://doi.org/10.1371/journal.pone.0167100.

Pabinger, S., Dander, A., Fischer, M. et al. (2014). A survey of tools for variant analysis of next-generation genome sequencing data. *Briefings in Bioinformatics* 15 (2): 256–278. https://doi.org/10.1093/bib/bbs086.

Patel, R.K. and Jain, M. (2012). NGS QC toolkit: a toolkit for quality control of next generation sequencing data. *PLoS One* 7 (2): e30619. https://doi.org/10.1371/JOURNAL.PONE.0030619.

Piñeiro-Yáñez, E., Reboiro-Jato, M., Gómez-López, G. et al. (2018). PanDrugs: a novel method to prioritize anticancer drug treatments according to individual genomic data. *Genome Medicine* 10 (1): 41. https://doi.org/10.1186/s13073-018-0546-1.

Poplin, R., Chang, P.C., Alexander, D. et al. (2018). A universal SNP and small-indel variant caller using deep neural networks. *Nature Biotechnology* 36 (10): 983. https://doi.org/10.1038/nbt.4235.

Quang, D., Chen, Y., and Xie, X. (2015). DANN: a deep learning approach for annotating the pathogenicity of genetic variants. *Bioinformatics* 31 (5): 761–763. https://doi.org/10.1093/bioinformatics/btu703.

Rausch, T., Zichner, T., Schlattl, A. et al. (2012). DELLY: structural variant discovery by integrated paired-end and split-read analysis. *Bioinformatics* 28 (18): 333–339. https://doi.org/10.1093/bioinformatics/bts378.

Rentzsch, P., Witten, D., Cooper, G.M. et al. (2019). CADD: predicting the deleteriousness of variants throughout the human genome. *Nucleic Acids Research* 47 (D1): D886–D894. https://doi.org/10.1093/nar/gky1016.

Rimmer, A., Phan, H., Mathieson, I. et al. (2014). Integrating mapping-, assembly- and haplotype-based approaches for calling variants in clinical sequencing applications. *Nature Genetics* 46 (8): 912–918. https://doi.org/10.1038/ng.3036.

Robbe, P., Popitsch, N., Knight, S.J.L. et al. (2018). Clinical whole-genome sequencing from routine formalin-fixed, paraffin-embedded specimens: pilot study for the 100,000 Genomes Project. *Genetics in Medicine* 20 (10): 1196–1205. https://doi.org/10.1038/gim.2017.241.

Roth, A., Ding, J., Morin, R. et al. (2012). JointSNVMix: a probabilistic model for accurate detection of somatic mutations in normal/tumour paired next-generation sequencing data. *Bioinformatics* 28 (7): 907–913. https://doi.org/10.1093/BIOINFORMATICS/BTS053.

Roy, S., Coldren, C., Karunamurthy, A. et al. (2018). Standards and guidelines for validating next-generation sequencing bioinformatics pipelines: a joint recommendation of the association for molecular pathology and the college of american pathologists." *Journal of Molecular Diagnostics.* 20 (1): 4–27. https://doi.org/10.1016/j.jmoldx.2017.11.003.

Ruffalo, M., Laframboise, T., and Koyutürk, M. (2011). Comparative analysis of algorithms for next-generation sequencing read alignment. *Bioinformatics* 27 (20): 2790–2796. https://doi .org/10.1093/bioinformatics/btr477.

Rumble, S.M., Lacroute, P., Dalca, A.V. et al. (2009). SHRiMP: accurate mapping of short color-space reads. *PLoS Computational Biology* 5 (5): e1000386. https://doi.org/10.1371/ JOURNAL.PCBI.1000386.

Sahraeian, S.M.E., Liu, R., Lau, B. et al. (2019). Deep convolutional neural networks for accurate somatic mutation detection. *Nature Communications* 10 (1): 1041. https://doi.org/ 10.1038/s41467-019-09027-x.

Salmela, L., Walve, R., Rivals, E. et al. (2017). Accurate self-correction of errors in long reads using de Bruijn graphs. *Bioinformatics* 33 (6): 799–806. https://doi.org/10.1093/ BIOINFORMATICS/BTW321.

Sandve, G.K., Nekrutenko, A., Taylor, J., and Hovig, E. (2013). Ten simple rules for reproducible computational research. *PLoS Computational Biology* 9 (10): e1003285. https:// doi.org/10.1371/JOURNAL.PCBI.1003285.

Saunders, C.T., Wong, W.S.W., Swamy, S. et al. (2012). Strelka: accurate somatic small-variant calling from sequenced tumor–normal sample pairs. *Bioinformatics* 28 (14): 1811–1817. https://doi.org/10.1093/bioinformatics/bts271.

Schmidt, B. and Hildebrandt, A. (2021). Deep learning in next-generation sequencing. *Drug Discovery Today* 26 (1): 173–180. https://doi.org/10.1016/j.drudis.2020.10.002.

Schmieder, R. and Edwards, R. (2011). Quality control and preprocessing of metagenomic datasets. *Bioinformatics* 27 (6): 863–864. https://doi.org/10.1093/BIOINFORMATICS/ BTR026.

Sedlazeck, F.J., Rescheneder, P., Smolka, M. et al. (2018). Accurate detection of complex structural variations using single-molecule sequencing. *Nature Methods* 15 (6): 461–468. https://doi.org/10.1038/s41592-018-0001-7.

Shafin, K., Pesout, T., Chang, P.-C. et al. (2021). Haplotype-aware variant calling with PEPPER-margin-DeepVariant enables high accuracy in nanopore long-reads. *Nature Methods* 2021 (November): 1–11. https://doi.org/10.1038/s41592-021-01299-w.

Sherry, S.T., Ward, M., and Sirotkin, K. (1999). DbSNP—Database for single nucleotide polymorphisms and other classes of minor genetic variation. *Genome Research* 9 (8): 677–679. https://doi.org/10.1101/GR.9.8.677.

Singer, J., Ruscheweyh, H.J., Hofmann, A.L. et al. (2018). NGS-Pipe: a flexible, easily extendable and highly configurable framework for NGS analysis. *Bioinformatics* 34 (1): 107–108. https://doi.org/10.1093/bioinformatics/btx540.

Smith, A.D., Chung, W.Y., Hodges, E. et al. (2009). Updates to the RMAP short-read mapping software. *Bioinformatics* 25 (21): 2841–2842. https://doi.org/10.1093/BIOINFORMATICS/ BTP533.

Smith, K.S., Yadav, V.K., Pei, S. et al. (2016). SomVarIUS: somatic variant identification from unpaired tissue samples. *Bioinformatics* 32 (6): 808–813. https://doi.org/10.1093/ BIOINFORMATICS/BTV685.

Sović, I., Šikić, M., Wilm, A. et al. (2016). Fast and sensitive mapping of nanopore sequencing reads with GraphMap. *Nature Communications* 7 (1): 11307. https://doi.org/10.1038/ncomms11307.

Spinella, J.F., Mehanna, P., Vidal, R. et al. (2016). SNooPer: a machine learning-based method for somatic variant identification from low-pass next-generation sequencing. *BMC Genomics* 17 (1): 912. https://doi.org/10.1186/s12864-016-3281-2.

Tarraga, J., Gallego, A., Arnau, V. et al. (2016). HPG pore: an efficient and scalable framework for nanopore sequencing data. *BMC Bioinformatics* 17 (1): 1–7. https://doi.org/10.1186/s12859-016-0966-0.

Tate, J.G., Bamford, S., Jubb, H.C. et al. (2019). COSMIC: the catalogue of somatic mutations in cancer. *Nucleic Acids Research* 47 (D1): D941–D947. https://doi.org/10.1093/NAR/GKY1015.

Teer, J.K., Zhang, Y., Lu, C. et al. (2017). Evaluating somatic tumor mutation detection without matched normal samples. *Human Genomics* 11 (1): 1–13. https://doi.org/10.1186/s40246-017-0118-2.

Tham, C.Y., Tirado-Magallanes, R., Goh, Y. et al. (2020). NanoVar: accurate characterization of patients' genomic structural variants using low-depth nanopore sequencing. *Genome Biology* 21 (1): 1–15. https://doi.org/10.1186/s13059-020-01968-7.

Thankaswamy-Kosalai, S., Sen, P., and Nookaew, I. (2017). Evaluation and assessment of read-mapping by multiple next-generation sequencing aligners based on genome-wide characteristics. *Genomics* 109 (3–4): 186–191. https://doi.org/10.1016/j.ygeno.2017.03.001.

The Cancer Genome Atlas Program - National Cancer Institute (n.d.). https://www.cancer.gov/about-nci/organization/ccg/research/structural-genomics/tcga.

UCSC Genome Browser Home (n.d.). https://genome.ucsc.edu/.

Vallania, F., Ramos, E., Cresci, S. et al. (2012). Detection of rare genomic variants from pooled sequencing using SPLINTER. *JoVE (Journal of Visualized Experiments)* 64: e3943. https://doi.org/10.3791/3943.

Wang, K., Li, M., and Hakonarson, H. (2010). ANNOVAR: functional annotation of genetic variants from high-throughput sequencing data. *Nucleic Acids Research* 38 (16): e164–e164. https://doi.org/10.1093/NAR/GKQ603.

Wang, J.R., Holt, J., McMillan, L., and Jones, C.D. (2018). FMLRC: hybrid long read error correction using an FM-index. *BMC Bioinformatics* 19 (1): 1–11. https://doi.org/10.1186/s12859-018-2051-3.

Wang, Y., Zhao, Y., Bollas, A. et al. (2021). Nanopore sequencing technology, bioinformatics and applications. *Nature Biotechnology* 2021: 1–18. https://doi.org/10.1038/s41587-021-01108-x.

Watson, M., Thomson, M., Risse, J. et al. (2015). PoRe: an R package for the visualization and analysis of nanopore sequencing data. *Bioinformatics* 31 (1): 114–115. https://doi.org/10.1093/BIOINFORMATICS/BTU590.

Wei, Z., Wang, W., Hu, P. et al. (2011). SNVer: a statistical tool for variant calling in analysis of pooled or individual next-generation sequencing data. *Nucleic Acids Research* 39 (19): e132. https://doi.org/10.1093/nar/gkr599.

Weischenfeldt, J., Symmons, O., Spitz, F., and Korbel, J.O. (2013). Phenotypic impact of genomic structural variation: insights from and for human disease. *Nature Reviews Genetics* 142 (2): 125–138. https://doi.org/10.1038/nrg3373.

Wratten, L., Wilm, A., and Göke, J. (2021). Reproducible, scalable, and shareable analysis pipelines with bioinformatics workflow managers. *Nature Methods* 2021, 18 (10): 1161–1168. https://doi.org/10.1038/s41592-021-01254-9.

Wu, C., Zhao, X., Welsh, M. et al. (2020). Using machine learning to identify true somatic variants from next-generation sequencing. *Clinical Chemistry* 66 (1): 239–246. https://doi.org/10.1373/clinchem.2019.308213.

Xu, H., DiCarlo, J., Satya, R.V. et al. (2014). Comparison of somatic mutation calling methods in amplicon and whole exome sequence data. *BMC Genomics* 15 (1): 1–10. https://doi.org/10.1186/1471-2164-15-244.

Xu, Z., Mai, Y., Liu, D. et al. (2021). Fast-bonito: a faster deep learning based basecaller for nanopore sequencing. *Artificial Intelligence in the Life Sciences* 1: 100011. https://doi.org/10.1016/J.AILSCI.2021.100011.

Yuan, Y., Shi, Y., Li, C. et al. (2016). DeepGene: an advanced cancer type classifier based on deep learning and somatic point mutations. *BMC Bioinformatics* 17 (Suppl 17): 243–256. https://doi.org/10.1186/s12859-016-1334-9.

Zarate, S., Carroll, A., Mahmoud, M. et al. (2021). Parliament2: accurate structural variant calling at scale. *GigaScience* 9 (12): giaa145. https://doi.org/10.1093/gigascience/giaa145.

Zarrei, M., MacDonald, J.R., Merico, D., and Scherer, S.W. (2015). A copy number variation map of the human genome. *Nature Reviews Genetics* 16 (3): 172–183. https://doi.org/10.1038/nrg3871.

Zeng, J., Cai, H., Peng, H. et al. (2020). Causalcall: nanopore basecalling using a temporal convolutional network. *Frontiers in Genetics* 10 (January): 1332. https://doi.org/10.3389/FGENE.2019.01332.

Zhou, J. and Troyanskaya, O.G. (2015). Predicting effects of noncoding variants with deep learning-based sequence model. *Nature Methods* 12 (10): 931–934. https://doi.org/10.1038/nmeth.3547.

Zhou, A., Lin, T., and Xing, J. (2019). Evaluating nanopore sequencing data processing pipelines for structural variation identification. *Genome Biology* 20 (1): 1–13. https://doi.org/10.1186/s13059-019-1858-1.

Zou, J., Huss, M., Abid, A. et al. (2019). A primer on deep learning in genomics. *Nature Genetics* 51 (1): 12–18. https://doi.org/10.1038/s41588-018-0295-5.

12

Artificial Intelligence: From Drug Discovery to Clinical Pharmacology

Paola Lecca

Faculty of Engineering, Computer Science and Artificial Intelligence Institute, Free University of Bozen-Bolzano, Bolzano, Italy

12.1 Artificial Intelligence and the Druggable Genome

Drug discovery is the process through which potential new medications are identified. It involves a wide range of scientific disciplines, including biology, chemistry, and pharmacology, and more recently also mathematics and artificial intelligence (AI). Already in a report from 2005, Paul L. Herrling of Novartis International AG Corporate Research reported that the tremendous progress in biomedical knowledge and technology since 1995 necessitated a complete redesign of the drug discovery process (Herrling 2005). The reasons that promoted this progress were an exponential increase in the number of therapeutic targets, and the discovery of very high levels of complexity of gene networks and their corresponding protein–protein network, as exemplified by the combinatorial interaction of proteins in signaling pathways.

In 2002, Hopkins and Groom (2002) coined the term *druggability* for proteins. Druggability of a protein is its potential to be modulated by drug-like molecules (Liu and Altman 2014). The most common approach for estimating druggability is to classify targets by whether they belong to gene families known to be druggable, such as G-protein-coupled receptors (Hopkins and Groom 2002).

In drug discovery, the ability to accurately predict protein druggability is of utmost importance, as it can capitalize on the huge investments made in structural genomics initiatives by identifying highly druggable proteins and using this information in target identification and validation campaigns (Hajduk et al. 2005). Herrling reported that in 1996, all existing therapeutic agents interacted with an estimated 500 drug targets, but the sequencing of the human genome revealed about 25,000–30,000 protein-coding genes. If also splicing and posttranslational modifications are taken into account, there must be more than 100,000 functionally different proteins assuming 25,000 protein-coding genes, and an average of five splice variants per protein. It is estimated that 57% of the human protein-coding genes display alternative splicing, and that they contain an average of 9 (8.94) exons, this would result in about 12,5000 proteins. Note that this number does not take into account posttranslational modifications such as proteolytic processing of larger proteins into smaller active ones or RNA editing. Some

Big Data Analysis and Artificial Intelligence for Medical Sciences, First Edition.
Edited by Bruno Carpentieri and Paola Lecca.
© 2024 John Wiley & Sons Ltd. Published 2024 by John Wiley & Sons Ltd.

estimates indicate that only 5000–10,000 of these proteins might be useful drug targets (or "drugable"). However, Herrling noted that this estimate was based on the subset of "disease" genes, and there might be many more proteins involved in disease processes than the number of "disease" genes (Herrling 2005). Similar estimates were reported by Hopkins et al. (Hopkins and Groom, 2002) that drug targets belong to ~130 protein families, which covers 10% of all genes in the genome. However, not all members of a given gene family are equally druggable, and more importantly, gene families not currently known to be druggable may still yield novel targets (Liu and Altman 2014).

The enormous increase in data digitalization experienced by the pharmaceutical sector over the past few years came with the twofold challenge of analyzing this huge amount of data and applying that acquired knowledge to solve complex clinical problems. This motivates the use of AI, since it has been proven to handle large volumes of data with enhanced automation. AI utilizes systems and software that can interpret and learn from the input data to make decisions for accomplishing specific objectives. Its applications are continuously being extended, as witnessed by a number of recent publications dealing and promoting the use of artificial intelligence techniques in drug design and development (Gupta et al. 2021; Hinkson et al. 2020; Jang 2019; Patel and Shah 2021; Zhavoronkov et al. 2020; Paul et al. 2021; Dara et al. 2021).

Involvement of AI in the development of a pharmaceutical product can aid drug design; propose a therapy for a patient, including personalized medicines; and process the clinical data generated and use it for future drug development. These four tasks can be completed if the drug–target interaction network can be predicted, and in turn, if this network is predicted, it can also be used to check the possibility of the effectiveness of drug repurposing. Recent, but already numerous articles deal with the use of machine learning and deep learning techniques for the prediction of drug–target interaction networks. As an example, we refer the reader to the references Kim et al. (2021), Doğan et al. (2021), Gallego et al. (2021), Ru et al. (2021), Ezzat et al. (2018), Ismail et al. (2021), D'Souza et al. (2020), Bagherian et al. (2020), Xu et al. (2021), Chen et al. (2018), Dara et al. (2021), Paul et al. (2021), Zhavoronkov et al. (2020), and Patel and Shah (2021).

Drug discovery is not only the process to identify interactions between drugs and targets (e.g. genes or proteins), but, specifically, it is process to identify interactions between drugs and targets which can be reliably performed by *in vitro* experiments (Bagherian et al. 2020). A significant reduction of the temporal and monetary costs can be achieved through *in silico* experiments to be carried out upstream of *in vitro* experiments. For example, instead of an exhausting *in vitro* search, virtual screening is initially performed and possible candidates are then experimentally verified. Generally, there are two approaches for *in silico* prediction of drug–target interaction: docking simulations and machine learning methods. In docking simulations, the 3D structure of drug molecules and targets are considered and potential binding sites are identified. As reported by Bagherian et al. (2020), this process cannot be applied if the 3D structure of the protein is unknown. For instance, it is known that for a class of proteins called G-protein-coupled receptors (GPCR), very few structures have been crystallized (orphan GPCR), so docking simulations cannot be applied. To tackle this issue, *chemogenomics* (Bredel and Jacoby 2004; Ezzat et al. 2018) was introduced as a way to aim at mining the entire space for interaction with the biological space (also referred to as genomic or proteomic space), instead of considering each protein target independently from other proteins. We report here the definition of chemigenomics given by Bredel et al. Bredel and Jacoby (2004): "Chemogenomics is the study of the genomic and/or proteomic response of an intact biological system to chemical compounds, or the ability of isolated molecular targets to interact with such compounds."

It is well known that even if the 3D structure were known, the docking simulation would still be time consuming (Bagherian et al. 2020). Nevertheless, chemogenomics provides a basis for machine-learning procedures. Indeed, chemogenomics research is to relate the chemical space of possible compounds with the genomic/proteomic space in order to identify potentially useful compounds such as imaging probes and drug leads. All the chemogenomics approaches (such as ligand based, target based, and target–ligand based, approaches) are based on similarities between members proteins and targets. In fact, it is precisely this point of view of chemogenomics that allows the machine learning algorithms to be suitable for prediction of drug–target interactions. The drug–target prediction problem can be categorized into four classes (Bagherian et al. 2020):

1) Known drug versus known target,
2) Known drug versus new target candidate,
3) New drug candidate versus known target, and
4) New drug candidate versus new target candidate.

In machine learning methods, knowledge about drugs, targets, and already confirmed drug–target interactions are translated into features that are used to train a predictive model, which in turn is used to predict interactions between new drugs and/or new targets. The main assumption of these studies is that if drug D is interacting with protein P, then

1) drug compounds similar to D are likely to interact with protein P,
2) proteins similar to P are likely to interact with drug D, and
3) drug compounds similar to D are likely to interact with proteins similar to P.

In sections 12.2, 12.3 and 12.4, we review the currently most used artificial intelligence methods based in drug discovery. We categorize them into

- feature-based methods,
- similarity/distance based methods,
- matrix factorization methods,
- network inference methods,
- network inference/reconstruction methods.

These four categories can in turn be grouped into two sets as illustrated in Figure 12.1 that can be used as a guide to the structure of the whole chapter. There are essentially two types of wiring diagrams for representing the drug–target network: the network of associations between drug and target reconstructed from descriptive data on the qualitative and quantitative physical and chemical features of the nodes, and the network of relations between drug and target reconstructed from knowledge of the metabolic and signaling networks of proteins and cellular components, among which would be the candidate drug targets. The two different types of data, i.e. node data and pathway data, are processed with algorithms

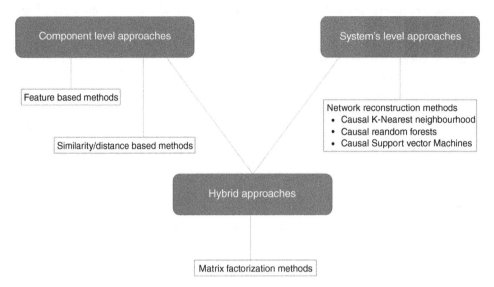

Figure 12.1 Classification of machine learning and AI methods for drug–target network construction. Component-level methods rely on physico chemical characteristics of the drug molecules and their putative targets to determinate associations between drugs and targets. System's level methods rely on the integration of gene or protein causal interaction networks inference/reconstruction and its usage in the identification of the drug effects on putative pathways.

belonging to component-level and system-level approaches, respectively. The essence of the network identified with the two approaches is also different: in the first case, it is a network of associations, while in the second case it is a network of causal relations. In system's level approaches, the concept of a drug–target network should more appropriately be replaced by the concept of a drug-pathway network, to express the fact that the action of a drug is carried out overall on a pathway rather than on a single component. In this chapter, therefore, we will make this distinction where appropriate. Finally, hybrid approaches have also been proposed, of which matrix factorization methods are the most popular (Ceddia et al. 2020a; Cobanoglu et al. 2013; Poleksic 2023). Reviews of the state of the art on these three categories of methods can be found in many research papers, e.g. Guvenilir and Doğan (2023), Selvaraj et al. (2021), Jiménez-Luna et al. (2020), Réda et al. (2020), Askr et al. (2022), Han et al. (2022), Gaudelet et al. (2021).

Sections 12.2, 12.3, and 12.4 will give an overview of the methodologies (rather than the methods) implemented by these approaches. From these methodologies have originated several context-specific methods and algorithms that the reader can consult by referring to the bibliography cited in this chapter and in review and perspective articles such as (Bender and Cortés-Ciriano 2021; Paul et al. 2021; Arabi 2021; Bagherian et al. 2020; Vamathevan et al. 2019; Fleming 2018). Among the machine learning network-based methods, we mention three classic machine learning algorithms that have been extended from classifiers to causality discovery methods, and we refer the reader to a more complete discussion in Lecca's work (Lecca 2021).

12.2 Feature-Based Methods

This is a broad range of methods including a number of machine learning methods. A comprehensive review can be found in Sachdev and Gupta (2019).

The general idea behind this category of methods is that any pairs of drugs and targets is represented by feature vectors with certain length (see for example) (Liu et al. 2021; Lin et al. 2022; Mesrabadi et al. 2023)). A feature space can be defined as F where

$$F = \{\mathbf{d} \oplus \mathbf{p} \mid \mathbf{d} = (d_1, d_2, \dots, d_n), \mathbf{p} = (p_1, p_2, \dots, p_m)\}, \tag{12.1}$$

where $\mathbf{p}$ and $\mathbf{d}$ denote the target protein and drug feature vectors of length n and m, respectively.

The drug feature vector $\mathbf{d}$ and the target feature vector $\mathbf{p}$ are calculated independently. These may be computed by selecting certain discriminative properties for encoding or using certain software packages or tools that can compute the descriptors automatically (Sachdev and Gupta 2019). Some methods also employ dimensionality reduction techniques to reduce feature dimensionality (Lin et al. 2022; Mahmud et al. 2021; Liu 2004), thereby improving the performance as well as the efficiency of the technique. The drug-target pair vector is then used in a classifier. For the purpose of classification, the entire dataset is divided into training and testing data. The data consists of two types of drug-target interaction pairs: positive and negative. The positive pair implies the drug-target pair that is known to interact. The negative pairs are those for which the interaction is not known. The drug-target pair vectors of the training data are then transferred to a classifier. Various classifiers like Support Vector Machines (SVM) (Steinwart and Christmann 2008), Relevance Vector Machines (RVM) (Saarela et al. 2010), Rotation Forest (Rodriguez et al. 2006) etc., have been used under different techniques. The classifier then predicts the label for the testing data i.e. whether the drug target pair interacts or not.

Once the feature space is defined, assorted machine learning methods can be established to perform the drug–target prediction tasks (Bagherian et al. 2020). However, in spite of the large use of feature-based methods, it should be noted that these methods are jeopardized by the lack of 3D structures of membrane proteins preventing the extraction of the main features, which would have yielded to better prediction performances.

12.3 Similarity/Distance-Based Methods

These methods rely on a distance function that defines how similar (or here "close") a new drug is with respect to the known pairs. There are several ways to define the closeness through a distance function for nearest neighbor (NN) algorithms. Among which the Euclidean distance is well known. For instance, in He et al. (2010) the distance $\text{dist}(v, w)$ between two samples v and w, respectively belonging to the sample spaces V and W, is

$$\text{dist}(v, w) = \frac{v \cdot w}{||v|| ||w||}, \tag{12.2}$$

where "·" denotes the inner product and $|| \, ||$ the vector norm.

In addition to mathematical models for the distance, the similarity/distance function could be also defined based on the pharmacological similarity of drugs and genomic similarity of protein sequences as well as the topological properties of a multipartite network of the existing drugs and protein targets (Boo 2000; Takarabe et al. 2012). To this end, Perlman et al. (2011) defined five drug–drug similarity measures as

- chemical based,
- ligand based,
- expression based,
- side effect based, and
- annotation based.

On this Bagherian et al. (2020) comment that the main disadvantage of this group of methods lies in the fact that only a small number of drugs and their interactions are known while there exists a noticeable amount of unlabeled data among the datasets. The presence of unlabeled data is challenging to similarity methods, and this challenge has not yet been overcome. An in-depth discussion of this point along with a list of the methods based on similarity/distance is provided in Bagherian et al. (2020).

12.4 Matrix Factorization

Let us consider the interaction matrix $X_{m,n}$

$$X_{m,n} = \begin{pmatrix} x_{1,1} & x_{1,2} & \cdots & x_{1,n} \\ x_{2,1} & x_{2,2} & \cdots & x_{2,n} \\ \vdots & \vdots & \ddots & \vdots \\ x_{m,1} & x_{m,2} & \cdots & x_{m,n} \end{pmatrix}$$

where for $i = 1, 2, \ldots, m$ and $j = 1, 2, \ldots, n$

$$x_{ij} = \begin{cases} 1, & \text{if drug } d_i \text{ interacts with target } t_j, \\ 0, & \text{in the absence of any known interaction.} \end{cases}$$

$X_{m,n}$ is decomposed into two matrices, $Y_{m,k}$ and $Z_{n,k}$, where $X = YZ^T$ with $k < n, m$. This decomposition provides a factorization of matrix $X_{m,n}$ into two matrices with lower orders (i.e. rank reduction), which make it easier to perform the matrix completion techniques (Johnson 1990; Laurent 2008) in order to handle the missing data.

Some matrix factorization methods do not rely on chemical similarity or drug similarities and instead utilize collaborative filtering algorithms (see as an example (Chen et al. 2022) on collaborative filtering algorithms for drug–target prediction), among which we recall the probabilistic matrix factorization (Salakhutdinov and Mnih 2007; Nafshi and Lezon 2021). We briefly describe here the framework and the question of the probabilistic matrix factorization. We adopt the notation of (Bottegal and Suykens 2017).

We consider a matrix $Z \in \mathbb{R}^{n \times m}$ resulting from the product of two unknown matrices $U \in \mathbb{R}^{n \times r}$ and $V \in \mathbb{R}^{m \times r}$, and a noise matrix $E \in \mathbb{R}^{n \times m}$ such that

$$Z = UV^T + E. \tag{12.3}$$

We assume that the entries of E are i.i.d. realizations of Gaussian random variables, i.e.

$$e_{ij} \sim N(0, \sigma^2) \tag{12.4}$$

where the variance σ^2 is unknown. Typically, the matrix Z is not directly measurable, but only an entry-wise quantized version is available. Denoting by Y this quantized version, we have that

$$y_{ij} = Q[z_{ij}] \tag{12.5}$$

where Q is a known map of the type

$$Q[x] = s_k \quad \text{if } x \in (q_{k-1}, q_k], \tag{12.6}$$

with $s_k \in \{s_1, \ldots, s_p\}$ and $q_k \in \{q_0, \ldots, q_p\}$, and typically $q_0 = -\infty$ and $q_p = +\infty$. The probabilistic matrix factorization method addresses the question of reconstructing from the data matrix Y, the matrices (Z, U, V) that best match the model (12.3).

Some other methods are inspired by the idea of low-rank embedding (Li et al. 2013) with the goal of finding a low-rank matrix R representing the dataset X by an optimization problem and then fixing R and minimizing the reconstruction error in the embedded space in a way that the point-wise linear reconstruction is preserved. These methods assume that the drugs and targets belongs to the same distance space such that the distance among drugs and targets can be used to measure the strength of their interactions.

As a concrete example of the use of factoring procedures, we report the work of Dai et al. (2015). The matrix factorization method is used in drug discovery not only to reconstruct the network of drug–target interactions, but also to reconstruct drug–disease associations. This second objective is also part of drug discovery, since it also includes the identification of (new) suitable drugs to combat certain diseases. The authors define the problem in the following way. They denote with $U = \{u_1, u_2, \ldots, u_{N_u}\}$ the set of drugs, with $S = \{s_1, s_2, \ldots, s_{N_s}\}$ the set of diseases, and with $G = \{g_1, g_2, \ldots, g_{N_g}\}$ the set of genes. They denote with Y the interaction data. Y^{US} is then a $N_u \times N_s$ binary matrix of labels drug–disease associations, in which only some entries are known. In the known entries, $Y^{US}_{ij} = 1$ if drug u_i and disease s_j are known to be associated with each other and $Y^{US}_{ij} = 0$ if drug u_i and disease s_j are known to be not associated with each other. The other entries are unknown as we are not sure whether they are associated or not. A second binary $N_u \times N_g$ binary matrix represents the drug–gene interaction, in such a way that $Y^{UG}_{ij} = 1$ if drug u_i and gene g_j interact, and $Y^{UG}_{ij} = 0$ if drug u_i and gene g_j do not interact. Finally, the $N_s \times N_g$ binary matrix Y^{SG} represents the gene–disease associations. In particularly, $Y^{SG}_{ij} = 1$ if disease s_i is associated with gene g_j, and $Y^{SG}_{ij} = 1$ otherwise. Finally, the gene interaction network, consisting of N_g genes, is adopted for exploiting genomic topology. To study the effect of the integration of genomic space, Dai et al. (2015) assume that all the N_u drugs and all the N_s diseases have interacting genes in the gene interaction network. The goal is to calculate a $N_u \times N_s$ matrix F, derived from the known interaction data, whose entries indicate the potential association between drug u_i and disease s_j, to predict scores for the unknown entries in Y^{US}.

In Dai et al. (2015) the genomic space is exploited to create low-rank feature vectors, which are used to describe the feature spaces of genes, drugs, and diseases. The gene–gene interaction networks has been considered and a gene closeness metric has been proposed as:

$$c_{ij} = c_1 e^{\frac{c_2}{d_{ij}}} \tag{12.7}$$

where d_{ij} is the shortest distance (measured as number of edges) between gene g_i and gene g_j, and c_1 and c_2 are real numbers. The gene closeness defined in Eq. (12.7) are the entries of the gene matrix C. Afterward, eigenvalue decomposition of the matrix C is applied to construct a unified space, which is a low-rank Euclidean space, so that all the N_g genes can be represented by sets of k-dimension feature vectors $\{\mathbf{p}_{g_i}\}_{i=1}^{N_g}$. The feature space is obtained in Dai et al. (2015) as follows:

1) Calculate the eigenvalues of C, and arrange them in descending order; calculate the corresponding eigenvectors.
2) Retrieve the first k eigenvalues to form the $k \times k$ diagonal matrix Λ; retrieve the first k eigenvectors to for the $N_g \times k$ matrix Γ, where each column is an eigenvector.
3) Calculate

$$P = \Gamma \Lambda^{\frac{1}{2}}.$$

4) Decompose C as

$$C \approx PP^T = \Gamma \Lambda^{\frac{1}{2}} \Lambda^{\frac{1}{2}} \Gamma^T.$$

5) Represent all the genes by using the row vectors of the matrix $P = (\mathbf{p}_{g_1}, \mathbf{p}_{g_2}, \dots, \mathbf{p}_{g_{N_g}})^T$.

Next, the feature spaces of drugs and diseases are, respectively, obtained according to the interaction matrices Y^{UG} and Y^{SG}. Dai et al. (2015) proposed to calculate the feature vectors of drugs and diseases, denoted as $\mathbf{p}_u$ and $\mathbf{p}_g$, respectively, using the following formulae:

$$\mathbf{p}_{u_i} = \frac{\sum_{j=1}^{N_g} Y_{ij}^{UG} \mathbf{p}_{g_j}}{\sum_{j=1}^{N_g} Y_{ij}^{UG}}, \quad i = 1, 2, \dots, N_u, \tag{12.8}$$

$$\mathbf{p}_{u_i} = \frac{\sum_{j=1}^{N_g} Y_{ij}^{SG} \mathbf{p}_{g_j}}{\sum_{j=1}^{N_g} Y_{ij}^{SG}}, \quad i = 1, 2, \dots, N_s. \tag{12.9}$$

This procedure is a particularly illustrative example of the spirit of hybrid approaches. Indeed, the feature vectors of genes, drugs, and diseases are integrated into a unified space of the same rank. The assumption under this integration is that the association between drug and disease is based on knowledge of the gene interaction network. Indeed, the authors assume that if a drug is known to be associated with a disease, then targets of the drug might be more highly interconnected with the disease genes in the interactome network.

The Y^{US} is then factorized into two low-rank matrices: $A = (\mathbf{p}_1, \mathbf{p}_2, \dots, \mathbf{p}_{N_u})^T$, that is a $N_u \times k$ feature matrix of the drugs, and $B = (\mathbf{p}_1, \mathbf{p}_2, \dots, \mathbf{p}_{N_s})^T$, that is a $N_s \times k$ feature matrix of the diseases. A and B in the matrix factorization, are chosen to minimize the squared error of the known drug–disease associations. The matrix $Y^{US} = A^T B$ reports the association between drug and disease.

To complete the above, it should be noted that matrix factorization methods are also used for the purpose of drug repurposing (Sadeghi et al. 2021; Ceddia et al. 2020b; Yang et al. 2019), predicting the effects of drug combinations (Nafshi and Lezon 2021), and predicting drug side effects (Fukuto et al. 2021). Finally, despite the increasing use and popularity of matrix factorization methods, we note that their strong limitation is that rapid growth in the quantity and variety of data related to a certain drug and/or a target often exceeds the capacity of matrix-based data representations of many current analysis algorithms.

12.4.1 Causal K-Nearest-Neighborhood

Zhou and Kosorok (2017) first and then Hitsch and Misra (2018) introduced a way to use KNN to causal discovery. In the application domain of precision medicine, they first proposed a causal k-nearest neighbor (CKNN) method to estimate the optimal treatment regime and the causal treatment effects within the nearest neighborhood. The purpose was to tailor treatments to individual patients to maximize treatment benefit and reduce bad side-effects. Nevertheless, Zhou and Kosorok (2017) method is also applicable to biological networks, such as gene networks or protein–protein networks, to identify nodes or pathways affected by drug treatments or to design drug repurposing strategies, or for drug combination prediction, and more in general to identify differences between networks of different patients. In this respect, we refer the reader to some significant recent studies such as (Feng et al. 2017; Cheng et al. 2019; Lu et al. 2020; Hasan et al. 2020; Ruiz et al. 2021; Somolinos et al. 2021; Adhami et al. 2021). In this context, the crucial step is the determination of optimal treatment regime. By "treatment regime," we mean a decision rule that assigns a treatment to a patient based on his or her clinical or medical characteristics. Similarly, for a drug-pathways network by "treatment regime," we mean a decision rule that assigns a therapeutic intervention to a network based on the state of the network or some of its pathways (e.g. altered pathways in disease state). In the next, we describe and comment on how the decision rule is constructed in a KNN method.

The KNN rule is a classification approach, where a subject is classified by a majority vote of its k neighbors. As noted by Zhou and Kosorok (2017), the rationale of nearest neighbor rule is that close covariate vectors share similar properties more often than not. We briefly summarize causal KNN method, using a notation similar to that of Zhou and Kosorok (2017).

Let us consider a randomized clinical trial with M treatment arms. Let $R \in \mathcal{R}$ denote the observed clinical outcome, $A \in \mathcal{A}$ denotes the treatment assignment received by the patient, and $X = (X_1, \ldots, X_p)^T \in \mathcal{X} \subset \mathcal{R}^p$, where X is compact, denotes the covariates, describing the feature of a node (e.g. the patient's clinical covariates in a network patients-treatments, or gene expression in a gene network, or protein concentration in a protein–protein network). Let

$$\pi_m(x) = \mathbb{P}(A = m | X = x) \tag{12.10}$$

denote the probability of being assigned treatment m for a node with covariates x. In the Zhou et al. framework this probability is assumed to be predefined in the design. Potential outcomes, denoted by $R^*(1), \ldots, R^*(M)$, are introduced and are defined as the outcomes that would be observed were a node to receive treatment $1, \dots, M$, respectively. Very often in literature, we find two assumptions regarding the potential outcomes:

1) **Consistency assumption:** The potential outcomes and the observed outcomes agree, i.e.:

$$R = \Pi_{m=1}^{M} R^*(m) \mathbb{I}(A = m)$$

where $\mathbb{I}(\cdot)$ is the indicator function;

2) **No unmeasured confounders assumption:** Conditional on covariates X, the potential outcomes $\{R^*(1), \dots, R^*(M)\}$ are independent of the treatment assignment A that has been actually received.

Let us make some remarks on these assumptions right away. We point out that it is often assumed that assumption 2 is valid in the case of randomized trials, but this belief is debatable. We consider it more prudent to state that in randomized trials the number of unmeasured confounders is reduced, but not completely eliminated and that, in any case, the influence on the predictive ability of the algorithm is not only given by the number of possible confounders, but also by their role in the system studied.

A treatment regime d is mathematically formalized by a function from covariates X to the treatment assignment A. For a treatment regime d, we can thus define its potential outcome. Let

$$R^*(d) = \sum_{m=1}^{M} R^*(m) \mathbb{I}(d(X) = m), \qquad (12.11)$$

be the potential outcome of a treatment regime d. Let us denote with $\mathbb{E}(R^*(d)|X = x)$ the expected potential outcome under any regime d. An optimal regime d_{opt} is a regime that maximizes $\mathbb{E}(R^*(d))$, i.e.:

$$d_{\text{opt}}(x) = \text{argmax}_{m=1, \dots, M} \mathbb{E}(R^*(d)|X = x). \qquad (12.12)$$

By the consistency assumption and non-unmeasured confounder assumption, we have that

$$\mathbb{E}(R^*(d)|X = x) = \mathbb{E}(R|X = x \text{ and } A = m).$$

The causal nearest neighbor algorithm implements the following steps (i) to find a neighborhood of x in $\mathcal{X}$, (ii) to find an estimate $\hat{m} = \mathbb{E}(R|X = x \text{ and } A = m)$ for each arm in this neighborhood, and (iii) to plug $\hat{m}$ into Eq. (12.12) to obtain the nearest neighbor estimate for the optimal treatment regime, i.e.:

$$d_{\text{opt}}^{\text{CKNN}}(x) = \text{argmax}_{m=1, \dots, M} \hat{m}. \qquad (12.13)$$

$d_{\text{opt}}^{\text{CKNN}}(x)$ is called the CKNN regime (Zhou and Kosorok 2017).

We refer the reader to the works of Zhou and Kosorok (2017), Hitsch and Misra (2018), Kricke and Peschenz (2019) for the models used to calculate $\hat{m}$ and to the technical algorithmic details. What is important to note here is that the causal nearest neighbor regimes are calculated as local averaging, and k is a tuning parameter. It is required that k be small enough so that local changes of the distribution can be detected. On the other hand, k needs to be large enough so that averaging over the arm is effective. This parameter can be estimated by a cross validation procedure to balance the two requirements, provided we have a (i) sufficiently large sample and (ii) sufficient computational resources to deal with large complex network. However, in many realistic situations biological network inference is an undetermined problem, since the size of the node covariate sample is small, whereas the size of the network is huge. However, even assuming that computational costs can be managed and optimal covariate sample size can be obtained, still we have to deal with the problem that the potential outcomes of any node only depends on their nearest neighbors. The concept of neighbor is defined through the concept of distance, so ultimately the results of a CKNN in terms of both interpretation and reliability depend on the definition of distance we use.

12.4.2 Causal Random Forests

A random forest (RF) algorithm consists of many decision trees, i.e. a "forest" generated by the algorithm itself. The RF algorithm establishes the outcome based on the predictions of the decision trees. A decision tree predicts by taking the mean of the output from various trees. In random forests, the data is repeatedly split in order to minimize prediction error of an outcome variable. Causal forests are built similarly, except that instead of minimizing prediction error, data are split in such a way to maximize the difference across groups in the relationship between an outcome variable and a "treatment" variable. "Outcome variable" and "treatment" are used here in the broadest sense of the term, which is then specified according to the context of application. Causal forests principally estimate heterogeneity in a causal effect. In fact, the term *causal* referring to random forest can be misleading, as causal forests can reveal heterogeneity in a causal effect, but they do not by themselves infer the causal effect. There have been interesting approaches to achieve this goal very recently, see for example the work of Li et al. (2020) which developed a causal inference model combining Granger causality analysis (Shojaie and Fox 2022) and a random forest learning model. In the same vein, we find the works of Schmidt et al. (2020) and Tsai et al. (2020), all these devoted to identify cause-effect relationships in climatic phenomena, and at the present still not easily generalizable to the inference of biological networks (Lecca 2021). Nevertheless, on the same methodological line, there have also been important achievements in this direction in gene regulatory networks in the recent past, such as the development of a random forest algorithm for gene regulatory network inference by Petralia et al. (2015), Furqan and Siyal (2016), Deng et al. (2017), Huynh-Thu and Geurts (2018), Kimura et al. (2020), Zhang et al. (2020), Cassan et al. (2021). The majority of the methods base on random forest for causal discovery in gene regulatory networks.

Most of these approaches implement upstream of the inference process the integration of large amounts of data of different natures that are indispensable for inferring causal relationships in structures as complex as biological networks. The complexity of a biological network, be it a gene regulatory network or a signaling network or a metabolic or biochemical network, lies in its size expressed by the number of nodes and the potential number of arcs and very often by the potential nonlinear relationships between nodes that challenge the reliability and the accuracy of the regression techniques. The big amount of heterogeneous data would require the RF algorithm to generate a large quantity of trees to improve its efficiency. However, it is well known that the main limitation of random forest is that a large number of trees can make the algorithm too slow and ineffective for real-time predictions.

Another limitation of a RF algorithm is its inability to extrapolate. A RF algorithm can only calculate an average of previously observed labels. This means that when applied to a regression problem, the algorithm provides a range of predictions that is bound by the highest and lowest labels in the training data. This behavior is regrettable when the training and prediction inputs differ in their range and/or distributions. This is called *covariate shift* and it is difficult for most models to handle (also to KNN) but especially for RF algorithms, because they only interpolate. The frequency with which the problem of covariate shift may be encountered is also very high when using heterogeneous biological data to aid causal inference in complex biological networks.

Although the current literature is promising regarding the applications of RF-based methods for causal inference in biological networks, the overcoming of these limitations is still far to come so how far is their applications to networks other than gene regulatory networks (Lecca 2021).

12.4.3 Causal Support Vector Machine

SVMs appeared in the early nineties as optimal margin classifiers in the context of Vapnik's statistical learning theory (Vapnik 1995). The SVM algorithm aims to find a hyperplane in an N-dimensional space (where N is the number of features) that optimally classifies the data points. SVMs can be used both for classification and regression tasks.

Moguerza and Muñoz (2006) highlights that an advantage of the support vector approach is that sparse solutions to classification and regression problems are usually obtained, i.e. only a few samples are involved in the determination of the classification or regression functions. This fact constitutes a facilitation of the application of SVMs to problems that involve a large amount of data. However, at the moment of writing their extension to causal inference tool has not yet been developed. In the literature we find some works in which SVMs are used in combination with other techniques in order to infer the structure of gene regulatory networks. In these regards, we report the Gillani et al. work (Gillani et al. 2014) who proposed CompareSVM a tool that can be used to infer gene regulatory network which is highly accurate for networks with less than 200 nodes. The tool employs SVM Gaussian kernel for biological datasets (knockout, knockdown, multifactorial, and all). Interestingly, they state that since there are variations in prediction accuracy in all inference methods, prediction should be limited for simple network, and it is not recommended to be done for large networks.

Another study, representative of the works using SVMs in biological network inference, is the paper of Vert et al. (2007), who deal with inferring network edges in a supervised way from a set of high-confidence edges, possibly characterized by multiple, heterogeneous data sets (protein sequence, gene expression, etc.). In this setting the authors distinguish between two modes of inference: direct inference based upon similarities between nodes joined by an edge, and indirect inference based upon similarities between one pair of nodes and another pair of nodes. Theirs is a supervised approach for the direct case consisting of learning a distance metric. In this framework, a relaxation of the resulting convex optimization problem leads to the a SVM algorithm with a particular kernel for pairs, that is called "the metric learning pairwise kernel." The proposed methods hold the promise of being used by most SVM implementations to solve problems of supervised classification and inference of pairwise relationships from heterogeneous data.

Finally, a recent work by Le Borgne et al. (2021) not specifically on biological networks, but on treatment–effect networks, found that SVM approach is competing with the most powerful recent methods, such as G-computation (Snowden et al. 2011) for small sample sizes with one hundred nodes when the relationships between the covariates and the outcome are complex. These findings may constitute important insights into the development of an efficient future causal version of SVMs.

12.5 Opportunities and Challenges

The current drug discovery approaches have to face several common challenges. First of all, they require a huge amount of funding to take a drug candidate from preclinical development to clinical trials, thereby remarkably reducing further funding for optimization or rediscovery (RoboticsBiz 2021). Second, drug efficacy depends on each patient's unique needs and their specific genetic background. Third, pharmaceutical companies need about 15 years for a successful drug development, which costs more than $1 billion (Hughes et al. 2011). Fourth, only 1 in 10 small molecule projects become candidates for clinical trials, and only about 1 in 10 of those compounds will then pass successfully through clinical trials.

AI and machine learning hold the promise to overcome these issues and make the drug discovery more efficient and more effective. The construction and analysis of the drug–target network is the core of the drug discovery process, and in this chapter, we have seen the most promising mathematical methods whose use is becoming increasingly widespread for this purpose. However, AI and machine learning techniques are not limited to support drug discovery in this specific task. They include methods of computer-aided organic synthesis, compound discovery, assay development, biomarker discovery, drug molecules design, clinical trial design (Paul et al. 2021; Gupta 2021; Dara et al. 2021; Carracedo-Reboredo et al. 2021; Lipinski et al. 2019). Paul et al. (2021) summarize in a sentence the good perspective of AI in drug discovery, saying that "Using the latest AI-based technologies will not only speed up the time needed for the products to come to the market, but will also improve the quality of products and the overall safety of the production process, and provide better utilization of available resources along with being cost-effective, thereby increasing the importance of automation."

Despite the enthusiasm that accompanies the use of artificial intelligence methods in the drug discovery process, there is no shortage of critical views, such as those expressed by Bender and Cortés-Ciriano (2021). The authors highlight a number of critical issues, of which we report the main three. First, the note that much of the current efforts of AI in drug discovery are focused on ligand discovery, and this can certainly help in validating a target with respect to its ability to recover the diseased phenotype. However – they note – in the context of drug discovery, a ligand is not (yet) a drug, and state: "if AI approaches for drug discovery only end up generating a ligand for a protein, then there is no evidence that this will help drug discovery as a whole, which hence is an important aim for the future. To validate AI systems in drug discovery, we need to move to more complex biological systems (and the clinic) earlier, and more often." The second issue is that there are often no control experiments being conducted when AI delivers new compounds (such as no baseline methods being applied in parallel). Consequently, it is hence often impossible to disentangle whether the end product is a result of the method applied or the result of subjective choices on which compound to test. This issue combined with a large chemical space (third issue) from which to pick possible validation compounds tends to lead to trivial validation examples.

AI techniques are not new, but the recent advancements and the increased computational power allow their use in many application domains. This increasingly widespread use has in fact constituted a new scientific paradigm in data processing and the processes of extracting new knowledge from it. Like all new scientific paradigms, also this splits the scientific community into groups with favorable positions and groups with more cautious if not critical views. Only the use of these techniques in continuous and close cooperation with experts in the medical, biological, and pharmaceutical fields will be able to justify one position over another. As the overview presented in this chapter already suggests, AI still cannot replace a human scientist entirely in the process of drug discovery. AI predictions are as good as the algorithms used to investigate a dataset. AI can suffer from algorithm bias, in the way information is processed to generate predictions, and in the ways feature space and similarity/distance measure are defined. Consequently, the process may be not entirely objective and context-free. It also worth to note that AI and machine learning aid the process of drug discovery, but it cannot replace the experimental activity. Ultimately, computer's predictions have to be verified experimentally by scientists.

Author Biography

Paola Lecca got a Master Degree in Theoretical Physics and a PhD in Computer Science and Telecommunication from University of Trento, Italy. She is Assistant Professor at the Faculty of Engineering of the Free University of Bolzano-Bozen (Italy). Her research lines include graph theory, dynamical networks modeling, and statistical inference. Paola Lecca has experience in applying these conceptual and algorithmic tools to bioinformatics and computational biology. Paola Lecca is Senior Professional Member of Association for Computing Machinery, New York, the United States, and member of the advisory board of the International Research Institute Foundation for Artificial Intelligence and Computer, Salamanca Spain.

References

Adhami, M., Sadeghi, B., Rezapour, A. et al. (2021). Repurposing novel therapeutic candidate drugs for coronavirus disease-19 based on protein-protein interaction network analysis. *BMC Biotechnology* 21(1): https://doi.org/10.1186/s12896-021-00680-z.

Arabi, A.A. (2021). Artificial intelligence in drug design: algorithms, applications, challenges and ethics. *Future Drug Discovery* 3(2): https://doi.org/10.4155/fdd-2020-0028.

Askr, H., Elgeldawi, E., Ella, H.A. et al. (2022). Deep learning in drug discovery: an integrative review and future challenges. *Artificial Intelligence Review*. https://doi.org/10.1007/s10462-022-10306-1.

Bagherian, M., Sabeti, E., Wang, K. et al. (2020). Machine learning approaches and databases for prediction of drug–target interaction: a survey paper. *Briefings in Bioinformatics* 22(1): 247–269. https://doi.org/10.1093/bib/bbz157.

Bender, A. and Cortés-Ciriano, I. (2021). Artificial intelligence in drug discovery: what is realistic, what are illusions? Part 1: Ways to make an impact, and why we are not there yet. *Drug Discovery Today* 26(2): 511–524. https://doi.org/10.1016/j.drudis.2020.12.009.

Boo (2000). *To Err Is Human*. National Academies Press. https://doi.org/10.17226/9728.

Bottegal, G. and Suykens, J.A.K. (2017). Probabilistic matrix factorization from quantized measurements. *2017 International Joint Conference on Neural Networks (IJCNN)*, 270–277. https://doi.org/10.1109/IJCNN.2017.7965865.

Bredel, M. and Jacoby, E. (2004). Chemogenomics: an emerging strategy for rapid target and drug discovery. *Nature Reviews Genetics* 5(4): 262–275. https://doi.org/10.1038/nrg1317.

Carracedo-Reboredo, P., Liñares-Blanco, J., Rodríguez-Fernández, N. et al. (2021). A review on machine learning approaches and trends in drug discovery. *Computational and Structural Biotechnology Journal* 19: 4538–4558. https://doi.org/10.1016/j.csbj.2021.08.011.

Cassan, O., Lèbre, S., and Martin, A. (2021). Inferring and analyzing gene regulatory networks from multi-factorial expression data: a complete and interactive suite. *BMC Genomics* 22(1): https://doi.org/10.1186/s12864-021-07659-2.

Ceddia, G., Pinoli, P., Ceri, S., and Masseroli, M. (2020a). Matrix factorization-based technique for drug repurposing predictions. *IEEE Journal of Biomedical and Health Informatics* 24(11): 3162–3172. https://doi.org/10.1109/JBHI.2020.2991763.

Ceddia, G., Pinoli, P., Ceri, S., and Masseroli, M. (2020b). Matrix factorization-based technique for drug repurposing predictions. *IEEE Journal of Biomedical and Health Informatics* 24(11): 3162–3172. https://doi.org/10.1109/jbhi.2020.2991763.

Chen, R., Liu, X., Jin, S. et al. (2018). Machine learning for drug-target interaction prediction. *Molecules* 23(9): 2208. https://doi.org/10.3390/molecules23092208.

Chen, R., Xia, F., Hu, B. et al. (2022). Drug–target interactions prediction via deep collaborative filtering with multiembeddings. *Briefings in Bioinformatics* 23(2): https://doi.org/10.1093/bib/bbab520.

Cheng, F., Kovács, I.A., and Barabási, A.-L. (2019). Network-based prediction of drug combinations. *Nature Communications* 10(1): https://doi.org/10.1038/s41467-019-09186-x.

Cobanoglu, M.C., Liu, C., Hu, F. et al. (2013). Predicting drug–target interactions using probabilistic matrix factorization. *Journal of Chemical Information and Modeling* 53(12): 3399–3409. https://doi.org/10.1021/ci400219z.

D'Souza, S., Prema, K.V., and Balaji, S. (2020). Machine learning models for drug–target interactions: current knowledge and future directions. *Drug Discovery Today* 25(4): 748–756. https://doi.org/10.1016/j.drudis.2020.03.003.

Dai, W., Liu, X., Gao, Y. et al. (2015). Matrix factorization-based prediction of novel drug indications by integrating genomic space. *Computational and Mathematical Methods in Medicine* 2015: 1–9. https://doi.org/10.1155/2015/275045.

Dara, S., Dhamercherla, S., Jadav, S.S. et al. (2021). Machine learning in drug discovery: a review. *Artificial Intelligence Review* https://doi.org/10.1007/s10462-021-10058-4.

Deng, W., Zhang, K., Busov, V., and Wei, H. (2017). Recursive random forest algorithm for constructing multilayered hierarchical gene regulatory networks that govern biological pathways. *PLoS ONE* 12(2): e0171532. https://doi.org/10.1371/journal.pone.0171532.

Doğan, T., Güzelcan, E.A., Baumann, M. et al. (2021). Protein domain-based prediction of drug/compound–target interactions and experimental validation on LIM kinases. *PLoS Computational Biology* 17(11): e1009171. https://doi.org/10.1371/journal.pcbi.1009171.

Ezzat, A., Wu, M., Li, X.-L., and Kwoh, C.-K. (2018). Computational prediction of drug-target interactions using chemogenomic approaches: an empirical survey. *Briefings in Bioinformatics* 20(4): 1337–1357. https://doi.org/10.1093/bib/bby002.

Feng, Y., Wang, Q., and Wang, T. (2017). Drug target protein-protein interaction networks: a systematic perspective. *BioMed Research International* 2017: 1–13. https://doi.org/10.1155/2017/1289259.

Fleming, N. (2018). How artificial intelligence is changing drug discovery. *Nature* 557(7707): S55–S57. https://doi.org/10.1038/d41586-018-05267-x.

Fukuto, K., Takagi, T., and Tian, Y.-S. (2021). Predicting the side effects of drugs using matrix factorization on spontaneous reporting database. *Scientific Reports* 11(1): https://doi.org/10.1038/s41598-021-03348-y.

Furqan, M.S. and Siyal, M.Y. (2016). Inference of biological networks using bi-directional random forest granger causality. *Springerplus* 5(1): https://doi.org/10.1186/s40064-016-2156-y.

Gallego, V., Naveiro, R., Roca, C. et al. (2021). AI in drug development: a multidisciplinary perspective. *Molecular Diversity*. https://doi.org/10.1007/s11030-021-10266-8.

Gaudelet, T., Day, B., Jamasb, A.R. et al. (2021). Utilizing graph machine learning within drug discovery and development. *Briefings in Bioinformatics* 22(6): https://doi.org/10.1093/bib/bbab159.

Gillani, Z., Akash, M.S.H., Rahaman, M.D.M., and Chen, M. (2014). CompareSVM: supervised, support vector machine (SVM) inference of gene regularity networks. *BMC Bioinformatics* 15(1): https://doi.org/10.1186/s12859-014-0395-x.

Gupta, R.R. (2021). Application of artificial intelligence and machine learning in drug discovery. In: *Artificial Intelligence in Drug Design*, 113–124. Springer US https://doi.org/10.1007/978-1-0716-1787-8_4.

Gupta, R., Srivastava, D., Sahu, M. et al. (2021). Artificial intelligence to deep learning: machine intelligence approach for drug discovery. *Molecular Diversity* 25(3): 1315–1360. https://doi.org/10.1007/s11030-021-10217-3.

Guvenilir, H.A. and Doğan, T. (2023). How to approach machine learning-based prediction of drug/compound–target interactions. *Journal of Cheminformatics* 15(1): https://doi.org/10.1186/s13321-023-00689-w.

Hajduk, P.J., Huth, J.R., and Tse, C. (2005). Predicting protein druggability. *Drug Discovery Today* 10(23-24): 1675–1682. https://doi.org/10.1016/s1359-6446(05)03624-x.

Han, K., Cao, P., Wang, Y. et al. (2022). A review of approaches for predicting drug–drug interactions based on machine learning. *Frontiers in Pharmacology* 12: https://doi.org/10.3389/fphar.2021.814858.

Hasan, M.R., Paul, B.K., Ahmed, K., and Bhuyian, T. (2020). Design protein-protein interaction network and protein-drug interaction network for common cancer diseases: a bioinformatics approach. *Informatics in Medicine Unlocked* 18: 100311. https://doi.org/10.1016/j.imu.2020.100311.

He, Z., Zhang, J., Shi, X.-H. et al. (2010). Predicting drug-target interaction networks based on functional groups and biological features. *PLoS ONE* 5(3): e9603. https://doi.org/10.1371/journal.pone.0009603.

Herrling, P.L. (2005). The drug discovery process. In: Herrling, P.L., Matter, A., Rudin, M. (eds). Imaging in Drug Discovery and Early Clinical Trials. Progress in Drug Research, vol. 62. Birkhäuser Basel. https://doi.org/10.1007/3-7643-7426-8_1.

Hinkson, I.V., Madej, B., and Stahlberg, E.A. (2020). Accelerating therapeutics for opportunities in medicine: a paradigm shift in drug discovery. *Frontiers in Pharmacology* 11: https://doi.org/10.3389/fphar.2020.00770.

Hitsch, G.J. and Misra, S. (2018). Heterogeneous treatment effects and optimal targeting policy evaluation. *SSRN Electronic Journal* https://doi.org/10.2139/ssrn.3111957.

Hopkins, A.L. and Groom, C.R. (2002). The druggable genome. *Nature Reviews Drug Discovery* 1(9): 727–730. https://doi.org/10.1038/nrd892.

Hughes, J.P., Rees, S., Kalindjian, S.B., and Philpott, K.L. (2011). Principles of early drug discovery. *Br J Pharmacol.* 162(6): 1239–1249. doi: 10.1111/j.1476-5381.2010.01127.x. PMID: 21091654; PMCID: PMC3058157.

Huynh-Thu, V.A. and Geurts, P. (2018). Unsupervised gene network inference with decision trees and random forests. In: *Methods in Molecular Biology*, 195–215. New York: Springer https://doi.org/10.1007/978-1-4939-8882-2_8.

Ismail, H., Malim, N.H.A.H., Zobir, S.Z.M., and Wahab, H.A. (2021). Comparative studies on drug-target interaction prediction using machine learning and deep learning methods with different molecular descriptors. *2021 International Conference of Women in Data Science at Taif University (WiDSTaif)*. IEEE, March 2021. https://doi.org/10.1109/widstaif52235.2021.9430198.

Jang, I.-J. (2019). Artificial intelligence in drug development: clinical pharmacologist perspective. *Translational and Clinical Pharmacology* 27(3): 87. https://doi.org/10.12793/tcp.2019.27.3.87.

Jiménez-Luna, J., Grisoni, F., and Schneider, G. (2020). Drug discovery with explainable artificial intelligence. *Nature Machine Intelligence* 2(10): 573–584. https://doi.org/10.1038/s42256-020-00236-4.

Johnson, C.R. (1990). Matrix completion problems: a survey. https://doi.org/10.1090/psapm/040/1059486.

Kim, J., Park, S., Min, D., and Kim, W. (2021). Comprehensive survey of recent drug discovery using deep learning. *International Journal of Molecular Sciences* 22(18): 9983. https://doi.org/10.3390/ijms22189983.

Kimura, S., Fukutomi, R., Tokuhisa, M., and Okada, M. (2020). Inference of genetic networks from time-series and static gene expression data: combining a random-forest-based inference method with feature selection methods. *Frontiers in Genetics* 11: https://doi.org/10.3389/fgene.2020.595912.

Kricke, M. and Peschenz, T. (2019). Applied Predictive Analytics Seminar - Causal KNN. https://humboldt-wi.github.io/blog/research/applied_predictive_modeling_19/blog_post_causal_knn/ (accessed 28 September 2023).

Laurent, M. (2008). Matrix completion problems. In: *Encyclopedia of Optimization* (ed. C. Floudas and P. Pardalos), 1967–1975. Springer US. https://doi.org/10.1007/0-306-48332-7_271.

Le Borgne, F., Chatton, A., Léger, M. et al. (2021). G-computation and machine learning for estimating the causal effects of binary exposure statuses on binary outcomes. *Scientific Reports* 11(1): https://doi.org/10.1038/s41598-021-81110-0.

Lecca, P. (2021). Machine learning for causal inference in biological networks: perspectives of this challenge. *Frontiers in Bioinformatics*. 1: https://doi.org/10.3389/fbinf.2021.746712.

Li, C.-G., Qi, X., and Guo, J. (2013). Dimensionality reduction by low-rank embedding. In: *Intelligent Science and Intelligent Data Engineering*, 181–188. Berlin, Heidelberg: Springer-Verlag. https://doi.org/10.1007/978-3-642-36669-7_23.

Li, L., Shangguan, W., Deng, Y. et al. (2020). A causal inference model based on random forests to identify the effect of soil moisture on precipitation. *Journal of Hydrometeorology* 21(5): 1115–1131. https://doi.org/10.1175/jhm-d-19-0209.1.

Lin, X., Xu, S., Liu, X. et al. (2022). Detecting drug–target interactions with feature similarity fusion and molecular graphs. *Biology* 11(7): 967. https://doi.org/10.3390/biology11070967.

Lipinski, C.F., Maltarollo, V.G., Oliveira, P.R. et al. (2019). Advances and perspectives in applying deep learning for drug design and discovery. *Frontiers in Robotics and AI* 6: https://doi.org/10.3389/frobt.2019.00108.

Liu, Y. (2004). A comparative study on feature selection methods for drug discovery. *Journal of Chemical Information and Computer Sciences* 44(5): 1823–1828. https://doi.org/10.1021/ci049875d.

Liu, T. and Altman, R.B. (2014). Identifying druggable targets by protein microenvironments matching: application to transcription factors. *CPT: Pharmacometrics & Systems Pharmacology* 3(1): 93. https://doi.org/10.1038/psp.2013.66.

Liu, G., Singha, M., Pu, L. et al. (2021). GraphDTI: a robust deep learning predictor of drug-target interactions from multiple heterogeneous data. *Journal of Cheminformatics* 13(1): https://doi.org/10.1186/s13321-021-00540-0.

Lu, H., Zhou, Q., He, J. et al. (2020). Recent advances in the development of protein–protein interactions modulators: mechanisms and clinical trials. *Signal Transduction and Targeted Therapy* 5(1): https://doi.org/10.1038/s41392-020-00315-3.

Mahmud, S.M.H., Chen, W., Jahan, H. et al. (2021). Dimensionality reduction based multi-kernel framework for drug-target interaction prediction. *Chemometrics and Intelligent Laboratory Systems* 212: 104270. https://doi.org/10.1016/j.chemolab.2021.104270.

Mesrabadi, H.A., Faez, K., and Pirgazi, J. (2023). Drug–target interaction prediction based on protein features, using wrapper feature selection. *Scientific Reports* 13(1): https://doi.org/10.1038/s41598-023-30026-y.

Moguerza, J.M. and Muñoz, A. (2006). Support vector machines with applications. *Statistical Science* 21(3): https://doi.org/10.1214/088342306000000493.

Nafshi, R. and Lezon, T.R. (2021). Predicting the effects of drug combinations using probabilistic matrix factorization. *Frontiers in Bioinformatics*. 1: https://doi.org/10.3389/fbinf.2021.708815.

Patel, V. and Shah, M. (2021). A comprehensive study on artificial intelligence and machine learning in drug discovery and drug development. *Intelligent Medicine*. https://doi.org/10.1016/j.imed.2021.10.001.

Paul, D., Sanap, G., Shenoy, S. et al. (2021). Artificial intelligence in drug discovery and development. *Drug Discovery Today* 26(1): 80–93. https://doi.org/10.1016/j.drudis.2020.10.010.

Perlman, L., Gottlieb, A., Atias, N. et al. (2011). Combining drug and gene similarity measures for drug-target elucidation. *Journal of Computational Biology* 18(2): 133–145. https://doi.org/10.1089/cmb.2010.0213.

Petralia, F., Wang, P., Yang, J., and Tu, Z. (2015). Integrative random forest for gene regulatory network inference. *Bioinformatics* 31(12): i197–i205. https://doi.org/10.1093/bioinformatics/btv268.

Poleksic, A. (2023). Hyperbolic matrix factorization improves prediction of drug-target associations. *Scientific Reports* 13(1): https://doi.org/10.1038/s41598-023-27995-5.

Réda, C., Kaufmann, E., and Delahaye-Duriez, A. (2020). Machine learning applications in drug development. *Computational and Structural Biotechnology Journal* 18: 241–252. https://doi.org/10.1016/j.csbj.2019.12.006.

RoboticsBiz, AI In Drug Discovery – Benefits, Drawbacks, And Challenges, Editorial, 9 April 2021, URL: https://roboticsbiz.com/ai-in-drug-discovery-benefits-drawback-and-challenges/, accessed: 2022-02-03.

Rodriguez, J.J., Kuncheva, L.I., and Alonso, C.J. (2006). Rotation forest: a new classifier ensemble method. *IEEE Transactions on Pattern Analysis and Machine Intelligence* 28(10): 1619–1630. https://doi.org/10.1109/TPAMI.2006.211.

Ru, X., Ye, X., Sakurai, T. et al. (2021). Current status and future prospects of drug–target interaction prediction. *Briefings in Functional Genomics* 20(5): 312–322. https://doi.org/10.1093/bfgp/elab031.

Ruiz, C., Zitnik, M., and Leskovec, J. (2021). Identification of disease treatment mechanisms through the multiscale interactome. *Nature Communications* 12(1): https://doi.org/10.1038/s41467-021-21770-8.

Saarela, M., Elomaa, T., and Ruohonen, K. (2010). An analysis of relevance vector machine regression. In: *Advances in Machine Learning I*, 227–246. Berlin, Heidelberg: Springer-Verlag https://doi.org/10.1007/978-3-642-05177-7_11.

Sachdev, K. and Gupta, M.K. (2019). A comprehensive review of feature based methods for drug target interaction prediction. *Journal of Biomedical Informatics* 93: 103159. https://doi.org/10.1016/j.jbi.2019.103159.

Sadeghi, S., Lu, J., and Ngom, A. (2021). A network-based drug repurposing method via non-negative matrix factorization. *Bioinformatics*. https://doi.org/10.1093/bioinformatics/btab826.

Salakhutdinov, R. and Mnih, A. (2007). Probabilistic matrix factorization. In: *Proceedings of the 20th International Conference on Neural Information Processing Systems*, NIPS'07, 1257–1264. Red Hook, NY: Curran Associates Inc. ISBN 9781605603520.

Schmidt, L., Heße, F., Attinger, S., and Kumar, R. (2020). Challenges in applying machine learning models for hydrological inference: a case study for flooding events across Germany. *Water Resources Research* 56(5): https://doi.org/10.1029/2019wr025924.

Selvaraj, C., Chandra, I., and Singh, S.K. (2021). Artificial intelligence and machine learning approaches for drug design: challenges and opportunities for the pharmaceutical industries. *Molecular Diversity* 26(3): 1893–1913. https://doi.org/10.1007/s11030-021-10326-z.

Shojaie, A. and Fox, E.B. (2022). Granger causality: a review and recent advances. *Annual Review of Statistics and Its Application* 9(1): 289–319. https://doi.org/10.1146/annurev-statistics-040120-010930.

Snowden, J.M., Rose, S., and Mortimer, K.M. (2011). Implementation of g-computation on a simulated data set: demonstration of a causal inference technique. *American Journal of Epidemiology* 173(7): 731–738. https://doi.org/10.1093/aje/kwq472.

Somolinos, F.J., León, C., and Guerrero-Aspizua, S. (2021). Drug repurposing using biological networks. *Processes* 9(6): 1057. https://doi.org/10.3390/pr9061057.

Steinwart, I. and Christmann, A. (2008). *Support Vector Machines*, Information Science and Statistics, 2008e. New York: Springer.

Takarabe, M., Kotera, M., Nishimura, Y. et al. (2012). Drug target prediction using adverse event report systems: a pharmacogenomic approach. *Bioinformatics* 28(18): i611–i618. https://doi.org/10.1093/bioinformatics/bts413.

Tsai, W.-P., Fang, K., Ji, X. et al. (2020). Revealing causal controls of storage-streamflow relationships with a data-centric bayesian framework combining machine learning and process-based modeling. *Frontiers in Water* 2: https://doi.org/10.3389/frwa.2020.583000.

Vamathevan, J., Clark, D., Czodrowski, P. et al. (2019). Applications of machine learning in drug discovery and development. *Nature Reviews Drug Discovery* 18(6): 463–477. https://doi.org/10.1038/s41573-019-0024-5.

Vapnik, V. (1995). *The Nature of Statistical Learning Theory*. New York: Springer New York. ISBN: 978-1-4757-2440-0.

Vert, J.-P., Qiu, J., and Noble, W.S. (2007). A new pairwise kernel for biological network inference with support vector machines. *BMC Bioinformatics* 8(S10): https://doi.org/10.1186/1471-2105-8-s10-s8.

Xu, L., Ru, X., and Song, R. (2021). Application of machine learning for drug–target interaction prediction. *Frontiers in Genetics* 12: https://doi.org/10.3389/fgene.2021.680117.

Yang, X., Zamit, L., Liu, Y., and He, J. (2019). Additional neural matrix factorization model for computational drug repositioning. *BMC Bioinformatics* 20(1): https://doi.org/10.1186/s12859-019-2983-2.

Zhang, Y., Chen, Q., Gao, D., and Zou, Q. (2020). GRRFNet: guided regularized random forest-based gene regulatory network inference using data integration. *2020 IEEE International Conference on Bioinformatics and Biomedicine (BIBM)*. IEEE, December 2020. https://doi.org/10.1109/bibm49941.2020.9313349.

Zhavoronkov, A., Vanhaelen, Q., and Oprea, T.I. (2020). Will artificial intelligence for drug discovery impact clinical pharmacology? *Clinical Pharmacology & Therapeutics* 107(4): 780–785. https://doi.org/10.1002/cpt.1795.

Zhou, X. and Kosorok, M.R. (2017). Causal nearest neighbor rules for optimal treatment regimes.

13

Using AI to Steer Brain Regeneration: The Enhanced Regenerative Medicine Paradigm

Gabriella Panuccio[1], Narayan P. Subramaniyam[2], Angel Canal-Alonso[3,4], Juan M. Corchado[3,4] and Carlo Ierna[5]

[1]*Enhanced Regenerative Medicine Lab, Istituto Italiano di Tecnologia, Via Morego 30, Genova 16163, Italy*
[2]*Computational Biophysics Lab, Faculty of Medicine and Health Technology and BioMediTech Institute, Tampere University, 33520, Tampere, Finland*
[3]*BISITE Research Group, University of Salamanca, Salamanca 37008, Spain*
[4]*Institute for Biomedical Research of Salamanca, University of Salamanca, Salamanca 37008, Spain*
[5]*Radboud University Nijmegen, Faculty of Philosophy, Theology, and Religious Studies, Center for the History of Philosophy and Science, Nijmegen 6500 HD, The Netherlands*

13.1 The Challenge of Brain Regeneration

The brain has been considered for centuries a perennial organ, i.e. an organ that cannot repair itself once damaged. However, pioneering discoveries in the 1960s and subsequent studies have demonstrated that regeneration may also occur within the brain, wherein stem cell niches provide a source for cell renewal and tissue repair (Takagi 2016; Bifari et al. 2017; Decimo et al. 2021). Nonetheless, the self-repairing ability of the brain is very limited compared to that of other organs of the human body, like the skin; thus, when its damage extends beyond the ability of self-repair, it leaves permanent lacunae that require an exogenous intervention.

Regenerative medicine is the latest frontier toward the breakthrough of healing brain damage. This is based on two primary approaches: (i) stimulating the endogenous neurogenic potential of the brain and (ii) grafting exogenous cellular elements or bioengineered brain tissue in the damaged region. While the former approach is limited by the neurogenic potential of the brain, the latter holds promise to surpass such limitations. As of today, the progress achieved in stem cell biotechnology, cell therapy, brain tissue, and brain organoid bioengineering provides a solid foundation for such a challenging undertaking. Pioneering studies have indeed demonstrated the feasibility of grafting cells (Cunningham et al. 2014) or tissue (Mansour et al. 2018; Shetty and Turner 1995, 1996, 1997) to repair brain damage or recover brain function. However, these studies have also highlighted the limitations of such approaches: while biological grafts promise to improve the neurological condition, none of such approaches has successfully managed to definitely *heal* brain damage; further, the unpredictable behavior of biological grafts might endanger the patient's safety unless adequately fine-tuned. Herein, the major challenge is understanding, predicting, and controlling how grafted cells or tissue develop, interact, and integrate within the host brain.

Big Data Analysis and Artificial Intelligence for Medical Sciences, First Edition.
Edited by Bruno Carpentieri and Paola Lecca.
© 2024 John Wiley & Sons Ltd. Published 2024 by John Wiley & Sons Ltd.

In fact, the uncontrolled growth of stem cells, which inherently possess a high proliferative potential, may originate a niche for tumor development (Peterson et al. 2016), while the intrinsic plasticity of neuronal grafts may yield a focus of pathological activity (Buzsaki et al. 1989). In this, the complex structural and functional organization of the brain adds significant uncertainties, since we are yet to fully understand them.

In this scenario, it is crucial to understand the advantages and limitations of mechanistic (first principles) and phenomenological (evidence-based) approaches to study and treat brain disorders. The mechanistic approach aims at pinpointing the exact mechanisms of brain function and dysfunction, which, in turn, supports the design of disease-specific therapeutic tools; however, a mechanistic understanding of the exact cause of a disease entails a long and winding quest, which hinders the fast discovery of such therapeutic tools. The phenomenological approach relies on the observation of phenomena to derive abstract rules for their occurrence and correlation, regardless of the exact underlying mechanisms; this permits to devise generalized therapeutic frameworks, which, in turn, are faster to achieve.

Artificial intelligence (AI) bridges both approaches, as witnessed by the increasing body of work wherein AI crosses the boundaries of experimental neuroscience and clinical research. These are fueled by the availability of large-scale data from diverse methods such as diffusion tensor imaging, magnetic resonance imaging (MRI), functional MRI (fMRI), functional near-infrared spectroscopy, electroencephalography (EEG), and magnetoencephalography. In addition, availability of genomic and proteomic data also offers an exciting opportunity toward multimodal analysis of neuroscience data. For instance, several neurodegenerative disorders are known to cause disruptions that span molecular pathways, synapses, and local as well as higher-order neural networks (Palop et al. 2006); thus, their treatment will immensely benefit from multimodal data analysis. AI approaches, particularly deep learning (DL) methods, have the potential to bridge such varied and large-scale datasets in a unifying framework, and with this, contribute a deeper and holistic understanding of the pathophysiology of brain disorders toward more effective treatments.

In this chapter, we focus on AI as the core of a holistic approach to brain regeneration, wherein we foresee that it will become an integral part of regenerative medicine to overcome its inherent biological bottlenecks. Specifically, we describe the role of AI within the novel paradigm of enhanced regenerative medicine, where it is used to aid the process of graft–host integration toward controlled, effective, and safe brain regeneration via exogenous cells/tissue grafts.

13.2 The *Enhanced* Regenerative Medicine Paradigm

It has been long known that interfering with brain bioelectricity can modulate its structure and function: electrical pulses can induce neural plasticity (e.g. long-term potentiation) and modulate brain function to rectify pathological electrical patterns (e.g. deep brain stimulation – DBS); further, neurons subjected to electric fields modify their shape and migrate along the electric field direction (galvanotaxis) (Rajnicek et al. 1992; Rajnicek et al. 2006; Rajnicek et al. 2006; Yao et al. 2008). While for decades neuroscientists have been using electrical pulses and electric fields exclusively to address brain plasticity, function modulation, and neuron migration and reshaping, their use in the neurosciences is no longer limited to these purposes: their ability to promote stem cell differentiation into functional neurons has indeed recently emerged as a novel surprising role for these tools (Tomaskovic-Crook et al. 2019; Chang et al. 2011; Kobelt et al. 2014; Zhang et al. 2018).

Along these lines, electrical stimulation can be deployed to guide the graft–host interaction and integration, thus controlling the brain regeneration process effectively and safely. In this view, an artificial counterpart (neuroprosthesis) can be coupled to the bioengineered brain tissue graft to serve three main purposes: (i) guiding the graft structural organization by controlling stem cell differentiation, neuronal plasticity, and galvanotaxis; (ii) modulating the graft function; (iii) preventing the graft from being entrained by pathological activity generated by the host brain while it is still being regenerated. However, our current knowledge gap in brain function and dysfunction imposes human preprogramming of the neuroprosthesis via a significant trial-and-error effort to devise the appropriate stimulation policy; this is particularly relevant for guided brain regeneration, given the constantly evolving dynamics of brain activity during the graft integration. Instead, it would be desirable to couple the brain tissue graft with an adaptive artificial counterpart, capable of understanding the evolving graft–host dynamics and adapting to it without requiring human intervention for its fine-tuning.

In this scenario, neuromorphic engineering presents the key to endow neuroprostheses with flexibility and adaptability. In fact, neuromorphic systems take inspiration from the working mode of the brain for brain-inspired computation; they can learn and adapt from experience, and are tolerant to errors. By virtue of these inherent features, they hold great promise to overcome the limitations of current implantable neuromodulators that are preprogrammed by humans (Vassanelli and mahmud 2016) and are emerging as the latest frontier in intelligent neuroprostheses to restore brain function (Buccelli et al. 2019; Serb et al. 2020). However, in the diseased brain, pathological activity might prevail and represent the strongest stimulus for the neuromorphic neuroprosthesis, which, in turn, might learn to reinforce rather than control pathological brain discharges. To counteract this potential drawback, AI can act as *super partes* teacher and coordinator supervising the biohybrid interplay by overseeing and training the behavior of the neuromorphic neuroprosthesis coupled to the graft.

The symbiotic coexistence of the biological brain tissue graft with a neuromorphic artificial counterpart coordinated by AI makes up biohybrid neuronics (neural electronics) and is the core of the enhanced regenerative medicine paradigm. The foundation of this paradigm stems from five core concepts defining the building blocks for brain repair, that should be simultaneously addressed but have so far been overlooked by other attempts to heal brain damage (Figure 13.1):

Rebuild – graft nervous tissue may rebuild/repair the damaged/dysfunctional brain circuits.

Function – the graft nervous tissue should exhibit the required functional features.

Interaction – graft and host nervous tissues should establish a functional dialogue.

Integration – the graft–host interaction should be precisely controlled.

Adaptation – the graft nervous tissue should adapt to the host without evolving toward nor being entrained by pathological behavior (functional stability).

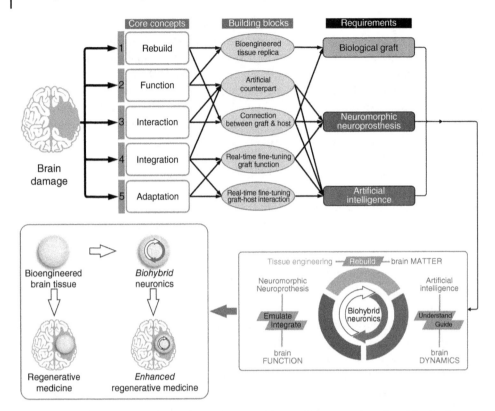

Figure 13.1 Core concept of the enhanced regenerative medicine paradigm. Repairing brain damage is a multifaceted problem: core concepts define intermingled building blocks underpinning the requirement for the convergence of biological and artificial components to biohybrid neuronics.

Ultimately, as opposed to current thinking in the biomedical field, it is expected that the correct functional integration of the graft into the host brain will eventually allow deactivation of the artificial components; thus, the patient will no longer depend on their operation for a lifetime (healing versus treating).

In the sections 13.3, 13.4 and 13.5, we will illustrate how the combined use of software and hardware AI can be brought forward to understand and guide graft–host interaction and integration aiming at repairing brain damage, bringing the case of epilepsy; lastly, in section 13.7 we analyze the use of AI under a philosophical perspective, considering relevant issues in ethics, patient and societal acceptance.

13.3 The Case of Epilepsy

Epilepsy is a chronic life-threatening neurological disorder characterized by the brain's enduring predisposition to generate recurrent and spontaneous seizures, i.e. abrupt and uncontrolled synchronous electrical discharges causing the loss of control of body function. Epilepsy is not a single nosological entity: several syndromes fall under the umbrella of this term. Classification of the epilepsies has important implications for the therapeutic

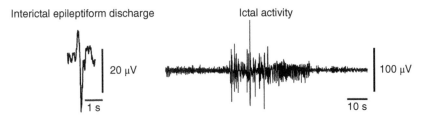

Figure 13.2 Electrographic features of epilepsy. EEG recording of a representative interictal spike and an ictal discharge from the hippocampus of a drug-refractory epileptic patient. Not the short duration of the interictal spike compared to the ictal event.

approach and management; however, it is a very complex task due to the polyhedral nature of the disorder. Epileptologists refer to the classification provided by the International League Against Epilepsy (ILAE) (Scheffer et al. 2017). The classification is periodically revised based on several criteria, such as the underlying etiopathogenesis, the involved brain regions, and their clinical manifestations.

The diagnosis of epilepsy relies on the combination of signs and symptoms, EEG recording, and brain imaging techniques. At the EEG level, a first distinction must be made between the abnormal electrographic patterns observed during the seizure and between seizures (Figure 13.2). The former is referred to as "ictal" activity (from the Latin term *ictus*), whereas the latter is referred to as "interictal." Thus, the seizure is the clinical manifestation of ictal activity seen at the EEG as a prolonged high-frequency synchronized discharge. Interictal epileptiform discharges are the typical sign of epileptic hyperexcitability and they appear in the form of short EEG transients.

Epilepsy affects 1% (~65 million people) of the global population (WHO 2006), it is often accompanied by cognitive impairment and psychiatric comorbidities, and by a significant social stigma (Fiest et al. 2014). Epilepsy is a dynamic disease, i.e. it causes abrupt transitions in brain activity (Lopes da Silva et al. 2003), and it is progressive in nature. These features make epilepsy treatment and management highly challenging. In fact, despite the advancements in antiepileptic drug development, ~30% of the patients are or become resistant to pharmacological therapy (Laxer et al. 2014), requiring surgical resection of the affected brain area. However, neurosurgery must be carefully evaluated on a case-by-case basis, also considering that it is not devoid of risks in terms of short-term postoperative morbidity, mortality, complications, and readmissions (Kerezoudis et al. 2018). The latter is also related to the emergence of secondary foci upon resection of the identified primary one. Furthermore, not all patients may be candidates for surgical intervention: while multifocal epilepsy or epileptic foci affecting eloquent areas cannot be addressed surgically, identifying the epileptic focus can be a challenge in itself. As a result, neurosurgery may still not guarantee a seizure-free life: patients truly benefitting of such an invasive solution are a fair but yet unacceptable ~50% (Berg 2004).

These issues are particularly emphasized in patients suffering from mesial temporal lobe epilepsy (MTLE), which is without any doubt the most common and most studied epileptic syndrome. In fact, MTLE represents ~40% of the epilepsies, and is the most often refractory to antiepileptic medications. MTLE affects mesial temporal lobe structures that are also part of the wider limbic system governing cognition and emotion. As a result, MTLE cannot be solely defined as a neurological disorder: it is a complex neuropsychiatric syndrome affecting the person body and mind as a whole. A hallmark of MTLE is the sclerosis of the hippocampus, an anatomopathological feature found in ~70% of drug-refractory MTLE patients (Prayson 2018). Hippocampal sclerosis may be unilateral or bilateral; in the latter case, surgical ablation is not possible, as it will leave permanent sequelae in terms severe cognitive impairment, as we have learned from the emblematic story of the H.M. patient (Squire 2009). In such cases, and in surgical epilepsy patients overall, regenerative medicine presents the key to rebuild the removed portion of the brain. However, as stated above, the regeneration process must be carefully controlled. This is particularly crucial when the hippocampus is to be rebuilt, given the plethora of complex functions it serves. Furthermore, the graft would be introduced in a pathological environment, here the epileptic brain, in which hyperexcitability and continuous aberrant reorganization of connectivity will likely invade the transplanted neurons/stem cells and promote their dysfunctional adaptation. Instead, achievement of the desired graft–host interaction requires that the graft nervous tissue exhibits specific structure/function relationship and that its connection to the host brain recapitulates native neuronal pathways.

In the *enhanced* regenerative medicine paradigm, an artificial neuromorphic counterpart is deployed to complement the pitfalls of a purely regenerative approach by providing adaptive control of the graft–host interaction through electrical stimulation. Adaptive control systems operate in response to the continuing feedback from the environment being controlled (here, the brain or the graft); they process and respond to several inputs, but their output response is not predetermined; rather, they are capable of real-time self-adjustment based on their past experience, a set of learning rules, performance evaluation or reward functions (Panuccio et al. 2018). By virtue of their learning capability, neuromorphic systems are inherently endowed with self-adaptive and self-evolving behavior; however, neuromorphic devices are not inherently capable of distinguishing between physiological and pathological activity; hence, if driven directly by pathological learning rules, they will likely learn to reinforce epileptic dynamics rather than preventing them, ultimately contributing to dysfunctional brain rewiring. Furthermore, epilepsy is a dynamic disease, i.e. brain states change over time with recurring yet unpredictable interictal-to-ictal transitions while the disease progression leads to ever-evolving changes in brain structure and function. Thus, neuromorphic devices for biomedical applications must be appropriately trained.

In this scenario, AI is crucial to supervise the biohybrid interplay at different levels of interaction: (i) the graft and its artificial neuromorphic counterpart, (ii) the graft and the host, (iii) and the behavior of the neuromorphic neuroprosthesis in response to brain patterns. This complex biohybrid interplay is illustrated in Figure 13.3: a biological brain tissue graft is coupled to a neuromorphic neuroprosthesis acting as artificial counterpart. This yields a biohybrid neural tissue conveying brain matter rebuild with function control. In the perspective of a fully integrated biohybrid neural tissue, the neuromorphic device can only read from its biological counterpart and cannot see the behavior of the host brain embedding the biohybrid neural tissue. Thus, an AI agent must first coordinate the interplay of the graft and its neuromorphic counterpart, and oversee the outcome of the biohybrid interaction in terms of effects on the host brain. This is attained by reading the biological signals of the graft, the actions (stimuli) taken by the neuromorphic device, and the electrical activity of the host brain. By overseeing the behavior of all the involved

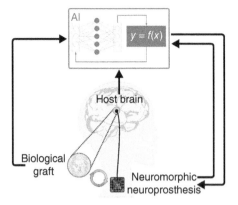

Figure 13.3 Biohybrid interplay and the role of AI as teacher and coordinator in the enhanced regenerative medicine paradigm. A biological graft is coupled to a neuromorphic neuroprosthesis acting as artificial counterpart, yielding a biohybrid neural tissue that conveys brain matter rebuild with function control. From the perspective of a fully integrated biohybrid neural tissue, the neuromorphic device can only read from its biological graft counterpart and cannot see the behavior of the host brain. Thus, an AI agent must first coordinate the interplay of the graft and its neuromorphic counterpart, and oversee the outcome of the biohybrid interaction in terms of effects on the host brain.

parties, the AI agent acts as *super partes* teacher and coordinator of the enhanced brain regeneration process, wherein it trains the neuromorphic device to adjust its parameters according to the ongoing (evolving) dynamics of the graft–host interaction.

To this end, the AI agent should be capable of recognizing an occurring seizure and the abnormal brain states heralding it; this would enable to rectify in real-time the suboptimal behavior of the neuromorphic counterpart while it is still learning until achievement of its appropriate training. Such a role for the AI agent implies three crucial features: (i) understanding brain dynamics from a network perspective, since epilepsy is a network phenomenon; (ii) the design of seizure detection and seizure prediction algorithms of high accuracy and sensitivity; and (iii) a reverse-engineering approach to DBS aimed at reverting pathological brain states based on mapped state-dependent evoked responses.

In section 13.4 we describe recently emerged AI methods for seizure type classification and the identification of the seizure onset zone (SOZ) for surgical purposes, as a relevant aspect of brain regeneration in epilepsy; we then focus on widely applied AI-based solutions for seizure detection and prediction, as well as AI-driven DBS approaches as an integral part of the operating mode of biohybrid neuronics. We offer some perspective on how the performance can be improved for each of these applications.

13.4 AI to Understand Epilepsy

As a starting point, we provide a brief overview of the bases of AI to guide the reader through its diverse applications described subsequently. For a more in-depth description, we remind the reader to (Handbook of Artificial Intelligence in Biomedical Engineering 2021) and (Artificial Intelligence in Bioinformatics 2022).

AI refers to systems or programs that can perform tasks that typically require human intelligence. Examples of such tasks include recognizing images, making decisions, and playing games. Machine learning (ML) algorithms are commonly used for implementing AI; ML involves the development and application of statistical methods that can learn from data and improve over time without being explicitly programmed (Nasser 2007; Gareth James et al. 2013). The different categories of learning tasks within ML can be summarized as follows:

- **Supervised learning** – This is based on providing an ML algorithm with many examples of input data and corresponding labels, with the goal of building a predictive model that can output the desired label when presented with new input data. This type of learning has been widely used in the context of epilepsy.
- **Unsupervised learning** – This deals with unlabeled data and aims to discover the structure hidden within the data to extract meaningful information. Clustering and dimensionality reduction, such as Principal Component Analysis, are examples of unsupervised learning techniques.
- **Reinforcement learning (RL)** – This method involves developing a system that can improve its performance based on its interaction with the environment, where feedback is provided in the form of a reward signal. The agent tries to learn a series of actions that maximize this reward via a trial-and -error approach or deliberate planning Examples of RL include gaming programs and recommendation systems.
- **Semi-supervised learning** – This approach is a mixed case that involves a small amount of labeled data inserted between a large amount of unlabeled data. Semi-supervised learning is quickly growing in the biomedical AI field because it tackles the problem of the lack of labeled data and the tedious process of labeling large datasets.

DL is a subfield of ML relying on algorithms loosely inspired by the function and structure of the biological brain to perform the learning tasks.

One key difference between traditional ML algorithms, such as linear regression or support vector machines (SVMs), and DL algorithms is that the latter can automatically extract features from the input data, whereas traditional ML algorithms require the features to be defined by the user. The relation between AI, ML, and DL is shown in Figure 13.4. Below, we provide the most salient features of DL; for a comprehensive introduction to the topic, the reader is referred to (Goodfellow et al. 2016; Nielsen 2015).

DL algorithms have a multi network architecture, i.e. they have several layers of artificial neural networks (ANNs) stacked between the input and output. This feature is what the term "deep" in DL refers to. In particular, the layers between the input and the output are termed "hidden layers" and they are used to extract higher-level features from input data and perform learning tasks. Each layer is composed of nodes (or artificial neurons); further, the connections between these layers carry defined weights. Figure 13.5 illustrates a DL network consisting of three hidden layers. Such a network is known as a fully connected, feedforward network as every node/neuron in a layer is connected to every other neuron in the next layer.

Each neuron in a layer computes the weighted sum of inputs received from neurons of the previous layer and applies what is known as the activation function. This is essentially a nonlinear transformation that determines whether the neuron should be activated or not.

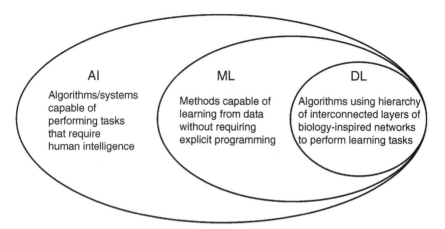

Figure 13.4 The relation between AI, ML, and DL.

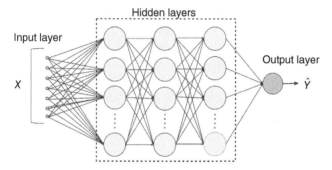

Figure 13.5 Fully connected feedforward DL network. The network includes three hidden layers, and every node/neuron in a layer is connected to every other neuron in the next layer.

Each neuron is also associated with a bias term, i.e. a threshold that needs to be exceeded by the nonlinear transformation output for the neuron to be activated. The commonly used activation functions are the sigmoid function and the rectified linear unit function. For a comprehensive introduction to the topic of DL, the reader is referred to (Goodfellow et al. 2016; Nielsen 2015).

Given several input data and the corresponding labels (desired output), the neural network is trained by adjusting the weights and biases of the network such that the actual output of the neural network obtained by feeding the input data matches as closely as possible to the desired output. This is also known as minimizing the error loss function. The backpropagation algorithm (and its variants) is commonly used for training such feedforward neural networks.

A particular mention must be made of transfer learning, first introduced by Stevo Bozinovski in the 1970's (Bozinovski 2020). This is an ML approach that uses knowledge gained while solving one task to another related task. In other words, knowledge derived from a learning problem is used ("transferred") to enhance learning on a related problem, like knowledge gained while learning to recognize cats can be applied to improve recognition of dogs.

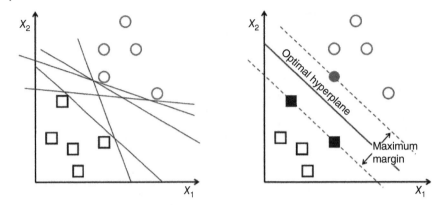

Figure 13.6 Optimal hyperplane according to SVM generalization. Source: Inspired by https://docs .opencv.org/2.4/doc/tutorials/ml/introduction_to_svm/introduction_to_svm.html.

13.4.1 Commonly Applied Learning Algorithms for Basic Neuroscience and Clinical Application in Epilepsy

The most commonly applied learning algorithms include traditional ML approaches, such as SVMs, and DL approaches, such as convolutional neural networks (CNNs) and recurrent neural networks (RNNs).

ML approaches: the SVM. Given a classification task, the SVM aims to find an optimal hyperplane (Figure 13.6), which acts as a decision boundary to distinguish between different classes. Such an optimal hyperplane has the farthest minimum distance to the training data. The SVM is a generalization of the maximal margin classifier. However, while the maximal margin classifier can only be applied to classes that can be separated by a linear boundary, the SVM can also accommodate nonlinear class boundaries by making use of various kernels (e.g. Gaussian radial basis function kernel, quadratic kernel). This makes SVM the popular choice for problems such as seizure type classification, seizure detection, and prediction, where the data may not be linearly-separable.

DL approaches: CNNs and RNNs. CNNs are one of the most popular DL architectures. Inspired by the layered architecture of neurons in the visual cortex of the mammals, CNNs are constructed using several layers of artificial neurons and can capture the rich spatial information in the data. Due to their deformation stability and translation invariance, CNNs are widely used for processing image and video data (LeCun et al. 2015; Mallat 2016). Most CNNs consist of a convolutional layer and a pooling layer. The convolutional layers consists of a large number of convolutional filters, which are convolved with the input image to produce feature maps to detect edges, shapes, textures, etc.; the pooling layer is responsible for reducing the size of the feature maps produced by convolutional layer via max pooling or average pooling. An example of CNN is illustrated in Figure 13.7.

Just as CNNs are suited to process image data, RNNs are the perfect fit for the processing of time series or other kinds of sequential data. RNNs are an extension of the fully connected neural networks, and present loops allowing hidden layers at one time instant to be used as input for the hidden layer at the next time instant (Figure 13.8a). Compared to fully-connected neural networks, which have separate parameters for each input feature,

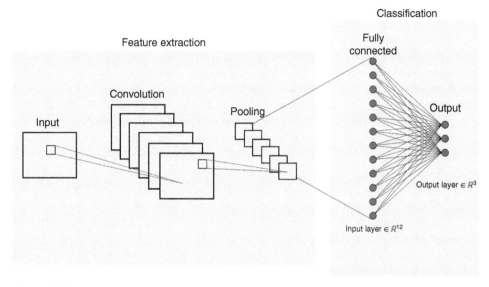

Figure 13.7 A simple CNN containing the convolution, pooling, and fully connected layers.

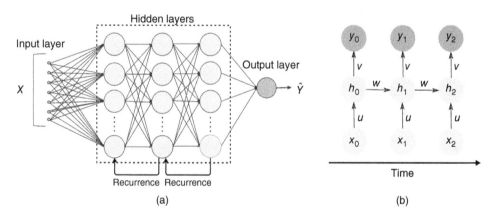

Figure 13.8 **Recurrent Neural Network (RNN).** (a) Schematic of a RNN with loops between hidden layers. (b) An unrolled RNN illustrating the concept of the same parameters (i.e. weights w, u, and v) shared across the time steps.

an RNN shares the same parameters (i.e. weights) across several time steps. It is this property that allows RNNs to generalize to sequence lengths not seen during training, and share statistical strength across different sequence lengths and across different positions in time (Figure 13.8b).

LSTM networks proposed by (Hochreiter and Schmidhuber 1997) are a special kind of RNN, capable of learning long-term dependencies. LSTMs are specifically designed to handle long-term dependency problems, i.e. situations where the output not only depends on the information from the recent past but also on the information from long periods of past time.

13.4.2   Seizure and Epilepsy Type Classification

Accurate classification of seizure and epilepsy type is fundamental for the successful treatment of epilepsy and for improving long-term patient care, including the choice of the most appropriate pharmacological therapy and its timely adjustments, and optimal patient selection for clinical trials (Harrer et al. 2019). Currently, clinicians classify the seizure and epilepsy types based on the clinical features and visual inspection of the EEG; however, this process is time-consuming, subjective, and prone to human error. Nonetheless, very little work has focused on the use of AI for the purpose of seizure and epilepsy-type classification compared to the problem of seizure detection and prediction (An et al. 2020). This is largely due to the unavailability of labeled EEG datasets and the complex nature of the task. Most of the studies focusing on seizure type classification have used the Temple University Hospital (TUH) EEG Seizure Corpus dataset (referred to as the TUH dataset hereafter) (Shah et al. 2018), which is the largest publicly available dataset (obtained from 239 patients so far), and includes annotations by experts.

Using CNNs, Asif et al. have proposed the SeizureNet framework to classify seizure types (Asif et al. 2020) in the TUH dataset using saliency-encoded spectrograms as input features. With this approach, they achieved a performance accuracy (weighted F1-score) of 98.4%. Other approaches have included transfer learning in combination with an SVM classifier (Raghu et al. 2020), SVMs (Dwi Saputro et al. 2019), bilinear model combining CNNs and RNNs (Liu et al. 2020), with the majority of them using the TUH dataset and showing acceptable performance accuracy (weighted F1-score) in the range of 88–97%.

13.4.3   Seizure Onset Zone Localization

Localization of the seizure onset zone (SOZ) is crucial to understand which brain area(s) should undergo surgical removal (and regeneration) and the feasibility of the neurosurgery. At present, surgical ablation of the SOZ is not practically feasible if this affects eloquent areas or in the case of multifocal epilepsy; however, the future perspective of remove-and-rebuild offered by regenerative medicine opens new possibilities for those epileptic patients who cannot benefit from any of the currently available treatments (medication, DBS, and ablative neurosurgery). In addition, understanding the spatial features of seizure onset and propagation is fundamental to establish which area(s) of the brain should be constantly monitored by the AI agent during the regeneration process. This is particularly relevant in the case of multifocal epilepsy, where the SOZs may not be removed all simultaneously, or to ensure that secondary SOZs unmasked by the removal of the primary one are timely identified and controlled to avoid damage to the grafted cells/tissue by their entrainment from a propagating seizure. Nonetheless, identification of the SOZ and the seizure propagation pattern is challenged by the limited spatial resolution of EEG recording, which may not unveil the whole brain dynamics with the required accuracy and sensitivity. In this respect, AI would greatly benefit the presurgical evaluation, but only a few studies have so far used AI to identify the SOZ and the seizure propagation pattern.

SVMs using phase locking value, which measures the phase synchronization between EEG signals (Lachaux et al. 1999), have been successfully employed to identify the SOZ.

The approach could correctly label 96% of the electrodes within the SOZ in 6 out of 10 patients, who became seizure-free post-neurosurgery (Elahian et al. 2017). An SVM classifier has also been used to extract various entropy measures such as approximate entropy, permutation entropy, and spectral entropy from EEG signals decomposed into multiple frequency bands pertaining to high-frequency oscillations (HFOs) via an array of band-pass filters (Akter et al. 2020). As HFOs are also observed during the interictal period, they provide more samples for training a classifier compared to the ictal segments.

13.4.4 Seizure Detection

Seizure detection refers to identification of the ictal period in EEG recording and can be classified in offline and online detection. Online seizure detection refers to real-time identification of seizures, whereas offline seizure detection refers to the task of identifying seizures in EEG data that has already been acquired over a period. In both cases, AI methods require EEG signals to be categorized according to the time-course of state transition to seizure (ictogenesis) in order to pinpoint state-specific features.

While offline seizure detection is extremely helpful to substitute the laborious task of EEG visual inspection for manual seizure labeling, online seizure detection is of greater interest from the viewpoint of brain regeneration in epilepsy. Online seizure detection can in fact be used as a trigger to initiate DBS to suppress the seizure or to prevent the invasion of seizure from the host into the implanted graft. Nonetheless, the vast majority of AI-based solutions for seizure detection have been proposed for offline use (Supratak et al. 2014; Acharya et al. 2015; Faust et al. 2015; Samiee et al. 2015; Lin et al. n.d.; Thodoroff et al. 2016; Johansen et al. 2016; Yuan et al. 2019). For online seizure detection, SVMs have been a popular choice due to their simple implementation and high accuracy (Seng et al. 2012; Zhang et al. 2016; Yoo et al. 2013; MAB et al. 2016; Wang et al. 2018). Nonlinear SVMs using radial basis function kernel have been commonly used to solve the binary classification task in online seizure detection (distinguishing between inter-ictal and ictal), with latency ranging from two to five seconds, sensitivity ranging from 83% to 100% and specificity ranging from 87% to 99%, with false alarms ranging from 0.3–1 per day. Nonetheless, a two to five seconds latency is still sub-optimal. In fact, at the time of seizure detection, it could already be too late to effectively suppress the seizure or prevent its invasion into the graft. In this sense, seizure prediction is more advantageous as it offers the possibility of intervention even before the seizure has started; as anticipated above, in the case of brain regeneration, this would offer the crucial feature of preventing the graft entrainment by seizure activity and so safeguarding it from becoming epileptic itself.

13.4.5 Seizure Prediction

The interictal period contains highly informative features for seizure prediction. In fact, as stated in Section 13.3, interictal epileptiform discharges are the hallmark of epileptic hyperexcitability; thus, their features, such as rate of occurrence, amplitude, duration, and frequency components, reflect the state of epileptic brain networks as seen from a dynamical systems perspective. As anticipated in Section 13.3, the epileptic brain can indeed be regarded as a dynamical system (Lopes da Silva et al. 2003), i.e. a system that changes its

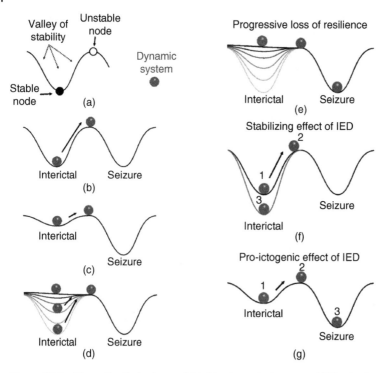

Figure 13.9 The epileptic brain as a bistable dynamical system. (a) The brain can be conceptualized as a dynamic system that can exist in the interictal or seizure state. Each state can be described by the valley of stability with its stable node at the bottom of the valley to which the system is attracted. Both states are separated by the unstable node (tipping point) where bifurcation occurs. (b) Seizure emerging from stable brain dynamics requires significant perturbation to shift to seizure. (c) Generalized epilepsies are characterized by low stability and low resilience to perturbation when even weak stochastic disruptions can easily initiate seizure. (d) The transition to seizure via critical slowing occurs when the system progressively loses stability and resilience. It manifests by increasing sensitivity to perturbation and delayed recovery from the perturbation with approaching seizure. (e) Changes in slow parameters result in progressive loss of resilience, which will end up in a spontaneous transition to seizure. (f) The IED perturbs the interictal dynamics and displaces the system (brain). During the stable state, even large perturbation is insufficient to shift the dynamic regime to seizure and the system rapidly recovers back. The perturbation may paradoxically stabilize the system. Such IED has an anti-ictogenic effect. (g) Similar IED perturbation that occurs during the low-resilience state can have pro-ictogenic effect and trigger seizure prematurely. Source: Adapted from Chvojka et al. (2021).

state over time, as opposed to static systems which constantly remain in a single state. Specifically, the epileptic brain can be regarded as a bistable dynamical system (Chvojka et al. 2021; de Curtis and Avanzini 2001; Lévesque et al. 2018; Chang et al. 2018), i.e. a dynamical system that transitions between two states, namely the interictal and ictal states (Figure 13.9a–d).

These transitions can be viewed as bifurcations, which, in complex systems dynamics occur when small perturbations in a system cause an abrupt dramatic shift in its behavior. From this dynamical standpoint, interictal epileptiform discharges can be thus regarded as a perturbation of brain dynamics, the outcome of which will depend on the dynamical state of the epileptic brain when the perturbation occurs. For this reason, interictal epileptiform discharges may promote the transition to seizure (pro-ictogenic effect) or reinforce brain network resilience to it (anti-ictogenic effect) – Figure 13.9e–g. Specifically, interictal epileptiform discharges may promote seizures when the epileptic brain is in a state of poor resilience to perturbations (Chang et al. 2018). At variance, when the brain is in a highly stable state, the interictal perturbation is not able to push the system closer to the bifurcation toward the seizure; in this case, the brain quickly recovers from the interictal discharge, and the refractory period that follows it may even shift the brain dynamics to a higher stability (and hence, toward a higher resilience to seizures) (Dorn and Witte 1995; de Curtis et al. 2001).

The interictal period can be further distinguished into pre-ictal (right before the seizure), post-ictal (after the seizure), and stable interictal (after the post-ictal and before the pre-ictal state). Based on the above definition of bistable dynamical system and the pro- or anti-ictogenic role of interictal epileptiform discharges, this subdivision does not solely reflect the time relative to a seizure: each period is characterized by specific signal features that can be used to pinpoint state transitions and thus predict an impending seizure.

Several studies have used traditional ML algorithms such as SVMs as well as more recently developed DL algorithms for seizure prediction, with most studies validating their algorithms on open source databases such as the Freiburg Hospital dataset (http://epilepsy.uni-freiburg.de), the CHB-MIT dataset from physionet (https://openreview.net/forum?id=S1WjLoZu-r), and the American Epilepsy Society Seizure Prediction Challenge (Kaggle) dataset (https://www.kaggle.com/competitions/seizure-prediction/data). SVM for seizure prediction has achieved sensitivity varying between 75% and100% depending on the features used, with an average false positive rate ranging from 0.0324–0.09 per hour, when tested on open-source databases (Li et al. 2013; Zheng et al. 2014; Zhang et al. 2016). Given the low computational complexity of most of SVM-based methods, the possibility of implementing them in an implantable device is exciting.

As explained in at the inception of Section 13.4, DL methods have the ability to automatically extract relevant features, and approaches such as CNNs, RNNs, and auto-encoders have also been used for seizure prediction (Truong et al. 2018; Daoud and Bayoumi 2019; Shahbazi and Aghajan 2018), with sensitivity reported in the range of 75–99.7% and false positive rates ranging from 0.06–0.21 per hour. Since CNNs were originally developed to handle image data, EEG signals are represented as images before being processed by CNNs. The most common approach has been to transform the EEG data into spectrograms (e.g. using Fourier transforms). The workflow in using CNNs for seizure prediction is similar to what is used for seizure detection: (i) obtain labeled EEG data, (ii) design a CNN architecture, (iii) transform EEG data to image, (iv) train the CNN model, and (v) measure the performance accuracy. Figure 13.10 shows an example of CNN architecture proposed in (Truong et al. 2018) to predict ictal activity from spectrograms obtained from raw EEG signals.

Another example where CNN and RNN were combined to perform seizure prediction can be found in (Shahbazi and Aghajan 2018) and is illustrated in Figure 13.11. Here, the image input to CNN (DCNN) is an EEG data matrix (number of channels X time points). The output of the CNN is fed to bidirectional LSTM to extract the temporal features. LSTM networks are used for their known property to maintain long-time sequence dependencies

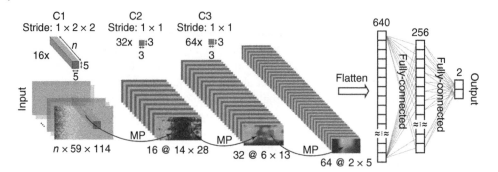

Figure 13.10 CNN architecture for seizure prediction. The input consists of short-time Fourier transform of 30-s windows of labeled raw EEG data. C1–C3 are convolutional blocks and MP refers to the max-pooling layers. The convolutional layers used a ReLU activation function and the features extracted by convolutional layers are flattened and connected to fully connected networks (using the sigmoid activation function and soft-max activation) for classification. Source: From (Truong et al. 2018) with permission. © 2018 Elsevier Ltd. All rights reserved.

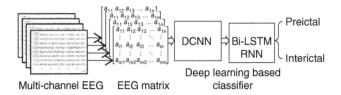

Figure 13.11 Seizure predictor combining CNN and bidirectional LSTM. The multichannel EEG signals are transformed into a data matrix (number of channels X time points). The output of the CNN is then fed to bidirectional LSTM, which uses information from both previous and next time instances to extract the temporal features and classify the signal in pre-ictal and interictal.

(as explained in Section 13.4), which helps in early seizure prediction. In the particular case proposed by (Shahbazi and Aghajan 2018), the bidirectional-LSTM uses information from both previous and next-time instances and hence is well suited to handle prediction problems.

13.4.6 Signal Feature Extraction for Seizure Detection and Prediction

The achievement of highly accurate and sensitive algorithms for seizure detection and prediction is inherently challenged by signal feature extraction, which is at the core of any such algorithms. Apart from the obvious signal preprocessing required to use a signal in computational neuroscience (filtering of spurious frequency components and removal of signal artifacts), almost any AI algorithm works with the raw signals as an input. The complex reality of time series analysis (as brain signals are) requires the extraction of some definitory characteristics as features of the signal, that can vary based on the goal of the algorithm that is being proposed. Among the plethora of classification criteria for the features that can be extracted from a signal, here, we focus specifically on statistical, morphological, nonlinear, spectral, and time-frequency features, which go beyond a mere use for signal analysis.

Statistical features track changes in the distribution of the brain signals (Tribbey 2007), the benefit of being very light in computational terms so they can be employed when fast computing is a requirement. They carry the drawback of not being able to capture the hidden information in the highly chaotic brain signals. Among the statistical features that can highlight some as mean, variance, skewness, kurtosis, phase correlation, and common spatial pattern (Grassberger and Procaccia 1983). All of those have been used with success to predict seizures and to analyze brain signals, either alone or in conjunction with other types of features (Goel et al. 2023).

Morphological features refer to the changes on the shape of the signal. They can be extremely powerful for some applications as peak detection and do not require any great computational effort. Some morphological features are the peak height, the zero-crossing rate, or the total area of the signal. They are more widely used for cardiac function studies but also have been deemed helpful in microelectrode array (MEA) and single cell electrophysiology analysis and EEG (Shanir et al. 2018).

Nonlinear features are the most widely used features in brain signal analysis. They reflect the chaos and complexity level of the signals (Rijlaarsdam et al. 2017). The robustness of nonlinear features relies on their ability to track changes in the hidden system dynamics, being able to detect even subtle changes that remain completely concealed for other feature extraction methods until the event that triggered the change appears in the raw signal. This enormous potential comes with a cost, nonlinear features require lots of computational power. If we dive in the plethora of nonlinear features that we can use to understand the mechanism of the brain we will find measurements of the similarity inside a signal (fractality dimension and Lempel-Ziv complexity) (Aarabi and He 2012), other features measure the complexity (correlation dimension) (Grassberger and Procaccia 1983) or the randomness inside the signal (spectral entropy and wavelet entropy) (Guo et al. 2009).

Spectral features, also called frequency domain features, drop the time parameters of the signal to rely on the frequency components. Those components usually are the phase and magnitude of the signal and can be extracted with Fourier transforms in their different modalities (Fractional Fourier transform, fast Fourier transform) (Ozaktas et al. 1996). Over these extracted features some additional calculations can be made to obtain the spectral density of the signal (Dressler et al. 2004).

Losing the time domain is sometimes an unacceptable condition due to the necessities of the research, in those cases using spectral features is relegated and time-frequency domain features are preferred. These features allow us to study and analyze the change in frequency components along the time scale of the signal, giving deeper information into signals whose characteristics vary with time. Wavelet transforms (Chui 1992) are usually one of the most widely used time-frequency components used in computational neuroscience, both in its continuous and discrete versions. Additionally, higher-order spectra can be used as a companion to nonlinear features to boost their capacities to extract hidden components from brain signals. In the same manner, variational mode decomposition offers a strong partnership with nonlinear features (Acharya et al. 2013). The decomposition process can be achieved also with bivariate empirical mode decomposition (BEMD) (Rilling et al. 2007) as a previous step before obtaining any other feature, upgrading the accuracy of the feature extraction.

13.4.7 Network Interactions and Evolving Dynamics in the Epileptic Brain: The Eye of AI

Epilepsy is a network phenomenon: complex interactions among local and global network dynamics underly the initiation, propagation, maintenance, and termination of seizures (Avoli et al. 2002; Panuccio et al. 2010). Thus, while cellular electrophysiology (e.g. patch-clamp) can pinpoint alterations in the biophysical properties of specific neuronal subpopulations, large-scale network recordings (e.g. stereo-EEG and microelectrode array) can provide the big picture of the global pathological dynamics in the epileptic brain. This approach entails high-dimensional paradigms, something that began to come to the fore in 2017 with the proposal of a multiclass SVM for seizure prediction in humans (Direito et al. 2017). Instead of using signal data from a single electrode, the aim is to combine information from different areas of the brain to obtain a network of points in which different features can be studied. Two main approaches can be distinguished here: (i) the study of the networks by creating mathematical models of them and (ii) the analysis of the common characteristics of the signals.

The modeling approach draws on connectivity studies in humans and animal models to get a faithful representation of the brain connectome, either at the global level or, more commonly, at the local level of the circuitry of interest, e.g. the SOZ. With the information provided by the *in vivo* studies (and by the knowledge base of neuroanatomy itself), a series of nodes (equivalent to electrodes or neuronal populations) and a series of connections between these nodes (assimilated to synapses or tracts) are established. Usually from this point onward, the network is analyzed using graph theory. A graph is a mathematical structure that represents a group of objects and the pairwise relations between them. Examples of graphs representing different types of network topologies are illustrated in Figure 13.12.

The graph-theoretic characterization of these networks is based on the assumption that the strength of a vertex connecting two nodes can be inferred from electrophysiological studies. If all possible connections between nodes are mapped, a connectivity matrix is obtained, which is the main tool on which properties such as the eigenvalue, eigenvector, and characteristic polynomial can be calculated, allowing the network to be analyzed in a simple way. In this way, it is possible to know if the network (the graph) is directed or undirected, what its modularity is, the centrality of a node, or the average path.

Graph theory helps studying how brain networks interact, thus entering in the field of connectivity. We can distinguish two different ways of analyzing interactions between brain regions: functional connectivity and effective connectivity (Feldt et al. 2011). Functional connectivity refers to the statistical dependencies between the activity of different brain regions, without necessarily implying any causal relationship between them. Functional connectivity is typically measured using fMRI or EEG/MEG signals, and it involves analyzing the temporal correlations or coherence between the signals recorded from different brain regions. Functional connectivity can reveal patterns of communication between brain regions that are active during a particular task or at rest and can be used to identify functional networks or modules in the brain.

Effective connectivity refers to the directed causal interactions between different brain regions, which can be inferred based on the observed changes in neural activity. Effective connectivity aims to identify the pathways of information flow within the brain and to

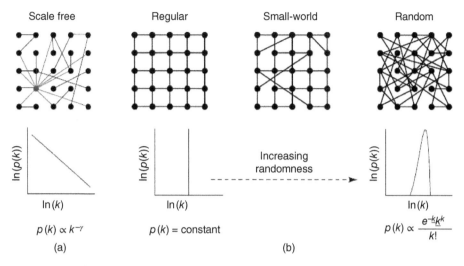

Figure 13.12 Graphs of different network topologies. Scale-free networks lack a characteristic scale, since the degree, k, of the nodes can span many orders of magnitude. Regular networks have an ordered arrangement and all their nodes have the same number of nearest neighbors. Random networks result from random processes, such that nodes can have different degrees, and the probability that a node has k connections is represented by a Poisson distribution Small-world networks share features with regular and random networks since they present a combination of dense local connections (like regular networks) and short characteristic path lengths (like random networks). Topologies commonly found in biological systems are scale-free and small-world. Source: From (Feldt et al. 2011), with permission. Copyright © 2011 Elsevier Ltd. All rights reserved.

determine the direction and strength of the causal relationships between different regions. Effective connectivity is typically estimated using dynamic causal modeling or structural equation modeling, which involves formulating a set of hypotheses about the underlying neural network and testing them against experimental data. However, the most widely used technique in effective connectivity analysis is, by far, Granger causality (Seth et al. 2015). To apply it, it is important to generate a model of the signal (instead of using the raw signal) in the form of a vector autoregressive vector. It is a robust and stable method that can be used on models generated from almost any functional neuroimaging or electrophysiology technique.

Once a hypothesis has been established about the connectivity between the different nodes of the network (thanks to Granger causality, for example), more targeted measurements can be carried out to test this hypothesis. One of the most widely used is dynamic causal modeling, which is based on Bayesian models to choose the network model that most faithfully represents reality. Although it is not intended for prospective studies, there is a current trend to carry out exploratory tests with different hypotheses.

When a similar analysis needs to be carried out but with a lower computational cost, it is advisable to use transfer entropy instead of Granger causality. It also has the advantage of being a model-independent measure, and, since it is nonlinear in nature, it can detect correlations or dependencies between signals that have varying time delays. However, it is a very general measure, so it is usually difficult to interpret the results when looking for a more functional approach.

Graphs as models on neural networks can also be used to measure and characterize parameters specific to the signal. The most commonly used are cross-correlation and coherence (either in the frequency or time domain). Both measurements require that a time delay be preset by the researcher in order to be calculated; traditionally, iterative studies were carried out with different delays resulting in large computational costs. Advances in the understanding of the epileptic brain signals now allow this time delay to be tuned without the need for trial-and-error, considerably reducing the computational time and cost of these measurements. Since the very physiological variations in the brain due to heart rate and breathing introduce a large amount of spurious correlation into these measurements, it is recommended that calculations be performed in the frequency domain rather than in the time domain.

Another method applicable to graphs is statistical parametric mapping, which works in more detail by analyzing local changes at each node of the network and making the necessary statistical inferences. Common clustering techniques (e.g. k-means, fuzzy c-means, and self-organizing maps) (Alashwal et al. 2019). can also be applied to these topological networks. Their high efficiency comes at the disadvantage of a high computational cost, which scales as the complexity of the network to be analyzed increases. For this reason, clustering techniques can be applied in the case of small networks, but are usually discarded in whole-brain connectivity studies.

Functional analysis of brain networks via graph theory provides a solid foundation for understanding the evolving dynamics of the epileptic brain. Along with informing the design of AI agents for SOZ identification, for seizure prediction, and DBS, it can be used to the advantage of brain regeneration for controlling the interaction between the grafted cells/tissue and the host brain, as explained in the section 13.5.

13.5 Artificial Intelligence to Guide Graft-Host Dynamics in Epilepsy

Guidance of graft–host dynamics is central in enhanced regenerative medicine. As explained in Section 13.2, the neuromorphic neuroprosthesis will serve as a read/write device monitoring the graft electrical activity and delivering electrical stimulation to it as required. This adaptive, state-dependent interplay (cf. Section 13.3) is necessary to meet the building blocks of enhanced brain regeneration, and, in particular, ensuring the graft structural and functional stability, as also addressed in Section 13.1. As the neuromorphic counterpart will read from the graft only, the latter will also serve as biological probe and modulator of the ongoing dynamics of the surrounding brain networks embedding it.

Graph theoretical analyses at mesoscopic scale (fMRI and EEG) have demonstrated *small-world networks* (clustering in functional modules) as key feature of the connectome (Bullmore and Sporns 2009), which, in MTLE, may contribute to aberrant synchronization (Ponten et al. 2007); further, large-scale modeling studies suggest that activation of only 1% of the neuronal population within small-world networks may trigger seizures (Morgan and Soltesz 2008); remarkably, evoked burst spiking in the single neuron can influence global brain dynamics (Li et al. 2009). Thus, deploying a biological graft both as reconstituting cellular component and biological neuromodulator holds an outstanding potential to advance to field of regenerative medicine for epilepsy and for brain disorders overall. However, an artificial counterpart inspired by current DBS devices would not achieve such challenging undertaking, and AI is thus a fundamental prerequisite. In fact, even the Food and Drug Administration (FDA)-approved NeuroPace device for responsive DBS (Sisterson et al. 2020; Morrell and Halpern 2016) implements a series of periodic stimulation frequencies and, even more importantly, it acts upon seizure detection, thus primarily aiming at halting rather than preventing seizures. As a result, establishment of the optimal parameters is still based on a trial-and-error approach, and the maximal seizure reduction rate is still <50% (Sisterson et al. 2020). Similarly, a proportional-integral-derivative (PID) controller has been recently deployed to achieve adaptive DBS (Wang et al. 2016). These loop controllers are vastly used in Internet of Things and other engineering applications and have recently gained considerable attention as a control solution in brain implants as opposed to other approaches such as radial basis function neural networks (Colic et al. 2011) and autoregressive models (Santaniello et al. 2011). However, while PID controllers allow for simple and robust control of devices, they must be preprogrammed for a specific input/output function (similarly to the NeuroPace system), not being able to learn on their own. Thus, they still require a first principles or a trial-and-error approach. These limitations are due to the fact that while basic neuroscience and clinical research have made outstanding advancement in the DBS field, the exact pathophysiology of epilepsy as well as the mechanism underlying DBS effect is still not fully understood; both the neuromorphic neuroprosthesis and AI are fundamental players in biohybrid neuronics, as they offer systems capable of learning from experience and of adapting to evolving brain dynamics. This view has been coming of age in recent years: while biohybrid systems using memristor-based neuromorphic neural interfaces have recently emerged (Serb et al. 2020), as also emphasized in (Dumpelmann 2019), closed-loop DBS devices should be conceived since the device design stage to implement ML techniques for early seizure detection and, ideally, prediction. However, in the latter case, the device's computational capability comes at the cost of hardware-related constraints such as size and power consumption. In this scenario, neuromorphic neural interfaces present the key to bypass bulky and power-consuming device architectures, while AI can become an integral part of their operation.

In this regard, software-based ML techniques have been successfully deployed to achieve an adaptive closed-loop strategy for seizure control in an vitro model of limbic ictogenesis, adopting either a reinforcement (Pineau et al. 2009) or a statistical approach (Panuccio et al. 2013). In both cases, the agent learned the optimal stimulation strategy, converging to the maximal seizure reduction rate while minimizing the number of delivered pulses, outclassing known effective periodic pacing frequencies. In parallel with this, great attentions is starting to arise around the applicability of the concept of "deep reinforcement learning" (Mnih et al. 2015) to the study of brain signals, as those algorithms are able to digest very large inputs before making a decision.

Along with the modulation of graft function and graft–host interaction, AI can solve parameter optimization problems for graft growth and thus its structural integration within the host brain. In fact, the use of nanoscale materials to modulate the extracellular matrix opens an enormous range of possible parameters in the topology domain (shape, roughness, and ordering of the materials), whereas tuning the graft culture parameters such as concentration of growth/differentiation/survival factors and their spatiotemporal gradients mimicking embryonic development is crucial to attain a realistic replica of the brain area to be replaced. However, this creates an excess of optimizable parameters that are not addressable with the standard research methods (making trials with all the virtually infinite possible combinations). In this regard, DL algorithms have been applied to predict the response of the stem cells in different growing conditions allowing for less time-consuming experiments (Mackay et al. 2020). Furthermore, the quality assessment of grafts can be automatically done by ML algorithms with the use of Artificial Vision and CNN (Orita et al. 2020).

Prediction of how the graft will behave once developed is also one of the challenges that regenerative medicine faces daily. With the help of mathematical models and AI, it is possible to understand and predict behaviors such as angiogenesis (Lemon et al. 2009), which is crucial for the graft survival once is implanted in the host brain (Mansour et al. 2018). This not only avoids the time investment required to perform the experiments but also reduces the number of experimental animals and the budget needed to develop these technologies, which undoubtedly represent the future of medicine. Along these lines, AI can be used to predict the outcome of grafting itself. In this regard, alternating decision trees (Pfahringer et al. 2001) have been successfully deployed to define the risk of graft-versus-host disease in allogenic hematopoietic stem cell transplants (Arai et al. 2019), and it is foreseen that their use can be extended to define graft–host integration dynamics by adapting the type of parameters to process (e.g. graft developmental stage, network connectivity, and cellular biophysical phenotype). This will help clinicians and researchers to assess the risk of individual experiments or interventions.

13.6 Challenges and Limitations

Although SVMs have shown impressive performance accuracy for the tasks of seizure classification, localization, detection, and prediction, they have several limitations. First, as is the problem with ML methods such as SVM, the performance depends heavily on the feature extraction method and the SVM kernel used. Extensive feature engineering, i.e. finding out what features best represent the EEG data is time-consuming and also requires domain expertise (thus resource-consuming), which is often not available and is thus undesirable. Extracting features from raw EEG recordings, which is also known as feature engineering, requires careful engineering and considerable domain expertise. The extracted feature vector must be highly related to the classification task. However, this strategy is difficult as various types of patterns appear during seizures. Moreover, many artifacts in the signal can have structures similar to the seizure patterns.

In contrast, DL methods have the ability to extract features from the EEG data and thus avoid the need for extensive feature engineering. However, there are other issues with DL methods that need to be solved before using in a clinical setting. For example, studies using CNN typically preprocess the EEG data and transform them to spectrograms as CNNs require images as an input. This could lead to information loss in terms of reduced temporal resolution as spectrograms are computed using sliding time windows (typically in window sizes of one to five seconds). Also, choosing appropriate window size is not a trivial task as EEGs are nonstationary signals and in this context how the window size affects the classification accuracy is not fully understood. For example, different seizure types have different spatiotemporal dynamics, and having the same window size for all might not be the most optimal.

Furthermore, specifically in the context of seizure prediction (or detection), most of the work has focused on building subject-specific models (SVM or DL models), given the high inter-subject variability of EEG data from epileptic patients. This might work well if tested on well-curated open-source databases, where adequate samples for each class may be present, but in a clinical setting that they do not offer a reliable solution for the problem when a patient has fewer seizure occurrences, leading to inadequate training samples (Dissanayake et al. 2021). Furthermore, since EEG is essentially a nonstationary signal, even training a subject-specific model using EEG at a certain time window might not well represent the data at another time interval in the same subject (Roy et al. 2019). For instance, when designing a real-time seizure detection system, the ML or DL model parameters are typically obtained during offline training, which may then be loaded into a chip to perform online seizure detection. However, due to the nonstationarity of EEG data, the seizure patterns of the patient are likely to change over a period of time, and thus the accuracy of the system might drop, remaining no longer clinically acceptable. This would then further require extraction of new features if necessary and retraining of the classifier, which is not desirable.

Building patient-independent models for seizure prediction (and also for other tasks such as classification of seizure types and SOZ localization) that have ability to solve these classification problems across multiple subjects in the dataset by learning a global predictive function would be highly desirable as it can generalize very well, but is a very complex task nonetheless. For example, in the task of localization of SOZ, very different locations of electrodes and subjects-specific nature of EEG would make it very challenging to implement such a system.

Another crucial issue is guaranteeing the patient's safety when an AI-enhanced construct is implanted in their brain. This calls for a mandatory technical robustness of the AI algorithms, herein included the neuromorphic neuroprosthesis operation (hardware AI). Thus, it is fundamental that researchers and clinicians understand the principles underlying the AI-enhanced system operation. In turn, this calls for the fundamental shift from AI to "explainable" AI.

13.6.1 From AI to Explainable AI

AI-based approaches such as DL have shown tremendous promise in several fields, including neuroscience, by performing at the level of human experts or even surpassing it in several fields, including neuroscience (Angelov et al. 2021). However, many such DL models are often built with a huge number of parameters (i.e. neural network weights ranging from millions to billions), making it hard to derive an explanation for the results obtained and to link the parameters to the problem being solved. AI solutions in addressing these problems have still remained as a "black box," hindering the routine use of these approaches in sensitive areas such as disease diagnosis and prediction (e.g. in epilepsy), and thus there is a growing need to make AI algorithms more transparent, understandable and explainable. Only when the decisions made by the AI system can be reasoned logically, trust will be gained in the AI system by its users, for example, medical practitioners and patients being directly interfaced with AI-based systems, like the AI-trained neuromorphic neuroprosthesis foreseen in enhanced regenerative medicine. Furthermore, making the model more explainable also gives opportunities to the developers to find justifiable ways to improve the model, rather than depending on ad hoc heuristics to optimize the models and achieve the desired accuracy (e.g. addition of extra layers, tweaking the learning rates and parameters) as is done presently.

It is important to note that the terms interpreting, understanding, and explaining in this context have different meanings. Briefly, understanding refers to functional understanding of the AI model, i.e. not the low-level mechanistic understanding of the algorithmic details, but an understanding of how the model arrived at a certain decision. Interpretability of a model can be described in terms of post hoc or intrinsic interpretability. In the case of intrinsic interpretability, the idea is to incorporate interpretability directly into the structure of the model by using simpler models such as linear models or decision trees that are easier to interpret. In contrast, post hoc interpretability refers to achieving interpretability after model training, where the goal is to understand what the model predicts in terms of the changes in the feature space. Finally, explanation refers to a collection of comprehensible features that have contributed toward a model arriving at a decision. For a detailed discussion of the meaning of these terms, the reader is kindly referred to (Montavon et al. 2018; Lipton 2018).

The field of explainable AI (XAI) aims to address these issues by developing AI models that not only achieve high accuracy, but are also explainable (Adadi and Berrada 2018; Fellous et al. 2019). Several techniques have already been developed toward explaining the decision-making process of deep neural networks with applications to EEG data emerging rapidly. Features based on image classification, such as deconvolution and class activation map (CAM), have been widely used to make the AI models more interpretable. CAMs produce heat-maps of the regions (feature space) that support the classification decision, thus making it intuitive for users to understand the decision made by AI (Baehrens et al. 2010). In addition to CAMs, several other methods have been proposed toward XAI and these are broadly divided into three categories known as (i) pre-modeling (characterizing the input data), (ii) modeling (developing explainable architectures and algorithms), and (iii) post-modeling approaches (extracting explanation from outputs) (Fellous et al. 2019).

Applications of XAI in epilepsy are just beginning to emerge. Gabeff et al. used XAI in seizure detection using a CNN architecture (Gabeff et al. 2021); to understand the decision the model makes, the work implemented a visualization method based on probability computed using model weights at the first layer to allow the user to infer if a frequency component is associated with the ictal or interictal period. Furthermore, the field of closed-loop stimulation can greatly benefit from the development of XAI methods, which can have major contributions to epilepsy treatment. Prevention of seizure activity using XAI-based predictions can activate an implanted neurostimulator in real-time, thereby improving the efficacy of brain stimulation devices (Fellous et al. 2019). However, there are several challenges: (i) how can the XAI algorithms detect the relevant biomarkers/brain states pertaining to an impending seizure? (ii) How can the XAI system be trained to generate the most effective stimulation pattern once the brain state corresponding to an impending seizure is detected? (iii) What would be the ethical and legal considerations of such a system? There are ambitious questions waiting to be answered.

13.7   A Philosophical Perspective on Enhanced Brain Regeneration

The enhanced regenerative medicine paradigm brings together technology and innovations from various domains: brain regeneration, AI, nanoscale electronics, neuromorphic computation, and bioengineered brain tissue grafts. It is not surprising that all of this would be needed in order to heal brain damage, since it is often remarked that the human brain might well be one of the most complex systems in the universe. On its own, the brain (and the central nervous system in general) is capable only of very limited self-repair after injury (see Section 13.1). As explained in Section 13.1, the process of brain regeneration must be adequately fine-tuned and well controlled in order to be effective and safe. The goal of the new biohybrid approach is to aid the process of brain regeneration and healing, in order to undo damage and restore normal function. To achieve this, it needs to be "enhanced" by AI. Here, we will address what "enhanced" means in this new paradigm and briefly indicate what this may imply for the philosophical and ethical concerns of identity, autonomy, and agency.

In various discussions about the ethics of (medical) technology, the term "enhanced" or "enhancement" is used to indicate that some normal, natural capability is being lifted to a new level (Ireni-Saban and Sherman 2021; Keskinbora 2019; Forlini and Hall 2016). Enhancement, therefore, is often considered as something "beyond human" (trans-humanist or post-humanist) and is in conflict with the idea of the natural capacities of a healthy body and simply restoring normal function. However, this is not the case for enhanced brain regeneration. In fact, while the approach of inserting AI in the brain might seem something from (dystopian) sci-fi, this does not all mean that its goal is to go beyond the limits of what a normal, healthy human body (or mind) can do; rather, it challenges and pushes forward the boundaries of medical technology, not those of human nature, as what is being enhanced is the process and technique of brain regeneration, not the brain itself.

An analogy might help to illustrate the issue. The human body is perfectly capable of recovering from a broken bone. Something like a greenstick fracture might heal completely on its own within a week or two. However, more complicated fractures do not. A surgeon might even need to re-break a misaligned bone. Then, temporarily, the bone might need extra support, a plaster cast, or external fixation with a metal rod. All of this is meant to help the bones heal and recover their function, not to replace or improve them. Despite all the medical interventions, ultimately the broken bones have to knit themselves together again. The external support is there so that they heal in the right way. One might say much the same about the medical intervention envisioned in the new biohybrid approach to brain regeneration. The function of the biohybrid graft with the neuromorphic chip and the AI is comparable to an external fixation that temporarily supports the self-healing capacity of the body. The AI guides the natural regeneration of the brain by helping the graft to integrate in the host brain in the right way and restore the normal function of the latter. It will not endow the patient with superhuman capabilities; it will not insert new knowledge in the brain like in Space Odyssey 3000; it will not extend their memory like in Johnny Mnemonic. In other words, what is being enhanced is not the human patient, but the medical procedure and the healing process.

What does this mean for ethical issues surrounding the identity, autonomy, and agency of the patient? These concerns are all closely interrelated, and all tie into further existential and moral debates about authenticity and responsibility. Autonomy, as the broadly defined capacity to decide on one's own good, weighing alternatives, and choose a plan of action, without coercion or manipulation (Pugh et al. 2018), is a central philosophical notion which plays a fundamental role also in social and political philosophy as well as economics. Hence, the implications of tampering with a patient's identity, autonomy, and agency are very far-reaching. Autonomy, in particular, has been the topic of much debate with respect to so-called closed-loop medical devices (Kellmeyer et al. 2016), such as neuroprostheses, which are an integral part of biohybrid neuronics.

Regarding identity, every invasive surgery and implant or even the simple use of a pill, glasses, or hearing aids can potentially give rise to feelings of alienation, toward one's own incapacitated body, perceived as a malfunctioning machine instead of a healthy organism, or the intervention itself, perceived as the insertion of a foreign body. Much depends on the subjective experience of the patient, their self-image, and their self-understanding as well as the communication of the medical team involved. Patients can just as well harmonize with an implant, seeing it as becoming part of their body or self, achieving a symbiosis, instead of experiencing it as foreign and in conflict with their body wholeness. In the case of the new class of biohybrid grafts several factors would contribute to a harmonious integration of the graft and the host, facilitating a more positive outlook on how the envisioned neuronic implant can integrate with the host and aid the healing process from within. The neural graft is cultivated from the hosts' own cells to be an autologous transplant, which contributes to preserve the identity in a biological sense. The neuromorphic computing system will contain artificial neurons and use an AI with a learning and training algorithm. In the case of epilepsy, the AI agent will learn to distinguish the healthy brain patterns from those leading to seizures. These are the patient's own brain patterns. The AI, therefore, does not replace, but simply reproduces the patient's own activation patterns, adapting and fitting in smoothly with the overall brain activity. The neuromorphic chip will model the structure and activation patterns of the host brain, instantiating an artificial Spiking Neural Network, which closely mimics the natural neural networks found in the brain. The only interventions it will make will be using electrical pulses to guide the graft neural plasticity and so its integration in the host brain and, as needed, counteract any pathological discharge impinging onto the graft from the host brain while this is still being regenerated (hence, still technically epileptic). In other words, the AI will simply act as intermediary for the brain itself, propagating its own patterns into the graft in order to tune it to better harmonize with the whole. What is being excluded and suppressed are precisely the harmful epileptic patterns, which would take away control, autonomy, and agency from the patient. The AI will serve as a tool to affirm and strengthen the autonomy and agency of the patient against the disease, by using and reinforcing the patient's own (healthy) activation patterns. Such intervention of the AI is moreover designed to decrease over time: less and less interventions will be required as the graft–host integration advances, the end result being that the role of the AI will be null and the reintegrated brain will be restored to a healthy, whole state. Likewise, at that point, the neuromorphic chip can also be removed, just like a cast or splint, having performed its temporary supporting function. The decisional autonomy of the patient is respected at every step of the healing process aimed at removing the interference of the epileptic seizures with the patient's agency. The patient is not "taken out of the loop" of any active decision-making process, given that the implant is trained by the patient's own brain, and, therefore, not "independent of the patient's will" (Gilbert et al. 2018). Unless we want to claim implicit volitional control over neuronal firing patterns, no decision is being preempted by the implant. Moreover, given that the patient does not choose or desire to undergo a seizure, the temporary intervention and training by the implant cannot be considered as suppressing "undesirable behavior" (Gilbert 2015), since a seizure is not "behavior." Unlike (extreme) emotional responses, a seizure is not a learned behavior, but the mere causal consequence of an illness. The autonomy of the patient is, therefore, not under the control of the implant, but the lack of autonomy due to the epileptic seizures is being remedied by the implant. At most, one could say that the autonomy of the patient is temporarily dependent on the implant, much as the ability to walk might be dependent on a crutch. However, just like in the case of the crutch, also the biohybrid neuronics implant is a temporary intervention aimed at restoring full autonomy by healing rather than treating the damaged brain.

Acknowledgments

This work was supported by the European Union under the Horizon 2020 FET-PROACTIVE project HERMES – Hybrid Enhanced Regenerative Medicine Systems, Grant Agreement n. 824164.

Acronyms

AI	artificial intelligence
ANN	artificial neural network
CNN	convolutional neural network
DBS	deep brain stimulation
DL	deep learning
EEG	electroencephalography
FDA	Food and Drug Administration
HFO	high-frequency oscillation
LSTM	long short term memory
MEA	microelectrode array
ML	machine learning
MRI/fMRI	magnetic resonance imaging/functional magnetic resonance imaging
MTLE	mesial temporal lobe epilepsy
PID	proportional-integral-derivative
RNN	recurrent neural network
SOZ	seizure onset zone
SVM	support vector machine
TUH	Temple University Hospital
XAI	explainable AI
CAM	class activation map

Author Biographies

Gabriella Panuccio, MD, and PhD graduated in Medicine and Surgery at Sapienza University of Rome and subsequently obtained the PhD in Biophysics from the same university. She has more than two decades of experience in mesial temporal lobe epilepsy research, and a polyhedral background acquired through extensive international experience in the fields of basic neuroscience, theoretical neurobiology, and neural engineering. Her research focuses on biohybrid approaches for brain regeneration and repair. She currently leads the Enhanced Regenerative Medicine laboratory at the Italian Institute of Technology.

Narayan Puthanmadam Subramaniyam received the MSc and PhD in Biomedical Engineering from Tampere University of Technology in 2009 and 2015 respectively. His research interests include statistical signal processing, complex systems, nonlinear dynamics, ML, and computational modeling with primary applications in neuroimaging data (EEG and MEG). He is a visiting researcher at Aalto University and postdoctoral fellow at Tampere University. He also serves as a research affiliate at Sapien Labs.

Ángel Canal-Alonso has been a researcher at the BISITE Research Group since 2019. He studied Biology at the University of Salamanca and worked initially at the Institute of Neurosciences of Castile and Leon. After three years, he shifted from cell biology to computational neuroscience and joined BISITE and the Artificial Intelligence Research Institute. He specializes in biological signal analysis and AI models. He was awarded the Young Researcher National Award in 2016.

Juan Manuel Corchado Rodríguez, PhD is a Professor at the University of Salamanca. He has been Vice-Rector for Research from 2013 to 2017 and Director of the Science Park of the University of Salamanca. Elected as Dean of the Faculty of Science twice, he holds a PhD in Computer Science from the University of Salamanca and a PhD in Artificial Intelligence from the University of the West of Scotland. He leads the renowned BISITE (Bioinformatics, Intelligent Systems and Educational Technology) Research Group, created in 2000.

Carlo Ierna, PhD holds a PhD in philosophy (Katholieke Universiteit Leuven) and an MSc in Cognitive Artificial Intelligence (Utrecht University). He is currently assistant professor at the Vrije Universiteit Amsterdam and researcher at the Radboud University Nijmegen. He has been the recipient of a Dutch NWO VENI grant and a Comenius Fellowship. His work focuses on the history of philosophy, cognition, and computation, with particular attention to the intersection of mathematics and psychology in the nineteenth century and the notion of symbolic intentionality in the School of Brentano.

References

Aarabi, A. and He, B. (2012). A rule-based seizure prediction method for focal neocortical epilepsy. *Clinical Neurophysiology* https://doi.org/10.1016/j.clinph.2012.01.014.

Acharya, U.R., Yanti, R., Zheng, J.W. et al. (2013). Automated diagnosis of epilepsy using CWT, Hos and texture parameters. *International Journal of Neural Systems* https://doi.org/10.1142/s0129065713500093.

Acharya, U.R., Fujita, H., Sudarshan, V.K. et al. (2015). Application of entropies for automated diagnosis of epilepsy using EEG signals: a review. *Knowledge-Based Systems* https://doi.org/10.1016/j.knosys.2015.08.004.

Adadi, A. and Berrada, M. (2018). Peeking inside the black-box: a survey on explainable artificial intelligence (XAI). *IEEE Access* https://doi.org/10.1109/ACCESS.2018.2870052.

Aggarwal, C.C. (2018). *Neural Networks and Deep Learning*. Springer. ISBN 978-3-319-94463-0.

Akter, M.S., Islam, M.R., Iimura, Y. et al. (2020). Multiband entropy-based feature-extraction method for automatic identification of epileptic focus based on high-frequency components in interictal iEEG. *Scientific Reports* https://doi.org/10.1038/s41598-020-62967-z.

Alashwal, H., Crouse, M.E.H.J.J. et al. (2019). The application of unsupervised clustering methods to Alzheimer's disease. *Frontiers in Computational Neuroscience* https://doi.org/10.3389/fncom.2019.00031.

An, S., Kang, C., and Lee, H.W. (2020). Artificial intelligence and computational approaches for epilepsy. *Journal of Epilepsy Research* https://doi.org/10.14581/jer.20003.

Angelov, P.P., Soares, E.A., Jiang, R. et al. (2021). Explainable artificial intelligence: an analytical review. *WIREs Data Mining and Knowledge Discovery* https://doi.org/10.1002/widm.1424.

Arai, Y., Kondo, T., Fuse, K. et al. (2019). Using a machine learning algorithm to predict acute graft-versus-host disease following allogeneic transplantation. *Blood Advances* https://doi.org/10.1182/bloodadvances.2019000934.

Cannataro, M. et al. (ed.) (2022). *Artificial Intelligence in Bioinformatics*. Elsevier.

Asif, U., Roy, S., Tang, J., and Harrer, S. (2020). *SeizureNet: Multi-Spectral Deep Feature Learning for Seizure Type Classification*. Cham: Springer International Publishing https://doi.org/10.1007/978-3-030-66843-3_8.

Avoli, M., D'Antuono, M., Louvel, J. et al. (2002). Network and pharmacological mechanisms leading to epileptiform synchronization in the limbic system in vitro. *Progress in Neurobiology* https://doi.org/10.1016/S0301-0082(02)00077-1.

Baehrens, D., Schroeter, T., Harmeling, S. et al. (2010). How to explain individual classification decisions. *Journal of Machine Learning Research*.

Berg, A.T. (2004). Postsurgical treatment of epilepsy. *Epilepsy Currents* https://doi.org/10.1111/j.1535-7597.2004.44001.x.

Bifari, F., Decimo, I., Pino, A. et al. (2017). Neurogenic radial glia-like cells in meninges migrate and differentiate into functionally integrated neurons in the neonatal cortex. *Cell Stem Cell* https://doi.org/10.1016/j.stem.2016.10.020.

Bozinovski, S. (2020). Reminder of the first paper on transfer learning in neural networks, 1976. *Informatica* https://doi.org/10.31449/inf.v44i3.2828.

Buccelli, S., Bornat, Y., Colombi, I. et al. (2019). A neuromorphic prosthesis to restore communication in neuronal networks. *iScience* https://doi.org/10.1016/j.isci.2019.07.046.

Bullmore, E. and Sporns, O. (2009). Complex brain networks: graph theoretical analysis of structural and functional systems. *Nature Reviews. Neuroscience* https://doi.org/10.1038/nrn2575.

Buzsaki, G., Bayardo, F., Miles, R. et al. (1989). The grafted hippocampus: an epileptic focus. *Experimental Neurology* https://doi.org/10.1016/0014-4886(89)90167-2.

Chang, K.-A., Kim, J.W., Kim, J.A. et al. (2011). Biphasic electrical currents stimulation promotes both proliferation and differentiation of Fetal neural stem cells. *PLoS One* https://doi.org/10.1371/journal.pone.0018738.

Chang, W.-C., Kudlacek, J., Hlinka, J. et al. (2018). Loss of neuronal network resilience precedes seizures and determines the ictogenic nature of interictal synaptic perturbations. *Nature Neuroscience* https://doi.org/10.1038/s41593-018-0278-y.

Chui, C.K. (1992). *An Introduction to Wavelets*. San Diego, CA: Academic Press.

Chvojka, J., Kudlacek, J., Chang, W.C. et al. (2021). The role of interictal discharges in ictogenesis - a dynamical perspective. *Epilepsy & Behavior* https://doi.org/10.1016/j.yebeh.2019.106591.

Colic, S., Zalay, O.C., and Bardakjian, B.L. (2011). Responsive neuromodulators based on artificial neural networks used to control seizure-like events in a computational model of epilepsy. *International Journal of Neural Systems* https://doi.org/10.1142/s0129065711002894.

Cunningham, M., Cho, J.H., Leung, A. et al. (2014). hPSC-derived maturing GABAergic interneurons ameliorate seizures and abnormal behavior in epileptic mice. *Cell Stem Cell* https://doi.org/10.1016/j.stem.2014.10.006.

de Curtis, M. and Avanzini, G. (2001). Interictal spikes in focal epileptogenesis. *Progress in Neurobiology* https://doi.org/10.1016/S0301-0082(00)00026-5.

de Curtis, M., Librizzi, L., and Biella, G. (2001). Discharge threshold is enhanced for several seconds after a single interictal spike in a model of focal epileptogenesis. *The European Journal of Neuroscience* https://doi.org/10.1046/j.0953-816x.2001.01637.x.

Daoud, H. and Bayoumi, M.A. (2019). Efficient epileptic seizure prediction based on deep learning. *IEEE Transactions on Biomedical Circuits and Systems* https://doi.org/10.1109/TBCAS.2019.2929053.

Decimo, I., Dolci, S., Panuccio, G. et al. (2021). Meninges: a widespread niche of neural progenitors for the brain. *The Neuroscientist* https://doi.org/10.1177/1073858420954826.

Direito, B., Teixeira, C.A., Sales, F. et al. (2017). A realistic seizure prediction study based on multiclass SVM. *International Journal of Neural Systems* https://doi.org/10.1142/S012906571750006X.

Dissanayake, T., Fernando, T., Denman, S. et al. (2021). Deep learning for patient-independent epileptic seizure prediction using scalp EEG signals. *IEEE Sensors Journal* https://doi.org/10.1109/JSEN.2021.3057076.

Dorn, T. and Witte, O.W. (1995). Refractory periods following interictal spikes in acute experimentally induced epileptic foci. *Electroencephalography and Clinical Neurophysiology* https://doi.org/10.1016/0013-4694(94)00214-6.

Dressler, O., Schneider, G., Stockmanns, G., and Kochs, E.F. (2004). Awareness and the EEG power spectrum: analysis of frequencies. *British Journal of Anaesthesia* https://doi.org/10.1093/bja/aeh270.

Dumpelmann, M. (2019). Early seizure detection for closed loop direct neurostimulation devices in epilepsy. *Journal of Neural Engineering* https://doi.org/10.1088/1741-2552/ab094a.

Dwi Saputro, I.R., Maryati, N.D., Solihati, S.R. et al. (2019). Seizure type classification on EEG signal using support vector machine. *Journal of Physics: Conference Series* https://doi.org/10.1088/1742-6596/1201/1/012065.

Elahian, B., Yeasin, M., Mudigoudar, B. et al. (2017). Identifying seizure onset zone from electrocorticographic recordings: a machine learning approach based on phase locking value. *Seizure* https://doi.org/10.1016/j.seizure.2017.07.010.

Faust, O., Acharya, U.R., Adeli, H., and Adeli, A. (2015). Wavelet-based EEG processing for computer-aided seizure detection and epilepsy diagnosis. *Seizure - European Journal of Epilepsy* https://doi.org/10.1016/j.seizure.2015.01.012.

Feldt, S., Bonifazi, P., and Cossart, R. (2011). Dissecting functional connectivity of neuronal microcircuits: experimental and theoretical insights. *Trends in Neurosciences* https://doi.org/10.1016/j.tins.2011.02.007.

Fellous, J.-M., Sapiro, G., Rossi, A. et al. (2019). Explainable artificial intelligence for neuroscience: Behavioral Neurostimulation. *Frontiers in Neuroscience* https://doi.org/10.3389/fnins.2019.01346.

Fiest, K.M., Birbeck, G.L., Jacoby, A., and Jette, N. (2014). Stigma in epilepsy. *Current Neurology and Neuroscience Reports* https://doi.org/10.1007/s11910-014-0444-x.

Forlini, C. and Hall, W. (2016). The is and ought of the ethics of Neuroenhancement: mind the gap. *Frontiers in Psychology* https://doi.org/10.3389/fpsyg.2015.01998.

Gabeff, V., Teijeiro, T., Zapater, M. et al. (2021). Interpreting deep learning models for epileptic seizure detection on EEG signals. *Artificial Intelligence in Medicine* https://doi.org/10.1016/j.artmed.2021.102084.

Gareth James, D.W., Hastie, T., and Tibshirani, R. (2013). An introduction to statistical learning with applications in R. In: *Springer Texts in Statistics*. Springer.

Gilbert, F.A. (2015). Threat to autonomy? The intrusion of predictive brain implants. *AJOB Neuroscience* https://doi.org/10.1080/21507740.2015.1076087.

Gilbert, F., O'brien, T., and Cook, M. (2018). The effects of closed-loop brain implants on autonomy and deliberation: what are the risks of being kept in the loop? *Cambridge Quarterly of Healthcare Ethics* https://doi.org/10.1017/S0963180117000640.

Goel, S., Agrawal, R., and Bharti, R.K. (2023). Epileptic seizure prediction and classification based on statistical features using LSTM fully connected neural network. *Journal of Intelligent Fuzzy Systems* https://doi.org/10.3233/JIFS-222745.

Goodfellow, I., Bengio, Y., and Courville, A. (2016). Deep learning. In: *Adaptive Computation and Machine Learning Series*. The MIT Press.

Grassberger, P. and Procaccia, I. (1983). Characterization of strange attractors. *Physical Review Letters* https://doi.org/10.1103/PhysRevLett.50.346.

Guo, L., Rivero, D., Seoane, J.A., and Pazos, A. (2009). Classification of EEG signals using relative wavelet energy and artificial neural networks. In: *Proceedings of the First ACM/SIGEVO Summit on Genetic and Evolutionary Computation*, 177–184. Shanghai, China: Association for Computing Machinery.

B. Surendiran, Saravanan Krishnan, Ramesh Kesavan, G. S. Mahalakshmi, Eds. *Handbook of Artificial Intelligence in Biomedical Engineering*, 1ste, 564. Apple Academic Press. 2021. ISBN 9781774637616.

Harrer, S., Shah, P., Antony, B., and Hu, J. (2019). Artificial intelligence for clinical trial design. *Trends in Pharmacological Sciences* https://doi.org/10.1016/j.tips.2019.05.005.

Hochreiter, S. and Schmidhuber, J. (1997). Long short-term memory. *Neural Computation* https://doi.org/10.1162/neco.1997.9.8.1735.

Ireni-Saban, L. and Sherman, M. (2021). Cyborg ethics and regulation: ethical issues of human enhancement. *Science and Public Policy* https://doi.org/10.1093/scipol/scab058.

Johansen, A.R., Jin, J., Maszczyk, T. et al. (2016). Epileptiform spike detection via convolutional neural networks. In: *2016 IEEE International Conference on Acoustics, Speech and Signal Processing (ICASSP)*. https://doi.org/10.1109/ICASSP.2016.7471776.

Kellmeyer, P., Cochrane, T., Müller, O. et al. (2016). The effects of closed-loop medical devices on the autonomy and accountability of persons and systems. *Cambridge Quarterly of Healthcare Ethics* https://doi.org/10.1017/S0963180116000359.

Kerezoudis, P., McCutcheon, B., Murphy, M.E. et al. (2018). Thirty-day postoperative morbidity and mortality after temporal lobectomy for medically refractory epilepsy. *Journal of Neurosurgery JNS* https://doi.org/10.3171/2016.12.JNS162096.

Keskinbora, K.H. (2019). Medical ethics considerations on artificial intelligence. *Journal of Clinical Neuroscience* https://doi.org/10.1016/j.jocn.2019.03.001.

Kobelt, L.J., Wilkinson, A.E., McCormick, A.M. et al. (2014). Short duration electrical stimulation to enhance neurite outgrowth and maturation of adult neural stem progenitor cells. *Annals of Biomedical Engineering* https://doi.org/10.1007/s10439-014-1058-9.

Lachaux, J.-P., Rodriguez, E., Martinerie, J., and Varela, F.J. (1999). Measuring phase synchrony in brain signals. *Human Brain Mapping* https://doi.org/https://doi.org/10.1002/(SICI)1097-0193(1999)8:4<194::AID-HBM4>3.0.CO;2-C.

Laxer, K.D., Trinka, E., Hirsch, L.J. et al. (2014). The consequences of refractory epilepsy and its treatment. *Epilepsy & Behavior* https://doi.org/10.1016/j.yebeh.2014.05.031.

LeCun, Y., Bengio, Y., and Hinton, G. (2015). Deep learning. *Nature* https://doi.org/10.1038/nature14539.

Lemon, G., Howard, D., Tomlinson, M.J. et al. (2009). Mathematical modelling of tissue-engineered angiogenesis. *Mathematical Biosciences* https://doi.org/10.1016/j.mbs.2009.07.003.

Lévesque, M., Salami, P., Shiri, Z., and Avoli, M. (2018). Interictal oscillations and focal epileptic disorders. *European Journal of Neuroscience* https://doi.org/10.1111/ejn.13628.

Li, C.Y., Poo, M., and Dan, Y. (2009). Burst spiking of a single cortical neuron modifies global brain state. *Science* https://doi.org/10.1126/science.1169957.

Li, S., Zhou, W., Yuan, Q., and Liu, Y. (2013). Seizure prediction using spike rate of intracranial EEG. *IEEE Transactions on Neural Systems and Rehabilitation Engineering* https://doi.org/10.1109/TNSRE.2013.2282153.

Lin, Q., Ye, S., Huang, X. et al. (2016). Classification of epileptic EEG signals with stacked sparse autoencoder based on deep learning. In: *Intelligent Computing Methodologies*. Cham: Springer International Publishing https://doi.org/10.1007/978-3-319-42297-8_74.

Lipton, Z.C. (2018). The mythos of model interpretability. *Communications of the ACM* https://doi.org/10.1145/3233231.

Liu, T., Truong, N.D., Nikpour, A. et al. (2020). Epileptic seizure classification with symmetric and hybrid bilinear models. *IEEE Journal of Biomedical and Health Informatics* https://doi.org/10.1109/JBHI.2020.2984128.

Lopes da Silva, F., Blanes, W., Kalitzin, S.N. et al. (2003). Epilepsies as dynamical diseases of brain systems: basic models of the transition between normal and epileptic activity. *Epilepsia* https://doi.org/10.1111/j.0013-9580.2003.12005.x.

MAB, A. and Yoo, J. (2016). A 1.83 microJ/classification, 8-channel, patient-specific epileptic seizure classification SoC using a non-linear support vector machine. *IEEE Transactions on Biomedical Circuits and Systems* https://doi.org/10.1109/TBCAS.2014.2386891.

Mackay, B.S., Praeger, M., Grant-Jacob, J.A. et al. (2020). Modeling adult skeletal stem cell response to laser-machined topographies through deep learning. *Tissue and Cell* https://doi.org/10.1016/j.tice.2020.101442.

Mallat, S. (2016). Understanding deep convolutional networks. *Philosophical Transactions of the Royal Society A: Mathematical, Physical and Engineering Sciences* https://doi.org/doi:10.1098/rsta.2015.0203.

Mansour, A.A., Gonçalves, J.T., Bloyd, C.W. et al. (2018). An in vivo model of functional and vascularized human brain organoids. *Nature Biotechnology* https://doi.org/10.1038/nbt.4127.

Mnih, V., Kavukcuoglu, K., Silver, D. et al. (2015). Human-level control through deep reinforcement learning. *Nature* https://doi.org/10.1038/nature14236.

Montavon, G., Samek, W., and Müller, K.-R. (2018). Methods for interpreting and understanding deep neural networks. *Digital Signal Processing* https://doi.org/https://doi.org/10.1016/j.dsp.2017.10.011.

Morgan, R.J. and Soltesz, I. (2008). Nonrandom connectivity of the epileptic dentate gyrus predicts a major role for neuronal hubs in seizures. *PNAS* https://doi.org/10.1073/pnas.0801372105.

Morrell, M.J. and Halpern, C. (2016). Responsive direct brain stimulation for epilepsy. *Neurosurgery Clinics of North America* https://doi.org/10.1016/j.nec.2015.08.012.

Nasser, M.N. (2007). Pattern recognition and machine learning. *Journal of Electronic Imaging* https://doi.org/10.1117/1.2819119.

Nielsen, M.A. (2015). *Neural Networks and Deep Learning*. Determination Press.

Orita, K., Sawada, K., Matsumoto, N., and Ikegaya, Y. (2020). Machine-learning-based quality control of contractility of cultured human-induced pluripotent stem-cell-derived cardiomyocytes. *Biochemical and Biophysical Research Communications* https://doi.org/10.1016/j.bbrc.2020.03.141.

Ozaktas, H.M., Arikan, O., Kutay, M.A., and Bozdagt, G. (1996). Digital computation of the fractional Fourier transform. *IEEE Transactions on Signal Processing* https://doi.org/10.1109/78.536672.

Palop, J.J., Chin, J., and Mucke, L. (2006). A network dysfunction perspective on neurodegenerative diseases. *Nature* https://doi.org/10.1038/nature05289.

Panuccio, G., D'Antuono, M., De Guzman, P. et al. (2010). In vitro ictogenesis and parahippocampal networks in a rodent model of temporal lobe epilepsy. *Neurobiology of Disease* https://doi.org/10.1016/j.nbd.2010.05.003.

Panuccio, G., Guez, A., Vincent, R. et al. (2013). Adaptive control of epileptiform excitability in an in vitro model of limbic seizures. *Experimental Neurology* https://doi.org/10.1016/j.expneurol.2013.01.002.

Panuccio, G., Semprini, M., Natale, L. et al. (2018). Progress in Neuroengineering for brain repair: new challenges and open issues. *Brain and Neuroscience Advances* https://doi.org/10.1177/2398212818776475.

Peterson, S.E., Garitaonandia, I., and Loring, J.F. (2016). The tumorigenic potential of pluripotent stem cells: what can we do to minimize it? *BioEssays* https://doi.org/10.1002/bies.201670915.

Pfahringer, B., Holmes, G., and Kirkby, R. (2001). Optimizing the induction of alternating decision trees. In: *Advances in Knowledge Discovery and Data Mining*. Berlin, Heidelberg: Springer.

Pineau, J., Guez, A., Vincent, R. et al. (2009). Treating epilepsy via adaptive neurostimulation: a reinforcement learning approach. *International Journal of Neural Systems* https://doi.org/10.1142/S0129065709001987.

Ponten, S.C., Bartolomei, F., and Stam, C.J. (2007). Small-world networks and epilepsy: graph theoretical analysis of intracerebrally recorded mesial temporal lobe seizures. *Clinical Neurophysiology* https://doi.org/10.1016/j.clinph.2006.12.002.

Prayson, R.A. (2018). Pathology of epilepsy. In: *Practical Surgical Neuropathology: A Diagnostic Approach*, 2e (ed. A. Perry and D.J. Brat), 617–632. Elsevier.

Pugh, J., Pycroft, L., Sandberg, A. et al. (2018). Brainjacking in deep brain stimulation and autonomy. *Ethics and Information Technology* https://doi.org/10.1007/s10676-018-9466-4.

Raghu, S., Sriraam, N., Temel, Y. et al. (2020). EEG based multi-class seizure type classification using convolutional neural network and transfer learning. *Neural Networks* https://doi.org/10.1016/j.neunet.2020.01.017.

Rajnicek, A.M., Gow, N.A., and McCaig, C.D. (1992). Electric field-induced orientation of rat hippocampal neurones in vitro. *Experimental Physiology* https://doi.org/10.1113/expphysiol.1992.sp003580.

Rajnicek, A.M., Foubister, L.E., and McCaig, C.D. (2006). Growth cone steering by a physiological electric field requires dynamic microtubules, microfilaments and Rac-mediated filopodial asymmetry. *Journal of Cell Science* https://doi.org/10.1242/jcs.02897.

Rajnicek, A.M., Foubister, L.E., and McCaig, C.D. (2006). Temporally and spatially coordinated roles for rho, Rac, Cdc42 and their effectors in growth cone guidance by a physiological electric field. *Journal of Cell Science* https://doi.org/10.1242/jcs.02896.

Rijlaarsdam, D., Nuij, P., Schoukens, J., and Steinbuch, M. (2017). A comparative overview of frequency domain methods for nonlinear systems. *Mechatronics* https://doi.org/10.1016/j.mechatronics.2016.12.008.

Rilling, G., Flandrin, P., Gonçalves, P., and Lilly, J.M. (2007). Bivariate Empirical Mode Decomposition. *IEEE Signal Processing Letters* https://doi.org/10.1109/LSP.2007.904710.

Roy, Y., Banville, H., Albuquerque, I. et al. (2019). Deep learning-based electroencephalography analysis: a systematic review. *Journal of Neural Engineering* https://doi.org/10.1088/1741-2552/ab260c.

Samiee, K., Kovacs, P., and Gabbouj, M. (2015). Epileptic seizure classification of EEG time-series using rational discrete short-time Fourier transform. *IEEE Transactions on Biomedical Engineering* https://doi.org/10.1109/TBME.2014.2360101.

Santaniello, S., Fiengo, G., Glielmo, L., and Grill, W.M. (2011). Closed-loop control of deep brain stimulation: a simulation study. *IEEE Transactions on Neural Systems and Rehabilitation Engineering* https://doi.org/10.1109/TNSRE.2010.2081377.

Scheffer, I.E., Berkovic, S., Capovilla, G. et al. (2017). ILAE classification of the epilepsies: position paper of the ILAE Commission for Classification and Terminology. *Epilepsia* https://doi.org/10.1111/epi.13709.

Seng, C.H., Demirli, R., Khuon, L., and Bolger, D. (2012). Seizure detection in EEG signals using support vector machines. In: *2012 38th Annual Northeast Bioengineering Conference (NEBEC)*. https://doi.org/10.1109/NEBC.2012.6207048.

Serb, A., Corna, A., George, R. et al. (2020). Memristive synapses connect brain and silicon spiking neurons. *Scientific Reports* https://doi.org/10.1038/s41598-020-58831-9.

Seth, A.K., Barrett, A.B., and Barnett, L. (2015). Granger causality analysis in neuroscience and neuroimaging. *The Journal of Neuroscience* https://doi.org/10.1523/JNEUROSCI.4399-14.2015.

Shah, V., Von Weltin, E., Lopez, S. et al. (2018). The Temple University Hospital seizure detection corpus. *Frontiers in Neuroinformatics* https://doi.org/10.3389/fninf.2018.00083.

Shahbazi, M. and Aghajan, H. (2018). A generalizable model for seizure prediction based on deep LEARNING USING CNN-LSTM ARCHITECTURE. In: *2018 IEEE Global Conference on Signal and Information Processing (GlobalSIP)*. https://doi.org/10.1109/GlobalSIP.2018.8646505.

Shanir, P.P.M., Khan, K.A., Khan, Y.U. et al. (2018). Automatic seizure detection based on morphological features using one-dimensional local binary pattern on long-term EEG. *Clinical EEG and Neuroscience* https://doi.org/10.1177/1550059417744890.

Shetty, A.K. and Turner, D.A. (1995). Enhanced cell survival in fetal hippocampal suspension transplants grafted to adult rat hippocampus following kainate lesions: a three-dimensional graft reconstruction study. *Neuroscience* https://doi.org/10.1016/0306-4522(95)00025-e.

Shetty, A.K. and Turner, D.A. (1996). Development of fetal hippocampal grafts in intact and lesioned hippocampus. *Progress in Neurobiology* https://doi.org/10.1016/s0301-0082(96)00048-2.

Shetty, A.K. and Turner, D.A. (1997). Development of long-distance efferent projections from fetal hippocampal grafts depends upon pathway specificity and graft location in kainate-lesioned adult hippocampus. *Neuroscience* https://doi.org/10.1016/S0306-4522(96)00413-7.

Sisterson, N.D., Wozny, T.A., Kokkinos, V. et al. (2020). A rational approach to understanding and evaluating responsive Neurostimulation. *Neuroinformatics* https://doi.org/10.1007/s12021-019-09446-7.

Squire, L.R. (2009). The legacy of patient H.M. For neuroscience. *Neuron* https://doi.org/10.1016/j.neuron.2008.12.023.

Supratak, A., Li, L., and Guo, Y. (2014). Feature extraction with stacked autoencoders for epileptic seizure detection. In: *36th Annual International Conference of the IEEE Engineering in Medicine and Biology Society*. https://doi.org/10.1109/EMBC.2014.6944546.

Takagi, Y. (2016). History of neural stem cell research and its clinical application. *Neurologia Medico-Chirurgica* https://doi.org/10.2176/nmc.ra.2015-0340.

Thodoroff, P., Pineau, J., and Lim, A. (2016). Learning robust features using deep learning for automatic seizure detection. *Proceedings of Machine Learning Research* 178–190.

Tomaskovic-Crook, E., Zhang, P., Ahtiainen, A. et al. (2019). Human neural tissues from neural stem cells using conductive biogel and printed polymer microelectrode arrays for 3D electrical stimulation. *Advanced Healthcare Materials* https://doi.org/10.1002/adhm.201900425.

Tribbey, W. (2007). *Numerical Recipes: The Art of Scientific Computing*, 3e (ed. W.H. Press, S.A. Teukolsky, W.T. Vetterling, and B.P. Flannery). Cambridge University Press, hardback, ISBN 978–0–521-88068-8, 1235 p. https://doi.org/10.1145/1874391.187410.

Truong, N.D., Nguyen, A.D., Kuhlmann, L. et al. (2018). Convolutional neural networks for seizure prediction using intracranial and scalp electroencephalogram. *Neural Networks* https://doi.org/10.1016/j.neunet.2018.04.018.

Vassanelli, S. and Mahmud, M. (2016). Trends and challenges in Neuroengineering: toward "intelligent" Neuroprostheses through brain-"brain inspired systems" communication. *Frontiers in Neuroscience* https://doi.org/10.3389/fnins.2016.00438.

Wang, J., Niebur, E., Hu, J., and Li, X. (2016). Suppressing epileptic activity in a neural mass model using a closed-loop proportional-integral controller. *Scientific Reports* https://doi.org/10.1038/srep27344.

Wang, H., Shi, W., and Choy, C.S. (2018). Hardware design of real time epileptic seizure detection based on STFT and SVM. *IEEE Access* https://doi.org/10.1109/ACCESS.2018.2870883.

WHO (2006). *Neurological Disorders: Public Health Challenges*. WHO.

Yao, L., Shanley, L., McCaig, C., and Zhao, M. (2008). Small applied electric fields guide migration of hippocampal neurons. *Journal of Cellular Physiology* https://doi.org/10.1002/jcp.21431.

Yoo, J., Yan, L., El-Damak, D. et al. (2013). An 8-channel scalable EEG acquisition SoC with patient-specific seizure classification and recording processor. *IEEE Journal of Solid-State Circuits* https://doi.org/10.1109/JSSC.2012.2221220.

Yuan, Y., Xun, G., Jia, K., and Zhang, A. (2019). A multi-view deep learning framework for EEG seizure detection. *IEEE Journal of Biomedical and Health Informatics* https://doi.org/10.1109/JBHI.2018.2871678.

Zhang, Z. and Parhi, K.K. (2016). Low-complexity seizure prediction from iEEG/sEEG using spectral power and ratios of spectral power. *IEEE Transactions on Biomedical Circuits and Systems* https://doi.org/10.1109/TBCAS.2015.2477264.

Zhang, C., Altaf, M.A.B., and Yoo, J. (2016). Design and implementation of an on-Chip patient-specific closed-loop seizure onset and termination detection system. *IEEE Journal of Biomedical and Health Informatics* https://doi.org/10.1109/JBHI.2016.2553368.

Zhang, Q., Beirne, S., Shu, K. et al. (2018). Electrical stimulation with a conductive polymer promotes neurite outgrowth and synaptogenesis in primary cortical neurons in 3D. *Scientific Reports* https://doi.org/10.1038/s41598-018-27784-5.

Zheng, Y., Wang, G., Li, K. et al. (2014). Epileptic seizure prediction using phase synchronization based on bivariate empirical mode decomposition. *Clinical Neurophysiology* https://doi.org/10.1016/j.clinph.2013.09.047.

14

Towards Better Ways to Assess Predictive Computing in Medicine: On Reliability, Robustness, and Utility

Federico Cabitza[1,2] and Andrea Campagner[2]

[1]*Department of Computer Science, Systems and Communication, University of Milano-Bicocca, Milan, Italy*
[2]*IRCCS Istituto Ortopedico Galeazzi, Milan, Italy*

14.1 Introduction

Computational classification systems built using machine learning (ML) techniques are increasingly being evaluated and employed in medical settings for a number of purposes and applications, including diagnosis, prognosis, and risk stratification. However, evaluation and validation practices that are commonly used and adopted in the application of ML to other disciplines are unlikely to be meaningfully applicable to medicine.

Indeed, these systems must be proven to bring clinical benefit when fed with real-world data (what we called pragmatic validation) and deployed in real-clinical settings (ecological validation), rather than just being "statistically valid" (what is usually done and reported in scientific reports and articles, in terms of accuracy measures like C-statistics or F-scores) (Cabitza and Zeitoun 2019).

In fact, otherwise, technically sound systems have been found to perform poorly in real settings, a concept that has been termed the "last mile of implementation" (Cabitza et al. 2020b; Coiera 2019) in the specialized literature. Unfortunately, despite its seeming shortness, this "final mile" is not a flat and uniform path, but rather has two chasms, as illustrated in Figure 14.1.

The chasm of human trust, in particular, is the most important impediment to the fulfillment of AI's promise at the point of care, since even the most accurate systems are harmed when clinicians do not trust them due to "prejudice against the machine" (Cabitza 2019). This chasm depicts medical AI's inability, despite its inherent correctness, to have a beneficial influence on clinicians' judgments. This can be due to a poor user interface, due to the fact that good advice arrives late or among several false alarms (Bezemer et al. 2019), or due to the fact that the decision maker is unable to take advantage of the AI due to the emergence of cognitive biases, including automation bias (Lyell and Coiera 2017) or automation complacency (Merritt et al. 2019).

The other chasm, which symbolizes how clinical experience from which ML models may learn is acquired and processed, by contrast, has often been overlooked. In fact, most data scientists would argue that this step is not even necessary: data scientists and ML developers typically assume that the datasets used to train their predictive models – dubbed

Big Data Analysis and Artificial Intelligence for Medical Sciences, First Edition.
Edited by Bruno Carpentieri and Paola Lecca.
© 2024 John Wiley & Sons Ltd. Published 2024 by John Wiley & Sons Ltd.

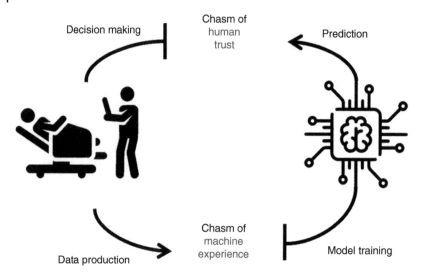

Figure 14.1 The chasms in the "last mile" between medical AI and human agency.

"ground truth" – are (i) accurate, (ii) dependable, and (iii) representative of the target population. This tripartite assumption, however, is seldom tenable and frequently ill-founded, at least to some extent (Cabitza et al. 2019).

As a result, the gap between machine experience and actual care as experienced by doctors represents the difference between actual care as experienced by doctors and its codified representation in the form of data, which is the only input for any machine, no matter how intelligent it is or may ever become. In this chapter, we will touch on three primary factors underlying the above mentioned chasms and discuss their impact on the effective development of medical ML, as well as propose possible solutions (in the forms of metrics, as well as validation practices and frameworks) to address them.

The first factor is that of noise or data reliability (Graber 2013). ML data are often thought of as good and reliable, in particular in regard to their ground truth annotations. This assumption however, ignores, or severely underestimates, the phenomenon of observer variability (also called inter-rater disagreement), that is the degree to which different expert clinicians can disagree in regard to the interpretation of the same cases. Obviously, this variability in data can severely impact and influence the actual reliability and validity of the ML models that are fed with them (Cabitza et al. 2020a). This necessitates the development of metrics that could be used to quantify the quality of data that is used to develop ML models, as well as to take into account the potential impact of data quality problems on ML performance. More in general, this problem implies the need for alternative solutions in ML development (Cabitza et al. 2023): possible such solutions include using different data sets or sets of annotators; carrying out data integration procedures; or renouncing to have a single ML model and instead adopting models that result from the integration of data sources that are given different credibilities based on different experimental evidences.

The second factor is that of meaning. Traditional error-based metrics distinguish between false-negative and false-positive errors, but they do not differentiate between instances on any other dimension[1], such as relevance, diagnostic difficulty, or rarity (Oakden-Rayner et al. 2019; Campagner et al. 2021); or whether accurate results were also found to be inter-pretable by experts (Vellido 2020). Furthermore, these metrics do not weigh results in terms of prediction risk (that is, confidence score): as a result, estimates are produced by assuming not only that the cases are all equivalent for the sake of simplicity, but also that the deci-sions are all equal, even though they are based on very different probability estimates (and often with unknown or low calibration) (Van Calster et al. 2019). All of this necessitates the development of sounder and more complete utility metrics that take these factors into account.

The third factor is that of replicability. Accuracy estimations are based on historical data with features that are often obtained from a single (or a few) institutions involved in the development of the ML model. Several studies have found that when used in different cir-cumstances, even very accurate models report relevant drops in their accuracy (McDermott et al. 2021). The models must then be validated externally, using data from a diverse set of sources that are distinct (in terms of work habits and equipment) from those participat-ing in the creation process (König et al. 2007). To achieve this goal, sound data similarity metrics must become more common and widely applied, allowing researchers to deter-mine whether validation data are similar or different from training and test data, and thus whether accuracy scores are strongly correlated with similarity or not: this means focusing on robustness rather than accuracy.

14.2 On Ground Truth Reliability

As it is well known, ML-based decision support is not directly grounded on rules or knowl-edge elicited by human specialists; rather, these frameworks ground their recommendation on examples and correlations to be detected by means of statistical algorithms within large datasets. By definition, human contribution is required to assemble and label these large datasets, called ground truths in the specialized literature (Beigman Klebanov and Beigman 2009; Beigman and Klebanov 2009; Rajkomar et al. 2019). These characteristics highlight that the the actual performance (i.e. the performance on the true, but unknown, labels) of any ML system is intrinsically connected with and directly depends on the reliability of the ground truth they have been trained on. While in the literature such ground truths are generally assumed to be 100% exact however, recent research work has called attention to that such a perfect ground truth is conceivable just in fictitious settings, as portrayed schematically in Figure 14.2.

As displayed in the Figure 14.2, a solitary, perfectly reliable rater would be adequate to get a 100% precise ground truth. Tragically, human specialists are however fallible: in diag-nostic assignments, the accuracy of clinical specialists goes from 70% to 90% (Brady 2017; Graber 2013; Pinto and Brunese 2010; Quekel et al. 1999). Accordingly, assuming we fully trust these appraisals, a simulation in view of these assessments (see Figure 14.3) confirms the instinctive thought that the more specialists are engaged in the annotation of cases, the

---

1 Here, with the term dimension, we denote some aspect of interest (of either the instances or the ML model) that can, in principle, be measured or quantified.

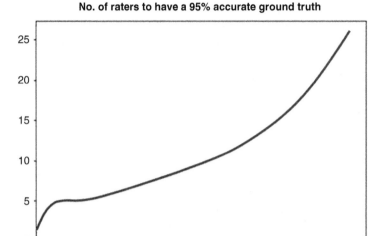

Figure 14.2 The figure depicts (on the *y*-axis) the number of raters that need to be involved to obtain a 95% accurate ground truth, as a function of the average accuracy of the raters involved (on the *x*-axis), if known. These estimates are obtained analytically, and, hence have general application.

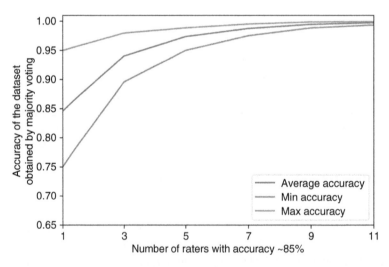

Figure 14.3 The figure depicts the average, minimum, and maximum accuracy of the datasets obtainable for a given number of raters, each with an average accuracy of 85% ± 1%, by simple majority voting among the raters for each case. The three estimates of accuracy were obtained by an analytical simulation, computed through random sampling from a simulated population of 100 individuals with the above mentioned characteristics and by computing, respectively, the average, minimum, and maximum observed value among the extracted samples.

more accurate the subsequent ground truth, when this latter is obtained by applying the strategy of majority (or, plurality) voting, that is essentially allotting to each case the label that has been chosen by most of the involved specialists.

Checking out Figures 14.2 and 14.3 invites a few reflections. To start with, the awful news is that ordinary (i.e. moderately precise) raters will not ever yield a 100% exact ground truth, albeit such a ground truth is commonly assumed to be available in any ML project. On a positive side, these observations confirm that unity is strength: the littlest group of annotators that is able to let a majority emerge (i.e. three raters) is able to improve the accuracy by 8%, compared to the accuracy of the single raters.

Consequently, it is easy to understand that the real accuracy of a ML model is distinct from the "hypothetical" accuracy that is assessed by expecting the ground truth to be perfect. For example, consider a 85% exact ground truth, which has been used to train and test a ML model that was found to be 98% accurate (with respect to the above mentioned, partially flawed, ground truth). While the hypothetical accuracy (that is, 98%) is near flawlessness, its real accuracy would be 83%, taking into account the flawedness of the ground truth: a much lower feat. This latter observation implies that the ML model, rather than being almost perfect, really commits errors nearly as frequently as a six can emerge by rolling a dice.

For the above reasons, determining how to evaluate how "solid" a ground truth is in ML settings is of critical importance, since this reliability influences and defines the reliability of the decision support. This is not an easy task, since this evaluation should be clearly made without any additional reference information. In the literature, the reliability of a ground truth is then understood as the precision or replicability of the process that created the data. In this way, in any multi-rater setting, the reliability of data can then be traced back to the agreement among the raters engaged with creating them.

Along these lines, it is natural to comprehend that the higher the agreement, anything it is, the "sounder" and more solid the ground truth. The simplest method for measuring the agreement in a group of raters is the percent of arrangement (Po), that is the proportion of times the raters concur with respect to the absolute number of joint evaluations. In any case, as is widely known and reported in the specialized literature (Gwet 2011; Hunt 1986), this rate can severely overestimate the agreement, in that raters can also concur by mere coincidence, and not on the grounds that they truly settle on the best way to label a particular case. We call this latter case genuine agreement and the former random agreement. To address this problem, several metrics have been proposed: here, we can recall the Cohen's kappa (for two raters) (Cohen 1960), the Fleiss kappa (for at least three raters) (Fleiss 1971), and Krippendorff's α (Krippendorff 2018). Albeit these measurements embrace a model of randomness so as to distinguish between genuine and random agreement, they present a few limitations, in regard to the types of data they can be applied to, their capacity to work with missing evaluations, or their being undefined for single cases. Besides, they are not exempt from so-called *paradoxes* (Feinstein and Cicchetti 1990; Cicchetti and Feinstein 1990): for example, it is known that the marginal distribution of labels could influence the value of the above mentioned metrics.

Furthermore, agreement is only a single component of reliability, that generally can be understood as a composite construct encompassing also confidence, that is the degree the involved raters are sure of their proposed labels, and competence, that is the performance and accuracy of the involved raters. To this purpose, in the following Section 14.2.1, we will discuss a reliability metrics (Cabitza et al. 2020a) that encompasses the above mentioned distinct dimensions of reliability.

14.2.1 Weighted Reliability

As expressed in the previous Section 14.2, ground truth's reliability can be understood as a composite concept containing the inter-rater agreement, the raters' confidence, and their competence (i.e. the capacity to settle on the ideal choice, overall).

Intuitively, an agreement happens when two raters assign the same label to the same case. We do not know whether a rating is correct, yet we expect that the more agreements (i.e. the more raters assign the same label to the same case) a rating gets, the higher the probability of it being correct, and thus the higher its reliability. However, not all agreements are equivalent, as some of them can arise purely out of coincidence and possibility.

To characterize this distinction, our metric uses the self-rated confidence of the raters in question. In the event that this confidence is high, we expect the raters to expressed their rating out of conviction. Thus, if two raters agree on a rating on which they are strongly confident, we expect their agreement to be genuine, that is, not due to mere chance. In any case, we should likewise think about the competence of the raters, as a method for discerning between agreements on a right label and agreements that are off-base. To this point, we think about the rater's expertise. This can be assessed in numerous ways, both subjectively and quantitatively. In this latter case, a possible proxy of the raters' competence is their average accuracy, e.g. as measured through a particular assessment test or by comparison to the majority voting of the other raters. Regarding Figure 14.4, our technique to measure

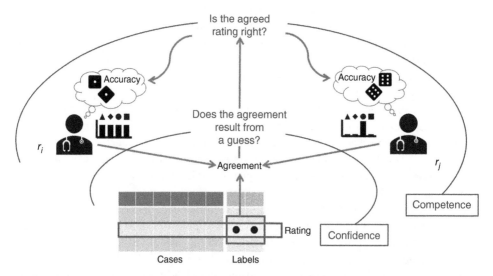

Figure 14.4 Graphical presentation of the general idea of the weighted reliability score, ϱ. This reliability score is multidimensional as it encompasses both the confidence of the raters and their competence. In this graphical example, rater r_i is much less competent than rater r_j, and hence, the probability that her/his rating is correct is lower.

the reliability can be portrayed as going in reverse from a rating on which two raters concur, i.e. an agreement: first, we assess whether, in view of the raters' confidence for the given rating, the agreement is genuine or simply due to chance; second, we consider whether or not the rating is correct, in light of the raters' competence.

Formally, we will assume the following setting: each rater in a group of k provides a label (from a given label set $C = \{1, \ldots, n\}$) to each case x in a dataset S. We denote rater's r_i labeling of case x as $r_i(x)$.

Furthermore, each rater r_i also reports the confidence $c_i(x)$, for each labeled case. Assuming that $c_i(x)$ represents the a-priori probability of having selected the reported label $r_i(x)$ by genuine conviction, the conditional estimate $P(r_i(x)$ genuinely $|r_i(x))$ can be estimated as:

$$\hat{c}_i(x) = \frac{c_i(x)}{c_i(x) + (1 - c_i(x))p(r_i(x))}. \tag{14.1}$$

Thus, given two raters r_i, r_j who have agreed on case x (i.e. $r_i(x) = r_j(x)$), their *Genuine Agreement* (GA) is defined as:

$$GA_x(r_i, r_j) = \begin{cases} 0 & r_i(x) \neq r_j(x) \\ \hat{c}_i(x)\hat{c}_j(x) & \text{otherwise} \end{cases}. \tag{14.2}$$

Then, the genuine agreement is defined as the average of GA both case-wise:

$$GA(x, R) = \binom{n}{2}^{-1} \sum_{r_i \neq r_j \in R} GA_x(r_i, r_j), \tag{14.3}$$

where the factor $\binom{n}{2}^{-1} = \frac{2(n-2)!}{n!}$ is the number of pairs of raters in R, and over the whole sample S (i.e. S is the set of all cases), that is:

$$GA(S, R) = \frac{1}{|S|} \sum_{x \in S} GA(x, R). \tag{14.4}$$

Thus far, we only considered the *agreement* aspect of our definition of reliability; we then have to discount the obtained reliability score by the raters' competence. To this aim, let $\widehat{acc}_i$ be an estimate of rater i accuracy. As previously mentioned, this latter can be set either on the basis of the empirical accuracy of the rater estimated on an another dataset sample, which would however provide the same value $\widehat{acc}_i$ for each x; or on the basis of a model-based estimation, such as the Rasch model (Rasch 1980). Thus, having an estimate of each rater's accuracy on each case, the probability that an observed agreement is correct is computed as $P(r_i(x), r_j(x) \text{ correct}) = \frac{\widehat{acc}_i * \widehat{acc}_j}{\widehat{acc}_i\widehat{acc}_j + (1 - \widehat{acc}_i)(1 - \widehat{acc}_j)}$.

Therefore, from the dataset-wise genuine agreement, we finally define the *weighted reliability score*, or ϱ, which also takes into account the accuracy of the raters and is defined at both the single case and whole dataset level:

$$\varrho(x, R) = \binom{m}{2}^{-1} \sum_{r_i \neq r_j \in R} GA_x(r_i, r_j) \cdot P(r_i(x), r_j(x) \text{ correct}), \tag{14.5}$$

$$\varrho(S, R) = \frac{1}{|S|} \sum_{x \in S} \varrho(x, R). \tag{14.6}$$

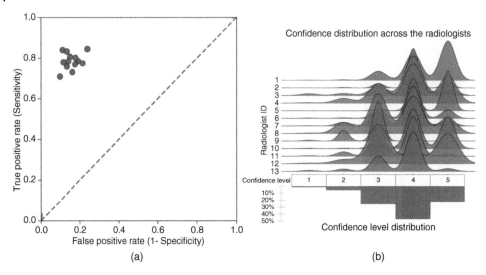

Figure 14.5 Results in graphical form. (a) The raters' performance in the ROC (receiver operating curve) space: Circles represent single raters. The red line represents random guessing. (b) Joyplot and histogram illustrating the raters' confidence distributions.

14.2.2 Example Application

To illustrate use of our metrics and depict the various aspects that could influence the ground truth quality in a multi-rater setting, we describe the results of a user study in which we involved radiology specialists in a ground truthing task, where they were invited to detect abnormalities in knee magnetic resonance imaging (MRI) images. In particular, we asked 13 radiologists in Italy to label 417 MRIs obtained from the MRNet dataset (Bien et al. 2018)[2]. For every one of these pictures, the doctors were approached to evaluate: the presence of abnormalities (hence, it was a binary classification setting) and their confidence in the provided diagnosis, on a five-levels ordinal scale. These information additionally used to assess the discriminative capability of the raters in terms of accuracy, by contrasting their evaluations and the MRNet ground truth.

The accuracy and distribution of the reported confidence values, for every one of the radiologists, are displayed in Figure 14.5a and b.

As respects the confidence communicated by the clinical specialists, we note that all the involved radiologists could be considered as experts in their profession, with some of them having over 20 years of day-to-day practice. Thus, it is not surprising that their confidence in the evaluations was by and large high, with four (out of five) being the level most often referenced (see Figure 14.5b). Nonetheless, as a first perception, we saw that being certain about a rating did not mean being also correct about it: Figure 14.6 shows this inconsistency, where 57% of wrong labels were related with the highest levels of confidence. This first result shows that confidence and accuracy are complementary aspects that can both affect the reliability of a multi-rater ground truth.

---

2 https://stanfordmlgroup.github.io/rivalries/mrnet/.

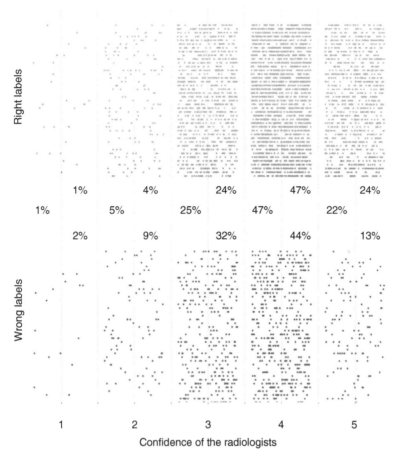

Figure 14.6 Results in graphical format: the distribution of the labels in terms of right/wrong annotation, with respect to the confidence levels. For each confidence level, the percentages in the left column indicate the confidence level proportion with respect to all the cases; the top and bottom percentages in the right column indicate the proportions of right (respectively wrong) labels in the corresponding confidence level.

In regard to agreement, we saw that for 322 cases (75%), the radiologists reached a statistically significant majority (i.e. 10 or more of them settled on the same rating, out of 13). In any case, as to 61 cases (14%), the majority of the raters picked the wrong label (w.r.t. the MRNet ground truth). In those cases, majority voting would prompt an error. Significantly more shockingly, in 41% of these last option cases (25 or 6% of the total amount of cases), the wrong majority was statistically significant. These results, similarly show that agreement and accuracy provide complementary information about the reliability of a multi-rater ground truth. The weighted reliability among the 13 radiologists ϱ was 0.58, when considering the reported and accuracy of the raters, and 0.45, when using the accuracy estimates based on the Rasch model (Rasch 1980). By contrast, both Krippendorff's α

(Krippendorff 2018) and Fleiss' k (Fleiss 1971) were significantly higher, with a value of 0.63, and closer to percent of agreement $P_o = 0.82$.

14.3 On Utility Metrics to Evaluate ML Performance

In the previous section, we focused on the concept of ground truth reliability: while this latter concept is mostly concerned with data quality, it also has an impact on the evaluation and validation of ML models, as we discussed in the previous Section 14.2. In this section, we will go further in details with respect to this latter aspect, by contesting that commonly used performance metrics are general enough to properly take into account all the relevant quality dimensions for clinical AI evaluation.

Indeed, in the literature, numerous metrics have been proposed for the purpose of evaluating ML models (Sokolova and Lapalme 2009; Vickers et al. 2016). In the clinical setting, the most widely recognized metrics depend on error rate: these include the accuracy, sensitivity, specificity, the $F1$ score, and the area under the receiver operating curve (AUROC or essentially AUC). Less ordinarily, utility-based metrics have also been proposed and applied: these are expected to display, as well as illuminate the human users about the ability of a ML system to limit harms (dually, boost benefits), in view of user-defined utility scales. In this light, here, we notice the net benefit (Vickers and Elkin 2006), and its standardized version (Kerr et al. 2016), as well as the relative utility (Baker et al. 2009).

Despite the fact that the previous class of metrics (and, specifically, the accuracy and the AUROC) have become progressively more well known for the assessment of ML-based emotionally supportive networks, there are issues with using them as quality criteria (Berner 2003). For example, error rate-based measurements can be misleading in imbalanced settings (Valverde-Albacete and Peláez-Moreno 2014; Briggs and Zaretzki 2008; Chicco et al. 2021). While utility-based metrics are more resistant to these issues, also these metrics nonetheless suffer from relevant limitations, as they disregard significant information that is nonetheless of critical relevance for quality assessment of ML systems: these include *hidden stratifications* (Oakden-Rayner et al. 2019) (i.e. subgroups of the data, whose characteristics are so different that a given ML model could perform differently on them); the perceptions and preferences of the clinicians and patients involved in the decision-making process; or the effects (both positive and negative) of the ML decision support on the whole decisional process: all these aspect could impact on the overall significance of accurately distinguishing various cases and, therefore, failing to take them into account could undermine the conclusions on the performance of a ML model. To address these limitations, in the following Section 14.3.1, we describe how to extend the net benefit to a more general utility-based metrics, called *weighted utility* (Campagner et al. 2021), that can better account for the above mentioned aspects.

14.3.1 Weighted Utility

Let $S = \langle x_1 \ldots, x_n \rangle$ be a dataset where $x_i \in X$ is an instance. As in the previous Section 14.2 on reliability, we assume that the dataset to be used to evaluate the ML model under consideration has been labeled by a set of raters $d_1, \ldots, d_m$, producing a set of binary annotations, denoted as $d_i^j \in \{0,1\}$: the label provided by rater d_j on case x_i. Note that we consider only binary classification problems: we associate *normality* with class 0, and *abnormality* (e.g. *presence of disease, treatment required*) with class 1. To each case x_i we also associate a target label $y_i \in \{0,1\}$, which represents the correct (i.e. the true) label for case x_i. We do not make any specific assumptions about how y_i is obtained: it could derive from an additional assessment (e.g. an objective examination) or could be obtained by majority voting from the raters' labels, as described in the previous Section 14.2.

Let h be a ML model that provides, for each x_i a confidence score $h(x_i)$, representing the probability that x_i belongs to the positive class.

Let $\mathbf{r} : X \mapsto [0,1]$ be a *relevance* function: intuitively, $\mathbf{r}(x_i)$ measures "how relevant it is that the model h correctly classifies x_i." While in practical contexts r could represent some specific properties of instances, e.g. their complexity or rarity, we assume a more general setting in which r is simply an abstract weight function.

Since, as we mentioned before, the metrics we discuss in this section starts from and extends the net benefit, for each decision maker d_j, we consider a *hesitation cutoff* $\tau_j : X \mapsto [0,1]$: the value $\tau_j(x_i)$ is the confidence score at which d_j would be uncertain between assigning any of the two labels to x. As a consequence, if $h(x) \geq \tau_j(x_i)$ then x_i is assigned to the positive class, while the opposite case (i.e. $h(x) < \tau_j(x_i)$) x_i would be assigned to the negative class. The hesitation cutoff can be associated with a utility-based interpretation, defined based on the the benefit (resp. cost) of the course of action associated with the positive class (e.g. in the medical case, further exams or any intervention), as estimated by the decision maker d_j, for case x_i (Vickers and Elkin 2006).

Grounding on the above defined elements, the *weighted utility* of a model h with respect to a ground truth S is defined as:

$$wU(\tau, \mathbf{r}, S, h, d_1, \dots, d_m) =$$

$$\frac{1}{m} \sum_{j=1}^{m} \left(\frac{1}{\Delta^j \mathbf{r}(\text{Pos})} \sum_{x_i : y_i = 1} \mathbf{r}(x_i) \cdot \mathbb{1}_{h(x_i) \geq \tau_j(x_i)} \cdot \delta_i^{j+} \right. \tag{14.7}$$

$$\left. - \frac{1}{\Delta^j \mathbf{r}(\text{Pos})} \sum_{x_i : y_i = 0} \mathbf{r}(x_i) \cdot \mathbb{1}_{h(x_i) \geq \tau_j(x_i)} \cdot \delta_i^{j-} \right).$$

where:

$$\mathbf{r}(\text{Pos}) = \sum_{x_i : y_i = 1} \mathbf{r}(x_i) \tag{14.8}$$

$$\delta_i^{j+} = \mathbb{1}_{d_i^j = y_i = 1} + \alpha \cdot \mathbb{1}_{d_i^j \neq y_i = 1} \tag{14.9}$$

$$\delta_i^{j-} = \frac{\tau_j(x_i)}{1 - \tau_j(x_i)} \cdot (\mathbb{1}_{d_i^j = y_i = 0} + \beta \cdot \mathbb{1}_{d_i^j \neq y_i = 0}) \tag{14.10}$$

$$\Delta^j = \sum_i \delta_i^{j+} \tag{14.11}$$

with $\alpha \geq 1$ and $0 \leq \beta < 1$, and $\mathbb{1}_P$ being the indicator function for the predicate P (i.e. the function which is equal to 1 when P is true and 0 otherwise). We note that $wU \in [-\infty, 1]$. Here, we describe the intuitive meaning of the different components in the definition of the wU:

- $\mathbf{r}(\text{Pos})$ represents the total relevance of the true positive instances;
- δ_i^{j+} represents the benefit that rater d_j would have, on case $(x_i, y_i = 1)$, by following the correct advice of the model on a positive case. In particular, if $d_i^j = y_i$ then this benefit is equal to 1, otherwise it is equal to $\alpha > 1$. Thus, intuitively, α represents the benefit of using a model that is able to correct the rater: the higher the value of α, the more we would consider the model useful;
- δ_i^{j-} represents the cost that rater d_j would incur on, for case $(x_i, y_i = 0)$, by following the incorrect advice of the model on a negative case. In particular, if $d_i^j = y_i$ then this cost is equal to 1, otherwise it is equal to $\beta < 1$. Thus, intuitively, $\frac{1}{\beta}$ represents the cost of automation bias: the lower the value of β, the more we penalize the model when it would deceive the decision maker into making a wrong decision;
- Δ^j, for rater j, is simply the sum of the terms δ_i^{j+}, for each case i. That is, Δ^j represents the total benefit of following the (correct) advice of the model on the positive cases. This factor is simply a normalization term to ensure that the range of wU is $[-\infty, 1]$.

In regard to the interpretation of the wU, we first note that the utility of h is essentially defined as the average of the utilities for the raters $d_1, \ldots, d_m$.

Second, as in the definition of the net benefit, utility is characterized as the difference between the normalized and weighted true positive rate and the normalized and weighted false positive rate: naturally a decision support is valuable assuming the times it is right is higher than the times it is wrong.

Furthermore, true positive cases are weighted for their (case-wise) relevance ($\mathbf{r}(x_i)$), as this is seen by the ground-truth raters. Cases are viewed as positive or negative as indicated by the confidence scores given by the classifier. A similar rationale applies likewise to the "false positive" part of the formula: to this regard, however, we additionally consider the impact (i.e. the cost) associated with following an incorrect advice, e.g. overdiagnosis and over-treatment, as determined by the hesitation cutoff (τ).

Lastly, the coefficients α and β (and, consequently $\delta_i^{j+}, \delta_i^{j-}$) represent one additional weighting, which depends on the *decisional impact* of the model (i.e. the impact that the model may have, and the costs that it could incur, based on actual decisions to be taken). With respect to α, it may be seen that the point of this coefficient is to value more cases for which a rater proposed a mistaken decision which was then amended by the ML model. In this manner, α quantifies the intuitive understanding that a model which can address the blunders of the raters is more valuable than one which just affirms their right decisions. On the other hand, β fills the need of further punishing incorrect suggestions provided by the ML model for which the decision maker's decision was rather right. Thus, β allows to model the notion of *automation bias*, that is the adverse impact that a support system could have on the decision making process.

With respect to the semantics of wU, we recall that wU is defined in the range $[-\infty, 1]$. As it is common in utility-based evaluation, if wU is greater than 0 than the evaluated model can provide at least some minimum benefit; while a value lower than 0 can be related with a model that has a negative impact 100% of the time.

14.3.2 Example Application

In this section, we report on an experiments that we directed to illustrate the applicability of the proposed metrics for model assessment. The experiment grounded on a user-study, by which we involved 13 board-certified radiologists to annotate a sample of 417 cases obtained from the MRNet dataset[3], that has been already described in the previous sections. We recall that we asked 13 radiologists to label the above mentioned MRNet cases in regard to whether these latter were affected by some abnormality (specifically, an anterior cruciate ligament (ACL) or meniscal tear), or not. The radiologists were additionally mentioned to survey each case in regard to its complexity, on a five-level ordinal scale, and the confidence with which they annotated the case, on a six-level ordinal scale.

The complexity and confidence evaluations of the elaborate clinicians were then utilized, respectively, to characterize the case-wise *relevance function* **r** and the case-wise likelihood threshold τ.

To show the use of the wU metric, we developed a deep learning model, namely a ResNet-50 convolutional neural network model to discriminate between abnormal cases and typical cases. The training set was an assortment of MRI tests taken from the MRNet dataset that were not given to the radiologists: the ML model was trained on 953 individual tests, every one of which was made out of a variable number of pictures. The ML model was then assessed on the 417 relabeled pictures utilizing various measurements, to be specific the accuracy, balanced accuracy, AUROC, (normalized) net benefit and the *weighted utility*.

As respects the *relevance*, we just utilized the average of the complexity ratings, for each case, standardized so to map their values in [0,1]. As respects the case-wise τ values, we adopted the following definition (based on the raters' reported confidence values), which requires the model's probability score to be higher than the probability that the raters assigned to the negative class:

$$\tau_j(x_i) = \begin{cases} \frac{c_j(x_i)+1}{2} & d_i^j = 0 \\ \frac{1-c_j(x_i)}{2} & d_i^j = 1 \end{cases}$$

where $d_i^j \in \{0,1\}$ is the label reported by rater d_j for case x_i, $c_j(x_i) \in [0,1]$ is the (normalized) confidence reported by rater d_j for case x_i.

The performance of the raters and of the ML model is reported in Figure 14.7. The average perceived case complexity was 0.70 (95% C.I [0.69, 0.71], IQR [0.63, 0.77]), the average τ was 0.55 (95% C.I. [0.52, 0.58], IQR [0.17, 0.85]). The performance of the AI model, in terms of wU and other metrics, is reported in Figure 14.8.

---

3 https://stanfordmlgroup.github.io/contests/mrnet/.

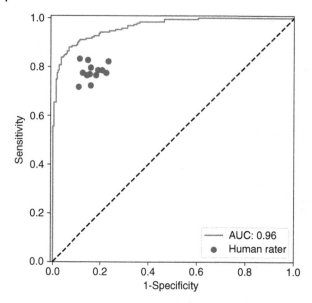

Figure 14.7 Performance of the raters and of the AI model, in the ROC space. The AI model outperforms the human raters on each operating point of the ROC space.

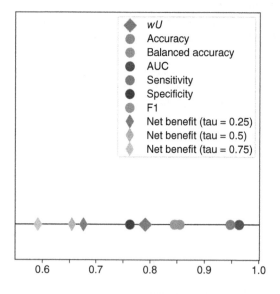

Figure 14.8 The performance of the AI model, in terms of the three different versions of *wU*, and a collection of other pertinent metrics.

14.4 On the Replicability of Clinical ML Models

In the last Section 14.3, we discussed the definition of a more comprehensive metrics for the validation of ML models, and we argued that its increased flexibility, in particular in regard to the ability to take into account different information about the validation setting, could provide a more reliable indication of a model's performance. Nonetheless, in our treatment we focused on the metrics itself, rather than on the validation process, which also must take into account the appropriateness of the data, that is used for validating the model with respect to the task at hand, and of the validation process itself.

In the expert writing, the validation of ML models is frequently intended and implemented as internal validation (Zhang et al. 2020): this alludes to validation conventions, including, for example hold-out testing, bootstrap or cross-validation, that aim to gauge the performance of the ML models by testing it on a part of the original dataset separate that was not used to develop the model itself (Kim 2009; Vabalas et al. 2019). This class of approaches has led the specialized literature to focus on but a single element to survey the sufficiency of the validation technique, in particular the size of the dataset utilized, or its cardinality (Riley et al. 2021). However, sample cardinality alone is not by itself adequate for understanding the dependability of a validation technique. Indeed, while internal validation techniques are generally utilized, particularly as a result of their convenience, they are not viewed as an adequate proof-of-validity in critical settings, similar to the clinical one (Bleeker et al. 2003; Steyerberg and Harrell Jr. 2016). In these settings, ML models should be robust, that is they should reliably work also in settings more or less similar to the one from which the training data has been obtained (Cabitza and Campagner 2021; Hernandez-Boussard et al. 2020). This necessity is expected either in light of the fact that the model should be deployed in a different (but related) setting, as it is the situation of clinical ML models that are to be sent in numerous medical clinics or nations (Futoma et al. 2020); or on the grounds that the data to be given as input to the model in day-to-day use could ultimately be affected by distribution shifts or drifts (Huggard et al. 2020).

Accordingly, in critical settings, external validation has been pushed as being of critical importance (Bleeker et al. 2003; Steyerberg and Harrell Jr. 2016). External data, in this setting, allude to the use of new data that come from different cohorts, facilities, or databases other than the data utilized for model creation. Frequently, performance on external datasets is largely worse than performance appraised on the development datasets, so that external validation practices aim to help users answer the following question about a ML model: will its performance be reproduced reliably across various settings?

In what follows, we will share an overall strategy to evaluate the sufficiency of an external validation procedure establishing on two ideas: dataset cardinality and dataset similarity.

14.4.1 Dataset Size

As described in the previous Section 14.4, high-quality ML studies expect that external validation is performed, to evaluate the ability of a current model to sum up across various destinations, and consequently to give a solid and reproducible estimate of its performance. To this aim, the sample size of the external validation datasets is an element of critical importance (Vergouwe et al. 2005): little sample sizes can bring about uncertain or excessively hopeful performance estimates.

Consequently, it is relevant to determine whether a sample size is adequately large to perform sound external validations, that is to decide a minimum sample size (MSS) adequate to ensure the generalizability of the consequences of an external validation strategy. In what follows, we portray the equations and calculation techniques for the MSS for the AUC, the Standardized Net Benefit and the Brier score. These three performance metrics aim to quantify three different aspects of model performance, to be specific discrimination power, utility and calibration (respectively). In particular, the AUC is a measure of discrimination power, which quantifies the average sensitivity of a model across different levels of specificity; the Standardized Net Benefit (Vickers et al. 2016) is a measure of utility, which quantifies a trade-off between true and false positives weighed by the cost of such errors; while the Brier score (Brier 1950) is a measure of calibration, which quantifies the deviation between predicted probabilities and actual, observed frequencies. Specifically, concerning the AUC and the Standardized Net Benefit, we take on the equations for MSS assessment proposed by Riley et al. (2021). Then again, for the Brier score, we take on the equation for MSS assessment proposed by Bradley et al. (2008). We note that we focus on the Standardized Net Benefit as a measure of utility, rather than the wU that we introduced in the previous sections: we decided to adopt the former in the following as the corresponding formulas for MSS assessment are available in the literature. Nonetheless, also the wU described in the previous section could be used for this purpose, e.g. by estimating the MSS via simulation approaches (Riley et al. 2021).

In regard to the AUC, let C be the AUC of the ML model on the external validation set, Φ be the proportion of the positive class in the external validation set, and SE(C) the targeted value of the standard error for C. Then, fixed a value for SE(C) (which determines the size of the confidence interval associated with the MSS), the MSS for the AUC can be computed according to the following formula (Riley et al. 2021):

MSS(AUC) = min $n \in \mathbb{N}$ s.t.

$$SE(C) \leq \sqrt{\frac{C(1-C)\left(1+(n/2-1)\frac{1-C}{2-C}+\frac{n/2-1}{1+C}\right)}{n^2\Phi(1-\Phi)}}. \tag{14.12}$$

In regard to the Standardized Net Benefit, let sNB_τ be the Standardized Net Benefit of the ML model on the external validation set (at fixed probability threshold τ), Φ be the proportion of the positive class in the external validation set, *Sens* (resp. *Spec*) the sensitivity (resp. specificity) of the ML model on the external validation dataset, SE(sNB_τ) the targeted valued of the standard error for sNB_τ, and $w = \frac{(1-\phi)\tau}{\phi(1-\tau)}$. Then, fixed a value for SE(sNB_τ) (which determines the size of the confidence interval associated with the MSS), the MSS for the Standardized Net Benefit can be computed according to the following formula (Riley et al. 2021):

$$MSS(sNB) = \frac{\frac{Sens(1-Sens)}{\phi} + \frac{w^2 Spec(1-Spec)}{1-\phi} + \frac{w^2(1-Spec)^2}{\phi(1-\phi)}}{SE(sNB_\tau)^2}. \tag{14.13}$$

Lastly, in regard to the Brier score, let B be the Brier score of the ML model on the external validation set, p_i the predicted probability score for the i-th case in the external validation set, y_i the true target class for the i-th case in the external validation set, n the cardinality of the external validation set, ϵ be the targeted size of the confidence interval associated with the MSS. Then, the SE(B) and the MSS can be estimated from the external validation dataset as:

$$SE(B) = \frac{1}{n}\sum_i p_i^4 - \frac{4}{n}\sum_i p_i^3 y_i + \frac{6}{n}\sum_i p_i^2 y_i - \frac{4}{n}\sum_i p_i y_i + \sum_i p_i - B^2, \tag{14.14}$$

$$MSS(B) = \left(\frac{2 \cdot t_\epsilon \cdot SE(B)}{0.05}\right)^2, \tag{14.15}$$

where t_ϵ is the ϵ-critical value for a Student's t distribution with $n-1$ degrees of freedom.

14.4.2 Dataset Similarity

The connection between data similarity and generalization properties of ML models was first proposed by Bousquet et al. Bousquet (2008), showing that data about similarity could be valuable to comprehend the reason why a ML model performs inadequately on an external validation set (Kouw et al. 2019). Here, we adopt the *Degree of Correspondance* (Ψ) proposed in Cabitza et al. (2020c), since this latter technique has been shown to be more robust compared to other proposed alternatives (Bousquet 2008; Schat et al. 2020). The procedure to compute the *Degree of Correspondance* is reported in Algorithm 1 as a reference. Intuitively, the Degree of Correspondance Ψ measures the similarity between two datasets by comparing the respective distributions of pairwise distances between instances distributions is defined as the p-value for a multi-variate topological test for equality of distributions. A Python implementation of this algorithm is available on GitHub[4] and a sandbox is provisionally running online[5].

Algorithm 14.1 The algorithm procedure to compute the similarity between the two dataset T and V, using the *Degree of Correspondance* (Ψ).

> **procedure** $\Psi(T, V$: datasets, d: distance, ∂ deviation metrics)
>> $d_T = \{d(t, t') : t, t' \in T\}$
>> For each $v \in V$, find $t_v \in T$, nearest neighbor of v in T
>> $T_{|V} = \{t \in T : \nexists v \in V \text{ s.t. } t = t_v\} \cup V$
>> $d_{T_{|V}} = \{d(t, t') : t, t' \in T_{|V}\}$
>> $\delta = \partial(d_T, d_{T_{|V}})$
>> Compute $\Psi = Pr(\delta' \geq \delta)$ using a permutation procedure
>> **return** Ψ
> **end procedure**

14.4.3 Meta-Validation Procedure

Grounding on both the dataset cardinality and the dataset similarity metrics discussed in the previous Section 14.4.2, here, we discuss a lean validation methodology, which encompasses two different steps. The initial step is pointed toward getting a first gauge of the robustness of the ML model, understood as the correlation between its performance and the dis(similarity) among training and (internal) test sets. Hence, the first step doesn't need an external validation dataset and could be performed by taking advantage of a cross validation, or bootstrap, strategy.

In this step, a linear regression should be derived by modeling the relationship between dataset similarity (as measured by the Degree of Correspondance presented above) as an explanatory variable and any balanced performance metric of choice (e.g. balanced accuracy, that is the average of sensitivity and specificity; F-score; AUC) as a dependent variable. The objective of this model is to give ML designers instructive clues about how data heterogeneity can impact on the performance of the model and, thus, its robustness. This information is conveyed by three different, however related, components of the linear model: the

---

4 https://github.com/AndreaCampagner/qualiMLpy/.
5 https://psicorrespondence.pythonanywhere.com/.

correlation coefficient (r, together with the associated p-value and statistical significance status); the coefficient of determination (that is, R^2); and the angular coefficient (b). The correlation coefficient quantifies the effect of dataset similarity on model generalizability: low correlation values suggest higher generalizability, while higher correlation values may be used to infer a more significant impact of dataset heterogeneity on the reproducibility of the model's outcomes. In this respect, one could adopt some commonly used convention to interpret correlation coefficients (Cohen 2013). The correlation coefficient can also be interpreted by means of its relationship with the coefficient of determination R^2, which is given by $R^2 = r^2$. Thus, making reference to the conventions described in Cohen (1960), strong correlations are those for which the linear model is able to clarify something like one fourth of the variation in model performance by variations in the similarity between datasets. Furthermore, the connection between r and b (given by the equation $b = r\frac{\sigma_y}{\sigma_x}$) can be utilized to determine a graphical portrayal of the "strength" of the connection between dataset similarity and model performance, as indicated by the chart addressed in Figure 14.9, which we call the potential robustness diagram, a kind of expanded scatterplot.

In this graph, the top half shows a scatterplot of the connection between dataset similarity and model performance, obtained through the previously mentioned methodology. The bottom half shows four "correlation regions," which permit to characterize the strength of the observed correlation: low angular coefficients can be understood as signs of model robustness against variability, as they correspond to either weak or absent correlation. Conversely, high angular coefficients would allude to a possibly significant effect of data variability on the performance and robustness of the ML model.

The second step of the meta-validation system, then again, relies on the availability of one of more external validation datasets (and the more datasets, the better). This step has the

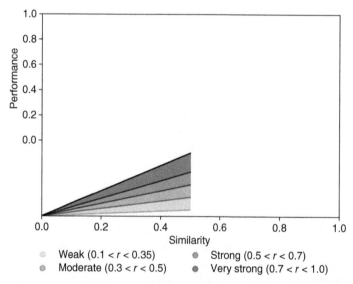

Figure 14.9 The *potential robustness diagram*, proposed to support the proposed meta-validation methodology at step 1. The empty top panel should represent a scatter plot of the similarity and performance relationship.

goal of providing a holistic view over the performance of the ML model, by considering two distinct aspects: dataset similarity (between the external validation dataset and the training set of the ML model); and dataset cardinality, in terms of adequacy of the size of the external validation datasets. The performance of the ML model is assessed in terms of discrimination power, calibration and utility, three elements of equivalent significance in the complete assessment of a model quality (Cabitza and Campagner 2021). This second step aims then to produce a meta-assessment of the validation procedure, so as to understand if this latter is sufficiently sound and conservative. This assessment is performed by means of a graphical portrayal of the previously mentioned data as displayed in Figure 14.10, that we call the external performance diagram. This diagram permits to portray, for any external validation dataset considered, whether or not the dataset meets (or surpasses) the MSS; together with

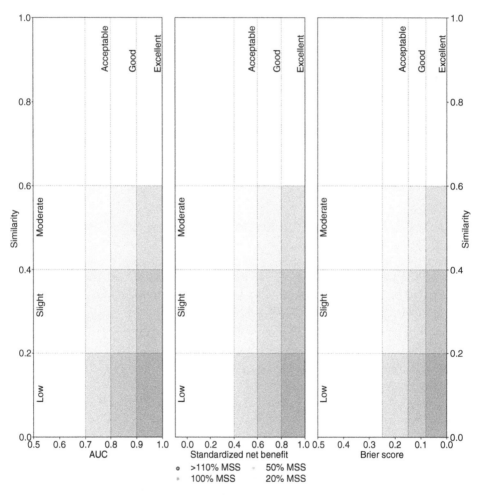

Figure 14.10 The *external performance diagram*, proposed to support the meta-validation procedure at step 2. Each panel represents the relationship between dataset similarity and a dimension of performance (discrimination power, in terms of AUC; utility, in terms of Standardized Net Benefit; and calibration, in terms of Brier score.

a quantitative measurement of the above mentioned quality dimensions (namely, discrimination power, in terms of the AUC; model utility, in terms of the Net Benefit; and model calibration, in terms of the Brier score) in light of the observed dataset similarity.

So as to adopt a consistent naming convention in regard to the dataset similarity, measured by means of the Degree of Correspondance, we adopt a nomenclature inspired by Landis and Koch Landis and Koch (1977), which is illustrated in the proposed diagram. Thus, a similarity higher than 60% (i.e. significant or fundamental) should make users and developers careful about the utility of such a validation strategy to inform about the genuine replicability of the model performance. Then again, great performance displayed by the model on external datasets that are under 40% similarity (slight or low similarity) should be viewed as adequate in providing a conservative estimate of model performance.

A similar terminology is likewise embraced concerning the model performance. Specifically, as for the AUC, values higher than 0.7 are considered acceptable [42]; while values higher than 0.8, or 0.9 as, respectively, good and excellent. Similar thresholds are also adopted for the (Standardized) Net Benefit and the Brier score.

All of these information pieces are represented in the external performance diagram. Specifically, in every one of the three figures in the diagram, the bottom regions correspond to the area of low similarity: if an external validation set falls into this area, the validation can be viewed as sufficiently conservative; in addition, if the performance of the model on this same dataset falls into the right-bottom region, the validation procedure can be considered as providing a good indication of model reproducibility.

14.4.4 Example Application

In what follows, we illustrate an experiment to illustrate the proposed meta-validation procedure. To this reason, we depict our experience on the external validation of a best in class COVID-19 analytic model (Cabitza et al. 2021a).

This ML model was created based on a training set incorporating 1736 cases and 21 features, gathered at the IRCCS Hospital San Raffaele (HSR) and IRCCS Istituto Ortopedico Galeazzi (IOG). The data were gathered between March 5, 2020, and May 26, 2020, that is during the main peak of the COVID-19 pandemic in Northern Italy.

We performed eight different external validations based on as many external datasets, to be specific:

- The Italy-1 dataset, gathered at the Desio Hospital in March/April 2020 and including 337 cases (163 positive, 174 negative);
- The Italy-2 dataset, gathered at the "Father Giovanni XXIII" Hospital of Bergamo in March/April 2020 and including 249 cases (104 positive, 145 negative);
- The Italy-3 dataset, gathered at the IRCCS HSR in November 2020 and including 224 cases (118 positive, 106 negative);
- The Spain dataset, gathered at the University Hospital Santa Lucia in Cartagena in October 2020 and including 120 cases (78 positive, 42 negative);
- The Brazil-3 datasets: The first dataset, Brazil-1, was gathered in the Fleury private clinics; while the other 2 datasets, Brazil-2 and Brazil-3, were gathered at the Albert

Einstein Israelite Hospital and the Hospital Sirio-Libanes. The datasets included, respectively, 1301 (352 positive, 949 negative), 2335 (375 positive, 1960 negative) and 345 (334 positive, 11 negative) cases, gathered between February 2020 and June 2020;

- The Ethiopia dataset, gathered at the National Reference Laboratory for Clinical Chemistry (Millenium COVID-19 Treatment and Care Center) of the Ethiopian Public Health Institute in Addis Ababa, between January and March 2021 and including 400 cases (200 positive, 200 negative).

The datasets, also in terms of their characteristics and features, are further described in Cabitza et al. (2021b) and are openly accessible on Zenodo[6].

In regard to the ML model, we validated a pipelined model including: a missing data imputation step (using K-Nearest Neighbors (Cover and Hart 1967)); a data standardization step; and a RBF support vector machine (Cortes and Vapnik 1995) classification model. As described in Cabitza et al. (2021a), this model was trained on a dataset including 1736 examples and 21 features, gathered at the HSR and IOG emergency clinics, and with an AUC of 0.76.

As mentioned above, the aim of the experiment was to illustrate the application of the proposed meta-validation procedure. To this reason, we performed two trials, to represent the two stages of the previously mentioned procedure. To start with, we thought about the initial step of the procedure, through a reproduction test in which we created from the first training dataset 100 random and 2 nonrandom (in particular, utilizing the data gathered at the HSR during March/April as training set, and the data gathered at the HSR during May, as well as the data gathered at the IOG, as test sets) hold-out parts. Second, we thought about the second step of the procedure, through the assessment of the above mentioned ML model on the eight external validation datasets.

As per the first step of the proposed system, we assessed the relationship between similarity and the accuracy of the ML model. The outcomes are accounted for in the potential robustness diagram, displayed in Figure 14.11.

The top portion of this chart reports a scatterplot of the 100 randomly sampled datasets: the average similarity was 0.43 ± 0.006, while the average was 0.76 ± 0.004. Specifically, the IOG portion of the dataset was viewed as significantly different from the remainder of the training set, with a similarity of only 0.1 and an accuracy of 0.70, while the data gathered at the HSR during May 2020 had a similarity of 0.43 and an accuracy of 0.82. The base portion of Figure 14.11 reports the regression line describing the relationship between accuracy and similarity. The dataset similarity and accuracy were moderately related (Pearson $\rho = 0.38$) and the connection was statistically significant ($p < 0.001$). The regression model had an angular coefficient of $b = 0.03$ and an intercept of $a = 0.76$, with $R^2 = 0.14$.

Concerning the second step of the procedure, we assessed the ML model on 8 external validation datasets. The performance of the ML model on the external validation datasets, in terms of the AUC, the Net Benefit and the Brier score, is reported in Figure 14.12.

The discriminative performance of the model (in terms of AUC) was generally good for most external datasets (for all datasets except the Spain dataset the AUC was higher

---

6 https://zenodo.org/record/4958146#.YMjK0kzONPY.

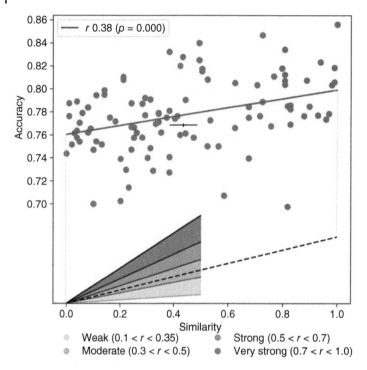

Figure 14.11 The *potential robustness diagram*, displaying the results of the "simulation of generalizability" step (i.e. step 1) for the study on the COVID-19 diagnosis. The correlation, shown by the dotted line, is moderate and statistically significant. Each circle represents a dataset from the repeated hold-out procedure; red circles represent two particular hold-out validation sets: the data collected at HSR in May 2020 (above) and the data collected at IOG (below). The black segment indicates the average similarity found among the partition datasets and its 95% confidence interval, indicating a "moderate" similarity.

than 75%). By contrast, while the calibration and utility (in terms of, respectively, Brier score and Standardized Net Benefit) were good on the datasets more similar to the training data (i.e. the three Italian dataset), the performance of the model with respect to these two quality dimensions was lower on the other external datasets. In particular, the connection between the AUC and the dataset similarity was very strong ($\rho = 0.74$) and significant ($p = 0.035$); the relationship between the Net Benefit and dataset similarity was moderate ($\rho = 0.39$) but not significant ($p = 0.345$); while the connection between the Brier score and dataset similarity was strong ($\rho = 0.66$) yet not significant ($p = 0.076$). Consequently, considering the observations reported for the first step of the procedure, we can see that data heterogeneity has a moderate effect on model performance.

In view of our meta-validation procedure, the model can be thought of as externally validated, as, for at least one external dataset associated with slight similarity the reported performance was acceptable (or better) for all the considered metrics. Moreover, most external validation datasets could be considered of adequate cardinality: all datasets except the Spain dataset surpassed the MSS for the three considered performance metrics.

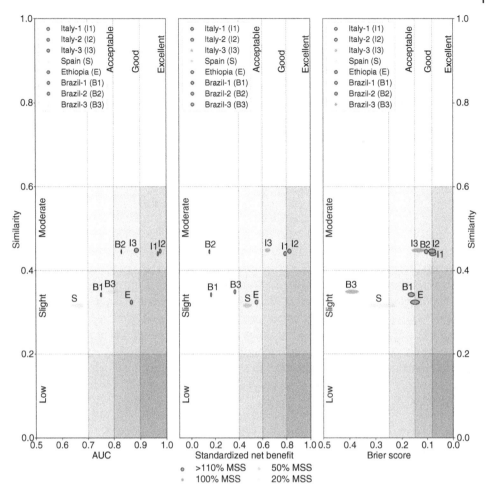

Figure 14.12 The *external performance diagram*, displaying the results from the external validation study on the COVID-19 diagnosis (second step of the meta-validation procedure). Information about the MSS is rendered in terms of hue brightness. The width of the ellipses is equal to the width of the 95% confidence interval w.r.t. the given performance metrics.

14.5 Conclusions and Future Outlook

In this chapter, we aimed to provide a general overview of several important, but still over-looked, ways to assess the quality of predictive models in medicine and healthcare with regards to reliability, robustness (as related to replicability and generalizability across new settings), and utility. The reliability of the ground truth data on which such predictive models are built, as well as the robustness of these latter are crucial factors for the success of AI and ML-based technologies in the medical domain. A reliable ground truth enables the creation of predictive models that are likewise reliable, as their development properly took into account, and controlled for, any observer variability in the data. Similarly, a robust model should perform well under a wide range of conditions, producing consistent results and generating accurate predictions across different populations and experimental setups. Finally, also utility is of practical importance, to ensure that the support provided by the predictive models is well aligned with the expectations and values of the involved actors. To illustrate the importance of these concepts, we reviewed metrics and frameworks to assess these different aspects and we also presented some example applications, through which we highlighted how the above mentioned tools can be applied and how they can inform the development and evaluation of ML models.

Future research in this field should focus on conducting more studies to determine the extent to which these metrics can improve the understanding of scholars and practitioners. Indeed, as we mentioned at the beginning of this chapter, despite the importance of these notions, their use and evaluation has so far been largely overlooked in the ML community. For this reason, we advocate for these metrics to be mentioned more frequently in assessment guidelines (Cabitza and Campagner 2021) and certification standards, so that they become more widespread and common and help raise the awareness about the centrality of the presented notions for the safe development and deployment of ML systems.

In conclusion, the assessment of predictive models in medicine and healthcare is a critical area that requires ongoing research and development. As predictive computing continues to play a vital role in the medical field, it is essential that the quality of predictive models is rigorously evaluated to ensure their reliability, robustness, and utility in providing accurate and trustworthy predictions. By promoting the use of metrics for measuring dimensions such as reliability, utility and robustness in assessments and certifications, we can ensure the continued advancement and widespread adoption of high-quality predictive models in medicine and healthcare.

Author Biographies

Federico Cabitza is an Associate Professor at the University of Milano-Bicocca (Milan, Italy) where he teaches various classes, including human-computer interaction, interaction design, information systems and decision support. He is head of the Laboratory of Uncertainty Models, Decisions and Interactions (MUDILab) in the department of Informatics at the above-mentioned university and is director of the local node of the CINI national laboratory "Computer Science and Society." Since 2016 he has been intensively collaborating with several hospitals, among which the IRCCS Hospital Galeazzi and Sant'Ambrogio in Milano (Italy), with which he is formally affiliated as senior researcher and where he co-founded the Medical AI laboratory. He is associate editor of the International Journal of Medical Informatics and a member of several editorial boards, including the Machine Learning and Knowledge Extraction journal, the Journal of Medical Artificial Intelligence, the Journal of Cross-disciplinary Research in Computational Law and Mondo Digitale, the official AICA journal. To date, he has published more than 150 research publications in international conference proceedings, edited books and high-impact scientific journals and is listed among the world's most influential scientists, according to Stanford's Top 2% Scientists list. He is the author with Prof. Luciano Floridi (former University of Oxford UK, now University of Bologna, Italy and Yale University, CT, USA) of the book "Artificial Intelligence, the use of the new machines".

Andrea Campagner is a Postdoc Researcher at the IRCCS Ospedale Galeazzi Sant'Ambrogio (Milan, Italy). He obtained his PhD in Computer Science in 2023 at the Department of Informatics, Systems and Communication of the University of Milano-Bicocca. His research interests lie at the intersection of uncertainty management, machine learning and human-AI interaction, as well as their applications in medicine and life science. He is an Associate Editor of the International Journal of Medical Informatics and the Soft Computing journal, a member of the Editorial Board of BMC Medical Informatics and Decision Making, and has been Program Chair of CD-MAKE 2023 and IJCRS 2023. He organized the special sessions on "Data Perspectivism in Ground Truthing and Artificial Intelligence", and "Machine Learning for Partially Labeled Data" at IPMU 2022, "Multi-perspectivist Data and Learning" at CD-MAKE 2023, and "Rough Sets: Theory, Applications, and Related Tools" at FLINS-ISKE 2024. He has also organized the workshop on "How to Assess Human Reliance on Artificial Intelligence in Hybrid Decision-Making" at HHAI 2023.

References

Baker, S.G., Cook, N.R., Vickers, A., and Kramer, B.S. (2009). Using relative utility curves to evaluate risk prediction. *Journal of the Royal Statistical Society* 172 (4): 729–748. https://doi.org/10.1111/j.1467-985X.2009.00592.x.

Beigman, E. and Klebanov, B.B. (2009). Learning with annotation noise. *Proceedings of the Joint Conference of the 47th Annual Meeting of the ACL and the 4th International Joint Conference on Natural Language Processing of the AFNLP: Volume 1-Volume 1*, 280–287. Association for Computational Linguistics.

Beigman Klebanov, B. and Beigman, E. (2009). From annotator agreement to noise models. *Computational Linguistics* 35 (4): 495–503. https://doi.org/10.1162/coli.2009.35.4.35402.

Berner, E.S. (2003). Diagnostic decision support systems: how to determine the gold standard? *Journal of the American Medical Informatics Association* 10 (6): 608–610. https://doi.org/10.1197/jamia.M1416.

Bezemer, T., De Groot, M.C.H., Blasse, E. et al. (2019). A human (e) factor in clinical decision support systems. *Journal of Medical Internet Research* 21 (3): e11732. https://doi.org/10.2196/11732.

Bien, N., Rajpurkar, P., Ball, R.L. et al. (2018). Deep-learning-assisted diagnosis for knee magnetic resonance imaging: development and retrospective validation of MRNet. *PLoS Medicine* 15 (11): e1002699. https://doi.org/10.1371/journal.pmed.1002699.

Bleeker, S.E., Moll, H.A., Steyerberg, E.W. et al. (2003). External validation is necessary in prediction research: a clinical example. *Journal of Clinical Epidemiology* 56 (9): 826–832. https://doi.org/10.1016/S0895-4356(03)00207-5.

Bousquet, N. (2008). Diagnostics of prior-data agreement in applied Bayesian analysis. *Journal of Applied Statistics* 35 (9): 1011–1029. https://doi.org/10.1080/02664760802192981.

Bradley, A.A., Schwartz, S.S., and Hashino, T. (2008). Sampling uncertainty and confidence intervals for the Brier score and Brier skill score. *Weather and Forecasting* 23 (5): 992–1006. https://doi.org/10.1175/2007WAF2007049.1.

Brady, A.P. (2017). Error and discrepancy in radiology: inevitable or avoidable? *Insights Into Imaging* 8 (1): 171–182. https://doi.org/10.1007/s13244-016-0534-1.

Brier, G.W. (1950). Verification of forecasts expressed in terms of probability. *Monthly Weather Review* 78 (1): 1–3.

Briggs, W.M. and Zaretzki, R. (2008). The skill plot: a graphical technique for evaluating continuous diagnostic tests. *Biometrics* 64 (1): 250–256. https://doi.org/10.1111/j.1541-0420 .2007.00781_1.x.

Cabitza, F. (2019). Biases affecting human decision making in AI-supported second opinion settings. *International Conference on Modeling Decisions for Artificial Intelligence*, 283–294. Springer. https://doi.org/10.1007/978-3-030-26773-5_25.

Cabitza, F. and Campagner, A. (2021). The need to separate the wheat from the chaff in medical informatics: introducing a comprehensive checklist for the (self-)assessment of medical AI studies. *International Journal of Medical Informatics* 153: 104510. https://doi.org/ 10.1016/j.ijmedinf.2021.104510.

Cabitza, F. and Zeitoun, J.-D. (2019). The proof of the pudding: in praise of a culture of real-world validation for medical artificial intelligence. *Annals of translational medicine* 7 (8): https://doi.org/10.21037/atm.2019.04.07.

Cabitza, F., Ciucci, D., and Rasoini, R. (2019). A giant with feet of clay: on the validity of the data that feed machine learning in medicine. In: *Organizing for the Digital World*, 121–136. Springer. https://doi.org/10.1007/978-3-319-90503-7_10.

Cabitza, F., Campagner, A., Albano, D. et al. (2020a). The elephant in the machine: proposing a new metric of data reliability and its application to a medical case to assess classification reliability. *Applied Sciences* 10 (11): 4014. https://doi.org/10.3390/app10114014.

Cabitza, F., Campagner, A., and Balsano, C. (2020b). Bridging the "last mile" gap between AI implementation and operation: "data awareness" that matters. *Annals of Translational Medicine* 8 (7): https://doi.org/10.21037/atm.2020.03.63.

Cabitza, F., Campagner, A., and Sconfienza, L.M. (2020c). As if sand were stone. New concepts and metrics to probe the ground on which to build trustable AI. *BMC Medical Informatics and Decision Making* 20 (1): 1–21. https://doi.org/10.1186/s12911-020-01224-9.

Cabitza, F., Campagner, A., Ferrari, D. et al. (2021a). Development, evaluation, and validation of machine learning models for COVID-19 detection based on routine blood tests. *Clinical Chemistry and Laboratory Medicine (CCLM)* 59 (2): https://doi.org/10.1515/cclm-2020-1294.

Cabitza, F., Campagner, A., Soares, F. et al. (2021b). The importance of being external. methodological insights for the external validation of machine learning models in medicine. *Computer Methods and Programs in Biomedicine* 208: 106288. https://doi.org/10.1016/j.cmpb .2021.106288.

Cabitza, F., Campagner, A., and Basile, V. (2023). Toward a perspectivist turn in ground truthing for predictive computing. *Proceedings of the AAAI Conference on Artificial Intelligence (AAAI 2023)*. AAAI.

Campagner, A., Conte, E., and Cabitza, F. (2021). Weighted utility: a utility metric based on the case-wise raters' perceptions. *International Cross-Domain Conference for Machine Learning and Knowledge Extraction*, 203–210. Springer. https://doi.org/10.1007/978-3-030- 84060-0_13.

Chicco, D., Tötsch, N., and Jurman, G. (2021). The Matthews correlation coefficient (MCC) is more reliable than balanced accuracy, bookmaker informedness, and markedness in two-class confusion matrix evaluation. *Biodata Mining* 14 (1): 1–22. https://doi.org/10.1186/ s13040-021-00244-z.

Cicchetti, D.V. and Feinstein, A.R. (1990). High agreement but low kappa: II. Resolving the paradoxes. *Journal of Clinical Epidemiology* 43 (6): 551–558. https://doi.org/10.1016/0895-4356(90)90159-M.

Cohen, J. (1960). A coefficient of agreement for nominal scales. *Educational and Psychological Measurement* 20 (1): 37–46. https://doi.org/10.1177/001316446002000104.

Cohen, J. (2013). *Statistical Power Analysis for the Behavioral Sciences*. Academic press.

Coiera, E. (2019). The last mile: where artificial intelligence meets reality. *Journal of Medical Internet Research* 21 (11): e16323. https://doi.org/10.2196/16323.

Cortes, C. and Vapnik, V. (1995). Support-vector networks. *Machine Learning* 20: 273–297.

Cover, T. and Hart, P. (1967). Nearest neighbor pattern classification. *IEEE Transactions on Information Theory* 13 (1): 21–27. https://doi.org/10.1109/TIT.1967.1053964.

Feinstein, A.R. and Cicchetti, D.V. (1990). High agreement but low Kappa: I. The problems of two paradoxes. *Journal of Clinical Epidemiology* 43 (6): 543–549. https://doi.org/10.1016/0895-4356(90)90158-L.

Fleiss, J.L. (1971). Measuring nominal scale agreement among many raters. *Psychological Bulletin* 76 (5): 378. https://doi.org/10.1037/h0031619.

Futoma, J., Simons, M., Panch, T. et al. (2020). The myth of generalisability in clinical research and machine learning in health care. *The Lancet Digital Health* 2 (9): e489–e492. https://doi.org/10.1016/S2589-7500(20)30186-2.

Graber, M.L. (2013). The incidence of diagnostic error in medicine. *BMJ Quality and Safety* 22 (Suppl 2): ii21–ii27. https://doi.org/10.1136/bmjqs-2012-001615.

Gwet, K.L. (2011). On the Krippendorff's alpha coefficient. *Manuscript submitted for publication. Retrieved October*, 2 (2011): 2011.

Hernandez-Boussard, T., Bozkurt, S., Ioannidis, J.P.A., and Shah, N.H. (2020). Minimar (minimum information for medical AI reporting): developing reporting standards for artificial intelligence in health care. *Journal of the American Medical Informatics Association* 27 (12): 2011–2015.

Huggard, H., Koh, Y.S., Dobbie, G., and Zhang, E. (2020). Detecting concept drift in medical triage. *Proceedings of the 43rd International ACM SIGIR Conference on Research and Development in Information Retrieval*, 1733–1736. https://doi.org/10.1145/3397271.3401228.

Hunt, R.J. (1986). Percent agreement, Pearson's correlation, and Kappa as measures of inter-examiner reliability. *Journal of Dental Research* 65 (2): 128–130. https://doi.org/10.1177/00220345860650020701.

Kerr, K.F., Brown, M.D., Zhu, K., and Janes, H. (2016). Assessing the clinical impact of risk prediction models with decision curves: guidance for correct interpretation and appropriate use. *Journal of Clinical Oncology* 34 (21): 2534. https://doi.org/10.1200/JCO.2015.65.5654.

Kim, J.-H. (2009). Estimating classification error rate: repeated cross-validation, repeated hold-out and bootstrap. *Computational Statistics & Data Analysis* 53 (11): 3735–3745. https://doi.org/10.1016/j.csda.2009.04.009.

König, I.R., Malley, J.D., Weimar, C. et al. (2007). Practical experiences on the necessity of external validation. *Statistics in Medicine* 26 (30): 5499–5511. https://doi.org/10.1002/sim.3069.

Kouw, W.M., Loog, M., Bartels, L.W., and Mendrik, A.M. (2019). Learning an MR acquisition-invariant representation using Siamese neural networks. *2019 IEEE 16th International Symposium on Biomedical Imaging (ISBI 2019)*, 364–367. IEEE.

Krippendorff, K. (2018). *Content Analysis: An Introduction to Its Methodology*. Sage Publications.

Landis, J.R. and Koch, G.G. (1977). The measurement of observer agreement for categorical data. *Biometrics* 33 (1): 159–174. https://doi.org/10.2307/2529310.

Lyell, D. and Coiera, E. (2017). Automation bias and verification complexity: a systematic review. *Journal of the American Medical Informatics Association* 24 (2): 423–431. https://doi.org/10.1093/jamia/ocw105.

McDermott, M.B.A., Wang, S., Marinsek, N. et al. (2021). Reproducibility in machine learning for health research: still a ways to go. *Science Translational Medicine* 13 (586): eabb1655. https://doi.org/10.1126/scitranslmed.abb1655.

Merritt, S.M., Ako-Brew, A., Bryant, W.J. et al. (2019). Automation-induced complacency potential: development and validation of a new scale. *Frontiers in Psychology* 10: 225. https://doi.org/10.3389/fpsyg.2019.00225.

Oakden-Rayner, L., Dunnmon, J., Carneiro, G., and Ré, C. (2019). Hidden stratification causes clinically meaningful failures in machine learning for medical imaging. *arXiv preprint arXiv:1909.12475*.

Pinto, A. and Brunese, L. (2010). Spectrum of diagnostic errors in radiology. *World Journal of Radiology* 2 (10): 377. https://doi.org/10.4329/wjr.v2.i10.377.

Quekel, L.G.B.A., Kessels, A.G.H., Goei, R., and van Engelshoven, J.M.A. (1999). Miss rate of lung cancer on the chest radiograph in clinical practice. *Chest* 115 (3): 720–724. https://doi.org/10.1378/chest.115.3.720.

Rajkomar, A., Dean, J., and Kohane, I. (2019). Machine learning in medicine. *New England Journal of Medicine* 380 (14): 1347–1358. https://doi.org/10.1056/NEJMra1814259.

Rasch, G. (1980). *Probabilistic Models for Some Intelligence and Attainment Tests. 1960.* Copenhagen, Denmark: Danish Institute for Educational Research.

Riley, R.D., Debray, T.P.A., Collins, G.S. et al. (2021). Minimum sample size for external validation of a clinical prediction model with a binary outcome. *Statistics in Medicine* 40 (19): https://doi.org/10.1002/sim.9025.

Schat, E., van de Schoot, R., Kouw, W.M. et al. (2020). The data representativeness criterion: predicting the performance of supervised classification based on data set similarity. *PLoS ONE* 15 (8): e0237009. https://doi.org/10.1371/journal.pone.0237009.

Sokolova, M. and Lapalme, G. (2009). A systematic analysis of performance measures for classification tasks. *Information Processing & Management* 45 (4): 427–437. https://doi.org/10.1016/j.ipm.2009.03.002.

Steyerberg, E.W. and Harrell, F.E. Jr. (2016). Prediction models need appropriate internal, internal-external, and external validation. *Journal of Clinical Epidemiology* 69: 245. https://doi.org/10.1016/j.jclinepi.2015.04.005.

Vabalas, A., Gowen, E., Poliakoff, E., and Casson, A.J. (2019). Machine learning algorithm validation with a limited sample size. *PLoS ONE* 14 (11): e0224365. https://doi.org/10.1371/journal.pone.0224365.

Valverde-Albacete, F.J. and Peláez-Moreno, C. (2014). 100% classification accuracy considered harmful: the normalized information transfer factor explains the accuracy paradox. *PLoS One* 9 (1): 1–10. https://doi.org/10.1371/journal.pone.0084217.

Van Calster, B., McLernon, D.J., Van Smeden, M. et al. (2019). Calibration: the Achilles heel of predictive analytics. *BMC Medicine* 17 (1): 1–7. https://doi.org/10.1186/s12916-019-1466-7.

Vellido, A. (2020). The importance of interpretability and visualization in machine learning for applications in medicine and health care. *Neural Computing and Applications* 32 (24): 18069–18083. https://doi.org/10.1007/s00521-019-04051-w.

Vergouwe, Y., Steyerberg, E.W., Eijkemans, M.J.C., and Habbema, J.D.F. (2005). Substantial effective sample sizes were required for external validation studies of predictive logistic regression models. *Journal of Clinical Epidemiology* 58 (5): 475–483. https://doi.org/10.1016/j.jclinepi.2004.06.017.

Vickers, A.J. and Elkin, E.B. (2006). Decision curve analysis: a novel method for evaluating prediction models. *Medical Decision Making* 26 (6): 565–574. https://doi.org/10.1177/0272989X06295361.

Vickers, A.J., Van Calster, B., and Steyerberg, E.W. (2016). Net benefit approaches to the evaluation of prediction models, molecular markers, and diagnostic tests. *BMJ* 352: i6.

Zhang, J.M., Harman, M., Ma, L., and Liu, Y. (2020). Machine learning testing: survey, landscapes and horizons. *IEEE Transactions on Software Engineering* 48 (1): 1–36.

15

Legal Aspects of AI in the Biomedical Field. The Role of Interpretable Models

Chiara Gallese

Department of Law, University of Turin, Italy

15.1 Introduction

In recent years, the development of artificial intelligence (AI) systems intended to be employed in the medical domain has greatly increased. Biomedical research has been trying to use them to improve analysis and treatment outcomes, producing an impressive number of publications (Rong et al. 2020), with the United States, China, and the United Kingdom publishing the highest number of studies in health care (Secinaro et al. 2021).

Following this rapid technological progress and the increment of the applications of AI models developed by researchers into actual clinical practice, many countries have started to regulate the use of personal data and AI systems, with particular attention to automated decision-making systems (ADM).

The enacting of the general data protection regulation (GDPR)[1] and the recently published European proposal for a Regulation on Artificial Intelligence (AI Act)[2] have changed the legal framework surrounding the development of AI systems. Legal scholars and the case law have started to face the issues of civil liability, discrimination, and medical malpractice, derived from the use of AI systems in everyday life.

GDPR, which is in force in all EU countries, introduced a general prohibition for the use of data concerning health (which are considered "special categories of data," i.e. sensitive data), providing for only a few exceptions and many mandatory conditions (Article 9). This had a significant impact not only on research in the medical field and in Computer Science, but also on the extent to which health care professionals are allowed to use AI systems on patients.

---

1 Regulation (EU) 2016/679 of the European Parliament and of the Council of 27 April 2016 on the protection of natural persons with regard to the processing of personal data and on the free movement of such data, and repealing Directive 95/46/EC (General Data Protection Regulation), text available here: https://eur-lex.europa.eu/eli/reg/2016/679/oj

2 Proposal for a Regulation of the European Parliament and of the Council laying down harmonized rules on Artificial Intelligence (Artificial Intelligence Act) and amending certain union legislative acts COM/2021/206 final, text available here: https://eur-lex.europa.eu/legal-content/EN/TXT/?uri=CELEX\%3A52021PC0206

Big Data Analysis and Artificial Intelligence for Medical Sciences, First Edition.
Edited by Bruno Carpentieri and Paola Lecca.
© 2024 John Wiley & Sons Ltd. Published 2024 by John Wiley & Sons Ltd.

Similarly, the AI Act will influence the way in which AI systems are developed and put into the market or into service by providing additional requirements and mandatory conditions, such as the examination of data sets in view of possible biases (Article 10).

In addition to these regulations, each country has different rules on medical practice, including liability issues and informed consent requirements, that regulate the boundaries within which health care professionals operate.

In this chapter, we will explain why understanding this complex legal framework is essential to be able to develop AI systems that can legally be employed on real patients, and to avoid fines and liability issues for both developers and health care professionals. On the other hand, we will see how complying with the existing legal framework is not only a matter of mere technical compliance, but it also means protecting the fundamental rights of patients and avoiding negative consequences on society as a whole.

We will also highlight the main legal principles surrounding AI systems employed in the medical domain, from the developing phase to the concrete application in the clinical practice.

The chapter starts with an overview of data protection law, which is always involved when it comes to the medical domain: personal data may be used to train a model (e.g. a data set composed of MRI scan fed to a neural network), or the model will be used by health care professionals on personal data (e.g. a doctor employs a system to analyze patients' vital parameters). Whichever is the case, GDPR and other privacy laws will be involved. The most important relevant principles, such as transparency, legal basis, right of explanation, accountability, fairness, and human oversight, are explained. Additional requirements provided by the recent proposal for a new Regulation on AI are also briefly addressed.

Both black box and white box AI models are considered in light of the legal principles, and the concepts of explainability and interpretability are introduced.

In section 15.9, the reasons in favor of employing interpretable models in the medical field are discussed.

15.2 Data Protection

According to GDPR, all kinds of data concerning an identifiable (living) person is considered personal data and only non-identifiable data falls outside the scope of GDPR.

Non-identifiable means that it is not possible to identify a person in any way. According to this definition, even when direct identifiers (e.g. names and surnames) are removed, it is still possible to identify the specific person linking different data sources (and GDPR then applies); therefore, in order to consider data anonymous, the anonymization process must be absolutely irreversible.

This is particularly difficult when hospitals are involved, because of the fact that they usually retain patients' data in their systems in order to carry out health care services; data possessed or provided by hospitals, therefore, can rarely be fully anonymous: most often, they are considered by GDPR as pseudonymized, as the hospital is able to match them back with patients' names and other personal details.

In addition to the problem of anonymization, there is also the problem of the prohibition to process special categories of data, as described in Article 9 of GDPR: according to the first paragraph,

> Processing of personal data revealing racial or ethnic origin, political opinions, religious or philosophical beliefs, or trade union membership, and the processing of genetic data, biometric data for the purpose of uniquely identifying a natural person, data concerning health or data concerning a natural person's sex life or sexual orientation shall be prohibited.

Health data, that is data related to a living person's body or mind, is in fact considered a "special category of data," therefore it falls under Article 9.

GDPR provides for some exceptions to the aforementioned prohibition, for example having the explicit consent of the patient (provided that the law does not prevent it),[3] or carrying out a project for scientific research purposes (provided that appropriate safeguards are in place).[4] Each State may, however, introduce additional requirements to be fulfilled, for example, allowing the processing of biometric data by public authorities by ordinary law.[5]

The fact that most data sets used to train or to make use of AI systems are considered special personal data means that particular care is needed in handling them, and that it is necessary to take additional measures prescribed by data protection laws. For example, a data protection impact assessment may be needed pursuant to Article of 35 GDPR, such as in cases in which big data is involved.

Even when a data set is going to be anonymized, a careful assessment is necessary before it is allowed to reuse it (European Data Protection Board 2019; European Medicines Agency 2020). In fact, the process of anonymization itself is considered a "processing," covered by GDPR. As a general rule, the processing of personal data for purposes other than those for which it was initially collected (that is, "reuse" or "secondary use") is allowed by GDPR only if it is *compatible* with the original purposes (that is, the reason for which the personal data were initially collected and of which the data subject has been properly informed). This means that patients should be informed in advance of the intention of reusing their data, and, where applicable, their prior explicit consent must be asked.

The assessment is needed because privacy is considered a fundamental human right, therefore personal data are non-disposable rights, *res extra commercium*, meaning that they

---

3 The second paragraph of Article 9 states: "Paragraph 1 shall not apply if one of the following applies: the data subject has given explicit consent to the processing of those personal data for one or more specified purposes, except where Union or Member State law provide that the prohibition referred to in paragraph 1 may not be lifted by the data subject."

4 Article 9 continues: "Paragraph 1 shall not apply if one of the following applies: [...] processing is necessary for archiving purposes in the public interest, scientific or historical research purposes or statistical purposes in accordance with Article 89(1) based on Union or Member State law which shall be proportionate to the aim pursued, respect the essence of the right to data protection and provide for suitable and specific measures to safeguard the fundamental rights and the interests of the data subject."

5 As allowed by the last paragraph of Article 9: "Member States may maintain or introduce further conditions, including limitations, with regard to the processing of genetic data, biometric data or data concerning health."

cannot be sold, rented, or gifted. The patients' consent that allows AI developers, doctors, or researchers to use their data, thus, only gives limited permission. Patients may give permission to have their bodies scanned in an MRI machine in order to allow doctors to find a disease, but they may not expect that their scan is used to train an AI model. They certainly do not expect that their scan is made available to insurance companies, banks, or public institutions that may use it to deny services, contracts, or rights to other patients suffering from the same disease.

If the data set is reused for scientific research, there is a presumption of compatibility, but, pursuant to Article 89 GDPR, appropriate technical and organizational safeguards must be in place and a careful assessment regarding compatibility is needed (European Data Protection Board 2020; Kindt et al. 2021). In addition, each state may have additional rules, such as France: the presumption of compatibility does not apply if the processing is used to make decisions about the data subject.[6]

Recital 156 of GDPR also notes that in case of further use a feasibility assessment should be carried out and appropriate safeguards should be granted:

> The further processing of personal data for archiving purposes in the public interest, scientific or historical research purposes or statistical purposes is to be carried out when the controller[7] has assessed the feasibility to fulfill those purposes by processing data which do not permit or no longer permit the identification of data subjects, provided that appropriate safeguards exist (such as, for instance, pseudonymisation of the data).

Additional safeguards with regards to special categories of data are prescribed by the AI Act in the last paragraph of Article 10: it is possible to process them to the extent that it is strictly necessary for the purposes of ensuring bias monitoring, detection, and correction in relation to high-risk AI systems, but appropriate safeguards are necessary (such as technical limitations on the reuse of data, and the adoption of state-of-the-art technical measures, including pseudonymization or encryption).[8]

GDPR and other types of law also contain general principles that must be respected altogether both when using data for the development of the model and later when applying the AI model on patients' data (for instance, in the hospital):

- **Lawfulness**: All applicable laws should be respected and data obtained illegally cannot be used. It must be assured that a proper legal basis for the processing is in place (e.g. that consent is given, or that a legitimate interest is present);

---

6 "Art, 4, par. 2, of the French "Loi n° 78-17 du 6 janvier 1978 relative Ã l'informatique, aux fichiers et aux libert's."
7 "Controller" is defined by GDPR as "the natural or legal person, public authority, agency or other body which, alone or jointly with others, determines the purposes and means of the processing of personal data."
8 "The concept is further explained in Recital 44: "In order to protect the right of others from the discrimination that might result from the bias in AI systems, the providers should be able to process also special categories of personal data, as a matter of substantial public interest, in order to ensure the bias monitoring, detection, and correction in relation to high-risk AI systems."

- **Purpose limitation**: Data can be used only for the specific purpose they were collected, which must be communicated to the data subjects;
- **Data minimization**: Only data strictly necessary to reach the specific purposes of the processing (e.g. answering the research questions; training the neural network) can be used;
- **Accuracy**: Data must be accurate as provided by the data subject or as collected. If an error in data is discovered, it should be promptly corrected;
- **Storage limitation**: Data can be kept only for the minimum necessary amount of time needed to reach each specific purpose;
- **Integrity and confidentiality**: Data cannot be accessed by unauthorized people and should be preserved from the risk of accidental (even if only temporary) loss, modification, or deletion.

Most of these principles are also present in the AI regulation. In the following, we will examine other relevant principles, such as fairness, transparency, and accountability, which are equally important.

Recital 171 of GDPR makes it clear that data processing activities initiated before 2018, or concerning data collected under the previous law, must comply with all GDPR requirements, even if past processing was compliant with the law at that time. Therefore, when using a dataset that relied on the legal basis of consent, if the privacy notice and consent were not up to GDPR standards then a new notice must be provided or consent must be requested again.

15.3 Transparency Principle

Transparency is a key principle and an overarching obligation both for GDPR and the new AI Act, but it is also an important ethical and legal requirement in the doctor-patient relationship. It is translated in many different areas: (i) right of explanation, (ii) right of information, and (iii) informed consent requirements.

15.3.1 Right of Explanation

Transparency is translated into a series of rights provided to the data subjects when profiling and ADM are involved.

In GDPR, *Profiling* is the collection of aspects of an individual's personality, behavior, interests, habits, and other elements, collected in order to analyze their behavior, make predictions, or take decisions about them through an automated process (GDPR, Recital 71 and Article 22). Because in some cases AI systems employed in health care collect a series of personal elements from the patients in order to build a medical profile (e.g. to provide personalized medicine services), they may fall within the definition of Profiling. Automated decisions can be made without profiling and profiling can take place without automated decisions.

Automated decision making is the process of taking a decision without human intervention, that produces legal effects or that has a significant impact on a person.

Article 22 of GDPR states:

1. The data subject shall have the right not to be subject to a decision based solely on automated processing, including profiling, which produces legal effects concerning him or her or similarly significantly affects him or her.
2. Paragraph 1 shall not apply if the decision:
    (a) is necessary for entering into, or performance of, a contract between the data subject and a data controller;
    (b) is authorized by Union or Member State law to which the controller is subject and which also lays down suitable measures to safeguard the data subject's rights and freedoms and legitimate interests; or
    (c) is based on the data subject's explicit consent.
3. In the cases referred to in points (a) and (c) of paragraph 2, the data controller shall implement suitable measures to safeguard the data subject's rights and freedoms and legitimate interests, at least the right to obtain human intervention on the part of the controller, to express his or her point of view and to contest the decision.
4. Decisions referred to in paragraph 2 shall not be based on special categories of personal data referred to in Article 9(1), unless point (a) or (g) of Article 9(2) applies and suitable measures to safeguard the data subject's rights and freedoms and legitimate interests are in place.

According to the definition, AI systems employed in health care are considered ADM whenever they are used to take a decision that has an impact on the patient (e.g. when employing tools that detect a certain type of disease to decide if a patient needs to start a certain treatment).

As explained in paragraph 4 of Article 22, there is a general prohibition of employing ADM systems to health data, unless there is the explicit informed consent of the patient, or the processing is necessary for reasons of "substantial public interest," and at the same time there are suitable measures in place as a guarantee.

In addition to those provisions, there is also the "right of explanation" to data subjects, which means that they have the right to have information about the rationale behind or the criteria relied on in reaching the decision, and about the significance and envisaged consequences of the processing of their data.

Before examining the different sources of law that contain the right of explanation, it is useful to consider the difference between explainability and interpretability. In the literature, there is great confusion about those concepts, and the two terms are often used interchangeably (Rudin et al. 2022), even if some scholars have tried to give a comprehensive definition of them (Köhl et al. 2019; Chazette and Schneider 2020; Chazette et al. 2021). In this paper, the two terms are considered as clearly distinct concepts.

If we consider the definition provided by Rudin (2019), explainability occurs when "a second (post hoc) model is created to explain the first black box model." In this scenario, then there are two models: the first is not transparent because it is not possible to understand why it gave a certain output, and the second, which has an output intelligible by a human, is employed to try to reconstruct the reasons behind the first model output.

According to the author, in certain circumstances explainability may not be a reliable method:

> Explainable ML methods provide explanations that are not faithful to what the original model computes. Explanations must be wrong. They cannot have perfect fidelity with respect to the original model. If the explanation was completely faithful to what the original model computes, the explanation would equal the original model, and one would not need the original model in the first place, only the explanation. (In other words, this is a case where the original model would be interpretable.) This leads to the danger that any explanation method for a black box model can be an inaccurate representation of the original model in parts of the feature space (Rudin 2019).

Babic et al. (2021) raise some concerns as well:

> Three points are important to note: First, the opaque function of the black box remains the basis for the AI/ML decisions because it is typically the most accurate one. Second, the white box approximation to the black box cannot be perfect, because if it were, there would be no difference between the two. It is also not focusing on accuracy but on fitting the black box, often only locally. Finally, the explanations provided are post hoc.

This highlights an important element that should be taken into account: black box models are usually more accurate than other models. Deep learning is nowadays outperforming white box models in several areas, such as imaging. However, interpretable models may have the same accuracy as black boxes in some areas (Christodoulou et al. 2019). Petch et al. (2021) propose a rule of thumb for the decision regarding the use of black boxes:

> From the outset, data scientists should train models using both interpretable and black-box methods to assess whether there is, in fact, an accuracy vs interpretability tradeoff in the specific case on which they are working. If there is no meaningful difference in accuracy between an interpretable model and a black box, an interpretable method should be used. However, if a black-box model does provide a higher degree of accuracy, the stakes of the decision should be considered. If the decision that will be informed by the model is a relatively low stake, a small improvement in accuracy may justify the use of a black box. However, if the stakes are high, it is reasonable to require a greater improvement in accuracy before sacrificing interpretability. Ideally, gains in accuracy from black-box methods should be sufficient to translate into meaningful improvements in clinical outcomes such as reduced morbidity or mortality. If the use of a black box model can be justified, explainability techniques should be employed to make the model and its predictions as transparent as possible, but clinicians should be aware of their limitations and be cautious of overinterpreting, which can lead to narrative fallacies.

On the other hand, interpretability refers to a model that is intelligible in a way that allows humans to understand the justification that led to a certain output. "Justifiable" might be a synonym: someone, whether the modeler, the domain expert, the final user, or the person who is subject to the output, must be able to understand the logic involved in the decision.

It is worth noting that the mere mathematical explanation and the understanding of how a model is built (e.g. being able to inspect the source code) is not enough, for humans, to justify why the model reached a certain conclusion: knowing the source code of a neural network, the number of parameters (weights), layers, or features, without knowing the reason why a relationship between data is found, may not enable humans to understand the output. As a simple example, we can imagine a classification model that, given a data set containing millions of physiological features of past patients, divides future patients of a certain disease into healthy or non-healthy. Doctors may insert data from a new patient in the system, such as blood levels, symptoms, anamnesis, genomic information, lifestyle choices, age, number of children, ethnicity, weight, height, number of sleep hours, job, place of birth, etc., to check if the system classifies that patient as healthy or ill. However, due to the high number and complexity of features, parameters, and layers involved in the process of reaching the output, the system is not able to tell *why* the patient is ill, e.g. because the blood levels are abnormal for a person of a certain age, ethnicity, weight, and daily amount of exercise. It is even possible that the system, by coincidence, relied on irrelevant elements, such as the ID number or the date of admission to the hospital. How could the doctor know? Not even the modeler is able to tell. Das and Rad (2020) explain that

> The large number of parameters in Deep Neural Networks (DNNs) make them complex to understand and undeniably harder to interpret. Regardless of the cross-validation accuracy or other evaluation parameters which might indicate a good learning performance, deep learning (DL) models could inherently learn or fail to learn representations from the data which a human might consider important. Explaining the decisions made by DNNs require knowledge of the internal operations of DNNs, missing with non-AI-experts and end-users who are more focused on getting accurate solution. Hence, often the ability to interpret AI decisions are deemed secondary in the race to achieve state-of-the-art results or crossing human-level accuracy.

Rudin (2019) notes that transparency is not a black and white concept, but rather a spectrum:

> There is a spectrum between fully transparent models (where we understand how all the variables are jointly related to each other) and models that are lightly constrained in model form (such as models that are forced to increase as one of the variables increases, or models that, all else being equal, prefer variables that domain experts have identified as important[…]).

There are differences in the literature about *what* should be explainable and in what context. Chazette et al. (2021) summarize the elements that, according to the literature and their own analysis, should be explained:

> the system in general, and, more specifically, its reasoning processes (e.g., inference processes for certain problems), its inner logic (e.g., relationships between the inputs and outputs), its model's internals (e.g., parameters and data structures), its intention

(e.g., pursued outcome of actions), its behavior (e.g., real-world actions), its decision (e.g., underlying criteria), its performance (e.g., predictive accuracy), and its knowledge about the user or the world (e.g., user preferences).

For example, if we consider a system that predicts the risk of being admitted to the ICU due to Covid-19, it would be considered interpretable only if it showed clearly what clinically relevant elements (e.g. saturation, age, comorbidities, weight, days since the symptom started, medications taken, etc.) were employed by the model to reach the output and which of them were weighted more than the others. Even if this explanation would be expressed in mathematical terms, the modellists would still be able to translate it in a way that would be intelligible by the doctors, and the doctors then would be able to explain it in simple words to the patients.

The concept of intelligibility is important because it carries many elements that should be taken into account, such as cultural differences,[9] mental capacity, age, education level, experience and expertise, and many other factors that may influence the ability to understand a certain output. As suggested by Article 13 of GDPR, adapting to the audience (the addressee) is crucial, even more when health is at stake. Many authors in the literature have highlighted that the addressee's understanding, which may vary depending on the context, is an important factor (Ribeiro et al. 2016; Carvalho et al. 2019; Miller 2019; Rosenfeld and Richardson 2019; Arrieta et al. 2020; Chazette et al. 2021).

As mentioned in Section 15.2, Articles 13 and 14 of GDPR grant the right to explanation regarding ADM and profiling to data subjects. Recital 71, par. 2, also specifies that:

> In any case, such processing should be subject to suitable safeguards, which should include specific information to the data subject and the right to obtain human intervention, to express his or her point of view, to obtain an explanation of the decision reached after such assessment and to challenge the decision.

According to the interpretation of GDPR, Controllers must provide meaningful information about the logic involved in the decision process, not necessarily a complex explanation of the algorithms used or the disclosure of the full source code,[10] but a "sufficiently comprehensive explanation that allows the data subject to understand the reasons for the decision" (Article 29 Data protection Working Party 2017). This concept is closer to interpretability than to explainability: it is more important that data subjects are able to understand what a model did than how it did it from a technical point of view.

---

9 Including language: different languages may have different ways of expressing a concept. Localization is an important element of the transparency principle.
10 Even consumer law does not require full disclosure of all the algorithms involved. Directive (EU) 2019/2161 requires transparency only regarding the main parameters used by the model: "Traders should not be required to disclose the detailed functioning of their ranking mechanisms, including algorithms. Traders should provide a general description of the main parameters determining the ranking that explains the default main parameters used by the trader and their relative importance as opposed to other parameters, but that description does not have to be presented in a customized manner for each individual search query" (Recital 23).

The right of explanation is present in the Council of Europe's Convention 108+ as well, a binding international instrument, as explained in the Explanatory Report, in Article 10:

> subjects should be entitled to know the reasoning underlying the processing of their data, including the consequences of such reasoning, which led to any resulting conclusions, in particular in cases involving the use of algorithms for automated decision making including profiling. For instance, in the case of credit scoring, they should be entitled to know the logic underpinning the processing of their data and resulting in a 'yes' or 'no' decision, and not simply information on the decision itself. Without an understanding of these elements, there could be no effective exercise of other essential safeguards such as the right to object and the right to complain to a competent authority.

The AI Act contains the principle of transparency and the right of explanation in Article 13: "High-risk AI systems shall be designed and developed in such a way to ensure that their operation is sufficiently transparent to enable users to interpret the system's output and use it appropriately. An appropriate type and degree of transparency shall be ensured."

As we have noted, the intended audience is an important element that should be taken into account when modeling the system: the output may be clear to computer scientists, but not to doctors or patients, therefore it would not meet the requirements of the right of explanation.

15.3.2 Right of Information

Transparency means that Controllers must provide to data subjects (e.g. patients) "relevant information related to fair processing, communicate and facilitate the exercise of their rights, enabling them to understand, and if necessary, challenge the data processing" (Article 29 Data protection Working Party 2018).

Articles 13 and 14 of GDPR list a series of mandatory elements that must be communicated to the data subjects within a reasonable period after obtaining the personal data, at the latest within one month from obtaining their data. These include, for example, information about what data processing is carried out, for what purposes, for how long, and under which legal basis, and information about their rights. The content of the communication varies if data is collected directly from data subjects (privacy notice pursuant to Art. 13) or if it is collected from a different source (privacy notice pursuant to Art. 14).

In the same Articles, it is required to disclose the existence of ADM, including profiling (Article 22), and to provide "meaningful information about the logic involved, as well as the significance and the envisaged consequences of such processing for the data subject." This requirement is explained in more detail in the subsection 15.3.3.

The whole set of information provided should be concise, transparent, intelligible, and in an easily accessible form, using clear and plain language, depending on the audience. In addition, GDPR requires that the way information is provided should be adapted to the age, mental ability, and education level of the data subjects.

Additional transparency requirements are drawn by the AI Act. In fact, Article 13 draws a list of information that should be provided to the users, and requires that they are also properly instructed: "High-risk AI systems shall be accompanied by instructions for use in an appropriate digital format or otherwise that include concise, complete, correct and clear information that is relevant, accessible and comprehensible to users." Articles 11 and 18 require that detailed technical documentation is created and kept up to date before the release of the system.

15.3.3 Informed Consent Requirements

If the legal basis that allows the processing of the patient's health data is consent, which is one of the exceptions provided by Article 9, then GDPR requires it to be both *explicit* and *informed*, other than freely given, specific, and unambiguous. However, national legislation[11] and international ethical guidelines also require a health care professional to provide additional information on the medical treatment, so that the meaning of *informed* consent is strengthened with respect to that of GDPR. This is based on the principle of self-determination as a fundamental human right.

Article 5 of The European Convention on Human Rights and Biomedicine (the "Treaty of Oviedo," 1997, which is legally binding) states that

> An intervention in the health field may only be carried out after the person concerned has given free and informed consent to it. This person shall beforehand be given appropriate information as to the purpose and nature of the intervention as well as on its consequences and risks. The person concerned may freely withdraw consent at any time.

The Charter of Fundamental Rights of the European Union also considers the rights of patients as a human right, clearly stating that

> Every individual has the right of access to all information that might enable him or her to actively participate in the decisions regarding his or her health; this information is a prerequisite for any procedure and treatment, including their participation in scientific research.

In addition, according to Article 3 of the charter doctors have the duty to only act with the consent of the patient:

> In the fields of medicine and biology, the following must be respected in particular: the free and informed consent of the person concerned, according to the procedures laid down by law.

In order to be considered valid, consent must also be *specific*. This means that it must be given to every specific medical treatment, but the law does not specify the exact degree of details required for the consent to be considered valid: it is the judge who makes a case-by-case evaluation (Rao 2008). For example, the Italian Court of Cassation has recently ruled that consent can be said to be valid only when the processing is clearly identified, that is, "well defined in its essential elements" Paolucci (2021).[12] It is clear,

---

11 Each country may have specific legislation regarding medical consent, e.g. the Italian Law no. 219/2017.
12 Corte di Cassazione, sez. I civ., 25 maggio 2021, n. 14381.

therefore, that it is crucial to sufficiently inform the patient in order to avoid liability if a Court is called upon to take a decision on the case.

The requirements regarding consent are not only legal obligations but also ethical (Bath and Watson 2009). Making the patient fully aware of the risks and consequences of medical treatments, procedures, and practices, is also a basic principle of ethics. When the treatment is experimental or the effects are unknown, additional ethical principles enshrined in the Helsinki Declaration[13] must also be respected.

With regard to A.I. ethics in the medical field, the World Medical Association (WMA) published a statement that recommends the enacting of the transparency principle:

> Developers and regulators of health care AI systems must ensure proper disclosure and note the benefits, limitations, and scope of appropriate use of such systems. In turn, physicians will need to understand AI methods and systems in order to rely upon clinical recommendations. Instruction in the opportunities and limitations of health care AI systems must take place both with medical students and practicing physicians, as physician involvement is critical to successful evolution of the field. AI systems must always adhere to professional values and ethics of the medical profession.[14]

This statement highlights the need of transparency whenever AI systems are employed in health care, and stresses the fact that doctors need to understand the system before relying on its output for clinical decisions. This further advocates for the use of interpretable models instead of black boxes.

15.4 Accountability Principle

The principle of accountability prescribes that Controllers must be able to demonstrate compliance in all aspects of the data processing at any time. The burden of proof is on them, and they are not only subject to fines from the Data Protection Authorities, but they are also liable for damages in Court (Article 82 of GDPR). When AI systems are in use in medical practice, the hospital, the clinic, and the doctor have a professional liability as well. It is in their interest, therefore, to comply with all applicable laws and regulations and to keep records that will allow them to demonstrate such compliance.

Considering all of the above, it is clear that when patients' data are involved the safest option is to use an interpretable model. Without knowing how data will be processed by the AI system, it is often impossible to inform sufficiently the data subjects involved and therefore to obtain their prior explicit consent for the data processing; it is also impossible

---

13 The Declaration of Helsinki is a document containing a set of ethical principles regarding human experimentation and was drafted in 1964 by the World Medical Association (WMA). After the first version in 1964, it has been revised many times. It is considered one of the most important documents on human research ethics.

14 WMA statement on augmented intelligence in medical care, Adopted by the 70th WMA General Assembly, Tbilisi, Georgia, October 2019, full text available at https://www.wma.net/policies-post/wma-statement-on-augmented-intelligence-in-medical-care/.

to meet the other transparency obligations regarding ADM as described in this chapter. In fact, from a technical point of view, only interpretable models are adequate to provide information about the logic involved in the decision process and the reasoning underlying the processing of their data. In addition, black box models may have a significant impact on medical malpractice liability claims (Nicholson Price II 2017), as it is not possible to justify and demonstrate in Court the reasons behind the decision of the AI system. The argument "the AI system said that the patient has cancer, and being more accurate than humans, I decided to suggest chemotherapy" does not hold in Court. This risk is mitigated only if the clinician has multiple reasons other than the output of the black-box AI system to justify the decision of administering a certain treatment.

From an accountability perspective, it is also more difficult to demonstrate compliance with applicable law when black boxes are involved, especially considering that, in addition to transparency obligations, fairness and non-discrimination principles need to be taken into consideration. We will explore these principles in the section 15.5.

15.5   Non-discrimination Principle and Biases

GDPR contains the principle of fairness and non-discrimination. Fairness means that personal data must be handled in ways that people would reasonably expect, and should not be used in ways that have unjustified adverse effects on them, for example in a discriminatory way. The principle of non-discrimination is also enshrined in the EU Charter of Fundamental Rights (Article 21), in many constitutions, and in multiple other legal sources.

Considering GDPR, Recital 71, par. 2, highlights that:

> In order to ensure fair and transparent processing in respect of the data subject, taking into account the specific circumstances and context in which the personal data are processed, the controller should use appropriate mathematical or statistical procedures for the profiling, implement technical and organizational measures appropriate to ensure, in particular, that factors which result in inaccuracies in personal data are corrected and the risk of errors is minimized, secure personal data in a manner that takes account of the potential risks involved for the interests and rights of the data subject and that prevents, inter alia, discriminatory effects on natural persons on the basis of racial or ethnic origin, political opinion, religion or beliefs, trade union membership, genetic or health status or sexual orientation, or that result in measures having such an effect. Automated decision-making and profiling based on special categories of personal data should be allowed only under specific conditions.

With relation to data sets, guidelines highlighted that:

> Controllers should carry out frequent assessments on the data sets they process to check for any bias, and develop ways to address any prejudicial elements, including any over-reliance on correlations. Systems that audit algorithms and regular reviews of the accuracy and relevance of automated decision-making including profiling are

other useful measures. Controllers should introduce appropriate procedures and measures to prevent errors, inaccuracies or discrimination on the basis of special category data. These measures should be used on a cyclical basis; not only at the design stage, but also continuously, as the profiling is applied to individuals. The outcome of such testing should feed back into the system design (Article 29 Data protection Working Party 2017).

The same concept is present in the AI Act as well. Because AI-based medical devices are considered "high-risk systems," the regulation sets strict requirements, such as the examination of data sets "in view of possible biases" and the fact that "training, validation and testing need to be relevant, representative, free of errors and complete, including appropriate statistical properties with regard to the persons or group of persons on which the system is intended to be used" (Article 10 and Recital 44), particularly in order to avoid perpetuating and exacerbating historical patterns of discrimination.

Deep learning and in general black box models are powerful methods that are very useful for patients and clinicians, for example in producing basic radiological findings, with high reliability (Stone et al. 2016). Their use in the medical practice is increasing despite a number of known issues (Challen et al. 2019; Babic et al. 2021), for example, the fact that they still carry a risk of introducing undetectable biases. In fact, if any bias is present in society, it will also be present in the data set, and machine learning algorithms will learn it and, in some cases, even exacerbate it (Panch et al. 2019). Mere feature and variable selection is not *per se* sufficient to reduce algorithmic bias (Rajkomar et al. 2018) also because small perturbations in the quality of data input can lead to relevant mistakes in output (Wang et al. 2020), and errors may occur if the systems is operating in an environment different from that of the training (Amodei et al. 2016) (a circumstance that is very frequent in the medical practice). Rudin and other scholars highlighted that explaining black boxes does not solve their problems but rather it may even worsen the issue because it might provide misleading or false characterizations (Rudin 2019; Laugel et al. 2019; Babic et al. 2021; Lakkaraju and Bastani 2020), or lead to use black boxes even when unnecessary (Rudin and Radin 2019).

Without an interpretable model, it is harder not only to explain the reason that lead to the biased output but also to detect the presence of an error or a bias in the first place (Challen et al. 2019).

Interpretability is also a prominent factor in generating trust in AI models (Wagstaff 2012; Rudin and Wagstaff 2014; Lo Piano 2020; Ashoori and Weisz 2019; Schmidt and Biessmann 2019; Thiebes et al. 2021; Spiegelhalter 2020; Rudin et al. 2022). Although trust is not a legal requirement, it is still very important for the success of technological applications. Even if doctors or patients know that a certain model is very accurate, they may not use it because of a lack of trust. On the opposite, there may be as well the risk that, with time, doctors may become so used to employing AI models in their everyday practice that they could trust them blindly, leading to mistakes, misdiagnosis, and the impossibility of meeting the human oversight requirement.[15]

---

15 Article 14, par. 4.b of the AI Act defines this risk as "automation bias."

15.6 High-Risk Systems and Human Oversight

Human oversight is required both by GDPR (with regards to ADM) and AI Act and it is considered a right of the data subject.

In fact, according to GDPR, data subjects have the right to obtain that the decision on them is made by a human being. This is particularly difficult in situations in which doctors strongly rely on automated means (e.g. because the number of data, parameters, or patients is too high to be processed by hand). In a recent study, it has been found that the output of an AI system may influence the decision of the clinician to treat a patient, up to the point that they decide to change the treatment (Somashekhar et al. 2019).

According to Article 14 of the AI Act, on the other hand, high-risks systems, such as medical devices,[16] should be provided with measures that enable the overseer to:

- (a) fully understand the capacities and limitations of the high-risk AI system and be able to duly monitor its operation, so that signs of anomalies, dysfunctions and unexpected performance can be detected and addressed as soon as possible;
- (b) remain aware of the possible tendency of automatically relying or over-relying on the output produced by a high-risk AI system ('automation bias'), in particular for high-risk AI systems used to provide information or recommendations for decisions to be taken by natural persons;
- (c) be able to correctly interpret the high-risk AI system's output, taking into account in particular the characteristics of the system and the interpretation tools and methods available;
- (d) be able to decide, in any particular situation, not to use the high-risk AI system or otherwise disregard, override or reverse the output of the high-risk AI system;
- (e) be able to intervene on the operation of the high-risk AI system or interrupt the system through a "stop" button or a similar procedure.

---

16 Article 1 of the Regulation on Medical Devices (Regulation (EU) 2017/745) defines a medical device as "any instrument, apparatus, appliance, software, implant, reagent, material or other article intended by the manufacturer to be used, alone or in combination, for human beings for one or more of the following specific medical purposes:

— diagnosis, prevention, monitoring, prediction, prognosis, treatment or alleviation of disease,
— diagnosis, monitoring, treatment, alleviation of, or compensation for, an injury or disability,
— investigation, replacement or modification of the anatomy or of a physiological or pathological process or state,
— providing information by means of in vitro examination of specimens derived from the human body, including organ, blood, and tissue donations, and which does not achieve its principal intended action by pharmacological, immunological, or metabolic means, in or on the human body, but which may be assisted in its function by such means."

The following products shall also be deemed to be medical devices:

— devices for the control or support of conception;
— "products specifically intended for the cleaning, disinfection or sterilization of devices as referred to in Article 1(4) and of those referred to in the first paragraph of this point." It is clear that a large number of AI models applied in the medical domain falls within this definition, and therefore must comply with the Regulation.

Recital 48 further specifies the concept, explaining that

> appropriate human oversight measures should be identified by the provider of the system before its placing on the market or putting into service. In particular, where appropriate, such measures should guarantee that the system is subject to in-built operational constraints that cannot be overridden by the system itself and is responsive to the human operator, and that the natural persons to whom human oversight has been assigned have the necessary competence, training and authority to carry out that role.

Human oversight is difficult when black boxes are employed in the health care practice, especially in complex cases, as doctors are unable to understand what factors lead to a certain decision and therefore cannot include it as part of a larger clinical assessment. With white boxes, on the contrary, clinicians can modify their assessment knowing that a certain output was or was not due to clinical factors (Wang et al. 2020). Interpretable models are, thus, more likely to satisfy this requirement.

15.7 Additional Requirements of the AI Act Proposal

The new proposal for a regulation of AI in Europe is providing for additional requirements for medical devices and other high-risk systems.[17]

One of the most important requirements is the risk management system, which is an overarching obligation throughout the whole phases of the AI life-cycle, including the post-release phase. Among different measures, it is worth noting paragraph 4 of Article 9: "In eliminating or reducing risks related to the use of the high-risk AI system, due consideration shall be given to the technical knowledge, experience, education, training to be expected by the user and the environment in which the system is intended to be used." As required by the transparency principle as well, this obligation is highlighting the importance of adapting the system to the peculiarities of the users according to their level of understanding, in order to reduce the risks. The degree of explanation given to the users needs to be modulated to their knowledge: a system intended for doctors will be designed differently than that intended for technicians, nurses, or patients. Figure 15.1 shows a summary of the envisaged measures. For high-risk systems, the AI Act proposal requires making an effort to foresee possible current and future risks, not only related to the correct use of the system, but also with a view to possible misuse. The evaluation of these risks must be carried out also after the release of the system in the market.

A complex system of data governance is required by Article 10 for "systems which make use of techniques involving the training of models with data." The novelty of the proposal is that it formally introduces technical measures meant to assure a good quality of the data

---

17 To make sure that an AI system is compliant with existing law, the Regulations on Medical Devices and on In-Vitro Diagnostic Devices (Regulation (EU) 2017/746) should also be taken into account, as they complement the requirements of the AI Act. However, the analysis of those regulations falls outside the scope of this work.

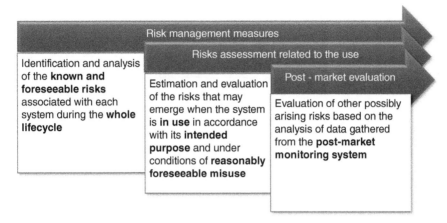

Figure 15.1 The risk management system prescribed by the AI Act proposal.

set and of the model itself.[18] For example, it requires testing the system and cleaning the data set, to assess whether biases are present. With regard to systems that continue to learn after being released, it must be ensured that 'possibly biased outputs due to outputs used as an input for future operations ("feedback loops") are duly addressed with appropriate mitigation measures' (Article 15). It is clear that the proposal is trying to promote a trustworthy AI framework at the European level. Considering the whole text of the AI Act, however, it is possible to say that in the medical field the requirements set by the proposal are hardly satisfiable by a black box system. Identifying biases is difficult even when it is clear why the system has given a particular output, but it may be impossible to detect them when it is not clear the reasoning underlying the output. Figure 15.2 shows a scheme of the obligations provided by the proposal throughout the different AI development phases.

15.8 Interpretability as a Standard

Many scholars have been arguing that, due to their inner opacity, black box algorithms should not be accepted as standard practice in fields like medicine, mainly because they

---

18 Paragraphs 2, 3, and 4 of Article 10 state that: "2. Training, validation and testing data sets shall be subject to appropriate data governance and management practices. Those practices shall concern in particular, (a) the relevant design choices; (b) data collection; (c) relevant data preparation processing operations, such as annotation, labeling, cleaning, enrichment, and aggregation; (d) the formulation of relevant assumptions, notably with respect to the information that the data are supposed to measure and represent; (e) a prior assessment of the availability, quantity, and suitability of the data sets that are needed; (f) examination in view of possible biases; (g) the identification of any possible data gaps or shortcomings, and how those gaps and shortcomings can be addressed. 3. Training, validation, and testing data sets shall be relevant, representative, free of errors, and complete. They shall have the appropriate statistical properties, including, where applicable, as regards the persons or groups of persons on which the high-risk AI system is intended to be used. These characteristics of the data sets may be met at the level of individual data sets or a combination thereof. 4. Training, validation, and testing data sets shall take into account, to the extent required by the intended purpose, the characteristics or elements that are particular to the specific geographical, behavioral, or functional setting within which the high-risk AI system is intended to be used."

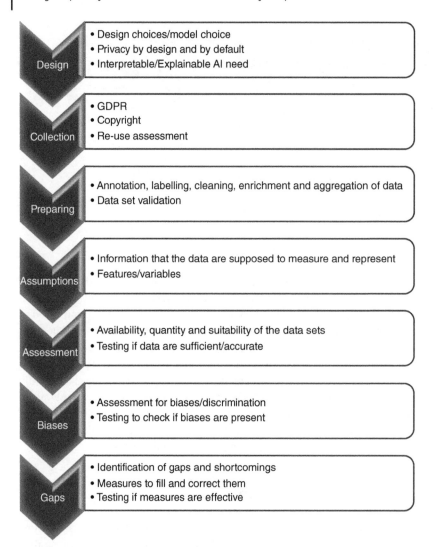

Figure 15.2 Data governance requirements.

cannot guarantee essential good medical practice features (Durán and Jongsma 2021). Some authors have even suggested that black box models should be totally excluded in high-sensitive domains such as the health care sector (Rudin 2019; Kundu 2021). (Das and Rad 2020) notes that

> Blindly trusting the results of a highly predictive classifier is, by today's standard, inadvisable, due to the strong influence of data bias, trustability, and adversarial examples in machine learning.

Regarding post hoc explainability, although it may be a useful tool, the limitations must be taken into account, as explained by Rudin (2019) and Babic et al. (2021). Vale et al. (2022) show

> the limitations of post-hoc explainability methods in demonstrating prima facie discrimination. Post-hoc explainability methods lack the orientation towards illustrating outcome parity, which is essential for EU non-discrimination law. Moreover, their technical shortcomings mean that they are in some cases unstable and suffer from low fidelity. Subsequently, they cannot faithfully demonstrate the absence of discrimination (the null hypothesis). Finally, the limited bias types unearthed through post-hoc explainability methods mean that their use must be confined and contextually appreciated. The utility of post-hoc explainability methods is useful, especially in model design and development, but they are possibly limited for regulatory or legal use. They, therefore, cannot be championed as silver bullets and/or can longer be appreciated alone in a void ignorant of broader fairness metrics. If post-hoc explainability methods cannot prima facie prove discrimination, the substantive legal weight they might be able to carry does not bode well. Accordingly, if one cannot guarantee the insights and/or inner workings of a black-box model, they ought not to use them in instances where its decisions can have long-lasting and/or dramatic effects.

It is worth mentioning that the European Commission has recently published a proposal for an AI Liability Directive, which interrelates with the AI Act and with the Product Liability Directive. Should discrimination arise from an AI system, civil liability for the producer or the user might lead to the compensation of damages.

Another fact that leads toward interpretable models in the medical field is that health is a fundamental human right that is protected both by international legal instruments and by most Constitutions; this implies that even a small risk of discrimination due to hidden biases is not tolerated by the legal system. Black boxes do not allow to have control over the model output, and it is not possible to review the reasoning process in order to check if it is based on discriminatory or irrelevant elements. In addition, it would be very difficult to ascertain if the biased output is a reflection of societal biases or of the modeler's own unconscious biases or beliefs, and, in some legal systems, that could lead to problems in ascertaining the liability (e.g. for gross negligence or willful misconduct in creating a biased model).

Considering the whole legal framework described in this chapter, it is possible to argue that interpretability should be used as a standard in the medical field and black boxes should be employed only in cases in which it is possible to take a decision evaluating other elements other than the AI output.

If part of a larger clinical assessment, for example, combined with interpretable models, or with other elements (such as physical examination, anamnesis, ultrasounds, etc.), black boxes can be an important resource. Multi-modal, heterogeneous systems,[19] however, are difficult to realize because it is complicated to have access to the relevant data from multiple sources and combine them consistently.

---

19 For example, combining a black box model that processes MRI scans with a model that processes additional data from the patients, which may be relevant for the clinical decision.

The Table below shows the main international sources of law cited in this chapter.

Name	Type	Year
AI Liability Directive proposal	EU Directive	2022
AI Act proposal	EU Regulation	2021
GDPR	EU Regulation	2016
Charter of Fundamental Rights of the European Union	EU Treaty	2000
Treaty of Oviedo	EU Convention	1994
Product Liability Directive	EU Directive	1985
Convention 108	International Convention	1981
Helsinki Declaration	International Guidelines	1964

15.9 Conclusion

The health care sector is inextricably linked to the processing of personal data. Both the persons creating an AI system intended for use in this field and the persons who will operate the system on real patients must abide by all the applicable laws and regulations, in particular complying with the principles enshrined in GDPR and in AI Act.

Complying with the principles of transparency, fairness, accountability, and human oversight is much easier with an interpretable model, while black boxes are very problematic because of their opacity.

The challenge of preserving accuracy while at the same time avoiding sacrificing transparency can be achieved through the use of heterogeneous systems, in which interpretable models work together with black boxes, in collaboration with human beings.

Future works in the fields of Law, Ethics, and Computer Science may give a better understanding of the use of post hoc explainability and the opportunities arising from interpretable models. Advances in research regarding bias detection and avoidance might mitigate the negative effects and outcomes arising from the use of AI systems in the biomedical field.

Author Biography

Chiara Gallese is Marie Sklodowska Curie Fellow at the Department of Law at Turin University (Italy), a guest researcher at the Department of Electrical Engineering at Eindhoven University of Technology (the Netherlands), and at the School of Engineering at Carlo Cattaneo University – LIUC (Italy). She is also a Fellow of the ISLC – Information Society Law Center, Milan (Italy) Her research interests include AI and Law, AI Ethics, and Privacy.

References

Amodei, D., Olah, C., Steinhardt, J. et al. (2016). Concrete problems in AI safety. *arXiv preprint arXiv:1606.06565*.

Arrieta, A.B., Díaz-Rodríguez, N., Del Ser, J. et al. (2020). Explainable artificial intelligence (XAI): concepts, taxonomies, opportunities and challenges toward responsible AI. *Information Fusion* 58: 82–115.

Article 29 Data protection Working Party (2017). Guidelines on automated individual decision-making and profiling for the purposes of regulation 2016/679. *WP215*, 1.

Article 29 Data protection Working Party (2018). Guidelines on transparency under regulation 2016/679. *WP260 rev*, 1.

Ashoori, M. and Weisz, J.D. (2019). In AI we trust? Factors that influence trustworthiness of ai-infused decision-making processes. *arXiv preprint arXiv:1912.02675*.

Babic, B., Gerke, S., Evgeniou, T., and Cohen, I.G. (2021). Beware explanations from AI in health care. *Science* 373 (6552): 284–286.

Bath, P.M.W. and Watson, A.R. (2009). Need for ethics approval and patient consent in clinical research. *Stroke* 40: 1555–1556.

Carvalho, D.V., Pereira, E.M., and Cardoso, J.S. (2019). Machine learning interpretability: a survey on methods and metrics. *Electronics* 8 (8): 832.

Challen, R., Denny, J., Pitt, M. et al. (2019). Artificial intelligence, bias and clinical safety. *BMJ Quality & Safety* 28 (3): 231–237.

Chazette, L. and Schneider, K. (2020). Explainability as a non-functional requirement: challenges and recommendations. *Requirements Engineering* 25 (4): 493–514.

Chazette, L., Brunotte, W., and Speith, T. (2021). Exploring explainability: a definition, a model, and a knowledge catalogue. *2021 IEEE 29th International Requirements Engineering Conference (RE)*, 197–208. IEEE.

Christodoulou, E., Ma, J., Collins, G.S. et al. (2019). A systematic review shows no performance benefit of machine learning over logistic regression for clinical prediction models. *Journal of Clinical Epidemiology* 110: 12–22.

Das, A. and Rad, P. (2020). Opportunities and challenges in explainable artificial intelligence (XAI): a survey. *arXiv preprint arXiv:2006.11371*.

Durán, J.M. and Jongsma, K.R. (2021). Who is afraid of black box algorithms? On the epistemological and ethical basis of trust in medical AI. *Journal of Medical Ethics* 47 (5): 329–335.

European Data Protection Board (2019). Opinion 3/2019 concerning the Questions and Answers on the interplay between the Clinical Trials Regulation (CTR) and the General Data Protection regulation (GDPR).

European Data Protection Board (2020). A Preliminary Opinion on data protection and scientific research.

European Medicines Agency (2020). The General Data Protection Regulation: Secondary Use of Data for Medicines and Public Health Purposes. Discussion Paper for Medicines Developers, Data Providers, Research-Performing and Research-Supporting Infrastructures. European Union.

Kindt, E., López, C.A.F., Czarnocki, J., and Kanevskaia, O. (2021). Study on the appropriate safeguards required under Article 89(1) of the GDPR for the processing of personal data for the scientific research. European Data Protection Board.

Köhl, M.A., Baum, K., Langer, M. et al. (2019). Explainability as a non-functional requirement. *2019 IEEE 27th International Requirements Engineering Conference (RE)*, 363–368. IEEE.

Kundu, S. (2021). Ai in medicine must be explainable. *Nature Medicine* 27 (8): 1328–1328.

Lakkaraju, H. and Bastani, O. (2020). "How do i fool you?" Manipulating user trust via misleading black box explanations. *Proceedings of the AAAI/ACM Conference on AI, Ethics, and Society*, 79–85.

Laugel, T., Lesot, M.-J., Marsala, C. et al. (2019). The dangers of post-hoc interpretability: unjustified counterfactual explanations. *Proceedings of the 28th International Joint Conference on Artificial Intelligence*, 2801–2807.

Lo Piano, S. (2020). Ethical principles in machine learning and artificial intelligence: cases from the field and possible ways forward. *Humanities and Social Sciences Communications* 7 (1): 1–7.

Miller, T. (2019). Explanation in artificial intelligence: Insights from the social sciences. *Artificial Intelligence* 267: 1–38.

Nicholson Price II, W. (2017). Medical malpractice and black-box medicine. Big Data, Health Law, and Bioethics (Cambridge University Press, 2018), University of Michigan Public Law Research Paper No. 536.

Panch, T., Mattie, H., and Atun, R. (2019). Artificial intelligence and algorithmic bias: implications for health systems. *Journal of Global Health* 9 (2): 020318.

Paolucci, F. (2021). Consenso, intelligenza artificiale e privacy. *MediaLaws –Rivista di diritto dei media*, 2/2021.

Petch, J., Di, S., and Nelson, W. (2021). Opening the black box: the promise and limitations of explainable machine learning in cardiology. *Canadian Journal of Cardiology* 38 (2): 204–213.

Rajkomar, A., Hardt, M., Howell, M.D. et al. (2018). Ensuring fairness in machine learning to advance health equity. *Annals of Internal Medicine* 169 (12): 866–872.

Rao, K.H.S. (2008). Informed consent: an ethical obligation or legal compulsion? *Journal of Cutaneous and Aesthetic Surgery* 1 (1): 33.

Ribeiro, M.T., Singh, S., and Guestrin, C. (2016). "Why should i trust you?" Explaining the predictions of any classifier. *Proceedings of the 22nd ACM SIGKDD International Conference on Knowledge Discovery and Data Mining*, 1135–1144.

Rong, G., Mendez, A., Assi, E.B. et al. (2020). Artificial intelligence in healthcare: review and prediction case studies. *Engineering* 6 (3): 291–301.

Rosenfeld, A. and Richardson, A. (2019). Explainability in human–agent systems. *Autonomous Agents and Multi-Agent Systems* 33 (6): 673–705.

Rudin, C. (2019). Stop explaining black box machine learning models for high stakes decisions and use interpretable models instead. *Nature Machine Intelligence* 1 (5): 206–215.

Rudin, C. and Radin, J. (2019). Why are we using black box models in AI when we don't need to? A lesson from an explainable AI competition. *Harvard Data Science Review* 1 (2): https://doi.org/10.1162/99608f92.5a8a3a3d.

Rudin, C. and Wagstaff, K.L. (2014). Machine learning for science and society. *Machine Learning* 95: 1–9.

Rudin, C., Chen, C., Chen, Z. et al. (2022). Interpretable machine learning: fundamental principles and 10 grand challenges. *Statistics Surveys* 16: 1–85.

Schmidt, P. and Biessmann, F. (2019). Quantifying interpretability and trust in machine learning systems. *arXiv preprint arXiv:1901.08558*.

Secinaro, S., Calandra, D., Secinaro, A. et al. (2021). The role of artificial intelligence in healthcare: a structured literature review. *BMC Medical Informatics and Decision Making* 21 (1): 1–23.

Somashekhar, S.P., Sepúlveda, M.-J., Shortliffe, E.H. et al. (2019). A prospective blinded study of 1000 cases analyzing the role of artificial intelligence: Watson for oncology and change in decision making of a multidisciplinary tumor board (MDT) from a tertiary care cancer center.

Spiegelhalter, D. (2020). Should we trust algorithms? *Harvard Data Science Review* 2 (1): https://doi.org/10.1162/99608f92.cb91a35a.

Stone, P., Brooks, R., Brynjolfsson, E. et al. (2016). Artificial intelligence and life in 2030: the one hundred year study on artificial intelligence.

Thiebes, S., Lins, S., and Sunyaev, A. (2021). Trustworthy artificial intelligence. *Electronic Markets* 31 (2): 447–464.

Vale, D., El-Sharif, A., and Ali, M. (2022). Explainable artificial intelligence (XAI) post-hoc explainability methods: risks and limitations in non-discrimination law. *AI and Ethics* 2: 815–826.

Wagstaff, K. (2012). Machine learning that matters. *arXiv preprint arXiv:1206.4656*.

Wang, F., Kaushal, R., and Khullar, D. (2020). Should health care demand interpretable artificial intelligence or accept "black box" medicine? *Annals of Internal Medicine* 172 (1): 59–60.

16

The Long Path to Usable AI

Barbara Di Camillo[1,2], Enrico Longato[1], Erica Tavazzi[1] and Martina Vettoretti[1]

[1]*Department of Information Engineering, University of Padova, Padua, Italy*
[2]*Department of Comparative Biomedicine and Food Science, University of Padova, Padua, Italy*

16.1 Promises and Challenges of Artificial Intelligence in Healthcare

There are a lot of expectations, nowadays, about artificial intelligence (AI) and its applications in medicine and healthcare in general. The hope and the promise are that these techniques will help integrate data automatically with the aim of revealing unknown patterns, risk factors, and diagnostic/prognostic variables, allowing us to predict the course of a disease. Aided by suitable technologies for data collection, data transfer, and computation/visualization of results, these methodologies promise to revolutionize medical care. The idea is that the outcome of AI models will help us define risk mitigation policies, promote behavioral changes, suggest diagnosis prognosis and treatment, optimize health cost analysis and distribution, and democratize medicine allowing access to quality healthcare.

However, the difficulties that separate us from the full exploitation of the so-called big data in healthcare are varied and manifold. First, there are difficulties in using and managing big data starting from their volume, which can make computing complex due to a lack of sufficient memory or computing power. The speed with which data is sometimes acquired (think, for example, of wearable sensors for continuous patient monitoring or the speed with which sequencing data is produced) sometimes leads to transmission problems or the need for real-time processing.

The healthcare data are then of a different type and nature. Typically, continuous, discrete, and categorical variables are available. Data of a completely different nature need to be integrated such as – omics data (RNA sequencing, DNA sequencing, protein data, etc.), clinical data, and environmental data. The available variables can also differ in terms of temporal availability, with data being available as a single time point or as time-series data, the latter often collected with a nonuniform sampling grid which might vary for different patients. Furthermore, healthcare data are often affected by significant technical and biological variability. Moreover, the change in clinical protocols or measurement tools might lead to variations in the scale or unit of measurement of the monitored variables without mentioning possible entry errors in databases. Given these premises, aspects such as data acquisition and storage, data cleaning, and data integration appear in all their complexity.

Big Data Analysis and Artificial Intelligence for Medical Sciences, First Edition.
Edited by Bruno Carpentieri and Paola Lecca.
© 2024 John Wiley & Sons Ltd. Published 2024 by John Wiley & Sons Ltd.

On a more organizational and regulatory level, there is the important issue of patient and citizen privacy and safety, and non-secondary aspects such as the ownership of data and results produced using the data, together with the data management and the possibility of sharing data to obtain more accurate and reliable results.

Based on fundamental rights and ethical principles, in April 2021 the European High-Level Expert Group on Artificial Intelligence made public a document (https://ec.europa.eu/futurium/en/ai-alliance-consultation.1.html), describing the seven key requirements that AI systems should meet in order to be trustworthy: (i) Human agency and oversight; (ii) Technical robustness and safety; (iii) Privacy and data governance; (iv) Transparency; (v) Diversity, non-discrimination, and fairness; (vi) Societal and environmental well-being; and (vii) Accountability.

AI should support humans in their decisions and tasks in a framework that allows humans fulfilling their goals and maintain autonomy in their interaction with AI systems. In this context, maintaining the ability of human self-determination, i.e. the ability to intervene in the decision and ultimately overrule it, requires a clear definition of the purposes of the AI systems and of their limits, of the domain of possible situations of use, and, finally, of the actions of humans in response to AI suggestions. This latter is strongly related to the capability of understanding the reasons of the AI-based suggestion.

A second important aspect of trustworthy AI is technical robustness. AI systems need to be protected by hacking and by data corruption that might lead to wrong decisions and harm. Cybersecurity practices necessary to prevent such events need to be adopted, together with backup strategies and the possibility of human intervention. The technical robustness also pertains the system accuracy, i.e. the ability to make correct predictions, together with AI systems reliability and reproducibility, i.e. the ability to make correct judgments with different data input in a well-defined domain of validity and in a reproducible way.

AI systems must guarantee privacy and data protection ensuring that data will not be used to infer aspects of private life that are out of the purpose of the specific tool and that might be used to discriminate. Quality and integrity of data must also be ensured together with data protocols governing data access so that duly qualified personnel with the competence and need to access individual's data should be allowed to do so.

An important aspect related to security and to human oversight is AI transparency. The data used for training the AI algorithms, their preprocessing, the algorithms themselves, and the process of model assessment should always be well described and documented. Possible prediction mistakes should be also traced, so to better understand the domain of validity and make possible corrective actions. On the other hand, AI must be explainable, i.e. decisions must be understandable by a human being so that, in case, the principle of human oversight can be advocated. It is important to note that the availability of AI systems also changes the organizational aspect. Think of a hospital where an automatic image analysis system is used as an aid to the doctors to enhance the number of screening exams and timely diagnosis. This will have an effect both on the physician's attitude toward the outcome of the examination (how much will he/she trust or be influenced by the suggestion of the algorithm) and on the increased number of interventions that the increased number of screening exams will lead to. It is important, from the point of view of explainability, also to make these aspects explicit, to clarify the impact of AI on the organization's decision-making processes.

Datasets used for AI model development might be biased in terms of lack of inclusiveness of subpopulations of interest. A typical example of bias starting from data collection is gender bias in medicine (Hamberg 2008). Indeed, removing bias starts with data collection and integration of meaningful variables and representative subjects. In this context, it is of mandatory importance to address data governance and data-sharing issues, so as to be able to integrate data from subjects of diverse gender, cultures, and ethnic groups.

Appropriate assessment of AI systems is also important: accuracy, precision, sensitivity, specificity, etc., need to be monitored using suitable train/validation/test frameworks and verifying the performance on subgroups of patients, less represented groups, and on different populations with respect to the ones initially used for training. Strategies to avoid unfair bias starts from the acknowledgment of the possible limitations stemming from the composition of the used data sets, but also include considering the diversity of users' needs and the availability of processes to test and monitor for potential biases during the assessment and the use of the system.

In line with the principles of fairness and prevention of harm, AI systems should ensure societal and environmental well-being. In the context of healthcare, we should make sure that AI tools do not negatively affect physical and mental well-being. For example, in the context of digital therapeutics, it has been shown that users might develop dependency on the tools (Jae-Yong 2019), that, despite the positive effect of the therapy, must be considered as a side effect and monitored as such. We should therefore envisage the need for prospective studies or even clinical trials to monitor effects on clinical decisions, patients' reactions, and possible side effects.

Finally, the last requirement, complementing the other six, is accountability and responsibility of AI systems both in the phase of assessment and in the phase of use. Responsibility is the acceptance of moral and legal consequences of a decision or action. Given the nature of AI, defining responsibility means defining a chain of actions and checks, which must be done at various levels, in which different individuals might be responsible for the different steps and these steps can be monitored and traced whenever necessary. As such, responsibility is strongly related to accountability and auditability, i.e. the possibility of deputed organizations to assess the system. Other measures ensuring accountability include assessment of risks, education of the users, documenting trade-offs, and mechanisms of redress in case of negative impact.

Research scientists, when developing AI methods and models, hardly take into consideration aspects related to trustworthy AI. However, if we want AI to realize its full potential, algorithms architecture should consider specific constraints already in the design phase.

In this chapter, we will focus on three different aspects related to AI applicability: (i) the need of taking into consideration model applicability from the very beginning in terms of the trade-off between costs and benefits, including data preprocessing issues; (ii) the advantage of considering longitudinal data to describe disease progression in time and how different variables concur in defining a temporal phenotype of a disease; (iii) the strategies applied to allow model generalisability and the need for recalibration when they are applied to new populations.

We start from considering a problem of data management and show an example of automatic data preprocessing based on deep learning. Indeed, despite model performance and transferability, AI usability is tightly connected to its possibility of cost-effective integration with user needs and laboratory practices. In particular, we address the problem of predicting major adverse cardiovascular events (MACEs) in people with diabetes using a year of pharmacy and hospitalization administrative claims, together with basic patient information. More specifically, our aim is to predict the first occurrence of death, heart failure, myocardial infarction, or stroke, with a variable prediction horizon of one to five years. The purpose here is to show a real-life application of predictive models at the institutional level using administrative claims with minimal data processing overhead. In this example, the possibility to preprocess the data in an automatic way is a central aspect to maintain limited costs, both in terms of money and time needed to synthesize disparate types of data into scalar features.

Next, we consider potentialities and challenges related to the use of longitudinal data, a data type commonly collected during the care delivery process. Despite the technical challenges, the temporal nature of the data provides a number of advantages related to the possibility of tracking the course of disease progression and exploring the effects of treatment or unknown adverse events. Focusing on longitudinal collections of clinical data from patients affected by amyotrophic lateral sclerosis (ALS), we show how dynamic Bayesian networks (DBNs) (Murphy 2002) can be used to model the course of ALS progression over time in a way that makes the conditional dependency relationships among variables explicit. Interestingly, these models can be used to simulate disease progression and to assess the effect of specific variables on the disease time course with a high level of explainability. As an additional example of use of longitudinal data in ALS, we show an application of process mining (PM) (van der Aalst and Adriansyah 2011). PM is a family of techniques originally developed in the business context to analyze, discover, monitor, and improve business processes, whose application to healthcare is still in its infancy. Here we show how PM techniques can be used to mine the evolution of diseases in terms of timing and probability of impairment of different functional domains.

Finally, we focus on barriers limiting the application of different predictive models for type 2 diabetes (T2D) onset in public health management. Namely, (i) the problem of model choice (some models are directly applicable only to certain ethnic groups because they have been trained exclusively on those groups); (ii) the presence of many missing input variables; and (iii) the need for recalibration in the population of interest. Cases (i) and (ii) limit the possibility of applying the models; case (iii) causes inaccurate and biased predictions. We also present a possible solution to the above problems, which is based on an integrated T2D risk model. The integrated model implements a simple recalibration strategy in which the risk scores are rescaled based on the T2D incidence in the target population and the applicable models are selected based on the available input variables. A global risk score is then calculated by averaging the single risk scores (a weighted average is used to give more weight to the most reliable models). It is important to note that the simple recalibration strategy based on risk scaling does not require retraining the models in the new populations, which would be expensive both in terms of money and time, and not always feasible since these types of models need retrospective longitudinal data, which are not always available. This example shows how appropriate validation of the domain of validity of available models is necessary on one hand and useful to increase usability on the other hand.

16.2   Deployment of Usable Artificial Intelligence Models

The effective deployment of an AI model into clinical practice typically hinges on a set of considerations surrounding the model itself and its relationship with its context of use. A sensible pipeline for the assessment of model usability would, then, start from verifying that the model exhibits adequate performance, in terms of both discrimination and calibration, to meet the clinical or public health needs that it was designed to address. It would, then, continue with a possible assessment of model transferability, i.e. the model's ability to adapt to a shift in covariates or in their relationship with the output across space (e.g. a model developed in a certain geographical area that we want to use elsewhere) and time (e.g. because of changing therapeutic guidelines). Finally, we would make sure that all technological requirements are met, e.g. in terms of run time or software availability.

On top of these purely technical considerations, we identify two additional layers of complexity, which we dub willingness to use and willingness to deploy. The former is, perhaps, the more intuitive concept. It boils down to the idea that, no matter how useful a model might be or how well it might perform, the degree to which it will be used in practice is directly proportional to how closely it is perceived to meet user needs, and how well it is integrated into their day-to-day operational toolbox (Shilo et al. 2020). In other words, willingness to use might take a hit when users, e.g. do not feel in control, do not see the point of querying the model instead of following established practices, or, more generally, are not satisfied with the return on the time investment needed, on their part, to operate the model. Willingness to deploy, instead, pertains to the perceived costs-benefits balance on the part of the institution (e.g. hospital, local government, insurance company) that would like to adopt the model and make it available within their organization. In the current technological landscape, dominated by scalable, on-demand computing power delivered via cloud infrastructure, this is has less to do with the technicalities of implementing a solid, production-grade version of the desired model than with the effort associated with creating and maintaining the entire data flow pipeline needed to feed it. Specifically, in the so-called era of big data, a perhaps surprisingly high amount of resources ends up being allocated to data management (Dash et al. 2019). Oftentimes, this is the result of an inevitable disconnect between the laboratory and real-life settings: rarely, if ever, model development in the lab happens by querying the real-life data source from which data will be eventually be ingested after deployment. This typically leads to a situation where entire preprocessing pipelines must be re-implemented from scratch to fit the security, data usage, and technological constraints of the data source. Additional effort is, then, needed to maintain the new pipeline, usually without the involvement of the original researchers, creating further overhead.

Within the machine learning and artificial intelligence communities, it is generally accepted that preprocessing is, in fact, part of the model. However, this is usually understood in terms of the purely methodological considerations with which we started this section (performance, robustness, etc.), leading to not placing the adequate emphasis on deployment during the development phase, and, thus, to the aforementioned mismatch between laboratory and real-life conditions. In the field of medical sciences, operating under the secondary use of data framework (Burton et al. 2017), we frequently encounter situations where clinical objectives are pursued via the best available data rather than the ideal data for the task. So, for instance, we might be missing critical variables, or we might be tied to unconventional data types that serve as proxy for the desired, but unavailable, clinical variables. An equally frequent scenario involves the mismatch between the inherently dynamic nature of the real-world data, which are ever-changing and continuously acquired, and the vast majority of machine learning techniques, which only accept static inputs. We are, then, faced with two conflicting problems, both of which are responsible for substantial increases of deployment costs: on the one hand, a scarcity of data informativeness, and, on the other, an almost paradoxical data abundance over time. Traditionally, solving these problems requires implementing complex data preprocessing steps to constrain the real-world data into the boundaries of the mathematical hypotheses underlying machine learning and artificial intelligence techniques.

In this section, we suggest a viable alternative to standard approaches, based on a combination of leveraging the implicit data processing capabilities of deep learning, and assuming a deployment-aware perspective. We believe that proceeding in this way, rather than procrastinating any considerations regarding willingness to deploy until it is possibly too late to make meaningful changes, might lead to generally more successful and usable AI models. We illustrate our proposal via a case study: the development of a deep learning model to predict the cardiovascular complications of diabetes using one year's worth of the administrative claims of Veneto, a populous region in NorthEast Italy (Longato et al. 2020b, 2021).

16.2.1 Case Study: Predicting the Cardiovascular Complications of Diabetes via a Deep Learning Approach

Cardiovascular disease (CVD), although it remains the first cause of death overall, has seen its incidence steadily decline within the general population. People with diabetes, however, have not been experiencing as rapid a decrease, with MACE rates remaining several times greater than hoped (Gregg et al. 2018). Given the compounding impact of CVD and all other comorbidities and healthcare needs of patients with diabetes, predicting instances of MACE is crucial on multiple levels, from individual quality of life to system-wide cost projections. It is, then, in the interest of healthcare providers to equip themselves with the most advanced analytical tools, including AI-powered models, able to meet this personal and public health need.

In Italy, healthcare is socialized and devolved, i.e. it is publicly funded by taxes and regulated by the central government's Ministry of Health, but managed at the regional level. Universal coverage is guaranteed for all citizens and foreign residents via a complex system of reimbursements that hinges upon consistent data exchanges between healthcare providers (e.g. hospitals, pharmacies, laboratories) and political institutions (e.g. local healthcare governance and, ultimately, the Ministry). Briefly, every time healthcare services are provided, be it in the form of a prescription medicine refill or of a long hospitalizations, a specific set of documents, called administrative claims, is generated and transmitted, reporting the exact type, amount, and cost of the service. Given the high emphasis placed on the economic value of healthcare, the amount of clinical information present in administrative claims is limited (e.g. there are no laboratory test results attached to laboratory test prescriptions), but their total coverage and ready availability at a governance level are extremely appealing for the possible deployment of integrated solutions aimed at predicting crucial (and costly) events of interest, such as MACE.

Having presented the context, let us now state the objective of our case study: we are tasked with developing a predictive model of MACE for people with diabetes, based on administrative claims, with the intention of deploying it within the eHealth ecosystem of the Veneto region, in Italy. Specifically, we predict a composite indicator of MACE, reflecting a wide array of possible manifestation of CVD, which are also the main drivers of healthcare expenditures, i.e. the 4-point MACE (4P-MACE) corresponding to the first event between: a hospitalization for (i) heart failure, (ii) myocardial infarction, or (iii) stroke, or (iv) all-cause death with or without a corresponding hospitalization.

The main challenge, here, stems from coaxing Veneto's administrative claims into a format that is manageable enough that deployment is still appealing, but, at the same time, compatible with state-of-the-art machine learning and artificial intelligence methodologies. In fact, originally, the data could not be farther from the typical input of a clinical prediction model. First, as previously mentioned, administrative claims do not capture clinical information unless it is necessary to justify expenditures. Second, their original format is that of a time stamped series of rows, comprising the temporal coordinates of each event and its details, rather than clean aggregated vectors of individual parameters; data quantity can also vary wildly between citizens. Third, they are stored in different tables, with different degrees of normalization, based on the legal requirements surrounding each individual type of claims (so, e.g. pharmacy claims and hospitalization claims wildly differ from a data organization perspective). Fourth, due to infrastructural constraints, they can only be accessed via a sequence of an SQL-like query and simple extract-transform-load operations.

In practice, we are dealing with three types of administrative data, of varying complexity and volume.

1. Basic patient information (age, sex, and diabetes duration) is available as a by-product of a published, validated algorithm for the identification of diabetes using Veneto's administrative claims; this is the same algorithm used to check for patient eligibility based on evidence of diabetes (further details in Longato et al. (Longato et al. (2020a))).
2. Hospitalization data record all hospital admissions and discharges, and all diagnoses accrued by the patient by the time they are discharged, up to a maximum of six (one primary, five secondary). Diagnosis codes follow the ICD-9-CM standard (ICD (year?)). Hospitalizations are thankfully rare, with only approximately 15% of patients experiencing one or more in any given year.
3. Pharmacy claims record all prescriptions refill happening in the Region's territory. Both prescription and refill timestamps are available; prescribed but never-refilled medications are not, and neither are over-the-counter medications. Data volumes are unpredictable, ranging from a few prescriptions a year (e.g. a metformin refill every few months) for relatively healthier patients to several hundred in severe multi-comorbidity scenarios.

To reduce both complexity and volume, and, especially, to guarantee a reasonable trade-off between applicability and reliability, we set a baseline period of one year, i.e. all data to be fed as input to the model must be gathered in the year prior to the start of the prediction horizon. In this way, we exclude only an exiguous minority of citizens who have come in contact with the regional healthcare system for less than a year (e.g. because of a recent move), but gain a lot in terms of input data homogeneity.

Let us, now, consider each data type individually, and explore our options for using them as model inputs.

1. Handling basic patient information is trivial: age, sex, and diabetes duration are well-defined variables, with obvious clinical significance. They are also given to us for free by a run of the same algorithm needed to identify a citizen as someone who has diabetes and for whom we would like to get a prediction of possible, future 4P-MACE. Thus, we simply use them as-is, in the form of a 3-dimensional vector.

2. Hospitalizations claims are relatively informative from a clinical standpoint, because they report all diagnoses that led to and happened during a given hospital stay. Hospitalizations are rare events, meaning that most patients will experience no hospitalizations (hence, no data management needed), while the 15% who do will most likely generate small volumes of data, bounded above by the reasonable, if unfortunate, assumption that a sequence of repeated hospitalizations within the same year is likely to be cut short by an early death. Thus, it would make sense to aggregate all diagnoses related to the same patient into a fixed vector, integrating over time. Blind aggregation on a code-by-code basis, however, would probably still be suboptimal, given the high degree of sparsity induced by coding full 5-digit ICD-9-CM codes as dummy variables. It would, then, be advisable to identify suitable ICD-9-CM code groups and conflate all diagnoses belonging to the same group so as to strike a satisfactory trade-off between the number and informativeness of input variables. In the case study at hand, a reasonable choice might be defining those code groups as the 19 ICD-9-CM chapters themselves. This would lead to a 19-dimensional vector, easily computed via the cascade of a simple 1 : 1 substitution of individual codes with their corresponding chapter and a GROUP BY query performed on the small (or, most of the times, even empty) set of hospitalization data belonging to each patient.

3. Pharmacy claims are by far the most complex type of data we need to deal with. A priori, they are highly predictive by virtue of their tight relationship with past health outcomes, current health status, and possible future ramifications (e.g. medications used in palliative care would signal past cancer, current rapidly deteriorating health, and likely impending death). In our real-life administrative claims repository, prescription medicines are identified via the ministerial equivalent of a bar code, i.e. in a way that identifies the medication down to commercial brand and packaging (e.g. blue box of 20 pills versus red box of 35). Given the economic nature of claims, it comes as no surprise that this coding scheme has no clinical significance. The Italian Ministry of Health, however, also provides official 1 : 1 mapping of these pseudo-bar codes to more meaningful anatomical therapeutic classification (ATC) codes (ATC (year?)), which identify all medications in terms of their active ingredients and biological effects. We found 1979 of these codes in the available data. At this point, we could consider a similar approach to the one detailed for hospitalizations, i.e. an aggregation over time of refilled prescriptions and a remapping to the 48 ATC classes (second therapeutic subgroups) identified by the first three alphanumeric characters of each ATC code. This approach comes with three obvious drawbacks: first, it is difficult to justify the definition of medication subgroups in a study on diabetes and medications, given the emphasis we are expected to

place on antidiabetic agents, which should be considered individually, to the full extent of their ATC codes; second, while hospitalizations are very consistent in the amount of expected data (at most one or two hospitalizations with at most 6 diagnoses each, often none), medication usage patterns vary greatly from individual to individual (or even, over time, for the same individual); third, the frequency with which prescriptions are refilled is high enough that it is difficult to justify the complete elimination of the time dimension when working with a one-year baseline (e.g. initiating or discontinuing a certain therapy regimen are indistinguishable after bag-of-word encoding, but are obviously two very different indicators in terms of overall health).

Overall, we can easily settle on the two well-characterized and easily computed vectors, namely, the 3-dimensional patient information vector and the 19-dimensional vector of hospitalizations, but, while it is certainly a serviceable first-order approximation, we have identified several limitations with applying simple aggregation to medications.

A possible alternative would be developing a complex preprocessing scheme to transform all medications and hospitalizations into meaningful pseudo-clinical variables, i.e. into composite variables that summarize all hints of a specific disease into a binary indicator (e.g. we can assume that a patient has hypertension if they are refilling prescriptions for antihypertensive or they were discharge from hospital with a hypertension-related diagnosis). For illustrative purposes, let us consider the following variables.

- **Pre-existing conditions (16)**: Hypertension, dyslipidaemia, anaemia, peripheral circulatory disease, remote ischaemic heart disease, remote CVD, neurological complications, ocular complications, renal complications, chronic kidney disease, peripheral circulatory complications, severe hypoglycaemia, chronic pulmonary disease, systemic inflammatory disease, cancer, Charlson index.
- **Glucose-lowering medications (12)**: Metformin, acarbose, any insulin, fast-acting, long-acting, inhalation insulin, pioglitazone, sulfonylureas, DPP4is, GLP-1RAs, SGLT2is, other antidiabetic agents.
- **Other therapies (11)**: Anticoagulants, platelet aggregation inhibitors, diuretics, antihypertensives, ACE inhibitors, beta-blockers, other antihypertensives, anti-lipemic agents, statins, PCSK9 inhibitors, ezetimibe.

Note how this approach solves the problems of arbitrary coding by defining clinically meaningful mapping rules, but still fails to capture the temporal relationships between prescriptions, which we have reason to believe are indicative of future cardiovascular outcomes. Furthermore, although this type of coding scheme is very popular (Young et al. 2018), it is also a detriment in terms of willingness to deploy, as it comes with a massive computational and data management overheard associated with having to pool and aggregate heterogeneous data from different claims data streams via a custom pipeline segment for each variable.

To overcome these limitations, we propose an innovative way to handle highly variable medication histories via a deep learning approach. We start from the observation that the (i) most natural, (ii) most informative, and (iii) least expensive (in terms of data management) format for medication data would be one that preserves precise ATC codes and temporal information, but does not require complex preprocessing. The ordered sequence of prescriptions refilled by each patient clearly meets these requirements: (i) it is a direct description of a subject's treatment regimens for various health conditions; (ii) does not sacrifice nuance or temporal relationships on the altar of simplifying the input; and (iii) is easily built via a simple SELECT-ORDER BY query after 1 : 1 mapping to ATC codes. The main caveat of this strategy, however, is that it produces a variable-length sequence corresponding to all the prescriptions refilled during the baseline year, and variable-length sequences are inherently incompatible with most predictive models, which, instead, require fixed-size input vectors similar to the basic patient information and hospitalization ones. In answer to that, we observe a striking similarity between variable-length sequences of medications and variable-length sequences of words: they are both comprised of meaningful tokens endowed with both an inherent and a positional meanings. We can, then, shift our perspective and think of our one-year baseline as a one-year-long sentence, which we can handle by following known best practices of natural language processing. A straightforward way to do so leverages the combination of an embedding layer and a recurrent layer to transform an opportunely padded and masked sequence of tokens (medications here; usually words) into a fixed-length vector that can be concatenated with other fixed-length vectors (basic patient information and hospitalizations grouped into ICD-9-CM chapters) and passed through a standard feed-forward subnetwork to obtain predictions. We can proceed as follows. For further implementation details please see Longato et al. (Longato et al. (2021)).

1. We start from the sequence of ATCs corresponding to the prescriptions refilled by the patient during the baseline year, and remap it to an integer index from 1 to 1979 (this can be done instead of mapping from pseudo-bar codes to ATCs, thus saving on computational time).
2. We zero pad the sequence to a fixed length of 300 (having noted that 272 was the maximum number of prescriptions refilled in a year in the development population; the extra 10% is for future proofing). The value 0, used only as padding, will be the masking value, elements of the sequences that are equal to zero will not contribute to the final prediction.
3. We feed the zero-padded sequence to an embedding layer, i.e. a layer that estimates a dense transformation from the (implicit) one-hot encoding signified by each integer index from 1 to 1979 to a dense matrix with 300 rows and a fixed number of columns. Each row corresponds to a medication, and the columns are the data-driven, dense representation of each ATC; rows corresponding to 0s in the original zero-padded sequence are still masked, i.e. for all intents and purposes, ignored.
4. We transform the dense sequences thus obtained into fixed-length vectors via a recurrent layer such as a gated recurrent unit (GRU) (Gal and Ghahramani 2016) and the long short-term memory (LSTM) unit (Gers et al. 1999). Intuitively, these types of layer perform a parametrized integral over time of the input dense sequence, retaining only the final value of the integral. The parameters to compute these special integrals depend on the flavor of recurrent layer, but are always learnt from the data to maximize predictive power, much like the sparse-to-dense transformation was.
5. We can now treat the resulting fixed-length, dense vector as any other input vector, the only difference being that it does not represent input variables directly (as a typical input vector would), but, rather, a data-driven transformation especially optimized to solve the 4P-MACE prediction problem. In other words, we can think of this fixed-length vector

as a compact, 1-dimensional representation of complex time-varying sequences, which can now be used as if they were static data. Hence, for instance, we can feed the vector to a dense subnetwork with four parallel branches, one for each component of 4P-MACE (heart failure, myocardial infarction, stroke, and death), all converging into a final prediction for the composite 4P-MACE indicator one to five years into the future.

Let us now evaluate a model built according to these principles and compare it to a series of benchmarks based on other input coding schemes to highlight the former's desirable properties. Table 16.1 shows a comparison between the following configurations.

- The deep learning model developed in Longato et al. (Longato et al. (2021)), which we have just described (input = patient information, hospitalization vector, sequence of medications) and whose high-level architecture is shown in Figure 16.1.
- The same deep learning model fed by an artificially inverted sequence of medications (input = patient information, hospitalization vector, inverted sequence of medications). With this configuration, we want to test the deep learning model's ability to follow the arrow of time (i.e. use the information): we hypothesize that using inverted sequences as an input the model should yield worse predictions.
- A Cox model (Cox 1972), (Therneau and Grambsch 2000) where medications are encoded via their time-aggregated ATC classes (input = patient information, hospitalization vector, ATC class vector). The Cox model is a semi-parametric model where the hazard (i.e. here, the instantaneous rate of occurrence of 4P-MACE) is represented as a linear combination of the input variables. It is the de facto standard for baseline survival analysis, and generally works well enough to represent a solid benchmark for comparison. In this configuration, the medication-related input to the Cox model is an ATC class vector such that each element is equal to 1 if and only if that medication was taken by the patient within the baseline period.
- A Cox model where pseudo-clinical variables, i.e. variables with a clinical meaning derived from administrative data, act as the input (input = patient information, pseudo-clinical variables).

The target metric was the cumulative/dynamic area under the receiver-operating characteristic curve (AUROC) (Bansal and Heagerty 2018) evaluated one to five years after the one-year baseline on a test set of 10,000 citizens of the Veneto region never used for training. The cumulative/dynamic AUROC is simply the AUROC computed with a ground truth representing the cumulative probability of the event having happened by a dynamic time point (i.e. the ground truth is the answer to a question such as "Has a 4P-MACE event happened before the 2-year mark?"). Results based on the concordance index (Longato et al. 2020c) are available in the original manuscript (Longato et al. 2021).

We note how the deep learning model exhibited consistently good performance at all prediction horizons, ranging from an AUROC of 0.812 (CI: 0.797–0.827) at one year to one of 0.792 (CI: 0.781–0.802) at five years. This is especially impressive, given that we are predicting cardiovascular complications of diabetes based on a year's worth of pharmacy and hospital bills, reporting minimal clinical information, after inexpensive preprocessing. The expected decrease in performance with longer prediction horizon was also very limited, showing both the short and long term power of artificial intelligence when dealing

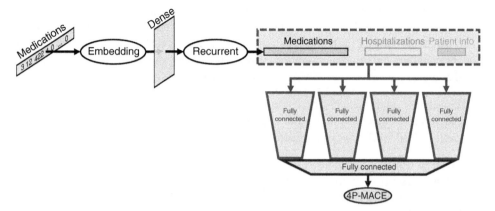

Figure 16.1 High-level view of the deep learning model's architecture. The figure represents the information flow through the model's internal components. From left to right, medication sequences are turned into fixed-length vectors by a cascade of embedding and recurrent layers; then, they are concatenated with hospitalizations and patient information; finally (top to bottom), a battery of parallel fully connected networks, one for each 4P-MACE components, converges into a single fully connected subnetwork to yield the final 4P-MACE prediction.

Table 16.1 4P-MACE prediction ($N = 10,000$).

Model	1 yr	2 yr	3 yr	4 yr	5 yr
Deep learning	0.812 (0.797–0.827)	0.808 (0.797–0.820)	0.804 (0.793–0.815)	0.799 (0.789–0.810)	0.792 (0.781–0.802)
Deep learning (inv.)	0.806 (0.791–0.822)*	0.804 (0.792–0.816)*	0.801 (0.790–0.812)*	0.797 (0.786–0.808)	0.791 (0.780–0.801)
ATC Cox	0.798 (0.783–0.814)*	0.794 (0.781–0.806)*	0.793 (0.782–0.804)*	0.788 (0.777–0.799)*	0.782 (0.772–0.793)*
Pseudo-clinical Cox	0.796 (0.781–0.811)*	0.793 (0.781–0.806)*	0.793 (0.782–0.804)*	0.789 (0.778–0.800)*	0.784 (0.774–0.795)*

"Deep learning" is the proposed model, "Deep learning (inv.)" is the model fed by inverted sequences, "ATC Cox" is the Cox proportional hazard model with ATC class codes, "Pseudo-clinical Cox" is the Cox proportional hazard model with pseudo-clinical variables. All results are reported together with 95% confidence intervals. Statistical significance at the 0.05 level is signaled by an asterisk.

with complex input data, including barely parsed, variable-length sequences. The predictive value of the sequences themselves is apparent by comparing the AUROC in the realistic scenario versus in the one where we artificially inverted the order of medications before running the model. If the order were irrelevant to model prediction, we would have expected not to see any difference in performance. Instead, we observed a statistically significant difference at one to three years, and a nominal difference at 4 and 5. This is consistent with the behavior of a model that is making use of medication order: initially, the direction of therapy changes can be extremely predictive (e.g. a patient starting or stopping therapy with morphine), whereas, as time goes on, which therapies were followed becomes more meaningful than their order.

Comparing the deep learning model to Cox models with traditional input schemes, we observe a stark superiority, in terms of raw performance, of the former: neither Cox model managed to yield an AUROC greater than 0.798, and all differences were significantly in favor of the deep learning model. It is also remarkable how pseudo-clinical variables and ATC classes were substantially indistinguishable in terms of predictive value, lending credibility to the ideas that (i) aggregating over time might have hidden important information from the model's learning mechanism, and (ii) higher preprocessing complexity does not correlate with better results. An argument could be made that simpler models are preferable in terms of interpretability. However, it is unclear exactly how much more interpretable pseudo-clinical variables might be, having been computed via administrative claims themselves, or out grouping ATCs according to their class might help understand model predictions any better than their ordered sequence.

Overall, our case study paints a pretty convincing picture to the effect that artificial intelligence, and, specifically, deep learning, might be instrumental in increasing the probability that models are, in fact, deployed. Indeed, it appears that planning for deployment from the onset, by carefully considering how a model might fit existing data flows and attempting to remove possible barriers to real-life usage, might not only lead to the removal of computational, maintenance, and data management overhead, but also yield comparable or even better performance than solutions rooted in traditional input-output schemes. So, almost paradoxically, solving a data ingestion problem might allow models to make use of more information, including some (e.g. order of medications) that might have been lost after expensive preprocessing steps.

16.3 Potential and Challenges of Employing Longitudinal Clinical Data in AI

AI technologies can take advantage of the increasing amount of clinical data nowadays produced in the healthcare routine. Multidimensional information (including a number of clinical parameters describing the patient's health status and recorded during clinical evaluations, through the use of testing machines, or performing laboratory tests) is progressively being structured and made available for both clinical and research purposes. These data can be stored in a variety of structures, including electronic health records, patient databases, clinical trial registers, medical imaging repositories, and laboratory information systems. Their use allows to directly acquire evidence-based insights into the patient condition with the aim of improving their care, as well as to improve the medical knowledge through broad applications within the health system, including the development of AI models.

When we have many acquisitions of a patient's health condition in time, we talk about *longitudinal* clinical data. This is the case, for example, of data collected over a follow-up period, such as in a sequence of screening visits for monitoring a chronic or progressive condition, or in consecutive clinical evaluations performed over multiple days of hospitalization. In general, this information can be captured as part of the standard care delivery process or during targeted activities such as research trials. In these cases, a dimension is added to the data, that is, *time*. By analyzing this information, clinicians can identify the advancement of a patient's health condition, assess the course of care, and plan the future health treatments. When longitudinal data from multiple patients are made available, we talk about longitudinal clinical data collection, an example among all being clinical registers of cohort studies. Representing one of the fundamental designs of epidemiology, these collections are widely used in medicine and in all related fields such as pharmacology, nursing, or biomedical engineering, where evidence-based investigations are performed.

In the framework of healthcare analytics, that is, the complex of quantitative and qualitative techniques applied to extract knowledge from the data made available in healthcare, longitudinally collected clinical data constitute an invaluable resource. Their temporal nature provides, indeed, a number of advantages. First, as briefly mentioned, the patient's clinical condition can be monitored in terms of evolution, tracking over time how their characteristics change as care progresses. Clinicians and researchers can inspect the effect of different treatments on patients with a similar medical history, assessing their improvement or the occurrence of adverse events. Notably, the time dimension not only lets us to focus on the observed values and how they change over time, but it also allows us to look at how much time passes between different occurrences. For example, the time between the administration of a certain treatment and the onset of a specific effect might be studied. When considering the data of more subjects, various potential targets can be investigated, moving the considerations from a single-patient to a population level and back, thus delineating subjective, overall, or individualized approaches. For example, we may want to delineate the progression trajectory for each patient, that is, the succession of events that characterize the path of care or disease pathway for that subject. Such a trajectory can be compared among patients, allowing us to detect similarities or deviations useful to identify clusters in the cohort. Then, by evaluating what clinically differentiates the patients, we may want to predict what the most likely progression trajectory will be for a new patient characterized by specific conditions. We will see an example of such analyses in a dedicated case study, in Section 16.3.2. Another example consists of the study of clinical conditions at the population level, where we can assess the occurrence of specific end points of interest and identify the effect of specific risk factors. Thanks to the dynamic nature of the longitudinal information, the influence or relationship of one or more variables on each other and on the outcomes at various time intervals can be examined. Section 16.3.1 reports a case study of such an analysis.

The benefits of such studies range from basic research to clinical and management applications, as they have the potential to significantly improve the lives of patients and benefit society as a whole ((Islam et al. 2018), (Nature Materials Editorial Board 2019)). From an economic point of view, the use of these strategies to improve the efficiency of practice leads to more affordable and high-quality healthcare. From a clinical standpoint, possible advances in medical knowledge, as well as diagnostic and prognostic capabilities, allow higher health standards. Survival analyses, for example, can uncover risk factors and detect the impact of certain treatments on illness progression and quality of life, paving the way for a more individualized healthcare system. Furthermore, an enhanced knowledge of diseases' mechanisms may be turned into computer-aided tools, providing doctors with increasingly reliable decision-making support systems.

However, even if longitudinal clinical data show different and excellent potential, handling their temporal dimension is not trivial, due to some characteristics of the data themselves that require specific attention. First, a longitudinal data collection could include not only dynamic variables, that is, those that are subsequently monitored; on the contrary, some information can refer to patient attributes that are constant throughout their clinical history (such as their demographic characteristics) and, therefore, can be coded as a static variable. Moreover, the features characterizing the patient's status may be of different types according to their nature, including continuous, categorical, and ordinal variables (such as age, sex, or the education level, respectively). This implies that the type of the variables constituting the dataset will be mixed both from a temporal and a type-based point of view. The tools selected for the analysis must therefore be able to appropriately manage this heterogeneity, or adapted to handle it. A second criticality emerges when we deal with data collected from a population of subjects and relates to the possible difference in the sampling times: apart from those cases for which the follow-up scheduling is strictly delineated, different subjects may have, in general, different observation times. This might be for instance due to the subject's specific monitoring needs, as well as to the availability calendar of the clinical center. Even for the same patient, the time that passes between two distinct pairs of acquisitions may be different. Related to this, another practical aspect concerns the possibility of having, at distinct time points, different sets of available variables according to the care the patient may have needed by then. From a data point of view, all these facts result in temporally sparse datasets, with patients being possibly described by observations collected at different time points, in a variable number, coded with heterogeneous variables and reporting diverse information: this implies that any analyses of interest will require an accurate, targeted preprocessing followed by the application of an analytic tool able to manage these data.

When approaching the use of longitudinal clinical data for developing AI models, we are confronted with a number of challenges. Most traditional mining techniques employ temporal data to determine the values of static outcomes only, such as the short- and long-term occurrence of end points of interest such as healing, adverse events, or death. Input variables are often limited to baseline values, thus preventing the identification and assessment of their dynamic influence on the outcomes, as well as the possible cross-relationships across time. Moreover, reducing the observation to static points precludes the chance of catching events that might be relevant, or determinant, for the evolution of the condition in a certain way. In addition, not all analytic techniques are capable of managing missing data and, therefore, a data imputation step is often required. When it comes to longitudinal data, the fact that each subject has, in general, multiple acquisitions is both a richness and a constraint. The sequentially collected information can, indeed, give indications on what the missing values might have been, but also set individual ranges or trends that have to be taken into account for not inserting nonphysiological values for that subject (take the example of body weight measurements for a subject with one specific missing acquisition). Specific imputation methodologies that take into account the dynamism of the data and exploit it to obtain complete datasets to be used for the analyses have been proposed (such as Daberdaku et al. (2020), Tavazzi et al. (2020a), and Xu et al. (2020)).

To sum up, longitudinal clinical data, although providing rich informative content for healthcare analytics applications, require appropriate management in their use due to their characteristics. If, on one side, data can be complex to handle, on the other hand, they can give insights on conditions both at an individual and population level, thus contributing in enhancing clinical practice and improving medical knowledge.

In the following of this section, we explore through two case studies how we can treat longitudinal clinical datasets to gain valuable knowledge from them for descriptive and predictive purposes. Focusing on longitudinal collections of clinical data from patients affected by a neurodegenerative disease, namely ALS, we take advantage of the data dynamics to investigate how this condition evolves over time. ALS is a rare condition caused by the degeneration of motor neurons that causes a progressive impairment of all functional abilities, which usually leads to death within a few years from the time of onset. Symptoms and progression rate can be heterogeneous between patients, causing difficulty in diagnosis and uncertainty in prognosis. AI models built on longitudinal clinical data can help shedding light on the manifestations of this disease, for instance highlighting progression patterns or suggesting prognostic factors.

In Section 16.3.1, we present an approach based on DBNs to model the course of ALS in terms of relationships among a number of clinical variables measured over time. We then use the DBN to simulate how the condition is expected to progress in a test population, thus assessing the ability of the model to predict the course starting from a baseline condition and based on the learned dynamics (Tavazzi et al. 2022a).

In Section 16.3.2 we explore the use of PM, a family of analytic techniques being increasingly applied to healthcare, for investigating the progression trajectories of a clinical trial ALS cohort. When mining the processes evolution of the disease through a process discovery algorithm, for each functional impairment we get insights on the timing and probability of experiencing it based on the subjects characteristics at baseline and the previously occurred disabilities (Tavazzi et al. 2022b).

In both case studies, we will highlight how the selected techniques as well as the choices behind the preprocessing allow us to gain insights on the inspected condition, preserving interpretability despite data and model complexity.

16.3.1 Case Study: Modeling the Progression of Amyotrophic Lateral Sclerosis Through a Dynamic Bayesian Network

DBNs are probabilistic graphical models that represent a set of variables and their conditional dependencies over time as a directed acyclic graph. Specifically, a DBN is defined by its structure (a set of parent-children nodes, each one representing a variable) annotated with a set of conditional probability distributions (CPDs), since each children node is a probabilistic function of its parents. The structure of a DBN is such that the directional relationships among its variables do not allow loops to be formed; the only exceptions are temporal variables, which are represented as distinct nodes at pairs of consecutive times (t) and ($t + 1$), and where loops and feedback are allowed when considering their relationships along different time slices.

Thanks to their ability of learning not only from data but also from domain literature and expert knowledge, DBNs are a well-suited methodology for modeling disease evolution, providing an explicit representation of the variable set and their interdependencies over time (Roversi et al. 2021).

In this case study, we employ this technique to model the progression of ALS using a longitudinal dataset (called from here on training set, since it is used for learning the model) that includes data from 3221 patients recruited from two Italian population-based ALS registers and four Italian and Israeli tertiary ALS clinics. For each patient, some demographic features and a series of observations, each corresponding to a screening visit, are included. Specifically, the available information can be subsetted into two main categories of variables according to their temporal nature:

- **Static variables**: Patient sex, site of onset (bulbar/spinal), age at onset, diagnostic delay, and the medical center that took care of the patient;
- **Dynamic variables**: The survival information (time from the onset of ALS to tracheostomy/death or censoring information), and the MiToS scores (Chiò et al. 2015), which are 4 Boolean variables – one for each functional domain among walking/self-care, breathing, communicating, and swallowing – which assume a value equal to 0 if the ability is preserved, 1 if impaired.

With the aim of modeling the passing of time, we introduced two additional derived variables, namely, the time between two consecutive visits and the time since the onset. These variables allow to account for different acquisition times, that may reflect the need of a different visit frequency as the disease progresses.

In our implementation, we employed the *bnstruct* R package (Franzin et al. 2017) that for learning a DBN requires data to be first discretized and then organized as couples of consecutive visits at time $(t-1)$ and time (t), respectively. Looking at them for all patients together, the DBN computes the conditional probability of each variable to assume a given value at time (t) given the values of the other variables at time $(t-1)$. More specifically, for each variable *child* at time (t), a set of *parents* at time $(t-1)$ is identified, that is, the variables that contribute in a joint way to probabilistically determine the value of the child. For more methodological details, please refer to Tavazzi et al. (Tavazzi et al. (2022a)). In this learning process, we can observe how the DBN uses the entire sequence of visits included in the data, thus accurately exploiting the longitudinal information provided.

Graphically, the learned model is a direct acyclic graph where each variable is represented by a node, and the conditional dependence over subsequent time steps of a node (the child) from one or more others (the parents) is reported as directed edges. On our training data, this results in the graph reported in Figure 16.2. By inspecting the network we can investigate the relationships among the variables emerging from the data: for instance, we can see how for a patient the probability of having the breathing ability impaired or not at the current visit jointly depends on the functionalities coded in the MiTos swallowing and walking/self-care domains at the previous visit, together with the breathing status itself at the previous time point, and on the time that has passed since the onset. The specific contribution of each parent variable to the conditional probability can be examined in tables (conditional probability tables) that are returned together with the graph when a DBN is learned. According to the data, such an analysis can identify both relationships previously known in literature and new ones emerging from the data.

Once a DBN model is learned, it can also be used to simulate how the disease can progress in new subjects. In this case, a static starting point is used as, in our case, the first recorded contact with the medical center providing the data. Based on the values of the variables measured at this baseline time, their values at successive instants (i.e. visits) can be simulated, one at a time, using the learned conditional dependencies and network structure.

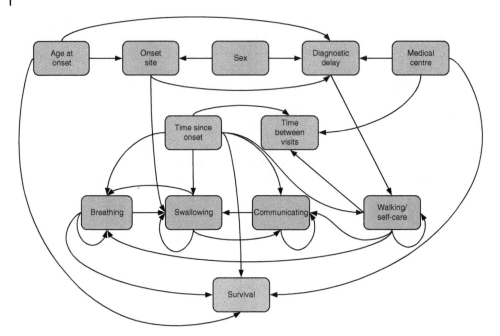

Figure 16.2 Graph of the DBN learned on the training set representing the conditional dependencies among the ALS variables over time. The loops on the four MiToS variables represent the dependency on the values of the same variable at the previous time-step. Source: Adapted from Tavazzi et al. (Tavazzi et al. (2022a)).

In this way, the evolution of ALS can be simulated step by step and followed in terms of progression trajectories.

The simulation can also be employed to assess the predicting ability of the model. Given a known set of visits of a subject, the real disease progression can be compared with the one predicted by employing the DBN, for instance in terms of real versus predicted occurrence of some endpoints of interest (here, the MiToS and the survival). Being the DBN a probabilistic model, to obtain probability estimates of the predicted follow-up and the corresponding outcomes' times, multiple simulations have to be run for each patient. It should be noted that, even if only some static information (the baseline values of the variables) is needed for the simulation, the complete patient history is required to learn the network in the training phase.

We used the DBN learned on the training set to predict the evolution of ALS in an independent test set (never used for training) consisting of 719 new subjects, performing 100 independent simulations each. We then assessed the model performance in terms of accuracy in predicting the occurrence of the 4 MiToS impairments and death, by first computing the AUROC for each clinical outcome at a 3-month step up to 96 months since the disease onset and then calculating its integral (iAUROC) at different time thresholds. Table 16.2 reports the iAUROC obtained at 24, 36, and 96 months from onset.

Moreover, the simulation procedure can be used to simulate cohorts of patients characterized by different phenotypes at baseline in order to assess the effect of one or more variables on the disease progression. More specifically, we can compare how the simulation

Table 16.2 Integral of the AUROC (iAUROC) computed up to 24, 36, and 96 months since the disease onset on the test set for the 4 MiTos and the survival outcomes.

Time since onset (mo)	MiToS walking/self-care	MiToS swallowing	MiToS communicating	MiToS breathing	Survival
$t = 24$	0.87	0.91	0.87	0.84	0.96
$t = 36$	0.85	0.87	0.84	0.80	0.93
$t = 96$	0.81	0.79	0.78	0.74	0.85

of cohorts that differentiate by the initial values of specific variables progresses, evaluating how the disease course is sensitive to this change and, therefore, determining the effect of these variables as progression risk factors. Here, we evaluated how the onset site affects the time at which a specific outcome, namely swallowing impairment, occurs by separately simulating the progression of the test set's subjects with a bulbar versus spinal onset. From this analysis, we were able to observe how subjects with bulbar onset have an increased risk of early impaired swallowing ability, with a cumulative probability 50 months after the onset of having already experienced the impairment equal to approximately 76% for the bulbar cohort versus 60% of the spinal cohort.

In this case study we have shown how DBNs are a technique that is able to model the disease progression in its entirety in a probabilistic fashion, exploiting all the longitudinal information provided in the data and without requiring one to focus on a single end point, differently from other predictive methods. Moreover, unlike other techniques that return a punctual prediction of the time of occurrence of an outcome, they are able to simulate a patient's whole progression trajectory from the first visit onward, thus providing a continuous estimate of the risk of experiencing several outcomes at the same time and allowing the investigation of the effect of different risk factors.

16.3.2 Case Study: Investigating Amyotrophic Lateral Sclerosis Progression Trajectories Leveraging Process Mining

PM is a family of analytic techniques arose in the process management context that provides methodologies to support the analysis of operational processes starting from the data recorded by an information system (van der Aalst and Adriansyah 2011). In PM, data are usually structured as an event log (EL), that is, a collection of activities (or events), each referred to a case and labeled with its occurrence time, together with an optional set of features (or attributes) characterizing the case or the activity. For each case, we can refer to its list of events as *trace*.

Different PM algorithms can be applied to the EL with the main goal of performing:

- **Process discovery**, that is, mining the process that produced the data observed in the EL;
- **Conformance checking** for assessing the compliance of the EL with regard to a given process model or vice versa;

- **Process enhancement**, which consists in improving process efficiency through problem diagnosis and prediction of delays, recommending process redesigns or supporting decision-making.

In all its forms, PM sits therefore between computational intelligence and data mining, on the one hand, and process modeling and analysis, on the other hand (van der Aalst and Adriansyah 2011).

PM is gaining popularity in a multitude of fields, including healthcare. In this setting, events include both clinical and nonclinical activities provided by different stakeholders, and may present different behaviors according to the specific organization (Mans et al. 2015). These processes are highly dynamic, complex, and increasingly multidisciplinary (Homayounfar 2012). Furthermore, they are often only partly structured and with many exceptional behaviors, due to their intrinsically required flexibility (Mans et al. 2015). Not least, most of the activities are often high-cost. All these characteristics make processes in healthcare both crucial to improve and interesting to analyze. Using PM techniques not only ensures that such procedures are better understood, but can also generate benefits associated with process efficiency and enhancement.

The type of processes in healthcare can be classified according to Lenz and Reichert (Lenz and Reichert (2007)), that distinguish between clinical processes and administrative or organizational processes. A recent review of PM in healthcare (De Roock and Martin 2022) highlights how clinical processes are the object of most of the state-of-the-art works, with applications including Primary Care (Williams et al. 2018; Litchfield et al. 2018), Emergency Care (Martinez-Millana et al. 2019; Mertens et al. 2020), Cardiology (Kusuma et al. 2018; Balakhontceva et al. 2018), and Oncology (Kurniati et al. 2016; Gerard et al. 2020; Tavazzi et al. 2020b), as well as the representation of clinical guidelines (Gatta et al. 2020).

In this case study, we explore how PM can provide means for gaining insights on the progression trajectories of patients affected by a ALS. Specifically, we employ a Process Discovery algorithm, namely the care flow miner (CFM) (Dagliati et al. 2018), on a longitudinal clinical dataset of 5389 clinical trial subjects extracted from the PRO-ACT dataset (Atassi et al. 2014).

First, we preprocessed the available measurement of the MiToS impairments at each visit as a string M_abcd consisting of four elements $\{a, b, c, d\}$, each corresponding to a functional domain in the following order: (a) Walking/Self-care, (b) Swallowing, (c) Communicating, and (d) Breathing, and assuming a value equal to 1 if the domain is impaired and 0 otherwise. In this way, a visit with no recorded impairments is coded by the string M_0000, while a visit with the only Walking/Self-care domain impaired corresponds to the string M_1000. Then, for each patient, we extracted and organized as an EL the following information:

- **Events:** The disease onset, the trial start, the status of the MiToS impairments at each visit coded as above, and the death or the censoring event;
- **Attributes:** The age at onset and the site of onset.

When applied to the EL, the CFM builds a graph that, starting from an event set as root node, creates a branch for each trace of the EL followed by at least one patient. The first level of the tree, just under the root, corresponds to the first event of each trace following the starting one, and the next levels sequentially correspond to the further ones. The resulting CFM graph can be represented as a tree where each node is labeled with the name of the corresponding event, together with some additional information such as the number of patients passing through that node or statistics about the time needed to reach it.

Here, we employed the implementation of the CFM available in the pMineR R package (Gatta et al. 2017), selecting as the root node the event M_0000, that is, the first (if available) visit of each patient where no impairments were recorded. For more methodological details, refer to Tavazzi et al. (Tavazzi et al. 2022b). The graph resulting from the CFM is reported in Figure 16.3. To avoid the so-called *spaghetti effect*, the graph has been thresholded for displaying only the pathways transitioned by at least 10 subjects.

By inspecting the CFM tree, we can observe, for instance, how in our population most of the patients without any recorded impairments then first loose the functional abilities in the Walking/Self-care domain (66%) and then die (10%). Another available analysis can be made on a temporal level, studying how much time passes from the root to each following event: for each node, the minimum, median, and maximum time of occurrence from the root are provided.

The version of the CFM available in pMineR not only shows the most frequent paths and characterizes the times needed to reach each node from the root, but also allows to investigate the effect of specific data features on the followed trajectories. Two CFM graphs built on cohorts characterized by different demographic or clinical characteristics, such as male versus female, can be compared, by automatically measuring node by node the time needed to move from a node to another, or differences in the patients' cardinality. This comparison is performed by implementing a Fisher's exact test or a χ^2 test (depending on the cardinality of patients passing through the node) for dichotomic categorical variables, or with a Wilcoxon–Mann–Whitney test for the continuous one, a nonparametric test of whether two mutually independent statistical samples are from the same population. In this way, we can inspect how specific subjects' characteristics impact on the progression trajectories.

Guided by clinical hypotheses, we explored how the distribution of the subjects in the nodes changes with respect to their site of onset. Figure 16.4 reports the resulting graph that compares the CFM trajectories of the bulbar versus spinal patients. We can observe a significant predominance of a first impairment in the Walking/Self-care domain for the subjects with spinal onset (M_1000, ratio spinal/bulbar equal to 1.3), and a significant predominance of first impairment in the Swallowing domain for the bulbar onset subjects (M_0100 with a ratio spinal/bulbar equal to 0.46), results that match with the expectations.

In this case study, we looked at how PM can provide a different viewpoint on the events that define a patient's clinical history. Starting from a selection of the main clinical events characterizing the disease progression for each patient, structured as an EL, we applied a modeling technique able to delineate the progression trajectory for each patient. In this way, for each event of interest (here the functional impairments) we get insights on the timing and probability of experiencing it both at a population level or based on the subject characteristics at baseline and/or the previous occurred disabilities. The analysis of the trajectories allows us to highlight the most followed paths, as well as unexpected sequences of events that merit a closer examination. The mined trajectories can be used not only to

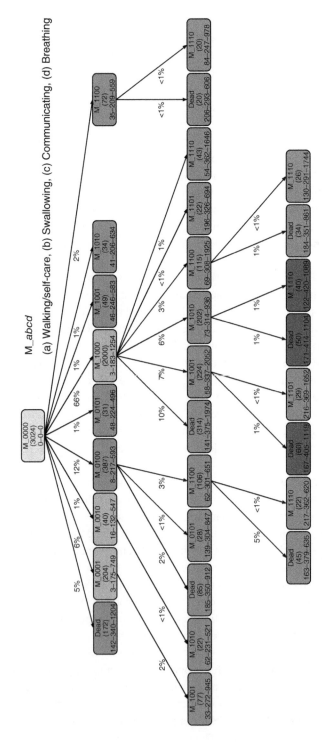

Figure 16.3 CFM graph built starting from M_0000. Each node reports the total number of patients passing through it (round brackets) and the min–median–max time, in days, needed to reach it from the root. Gray levels are graded on the median times, with intervals: <100, 101–200, 201–400, and >401 days. The edges report the percentage of patients passing through the child node with respect to the entire population (below). The graph has been thresholded for displaying only the pathways transitioned by at least 10 subjects. Source: Adapted from Tavazzi et al. (Tavazzi et al. (2022a)).

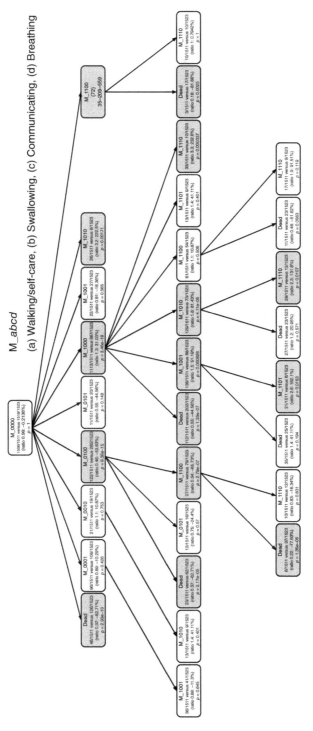

Figure 16.4 CFM graphs built starting from M_0000 and stratified for onset site. Each node reports the number of patients passing trough it for each cohort (spinal/bulbar onset, respectively). Moreover, the ratio of the two cardinalities with respect to the initial populations is reported in the round brackets, followed by the *p*-value for the Fisher's exact/χ^2 test. The node box is colored in gray if the *p*-value is lower than a given threshold (here 0.05). Both the graphs have been thresholded for displaying only the pathways transitioned by at least 10 subjects. Source: Adapted from Tavazzi et al. (Tavazzi et al. (2022a)).

describe the population, but also with predictive aims, such as the forecasting of the most likely progression pathway for a new patient characterized by specific conditions.

Such a process-oriented approach intrinsically allows to exploit the temporal nature of the data: PM offers a portfolio of techniques to treat the available information either in an agnostic way or integrating some domain knowledge. Recent tools integrate functions to perform investigations typical of the clinical context, such as survival analysis. In addition, this approach provides important self-consistency checks for data and allows to inspect patterns at different levels of abstraction, together with the associated outcomes. Moreover, the visualizations provided when implementing most of PM algorithms constitute an easy-to-understand and communicative resource able to boost dialogue and discussion among the working team and the scientific community in general, suggesting or confirming worthy research directions.

16.4 Enhancing the Applicability of AI Predictive Models by a Combined Model Approach: A Case Study on T2D Onset Prediction

The increasing availability of large amounts of heterogeneous health and well-being data has stimulated the application of AI techniques for new models for personalized and preventive medicine. In particular, AI techniques, such as supervised machine learning techniques, have been increasingly adopted for developing predictive models to predict ahead of time relevant clinical outcomes, such as the onset of a new disease or the prognosis of an already-diagnosed disease. Such AI-based predictive models have the ambitious goal to change the paradigm of healthcare, passing from a reactive system, focused on the treatment of already-diagnosed diseases, to a proactive system focused on disease prevention and maintaining individuals healthy as long as possible.

16.4.1 The Problem of Type 2 Diabetes Prediction

One interesting research area for the application of AI predictive models is the prediction of T2D onset. Diabetes is one of the greatest epidemiological challenges of our era, with more than 400 million people suffering from this disease worldwide, a number that is expected to further increase in the next years. T2D represents about 90% of all diabetes cases. It is a multifactorial disease that commonly appears in adulthood as a result of a combination of genetic and lifestyle factors. Common lifestyle risk factors include obesity, lack of physical activity, poor diet and stress. Several studies demonstrated that T2D can be prevented or at least delayed by early interventions on such modifiable risk factors ((Li et al. 2014), (Lindström et al. 2006)). An early identification of individuals at risk of developing T2D would then allow to deliver targeted prevention measures, e.g. lifestyle changes, that potentially can reduce the incidence and prevalence of T2D, and its long-term complications, with great reduction of healthcare costs.

Over the past two decades, several predictive models to identify subjects at risk of developing T2D based on multiple factors were developed. These models provide a risk score representing the individual's probability of developing T2D in the future, e.g. in the next 5–10 years (Noble et al. 2011). Some models only require easily accessible information which can be self-reported by the patient. Others require laboratory test results (e.g. fasting plasma glucose), which generally result in better predictive performance, but not always are available.

16.4.2   Potential Applications of T2D Predictive Models

T2D predictive models can have many important applications. General practitioners can use T2D predictive models to identify patients with high risk of diabetes who may require specific screening tests and preventive lifestyle change. Local health departments can apply these models to identify local communities with increased risk of diabetes and develop public health policies to mitigate this risk. Health departments may use the models to assess the risk of diabetes in different regions, predict diabetes-related health costs by region, and more efficiently plan the distribution of resources. Finally, T2D predictive models can be integrated in mobile health applications as tools to provide the users with a feedback about their health status (e.g. a diabetes risk indicator) and recommendations on how to improve it, also resorting to gamification strategies to promote healthy behaviors. Although the many potential users, T2D predictive models are scarcely used in real life.

16.4.3   Barriers to the Adoption of T2D Predictive Models

Some practical issues currently limit the application of T2D predictive models in clinical practice and public health (Nowak et al. 2015). First, most of the available models have been developed for specific populations. Therefore, the investigator must first choose the model that is most suitable for the target population. For example, some models can only be applied to specific race/ethnic groups that were represented in the development cohort. If the target population is heterogeneous, the investigator is forced to choose a general model, not having an input variable for race/ethnicity, although this might imply the choice of a model with lower performance.

Then, the investigator must check that all the features required by the selected model are available for the target population. In practical applications of the models, variables derived from invasive samples (e.g. blood test) are frequently missing. Missing values are also common for waist circumference, although not as common as body mass index (BMI) for measuring obesity, and family history of diabetes (often is not easy to retrieve information on family members), two variables commonly used by T2D predictive models. The presence of some missing values for a given subject forces the investigator to either not calculate the risk score (this generates a missing prediction), or to impute the missing values. A simple imputation method consists in substituting the missing values with the average or the most frequent values in the population. However, this method would drive to an underestimation of diabetes risk in at risk individuals. Alternatively, more sophisticated imputation algorithms may be applied, although such methods require the availability of a large training set and they are generally applicable only when missing values occur randomly. Therefore, missing data imputation is not always doable in practice.

The last issue is related to the possible lack of calibration of the model for the target population (Vettoretti et al. 2018). Although T2D predictive models usually perform very well in the populations in which they were developed, they often present suboptimal performance when applied to new populations, mainly because of differences in the variable definition and different population characteristics. In this case, predictive models need to be recalibrated, i.e. their parameters need to be updated to describe the new population. A full recalibration consists in reestimating all the model parameters on the new population. However, such a strategy can be applied only when a sufficiently large dataset for parameter reestimation is available which contains not only the values of predictors at baseline but also the information about T2D incidence during the follow-up.

16.4.4 Addressing Practical Issues by Combining Multiple T2D Predictive Models

To address these three practical issues, i.e. the problems of model choice, missing variables and recalibration, Vettoretti et al. (Vettoretti et al. (2020)) proposed a new prediction approach that combines eight existing T2D models, in a smart way, and provides in output a consensus T2D risk prediction. This combined model aims to extend the applicability of the existing T2D predictive models, by integrating multiple models independently developed on different populations.

The combined model requires in input the subject's variables (missing values are allowed) and the expected T2D incidence in the target population. Then the risk score for T2D onset is derived in three steps (Figure 16.5). In the first step, the combined model automatically selects for each subject the applicable models based on the subject's ethnicity and excludes the theoretically-applicable models for which some variables are missing. In the second step, the combined model calculates the risk scores of the selected models by using the original model equations. In the third step, such risk scores are rescaled according to the expected diabetes incidence as proposed in Janssen et al. (Janssen et al. (2009)) and Kengne et al. (Kengne et al. (2014)). Finally, in the last step, the combined model computes the weighted average of the rescaled risk scores, using different weights based on the level of information the models require. In particular, the models that use only easily accessible information that can be collected by questionnaires (scenario 1; Sc1) were assigned weight 1, the models that also require some noninvasive measurements collected by medical instruments, e.g. heart rate and blood pressure, (scenario 2; Sc2) were assigned weight 2, whereas the models requiring invasively-collected biomarkers (scenario 3; Sc3) were assigned weight 3. This weighting schema was designed to provide more relevance to the models that use variables collected by medical instrumentation, which generally have higher predictive ability than self-reported variables.

In summary, the combined model is designed to facilitate the investigators when applying existing models to new populations by:

- automatically performing the model choice
- bypassing the problem of missing values by integrating multiple models (if at least one model is applicable then there will be no missing prediction)
- automatically recalibrating the risk scores by a simple scaling method that does not require to retrain the models.

The current implementation of the combined model includes eight public models, two of Sc1, three of Sc2, and four of Sc3. Six models are based on logistic regression: the concise

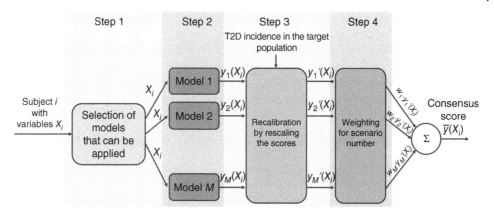

Figure 16.5 Schematic representation of the combined T2D model proposed by Vettoretti et al. (Vettoretti et al. (2020). In the first step, the applicable models are selected; in the second step, each applicable model is applied to compute the subject's risk of T2D; in the third step, the calculated risk scores are rescaled according to the T2D incidence in the target population; finally, in the fourth step, the consensus score is obtained as a weighted average of the rescaled risk scores.

version of the Finnish Diabetes Risk Score (FINDRISC; Sc1) (Lindström and Tuomilehto 2003), the Atherosclerosis Risk in Communities simple model (ARIC 1; Sc2) (Schmidt et al. 2005), the ARIC clinical model without lipids (ARIC 2; Sc3) (Schmidt et al. 2005), the ARIC clinical model with lipids (ARIC 3; Sc3) (Schmidt et al. 2005), the model published in Stern et al. (Stern et al. (2002)) (STERN; Sc3) and the Framingham model (FRAMINGHAM; Sc3) (Wilson et al. 2007). The other two models are based on Weibull survival model, i.e. the Diabetes Population Risk Tool (DPoRT; Sc1) (Rosella et al. 2011) and the basic model by published in Kahn et al. (Kahn et al. (2009)) (KAHN; Sc2). In the following, some details about each model are provided.

The concise FINDRISC model was developed in a Finnish population considering age, sex, use of hypertension medications, BMI and waist circumference as predictors of the risk of T2D onset. The ARIC models were developed on an American population including white and African American subjects. In total three ARIC models were developed, which use different input variables: a simple model (ARIC 1) with ethnicity, parental history of diabetes, age, waist circumference, height, and systolic blood pressure as input variables; a second model (ARIC 2) that, in addition to the variables of ARIC 1, also includes fasting plasma glucose concentration; and a third model (ARIC 3) that, in addition to the variables of ARIC 2, also includes high-density lipoprotein (HDL) cholesterol and triglycerides concentration. The STERN model was developed on a population including Mexican-Americans and non-Hispanic whites. This model included 8 input variables, i.e. age, sex, ethnicity, family history of diabetes, BMI, systolic blood pressure, fasting plasma glucose concentration, and HDL cholesterol. The FRAMINGHAM model was developed on data of the Framingham Offspring Study collected on white Americans. The input variables of this model includes age, sex, parental history of diabetes, BMI, blood pressure, HDL cholesterol, triglycerides concentration, waist circumference, and fasting plasma glucose concentration. The DPoRT model was developed on a Canadian cohort. It consists of two Weibull models, one for women, one for men. The women model includes the following input variables: age, BMI, ethnicity, immigrant status, education level, and hypertension. The men model requires age, BMI, ethnicity, education level, heart disease, hypertension, and smoking as input variables. Finally, the KAHN model was developed on the same population of the ARIC models, and it includes two scoring systems, for women and men, which use the following input variables: age, ethnicity, parental history of diabetes, smoking, waist circumference, height, weight, resting heart rate, and hypertension.

16.4.5 The Combined Model Achieves High Prediction Performance with High Coverage

The combined model was assessed on two datasets not used for training any of the models included in the combined model: the Multi-Ethnic Study of Atherosclerosis (MESA) dataset (Bild et al. 2002) (accessible upon submission of a research proposal) and the English Longitudinal Study of Ageing (ELSA) dataset (Steptoe et al. 2013) (accessible upon registration on the United Kingdom Data Service website: https://ukdataservice.ac.uk). In particular, Vettoretti et al. (Vettoretti et al. (2020)) evaluated the discrimination and calibration performance of the combined model for predicting the eight-year incidence of T2D in a MESA test set ($n = 1031$) and an ELSA test set ($n = 4820$). The two datasets present different characteristics: MESA includes a multiethnic US population, while ELSA includes a mostly White English population.

On the MESA dataset, Vettoretti et al. (Vettoretti et al. (2020)) first compared the existing T2D predictive models in their original form versus the models recalibrated with the rescaling approach versus the models fully recalibrated with all parameters re-estimated on the MESA dataset. Results demonstrated that (i) model discriminatory ability was good even without recalibration; (ii) the original models suffered from a lack of calibration when applied to different populations; and (iii) risk score rescaling achieved a good incidence prediction, comparable to that of the full recalibration. These results suggest that risk score rescaling is an effective technique to tackle lack-of-calibration issues. This technique simply relies on an estimate of the T2D incidence in the target population, without requiring the availability of a training set for parameter estimation, and it allows to achieve good calibration performance, comparable to that of the full recalibration. For this reason, the risk score rescaling was embedded in the combined model, as a much more practical, but equally effective, recalibration procedure than the full recalibration.

In particular, on the MESA test set, the model with best coverage was FINDRISC (0% missing predictions) which presented C-index = 0.72, while the models with highest C-index were the Sc3 models (C-index = 0.81–0.83) that, however, presented a percentage of missing predictions between 17% and 45%. The combined model was able to achieve both high coverage (0% missing predictions), like FINDRISC, and high discrimination performance (C-index = 0.83), like the Sc3 models. In the ELSA dataset, achieving good prediction performance with high coverage was even more challenging because of the high levels of missingness in some important features (e.g. fasting plasma glucose and family history of diabetes). In such a challenging scenario, the existing model with best coverage (FINDRISC) presented 19% missing predictions and C-index = 0.72; the combined model was able to achieve an excellent coverage (4% missing predictions) with discrimination performance comparable to the Sc3 models (C-index = 0.77 versus C-index = 0.77–0.82).

In the subset of the test sets without missing values, i.e. for those subjects for whom all the eight original models were applicable, the discrimination performance of the combined model was equivalent to that of the model with best discrimination performance (in this case ARIC 3 for MESA, FRAMINGHAM for ELSA). The combined T2D model also presented calibration performance similar to the best-performing rescaled model (in this case ARIC 3 for MESA, FINDRISC for ELSA). This further analysis proved that the discrimination and calibration performance of the combined model are not deteriorated by the averaging of risk scores of models with different performance, and thus the specific weighting strategy adopted is effective. Note that in general the model that will show the best performance on a new population is not known a priori. Thus, another remarkable advantage of the combined model is that it allows to achieve the performance of the best model, without knowing it a priori.

16.5 Conclusions and Future Outlook

In this contribution we have focused on different aspects of AI applicability and have presented: (i) the development of a deep learning model to predict the cardiovascular complications of diabetes using administrative claims by carefully considering how a model might fit existing data flows and attempting to remove possible barriers to real-life usage; (ii) the development of a DBN model that predicts and simulates the progression of a medical condition by taking advantage of all the longitudinal information provided by the data; (iii) the use of PM techniques that exploit the temporal nature of the data in an agnostic way or by integrating domain knowledge; and (iv) the integration of eight existing T2D predictive models by risk-score rescaling and averaging to address issues such as poor model calibration on the target population, resulting in a combined model of T2D onset prediction. The presented approaches help appreciate the different facets and challenges of AI usability, addressing the costs of data preprocessing, the needs and advantages of managing longitudinal data and the generalizability issue in practical contexts.

First, in Section 16.2, we exploited the implicit feature mapping capabilities of deep learning to automatically preprocess one year's worth of data of the administrative claims of Veneto, a populous region in NorthEast Italy, to predict the cardiovascular complications of diabetes (Longato et al. 2020b, 2021). The automatic preprocessing allowed making use of more information, including the temporal order of medications, that might have been lost using classical, non-automatized preprocessing approaches.

In Section 16.3, we presented two case studies in which, despite the complexity of the data and of the employed modeling techniques, we demonstrated how information can be extracted by longitudinal data promoting the interpretability of results. In Section 16.3.1, we showed how DBNs allow modeling the progression of a medical condition by taking advantage of all the longitudinal information provided by the data, considering multiple end points at the same time, and inspecting related risk factors. We also illustrated how this approach represents a tool to continuously simulate disease progression in populations with different clinical characteristics. In Section 16.3.2, we explored the use of PM techniques that exploit the temporal nature of the data in an agnostic way or by leveraging a process-oriented approach; and we performed typical investigations in the clinical setting, such as survival analysis and stratification studies, inspecting and characterizing patterns of progression at different levels of abstraction, along with associated outcomes, visualizing them effectively in communicative graphs.

Finally, in Section 16.4, we addressed the use of T2D predictive models in real-world applications, in which the investigators have to struggle with some practical issues, e.g. model choice, missing values in the model input variables, and poor model calibration on the target population. Vettoretti et al. (Vettoretti et al. (2020)) proposed a new strategy which consists in combining different existing T2D predictive models by rescaling and averaging the risk scores given as output by each model. This has the advantage of avoiding retraining the models on different populations, which is time-consuming and might be unfeasible if retrospective data are lacking. Moreover, the methodology adopted to develop the combined T2D model is general and can be applied to the prediction of other outcomes.

In conclusion, we believe that developing and implementing models addressing the problem of their deployment in real scenarios is the first step on the long journey of usable AI. We think that embedding the design of certain aspects in AI tools within the phase of model development will be an increasingly important aspect to address explainability and accountability, as well as usability and generalizability.

Author Biography

Barbara Di Camillo is Full Professor of Computer Science at the Department of Information Engineering, University of Padova, Italy. Her research activity is centered on the development and application of advanced modeling, data mining, and machine learning methods for high-throughput biological and clinical data analysis in the field of Bioinformatics and Health Informatics. She has authored more than 150 peer-reviewed scientific works. She has been involved in numerous national and international projects, and is currently the scientific coordinator of the Horizon project BRAINTEASER (Bringing Artificial Intelligence Home for a Better Care of Amyotrophic Lateral Sclerosis and Multiple Sclerosis).

Enrico Longato is Assistant Professor at the Department of Information Engineering, University of Padova, Italy, where he got his PhD in Information Engineering, curriculum Bioengineering, 2021. His research interests revolve around the fields of healthcare big data analytics and predictive modeling via routinely acquired biomedical data, and specifically models for non-transmissible chronic diseases, adverse outcomes, and deep learning for longitudinal data analysis. He has worked on four European projects on the development of predictive models of diabetes, asthma, sudden cardiac death after myocardial infarction, amyotrophic lateral sclerosis, and multiple sclerosis; retrospective observational studies via real-world evidence; and data simulation.

Erica Tavazzi is post-doctoral researcher at the Department of Information Engineering, University of Padova, Italy, where she got her PhD in Information Engineering, curriculum Information & Communication Technologies, in 2021. Her scientific activity is in the health informatics domain and is mainly devoted to the development of computational models of disease progression on dynamic clinical data, with a specific focus on the management and exploitation of longitudinally collected information. She has been involved in several European and international projects, with a particular focus on the development and application of probabilistic graphical models to neurological and gastrointestinal diseases, and aging.

Martina Vettoretti is Assistant Professor at the Department of Information Engineering, University of Padova, Italy, where she got her PhD in Information Engineering, curriculum Bioengineering, in 2017. Her research interests include artificial intelligence, machine learning, signal processing, modeling and simulation techniques in various applications regarding the prevention and treatment of chronic diseases (neurodegenerative, metabolic, and respiratory diseases). She has recently been contributing to several European projects on predictive and signal modeling, and on the enhancement of clinical trials with real-world data. She has considerable experience in the fields of diabetes technology and research.

References

van der Aalst, W. and Adriansyah, A. (2011). Process mining manifesto. In: *International Conference on Business Process Management*, 169–194. Springer.

Atassi, N., Berry, J., Shui, A. et al. (2014). The PRO-ACT database design, initial analyses, and predictive features. *Neurology* 83 (19): 1719–1725.

ATC (n.d.) https://www.whocc.no/ (accessed 30 September 2023).

Balakhontceva, M.A., Funkner, A.A., Semakova, A.A. et al. (2018). Holistic modeling of chronic diseases for recommendation elaboration and decision making. *Procedia Computer Science* 138: 228–237.

Bansal, A. and Heagerty, P.J. (2018). A tutorial on evaluating the time-varying discrimination accuracy of survival models used in dynamic decision making. *Medical Decision Making* 38 (8): 904–916. https://doi.org/10.1177/0272989X18801312.

Bild, D.E., Bluemke, D.A., Burke, G.L. et al. (2002). Multi-ethnic study of atherosclerosis: objectives and design. *American Journal of Epidemiology* 156 (9): 871–881.

Burton, P.R., Banner, N., Elliot, M.J. et al. (2017). Policies and strategies to facilitate secondary use of research data in the health sciences. *International Journal of Epidemiology* 46 (6): 1729–1733. https://doi.org/10.1093/ije/dyx195.

Chiò, A., Hammond, E.R., Mora, G. et al. (2015). Development and evaluation of a clinical staging system for amyotrophic lateral sclerosis. *Journal of Neurology, Neurosurgery & Psychiatry* 86 (1): 38–44.

Cox, D.R. (1972). Regression models and life-tables. *Journal of the Royal Statistical Society. Series B (Methodological)* 34 (2): 187–220.

Daberdaku, S., Tavazzi, E., and Di Camillo, B. (2020). A combined interpolation and weighted K-nearest neighbours approach for the imputation of longitudinal ICU laboratory data. *Journal of Healthcare Informatics Research* 4: 174–188.

Dagliati, A., Tibollo, V., Cogni, G. et al. (2018). Careflow mining techniques to explore type 2 diabetes evolution. *Journal of Diabetes Science and Technology* 12 (2): 251–259.

Dash, S., Shakyawar, S.K., Sharma, M., and Kaushik, S. (2019). Big data in healthcare: management, analysis and future prospects. *Journal of Big Data* 6 (11): 1–25. https://doi.org/10.1186/s40537-019-0217-0.

De Roock, E. and Martin, N. (2022). Process mining in healthcare–an updated perspective on the state of the art. *Journal of Biomedical Informatics* 127: 103995.

Franzin, A., Sambo, F., and Di Camillo, B. (2017). bnstruct: an R package for Bayesian Network structure learning in the presence of missing data. *Bioinformatics* 33 (8): 1250–1252.

Gal, Y. and Ghahramani, Y. (2016). A theoretically grounded application of dropout in recurrent neural networks. In: *Advances in Neural Information Processing Systems 29 (NIPS 2016)*. https://proceedings.neurips.cc/paper/2016/hash/076a0c97d09cf1a0ec3e19c7f2529f2b-Abstract.html (accessed 30 September 2023).

Gatta, R., Lenkowicz, J. et al. (2017). pMineR: an innovative R library for performing process mining in medicine. In: *Conference on Artificial Intelligence in Medicine in Europe*, 351–355. Springer.

Gatta, R., Vallati, M., Fernandez-Llatas, C. et al. (2020). What role can process mining play in recurrent clinical guidelines issues? A position paper. *International Journal of Environmental Research and Public Health* 17 (18): https://doi.org/10.3390/ijerph17186616.

Gerard, C.L., Tavazzi, E., Gatta, R. et al. (2020). A process mining approach to real-world advanced melanoma treatments. *Proceedings of the 55th the American Society of Clinical Oncology (ASCO) Conference*.

Gers, F.A., Schmidhuber, J., and Cummins, F. (1999). Learning to forget: continual prediction with LSTM. *Neural Computation* 12: 2451–2471.

Gregg, E.W., Cheng, Y.J., Srinivasan, M. et al. (2018). Trends in cause-specific mortality among adults with and without diagnosed diabetes in the USA: an epidemiological analysis of linked national survey and vital statistics data. *Lancet (London, England)* 391 (10138): 2430–2440. https://doi.org/10.1016/S0140-6736(18)30314-3.

Hamberg, K. (2008). Gender bias in medicine. *Women's Health* 4 (3): 237–243.

Homayounfar, P. (2012). Process mining challenges in hospital information systems. *2012 Federated Conference on Computer Science and Information Systems (FedCSIS)*, 1135–1140. IEEE.

ICD (n.d.) https://www.cdc.gov/nchs/icd/icd9cm.htm (accessed 30 September 2023).

Islam, M.S., Hasan, M.M., Wang, X. et al. (2018). A systematic review on healthcare analytics: application and theoretical perspective of data mining. In: *Healthcare*, vol. 6, 54. MDPI.

Jae-Yong, C. (2019). Digital therapeutics and clinical pharmacology. *Transl Clin Pharmacol* 27 (1): 6–11.

Janssen, K.J.M., Vergouwe, Y., Kalkman, C.J. et al. (2009). A simple method to adjust clinical prediction models to local circumstances. *Canadian Journal of Anesthesia/Journal canadien d'anesthésie* 56 (3): 194. https://doi.org/10.1007/s12630-009-9041-x.

Kahn, H.S., Cheng, Y.J., Thompson, T.J. et al. (2009). Two risk-scoring systems for predicting incident diabetes mellitus in U.S. adults age 45 to 64 years. *Annals of Internal Medicine* 150 (11): 741–751.

Kengne, A.P., Beulens, J.W.J., Peelen, L.M. et al. (2014). Non-invasive risk scores for prediction of type 2 diabetes (EPIC-InterAct): a validation of existing models. *The Lancet Diabetes & Endocrinology* 2 (1): 19–29. https://doi.org/10.1016/S2213-8587(13)70103-7.

Kurniati, A.P., Johnson, O., Hogg, D., and Hall, G. (2016). Process mining in oncology: a literature review. *2016 6th International Conference on Information Communication and Management (ICICM)*, 291–297. IEEE.

Kusuma, G., Hall, M., and Johnson, O. (2018). Process mining in cardiology: a literature review. *International Journal of Bioscience, Biochemistry and Bioinformatics* 8: 226–236.

Lenz, R. and Reichert, M. (2007). It support for healthcare processes–premises, challenges, perspectives. *Data & Knowledge Engineering* 61 (1): 39–58.

Li, G., Zhang, P., Wang, J. et al. (2014). Cardiovascular mortality, all-cause mortality, and diabetes incidence after lifestyle intervention for people with impaired glucose tolerance in the Da Qing Diabetes Prevention Study: a 23-year follow-up study. *The Lancet Diabetes & Endocrinology* 2 (6): 474–480. https://doi.org/10.1016/S2213-8587(14)70057-9.

Lindström, J. and Tuomilehto, J. (2003). The diabetes risk score: a practical tool to predict type 2 diabetes risk. *Diabetes Care* 26 (3): 725–731. https://doi.org/10.2337/diacare.26.3.725.

Lindström, J., Ilanne-Parikka, P., Peltonen, M. et al. (2006). Sustained reduction in the incidence of type 2 diabetes by lifestyle intervention: follow-up of the Finnish Diabetes Prevention Study. *The Lancet* 368 (9548): 1673–1679.

Litchfield, I., Hoye, C., Shukla, D. et al. (2018). Can process mining automatically describe care pathways of patients with long-term conditions in uk primary care? A study protocol. *BMJ Open* 8 (12): e019947.

Longato, E., Di Camillo, B., Sparacino, G. et al. (2020a). Diabetes diagnosis from administrative claims and estimation of the true prevalence of diabetes among 4.2 million individuals of the Veneto region (North East Italy). *Nutrition, Metabolism and Cardiovascular Diseases* 30 (1): 84–91. https://doi.org/10.1016/j.numecd.2019.08.017.

Longato, E., Fadini, G.P., Sparacino, G. et al. (2020b). Prediction of cardiovascular complications in diabetes from pharmacy administrative claims. *Proceedings of the 2020 20th IEEE Mediterranean Electrotechnical Conference (MELECON)*, 315–320. tex.ids: Longato Prediction Cardiovascular Complications 2020.

Longato, E., Vettoretti, M., and Di Camillo, B. (2020c). A practical perspective on the concordance index for the evaluation and selection of prognostic time-to-event models. *Journal of Biomedical Informatics* 103496. https://doi.org/10.1016/j.jbi.2020.103496.

Longato, E., Fadini, G.P., Sparacino, G. et al. (2021). A deep learning approach to predict diabetes' cardiovascular complications from administrative claims. *IEEE Journal of Biomedical and Health Informatics* 25 (9): 3608–3617. https://doi.org/10.1109/JBHI.2021.3065756. tex.ids: Longato Deep Learning Approach 2021.

Mans, R.S., van der Aalst, W.M.P., and Vanwersch, R.J.B. (2015). *Process Mining in Healthcare: Evaluating and Exploiting Operational Healthcare Processes*. Springer.

Martinez-Millana, A., Lizondo, A., Gatta, R. et al. (2019). Process mining dashboard in operating rooms: analysis of staff expectations with analytic hierarchy process. *International Journal of Environmental Research and Public Health* 16 (2): 199.

Mertens, S., Gailly, F., Van Sassenbroeck, D., and Poels, G. (2020). Integrated declarative process and decision discovery of the emergency care process. In: *Information Systems Frontiers*, 1–23.

Murphy, K.P. (2002). Dynamic Bayesian networks: representation, inference and learning.

Nature Materials Editorial Board (2019). Ascent of machine learning in medicine. *Nature Materials* 18 (407): https://doi.org/10.1038/s41563-019-0360-1.

Noble, D., Mathur, R., Dent, T. et al. (2011). Risk models and scores for type 2 diabetes: systematic review. *BMJ (Clinical Research Edition)* 343: d7163. https://doi.org/10.1136/bmj.d7163.

Nowak, C., Ingelsson, E., and Fall, T. (2015). Use of type 2 diabetes risk scores in clinical practice: a call for action. *The Lancet Diabetes & Endocrinology* 3 (3): 166–167. https://doi.org/10.1016/S2213-8587(14)70261-X.

Rosella, L.C., Manuel, D.G., Burchill, C., and Stukel, T.A., and for the PHIAT-DM team(2011). A population-based risk algorithm for the development of diabetes: development and validation of the Diabetes Population Risk Tool (DPoRT). *Journal of Epidemiology & Community Health* 65 (7): 613–620. https://doi.org/10.1136/jech.2009.102244.

Roversi, C., Tavazzi, E., Vettoretti, M., and Di Camillo, B. (2021). A dynamic Bayesian network model for simulating the progression to diabetes onset in the ageing population. *2021 IEEE EMBS International Conference on Biomedical and Health Informatics (BHI)*, 1–4. IEEE.

Schmidt, M.I., Duncan, B.B., Bang, H. et al., and for the Atherosclerosis Risk in Communities Investigators(2005). Identifying individuals at high risk for diabetes: the atherosclerosis risk in communities study. *Diabetes Care* 28 (8): 2013–2018. https://doi.org/10.2337/diacare.28.8.2013.

Shilo, S., Rossman, H., and Segal, E. (2020). Axes of a revolution: challenges and promises of big data in healthcare. *Nature Medicine* 26 (11): 29–38. https://doi.org/10.1038/s41591-019-0727-5.

Steptoe, A., Breeze, E., Banks, J., and Nazroo, J. (2013). Cohort profile: the English longitudinal study of ageing. *International Journal of Epidemiology* 42 (6): 1640–1648.

Stern, M.P., Williams, K., and Haffner, S.M. (2002). Identification of persons at high risk for type 2 diabetes mellitus: do we need the oral glucose tolerance test? *Annals of Internal Medicine* 136 (8): 575–581. https://doi.org/10.7326/0003-4819-136-8-200204160-00006.

Tavazzi, E., Daberdaku, S., Vasta, R. et al. (2020a). Exploiting mutual information for the imputation of static and dynamic mixed-type clinical data with an adaptive k-nearest neighbours approach. *BMC Medical Informatics and Decision Making* 20 (5): 1–23.

Tavazzi, E., Gerard, C.L., Michielin, O. et al. (2020b). A process mining approach to statistical analysis: application to a real-world advanced melanoma dataset. In: *ICPM Workshops Proceedings 2020*, Lecture Notes in Business Information Processing (ed. S. Leemans and H. Leopold). Germany: Springer-Verlag.

Tavazzi, E., Daberdaku, S., Zandonà, A. et al. (2022a). Predicting functional impairment trajectories in amyotrophic lateral sclerosis: a probabilistic, multifactorial model of disease progression. *Journal of Neurology* 269: 3858–3878.

Tavazzi, E., Gatta, R., Vallati, M. et al. (2022b). Leveraging process mining for modeling progression trajectories in amyotrophic lateral sclerosis. *BMC Medical Informatics and Decision Making* 22: 346.

Therneau, T.M. and Grambsch, P.M. (2000). *Modeling Survival Data: Extending the Cox Model*, Statistics for Biology and Health. New York: Springer New York. doi: 10.1007/978-1-4757-3294-8.

Vettoretti, M., Longato, E., Di Camillo, B., and Facchinetti, A. (2018). Importance of recalibrating models for type 2 diabetes onset prediction: application of the diabetes population risk tool on the health and retirement study. *2018 40th Annual International*

Conference of the IEEE Engineering in Medicine and Biology Society (EMBC), 5358–5361. https://doi.org/10.1109/EMBC.2018.8513554.

Vettoretti, M., Longato, E., Zandonà, A. et al. (2020). Addressing practical issues of predictive models translation into everyday practice and public health management: a combined model to predict the risk of type 2 diabetes improves incidence prediction and reduces the prevalence of missing risk predictions. *BMJ Open Diabetes Research & Care* 8 (1): https://doi .org/10.1136/bmjdrc-2020-001223.

Williams, R., Rojas, E., Peek, N., and Johnson, O.A. (2018). Process mining in primary care: a literature review. *Studies in Health Technology and Informatics* 247: 376–380.

Wilson, P.W.F., Meigs, J.B., Sullivan, L. et al. (2007). Sr. Prediction of incident diabetes mellitus in middle-aged adults: the Framingham offspring study. *Archives of Internal Medicine* 167 (10): 1068–1074. https://doi.org/10.1001/archinte.167.10.1068.

Xu, X., Liu, X., Kang, Y. et al. (2020). A multi-directional approach for missing value estimation in multivariate time series clinical data. *Journal of Healthcare Informatics Research* 4 (4): 365–382.

Young, J.B., Gauthier-Loiselle, M., Bailey, R.A. et al. (2018). Development of predictive risk models for major adverse cardiovascular events among patients with type 2 diabetes mellitus using health insurance claims data. *Cardiovascular Diabetology* 17 (1): 118. https://doi.org/ 10.1186/s12933-018-0759-z.

Index

Big Data Analysis and Artificial Intelligence for Medical Sciences, First Edition.
Edited by Bruno Carpentieri and Paola Lecca.
© 2024 John Wiley & Sons Ltd. Published 2024 by John Wiley & Sons Ltd.